Study Surgery

Haifa Alotaibi

Study Surgery

A Guidance to Pass the Board Clinical Exam

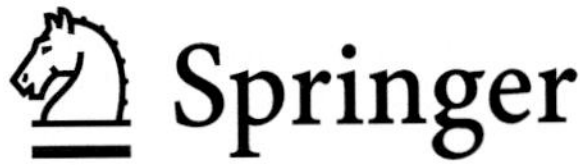

Haifa Alotaibi
Department of Surgery
College of Medicine Taif University (TU)
Taif
Saudi Arabia

ISBN 978-981-16-2307-3 ISBN 978-981-16-2305-9 (eBook)
https://doi.org/10.1007/978-981-16-2305-9

This Springer imprint is published by the registered company Springer Nature Singapore Pte Ltd.
The registered company address is: 152 Beach Road, #21-01/04 Gateway East, Singapore 189721, Singapore

To my daughter, Malak, you have made me stronger, better, and more fulfilled than I could have ever imagined.

Preface

"STUDY SURGERY, a guidance to pass the clinical board exam" is an organized single reference that any surgical trainee needs to prepare for the clinical board exam. It is a creative book that includes many mind maps and illustrations to help understand and memorize information. It enhances the knowledge and focuses on the required information in clinical exams. It teaches the resident how to approach patients with common surgical complaints and describes the management of common surgical disorders. Moreover, it guides the surgical trainees through the preoperative preparation, intraoperative steps of common operations, postoperative, follow-up, and management of complications. While the presented information was evidence-based and up to date, it was explained very simply. Helpful tools like algorithms and illustrations are provided to help understand and clarify any confusion that might be an area of misdiagnosis and mismanagement, which I believe is where/why most candidates struggle during exams. It also allows them to practice what they know using multiple case scenarios and questions to discuss their answers. They can test their solutions using the provided checklist. It empowers their knowledge and learns the common exam tricks. It is not a boring book, as I know from my recent experience preparing for the board exam how it feels when the trainees have to study; however, their energy is consumed by the amount of information that needs to be reviewed. So, I added many motivational and inspirational quotes said by surgeons in the field and famous successful people that will help and keep them motivated.

Taif, Saudi Arabia

Haifa Alotaibi

Acknowledgment

There are plenty of people who helped me bring this book to reality, and I am grateful to all of them. Once this book started to go from notes on my desk to a manuscript, there were many people involved who deserve to be acknowledged and thanked.

First and foremost, I would like to thank my mother for believing in me and has continuously encouraged me to keep working and pursue my dreams. I cannot thank her enough for being my source of inspiration to challenge myself and achieve more.

Additionally, I am so grateful to my friends who are behind this book's idea and helped me take it well above the level of simplicity into an organized work. They encouraged me to get it done and also helped in typing parts of some chapters.

Having an idea and turning it into a book is as hard as it sounds. The experience is both internally challenging and rewarding. I want to thank my colleagues in the surgical department, Taif University, especially Prof. Mohammed Alsaeed, as my teacher and mentor; he has taught me more than I could ever give him credit for here. He has shown me, by his example, what a good educator should be. I also would like to thank Dr. Abdullah Alsawat for reviewing and critiquing my illustrations; his recommendations have always been helpful.

I owe an enormous debt of gratitude to those who gave me detailed and constructive comments by reviewing the chapters, including Prof. Mohammed Alsaeed, Prof. Bilal Aljiffry, Dr. Nora Trabulsi, Dr. Majed Almourgi, Dr. Basem Alshareef, Dr. Abdulaziz Saleem, Dr. Hafiz Hamdi, Dr. Khalid Alzahrani, Dr. Abdullah Alsawat, Dr. Sahar Alnefaie, Dr. Ghader Jamjoum, Dr. Arif Khurshid, and Dr. Ahmed Alzahrani. They gave freely of their time not just to read my draft chapters but send detailed comments and feedback.

I want to express my special thanks to my colleague Dr. Ahmed Althobity for helping and writing the urology chapter. It would not be possible to include that chapter without his generous help.

Finally, I want to thank my publisher, Springer Nature, Dr. Jagjeet Kaur Saini and Dr. Naren Aggarwal for their editorial support and guidance, and Ms. Kripa Guruprasad for her coordination and following the manuscript preparation.

Contents

About the Author

Haifa Alotaibi is an Umm Alqura University graduate (UQU) with an excellent GPA and honor degree. She developed an early interest in education. When she was a medical student, her notes had been helpful to her colleagues, and she was known for her works among her college graduates.After graduation, she wanted to pursue an academic job in addition to her surgical training, so she joined Taif University (TU) as a lecturer. Her teaching ability was recognized by her seniors and appreciated by her students.Recently, she finished her surgical training and certified as a surgeon by the Saudi Commission for Health Specialties. During her residency, she was responsible for her training program's academic activities and always taught and educated her junior colleagues.She likes to simplify difficult information, making it easy to digest and memorize without compromising its depth and importance. In addition to that, she is an artist who implemented her talent in demonstrating and illustrating surgical anatomy and explaining the steps of surgical operations. She used her academic potentials and drawing talent to make this book a single most crucial source in preparing for clinical board exams for either local or international surgical trainees.For her, surgery is art, and surgeons work in the human body with diligence and care as the artist does on his/her canvas. She enjoyed joining science and art in her book. Her book is a creative work that helped her, and her friends successfully passed the board exam, and she is sure that it will help her junior colleagues.

Surgical Aspects of Breast Diseases for Clinical Board Exams

1

1.1 Part I: Knowledge

The river of knowledge has no depth.
—Chinonye J. Chidolue

Breast complaint could be one of the following:

- Lump
- Pain
- Nipple discharge
- Skin changes
- Eczematous rash around the nipple
- Abnormal finding on a screening image

Differential diagnosis: Table 1.1
Breast Anatomy: Fig. 1.1

Table 1.1 Differential diagnosis of common breast complaints

Lump	Discharge	Pain
Cyst Fibroadenoma Cancer Fat necrosis Abscess Granulomatous disease Phyllodes	Papilloma Cancer DCIS Duct ectasia Fistula	Cyclical mastalgia Mastitis Abscess Mondor's disease Cancer Muscular pain Fibrocystic changes

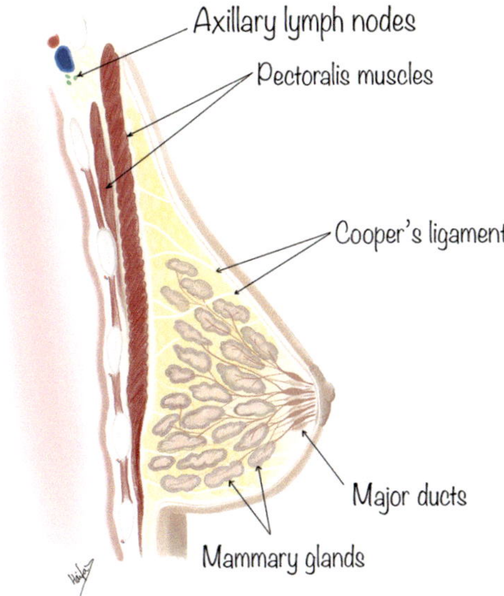

Fig. 1.1 The lateral view of the human female breast

1.1.1 Approach to Patient with Breast Lesion

Triple Assessment:

A. Clinical (history and physical examination)
B. Imaging
C. Histological assessment

H. Alotaibi, *Study Surgery*, https://doi.org/10.1007/978-981-16-2305-9_1

A) **Clinical assessment:**

History of Breast Complaint

- **Introduce yourself to the patient**
- **Personal data**
- **Chief complaint and duration**
- **History of presenting illness**
  - *Analysis of the chief complaint*

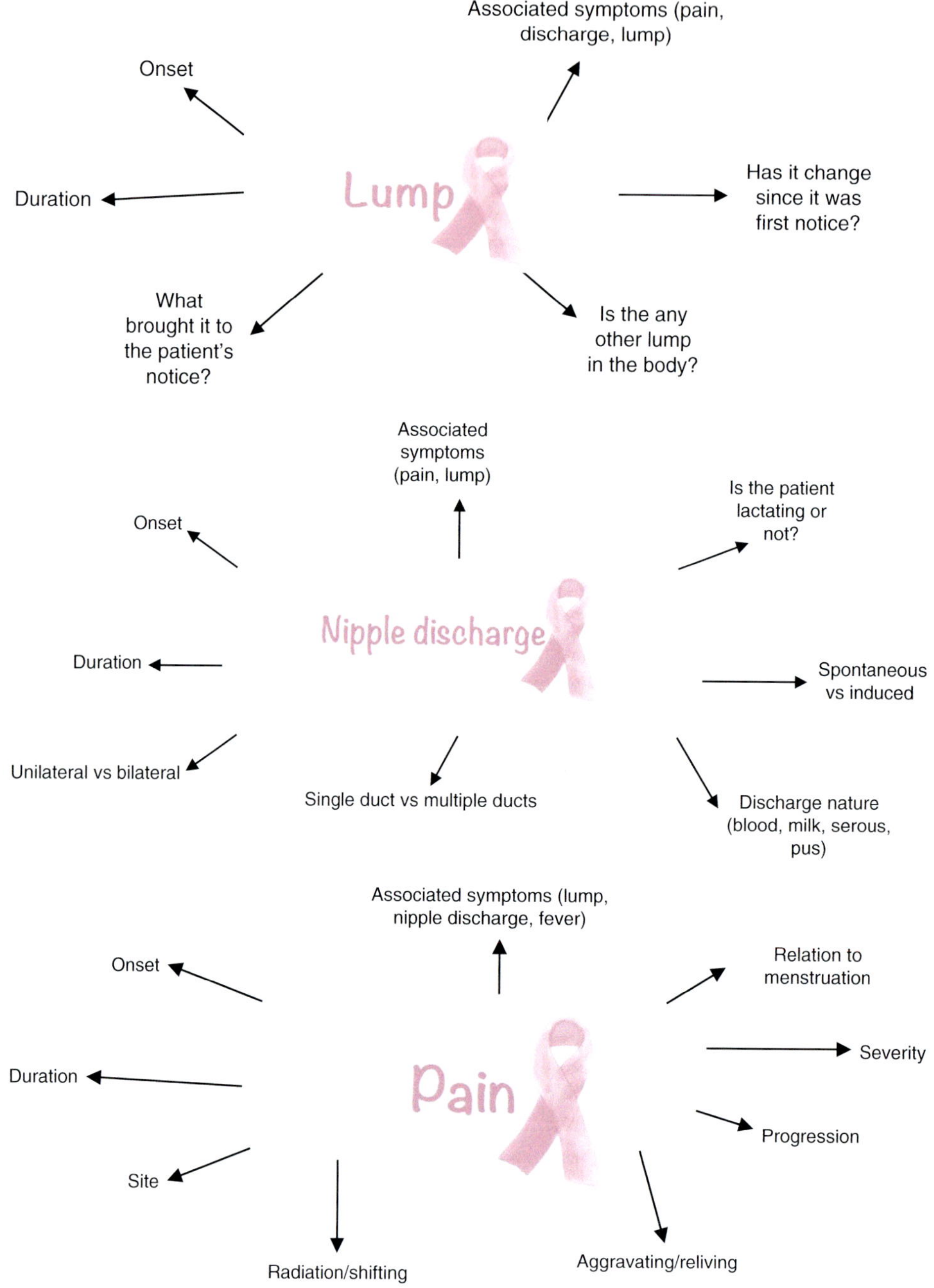

- **Associated symptoms:** fever, discharge, arm swelling
- **Constitutional symptoms:** weight loss, decrease appetite, night sweating
- **Risk factors:**
  Age of menarche/menopause
  Number of pregnancies
  Breast feeding
  History of chest wall radiation
  Age at first childbirth
  Hormonal treatment (OCP, HRT), duration of usage
  Family history of breast cancer, colon cancer, ovarian cancer, and prostate cancer and degree of relationship and age at the diagnosis if yes
  Personal history of breast or other cancers
- **Differential diagnosis:**
  History of trauma (fat necrosis)
  History of lactation (abscess, galactocele)
- **Symptoms of metastasis:** bone pain, abdominal pain, shortness of breath, cough
- **Previous similar attack**, previous investigation (mammogram, ultrasound, biopsy)
- **Systemic review of related system**

- **Past medical history**
- **Past surgical history**
- **Family history**
- **Social history**
- **Medication**
- **Allergy**
- **Transfusion**
- **Systemic review (general)**
  - **CNS:** headache, visual disturbance, seizure, numbness
  - **CVS:** dyspnea, chest pain, palpitation, limb swelling
  - **Respiratory system:** cough, hemoptysis, shortness of breath
  - **GIT:** dysphagia, heartburn, nausea, vomiting, changes in bowel habit
  - **Urological:** flank pain, dysuria, hematuria
  - **Musculoskeletal:** weakness, arthritis, bone pain

Physical Examination of the Breast:

- **Introduce yourself to the patient**
- **Obtain permission**
- **Assure privacy**
- **Wash hands**
- **Position**: 45 degree
- **Exposure**: upper trunk up to the waist
- **General examination**
  - Appearance
  - Body built
  - Color: jaundice, pale
  - Distress
  - Environment
- **Vital signs**
- **Breast**:
  - **Inspection:**
    Look for size, symmetry, skin (Peu d'orange, ulcers, erythema), and nipple areola (inversion, eczematous lesions, any accessory nipple, or obvious discharge).
    Ask the patient to slowly raise arm above the head and look for any skin changes or tethering.
    Ask the patient to press her hands over her hips to tense the pectoralis muscle, and this may reveal previously invisible lumps.
    Inspect the axilla, arms, and supraclavicular fossa for any grossly enlarged lymph node or lymphedema.
  - **Palpation:**
    Begin with normal side.
    Do not forget the axillary tail!
    If you palpate a lump, ascertain its size, shape, surface, edges, consistency, and mobility.
    Assess the relation to skin and chest wall.
    Palpate the nipple and ask the patient to squeeze to see if there is any discharge.
    Palpate the axilla, arm for lymph node, and lymphedema.
    Palpate the supraclavicular fossa and neck.
    Palpate the abdomen for hepatomegaly and ascites.
    Examine the spine.

B) **Imaging:**

- **Mammogram**:
  - Diagnostic mammogram if the patient has breast complaint.
  - Views: craniocaudal (CC), mediolateral (MLO), 90° lateral, and spot compression.
  - Screening mammogram if the patient has no symptoms.
  - Screening image consists of two views CC and MLO.
  - If any abnormality detected in screening mammogram, the patient should be called back for diagnostic mammogram.
  - Interpretation: using BI-RADS system (Table 1.2).
  - Mammographic features that suggest diagnosis of breast cancer:
    - Solid mass ± stellate features
    - Asymmetric thickening
    - Clustered microcalcification

Table 1.2 BIRADs system for breast imaging [1]

Grade	Interpretation	Action needed	Likelihood of malignancy
0	Need additional imaging	Recall for additional imaging	
I	Negative	Routine screening	Essentially 0%
II	Benign	Routine screening	Essentially 0%
III	Probably benign	Short interval follow-up (every 6 months)	>0% but <2%
IV	Suspicious (a) Low suspicion (b) Moderate suspicion (c) High suspicion	Need tissue biopsy	(a) 2–10% (b) 10–50% (c) 50–95%
V	Highly suggestive of malignancy	Need tissue biopsy	>95%
VI	Known, biopsy-proven malignancy	Surgical excision when clinically appropriate	

- **Ultrasound**
  - To resolve mammographic finding
  - To define cystic lesion
  - To demonstrate the echogenicity of specific solid mass
  - To assess the vascularity around the lesion
  - To guide trucut biopsy, wire localization
  - To assess the axilla
  - Features of suspicious lymph node:
    - Cortical thickening >3 mm
    - Size >10 mm
    - More circular appearance
    - Absence of fatty hilum and hypoechoic internal echoes [1]
- **MRI:** Table 1.3

C) **Biopsy:**

- Trucut needle biopsy: palpable or ultrasound detected lump, BIRADs IV, or more

Table 1.3 Indications of screening and diagnostic MRI

Indications of screening MRI [2]	Indications of diagnostic MRI
Based on evidence ▪ First-degree relative of breast cancer genetic mutation carrier, but untested ▪ Lifetime risk 20% or greater, as defined by models that are largely dependent on family history. Consider referral for genetic counseling for affected first-degree relatives. If testing declined or not recommended, recommend MRI **Based on expert consensus** ▪ Radiation to the chest between age 10 and 30 years **Consider MRI screening if lifetime risk >20% for:** ▪ LCIS/ALH ▪ ADH [2]	**Noncontroversial** ▪ Occult primary breast cancer ▪ Considering neoadjuvant chemotherapy **Controversial** ▪ Specific tumor type ILC ▪ Multifocality, multicentricity by ultrasound and mammogram ▪ Patient with dense breast ▪ Young patient <40 years old ▪ To assess contralateral breast in case of planned bilateral mastectomy ▪ BRCA positive or patient with family history suggestive gene mutation ▪ Paget's disease to rule out underlying primary if not detected by other imaging modalities [1]

- Stereotactic: for suspicious microcalcification, architectural distortion, lesions not seen on ultrasound
- Contraindications to stereotactic biopsy:
  – Unable to lie in prone position
  – Patient weight
  – Lesions near the nipple, too superficial or too posterior locations
  – Mammographically occult lesions
- MRI-guided trucut biopsy: for lesions not detected by ultrasound or mammogram

Note: Do not forget the clip if considering breast-conserving surgery, neoadjuvant systemic therapy, or after stereotactic biopsy.

Information you need to know from the biopsy:

- Cancer or not
- Invasive or in situ
- Pathological subtype if invasive (e.g., ductal, lobular, mucinous, tubular, medullary)
- Histological pattern if DCIS (e.g., comedo, cribriform, mixed) and the grade of necrosis
- Hormone status (ER, PR)
- HER2neu status
  – +1 = negative
  – +2 = equivocal, do FISH
  – +3 = positive
- Grade
- Ki 67 [1]

1.1.2 Management of Benign Breast Lesions

Cyst:

- Aspirate symptomatic/large cysts: if the fluid is not bloody or no mass after aspiration, discard the fluid.
- If there is mass or the fluid is blood, biopsy the mass or send the fluid for cytology.
- Indications for surgery:
  – Recurrence multiple times
  – If the result of the biopsy indicates surgical removal [3]

Fibroadenoma:

- Follow up generally
- Indications for surgical excision:
  – Continuous increase in size.
  – Cosmetic or the patient wants surgery (e.g., painful).
  – >2 cm in size.
  – If the mass is large >5 cm, biopsy it first to rule out phyllodes [3].

Breast abscess:

- Aspiration (ultrasound guided) if small size and antibiotics.
- If recurrence or the size is large, do incision and drainage in addition to antibiotics.
- If multiple recurrence, rule out other condition like granulomatous mastitis or inflammatory breast cancer [3].

Atypical ductal hyperplasia/atypical lobular hyperplasia:

- If found on biopsy, do excision to ensure no adjacent carcinoma is present [4].

Lobular carcinoma in situ:

- Triple assessment
- For classic LCIS, the options are:
  – Close observation
  – Chemoprevention with Tamoxifen or Raloxifene
  – Prophylactic bilateral mastectomy
- Pleomorphic LCIS: to be treated more like DCIS, with excision to negative margin [5]

Management of Ductal CarcinomaIn Situ

Mastectomy + SLNB

Indications of mastectomy:

- Multicentric (extensive) calcification.
- Large area of DCIS in relation to breast size.
- Clear margin can't be obtained with breast conserving surgery (BCS).
- Contraindication to BCS.

Indication of post mastectomy radiation therapy (XRT):
Margin closed to skin or chest wall

Indication of adjuvant endocrine therapy (for ER/ PR positive lesions):

- ≥ 4cm
- Positive margin that can't be revised
- High grade / comedo necrosis
- Strong family history (6)

Breast conserving surgery ± radiation therapy ± SLNB

Indicationsof SLNB:

- Presence of palpable mass
- Nipple discharge
- High grade/ comedo necrosis
- Large size > 4cm

Margin: 2mm (4)

When you can ommit radiation therapy post BCS?
Based on Van Nuys (table 1-4)

Table-4Van Nuys classification(6)

	I	II	III
Tumor size	< or = 15 mm	16-40 mm	>40 mm
Margin	= or > 10 mm	1-9 mm	< 1mm
Nuclear grade & necrosis	Non high grade / non comedo	Non high grade / comedo	High grade / comedo
Age	>60 years	40-60 years	<40 years

4-6 points: Radiation therapy can be omitted
10-12 points: may benefit from mastectomy

Indicationsof adjuvant endocrine therapy (for ER/ PR positive lesions):

- ≥ 4cm
- Positive margin
- High grade / comedo necrosis
- Strong family history (6)

1.1.3 Management of Invasive Breast Cancer

Molecular subtype: Table 1.5 [4]

Staging:
Refer to the TNM staging system from AJCC

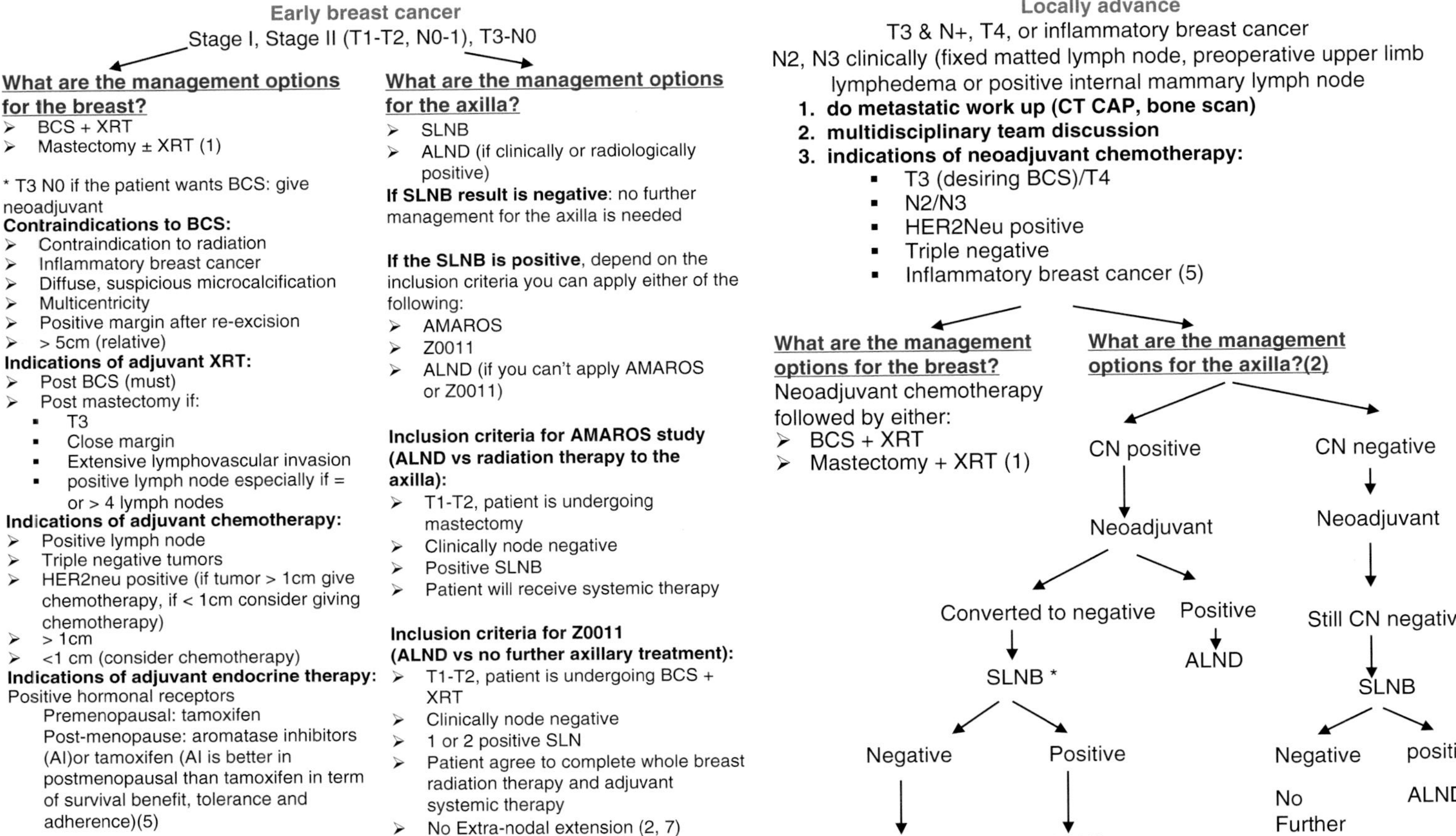
Management of breast cancer
Early breast cancer
Stage I, Stage II (T1-T2, N0-1), T3-N0
What are the management options for the breast?
➢ BCS + XRT
➢ Mastectomy ± XRT (1)
* T3 N0 if the patient wants BCS: give neoadjuvant
Contraindications to BCS:
➢ Contraindication to radiation
➢ Inflammatory breast cancer
➢ Diffuse, suspicious microcalcification
➢ Multicentricity
➢ Positive margin after re-excision
➢ > 5cm (relative)
Indications of adjuvant XRT:
➢ Post BCS (must)
➢ Post mastectomy if:
▪ T3
▪ Close margin
▪ Extensive lymphovascular invasion
▪ positive lymph node especially if = or > 4 lymph nodes
Indications of adjuvant chemotherapy:
➢ Positive lymph node
➢ Triple negative tumors
➢ HER2neu positive (if tumor > 1cm give chemotherapy, if < 1cm consider giving chemotherapy)
➢ > 1cm
➢ <1 cm (consider chemotherapy)
Indications of adjuvant endocrine therapy:
Positive hormonal receptors
Premenopausal: tamoxifen
Post-menopause: aromatase inhibitors (AI)or tamoxifen (AI is better in postmenopausal than tamoxifen in term of survival benefit, tolerance and adherence)(5)
What are the management options for the axilla?
➢ SLNB
➢ ALND (if clinically or radiologically positive)
If SLNB result is negative: no further management for the axilla is needed
If the SLNB is positive, depend on the inclusion criteria you can apply either of the following:
➢ AMAROS
➢ Z0011
➢ ALND (if you can't apply AMAROS or Z0011)
Inclusion criteria for AMAROS study (ALND vs radiation therapy to the axilla):
➢ T1-T2, patient is undergoing mastectomy
➢ Clinically node negative
➢ Positive SLNB
➢ Patient will receive systemic therapy
Inclusion criteria for Z0011 (ALND vs no further axillary treatment):
➢ T1-T2, patient is undergoing BCS + XRT
➢ Clinically node negative
➢ 1 or 2 positive SLN
➢ Patient agree to complete whole breast radiation therapy and adjuvant systemic therapy
➢ No Extra-nodal extension (2, 7)
Locally advance
T3 & N+, T4, or inflammatory breast cancer
N2, N3 clinically (fixed matted lymph node, preoperative upper limb lymphedema or positive internal mammary lymph node
1. do metastatic work up (CT CAP, bone scan)
2. multidisciplinary team discussion
3. indications of neoadjuvant chemotherapy:
▪ T3 (desiring BCS)/T4
▪ N2/N3
▪ HER2Neu positive
▪ Triple negative
▪ Inflammatory breast cancer (5)
What are the management options for the breast?
Neoadjuvant chemotherapy followed by either:
➢ BCS + XRT
➢ Mastectomy + XRT (1)
What are the management options for the axilla?(2)
CN positive
Neoadjuvant
Converted to negative
SLNB *
Negative
No further treatmet
Positive
ALND
Positive
ALND
CN negative
Neoadjuvant
Still CN negative
SLNB
Negative
No Further treatment
positive
ALND
*Dual tracer, at least 2 lymph nodes, expert pathologist, use immune histochemistry to identify micrometastasis. CN: clinical node

Table 1.5 Molecular subtype [4]

Luminal A	Low grade, high ER 50% of breast cancer	ER+, PR+, HER2Neu+ CK 8+, CK 18+
Luminal B	Higher grade, low ER 10% of breast cancer	ER+, PR± HER2 Neu±
HER 2	High grade, P53 mutation 5–10% of breast cancer	ER−, PR−, HER2+
Basal	High proliferation CK5+, CK14+, CK 17+ EGFR+	ER−,PR−,HER2−

Contraindications for Breast-Conserving Therapy Requiring Radiotherapy Include [2]:
Absolute

- Radiotherapy during pregnancy
- Diffuse suspicious or malignant appearing microcalcifications
- Widespread disease that cannot be incorporated by local excision of a single region or segment of breast tissue that achieves negative margins with a satisfactory cosmetic result
- Diffusely positive pathologic margins
- Homozygous (biallelic inactivation) for *ATM* mutation

Relative

- Prior RT to the chest wall or breast; knowledge of doses and volumes prescribed is essential
- Active connective tissue disease involving the skin (especially scleroderma and lupus)
- Persistently positive pathologic margin
- Patients with a known or suspected genetic predisposition to breast cancer:
  – May have an increased risk of ipsilateral breast recurrence or contralateral breast cancer with breast-conserving therapy
  – May be considered for prophylactic bilateral mastectomy for risk reduction
  – May have known or suspected Li-Fraumeni syndrome [2]

Recurrent Breast Cancer:

- Start all over again.
- Re-biopsy as luminal type can change.
- Staging (CT CAP, bone scan).
- Repeat everything except radiation therapy.
- Multidisciplinary team discussion [11].

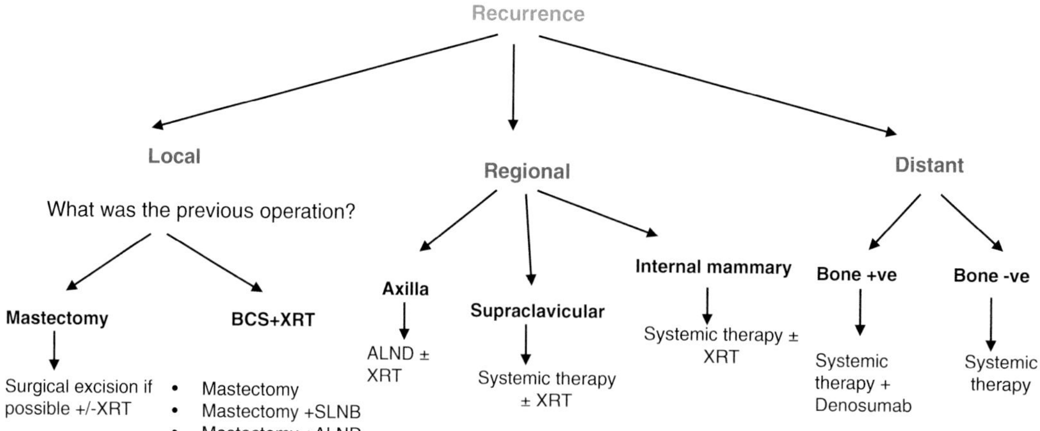

Inflammatory Breast Cancer:
Aggressive cancer and has poor prognosis

- Always neoadjuvant therapy.
- Always MRM regardless of response to neoadjuvant chemotherapy.
- If no response to chemotherapy, try second line and radiation therapy [12].

Stage IV Breast Cancer [2]:

- History and physical exam.
- Discuss goals of therapy, adopt shared decision-making, and document course of care.
- CBC.
- Comprehensive metabolic panel, including liver function tests and alkaline phosphatase.
- Imaging for systemic staging:
  - Chest diagnostic CT with contrast
  - Abdominal ± pelvic diagnostic CT with contrast or MRI with contrast
  - Brain MRI with contrast if suspicious CNS symptoms
  - Spine MRI with contrast if back pain or symptoms of cord compression
  - Bone scan or sodium fluoride PET/CT
  - FDG PET/CT (optional)
  - X-rays of symptomatic bones and long and weight-bearing bones abnormal on bone scan
- Biomarker testing:
  - Biopsy of first recurrence of disease
  - Evaluation of ER/PR and HER2 status to differentiate recurrent disease from new primary
  - Comprehensive germline and somatic profiling to identify candidates for additional targeted therapies
- Genetic counseling if patient is at risk for hereditary breast cancer.
- Assess for distress.
- National Comprehensive Cancer Network® (NCCN®) recommends metastatic disease at presentation or first recurrence of disease should be biopsied as a part of the work up.
- Genetic counseling if the patient is considered to be high risk.
- The primary treatment approach recommended by the NCCN Panel for women with metastatic breast cancer and an intact primary tumor is systemic therapy, with consideration of surgery after initial systemic treatment for those women requiring palliation of symptoms or with impending complications, such as skin ulceration, bleeding, fungation, and pain.
- Alternatively, radiation therapy may be considered as an option to surgery.
- The systemic treatment of breast cancer recurrence or stage IV disease prolongs survival and enhances quality of life but is not curative.
- The NCCN Panel recommends treatment with a bone modifying agent such as zoledronic acid, pamidronate, or denosumab in addition to chemotherapy or endocrine therapy if bone metastasis is present [2].

Pregnant Patient with Breast Cancer:

- Triple assessment
- Staging: chest X-ray with abdominal shield, abdominal ultrasound if indicated, non-contrast MRI to assess bone metastasis
- Multidisciplinary team discussion
- Contraindications during pregnancy: blue dye, XRT, anti HER2 [2]

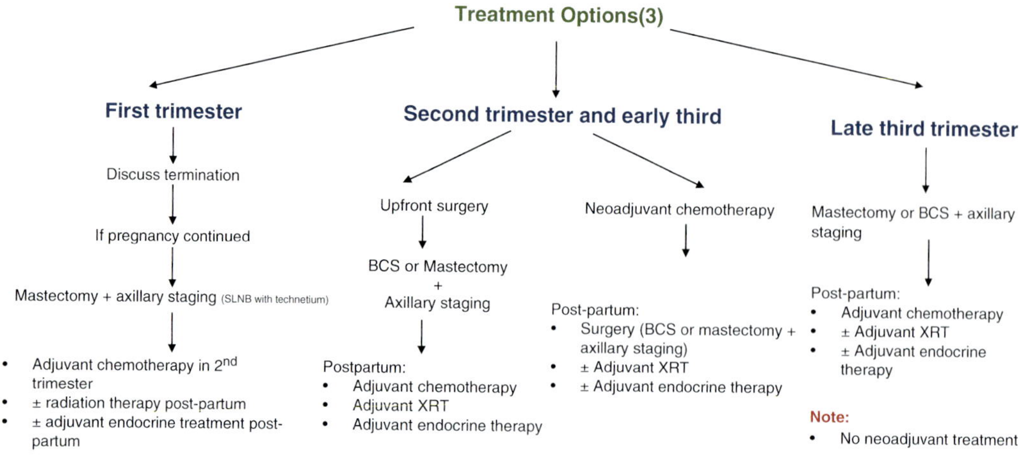

Note:
- No neoadjuvant chemotherapy in the first trimester
- No BCS

Occult Breast Cancer:
(patient presents with axillary lymph node but clinically and mammography are negative)

Follow these three main steps:

Step 1: confirm the diagnosis

Biopsy the lymph node (trucut) to confirm the tumor is of a breast origin (test the tissue for ER, PR, HER2Neu, cytokeratin 7 and 20, mammoglobulin, CEA and Ca-125).

Step 2: assess for another metastasis

CT CAP, bone scan.

Step 3: further assess the breast

Bilateral breast MRI. If it is positive for any lesion, do MRI guided biopsy and insert a clip! [9].

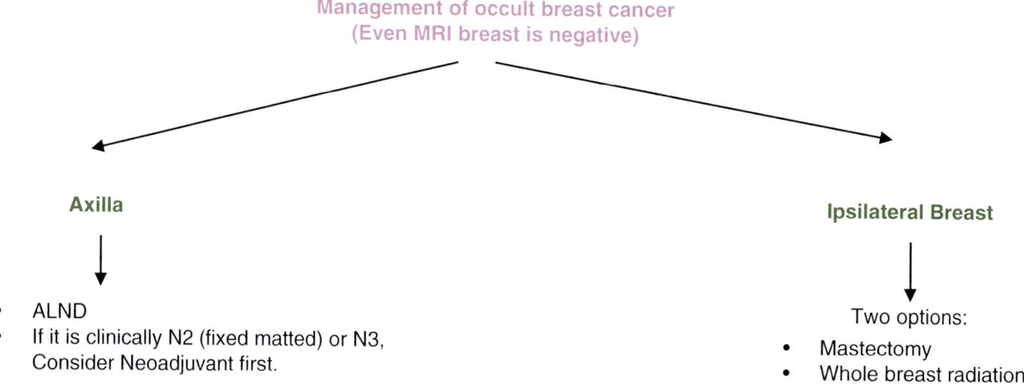

Male Breast Cancer:

- Triple assessment.
- Staging (similar to female breast cancer, if clinically stage III).
- Multidisciplinary team.
- Indication for neoadjuvant chemotherapy (similar to female breast cancer, the limitation in male breast cancer is almost always ER positive and has poor response to chemotherapy).

- Breast: mastectomy is the standard of care although BCS is possible at least theoretically.
- Axilla: Management of axilla is similar to female breast cancer except male patients are not eligible for AMAROS or Z0011 trials. So, if positive SLNB, do ALND [13].
- Postoperative:
  - Refer for genetic counselling.
  - Adjuvant chemotherapy similar to female breast cancer.
  - Follow up similar to female breast cancer but no need for screening mammogram of the contralateral breast.
  - For hormone positive tumor, use tamoxifen as adjuvant endocrine therapy.

Phyllodes Tumors:

- Triple assessment.
- Chest imaging to assess for any metastasis.
- Multidisciplinary team approach.
- Management includes complete surgical excision with 1 cm margin of normal breast tissue.
- Large tumor may require mastectomy.
- Axillary staging is not recommended [4].

Paget's Disease [2]**:**

- Up to 90% associated with cancer elsewhere in the breast; the associated cancer not necessarily located adjacent to nipple areola complex (NAC) and may be either DCIS or invasive cancer.
- Clinical assessment (history and physical examination).
- Breast imaging: if there is any breast lesion identified, it should be evaluated according to the guidelines.
- The skin of NAC should undergo surgical biopsy including the full thickness of the epidermis including at least a portion of any clinically involved NAC.
- If the biopsy is positive for Paget's disease, breast MRI is recommended to define the extent of the disease and identify any additional disease [2, 4].

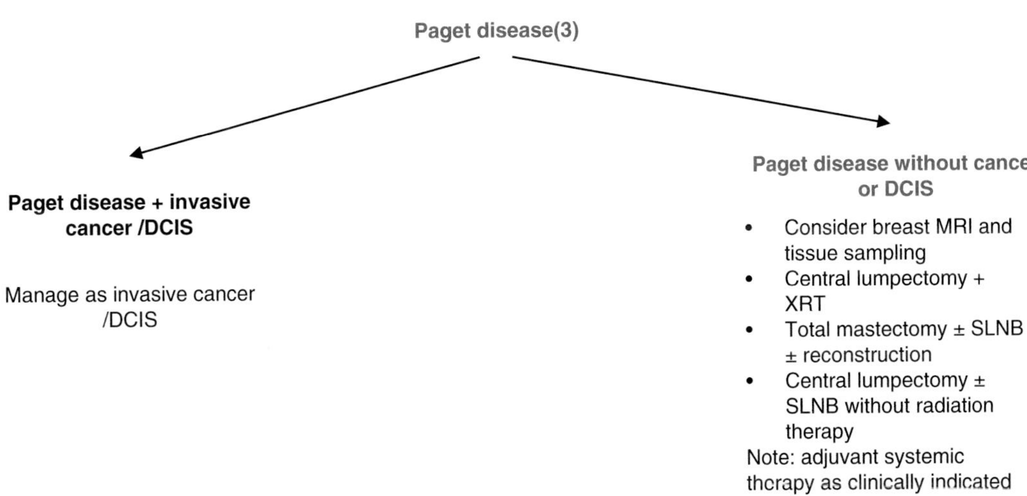

Adjuvant Treatment Common Side Effects:

- **Anthracycline;** Doxorubicin and Epirubicin: cardiotoxic
- **Texans**; Docetaxel and Paclitaxel: motor and sensory neuropathy, flushing and alopecia.
- **Anti HER2;** Trastuzumab (Herceptin): decreases left ventricle ejection fraction
- **Antiestrogen;** Tamoxifen: endometrial cancer 1%, DVT, PE 1%, vasomotor symptoms (hot flashes, sleep disturbance, headache)
- **Antiestrogen;** Raloxifene: vasomotor symptoms
- **Aromatase inhibitors;** Anastrozole: vasomotor symptoms, arthritis [8]

1.1.4 Operations for Breast Cancer

Preoperative:

- Review the clinical data.
- Evaluate the cardiopulmonary system.
- Review the following investigation:
  - Radiological imaging
  - Histopathology of the breast lesion
- If there is a plan regarding reconstruction, the patient needs to be evaluated by plastic surgery.
- Preoperative usual laboratory investigation: CBC, ECG, CXR, coagulation profile, LFT, RFT, blood group.
- Surgical site marking and shave the axilla if indicated.
- Informed consent.

Consent for Mastectomy:

- *Mention the procedure:*

  Removal of the breast through elliptical incision including the nipple and skin.

  If SLNB will be done, sample from axillary lymph node will be sent for pathological assessment with help of blue dye, sulfur colloid, or both.

  If ALND will be done, add with removal of most of the axillary lymph node and insertion of drainage tube.

  If immediate reconstruction will be done, explain if it is a flap or implant.
- *Mention if any other alternative is possible.*
- *Mention the risks and complications:*
  - General complications: DVT, PE, MI
  - Specific complications: bleeding, wound infection, seroma, flap necrosis, nerve injury (numbness on the medial aspect of the arm, or injury to the motor nerves leading to inability to raise the arm above the head for example, to comb her hair or winging of the scapula), lymphedema, complication of reconstruction if it is done, and the need for re-excision if margin is positive

1.1.5 Modified Radical Mastectomy

Mastectomy:

- Under general anesthesia and after endotracheal intubation.
- Confirm that antibiotic or DVT prophylaxis is given if indicated.
- Time out and confirm patient, procedure, and side, if special equipment is needed.
- Position:
  - Supine position with ipsilateral arm at 90°.
  - The skin is prepped and draped from the neck down to the costal margin with the arm freely draped.
- The surgeon stands on the side of the mastectomy to be performed and the first assistant on the opposite side.
- Incision: transverse elliptical incision with about 3 cm clearance around the tumor. The incision extended from lateral edge of the sternum medially to the mid axillary line laterally and should include the biopsy site. The incision should be below the hair line of the axilla (Fig. 1.2).
- Exposure: the skin incised until the subcutaneous tissue is identified, several Allis clamps are placed along the upper incision to provide vertical traction by the assistant.

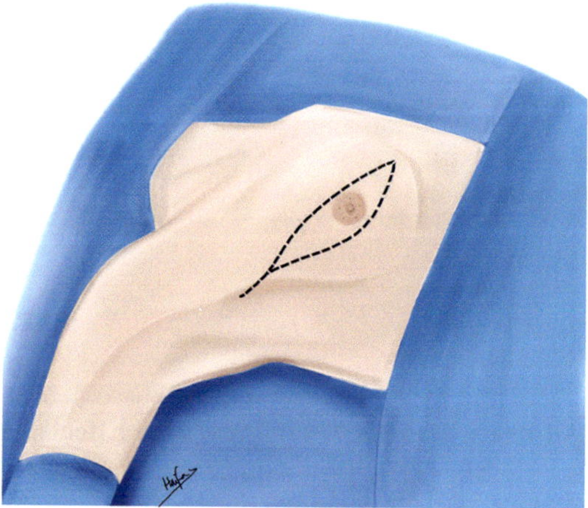

Fig. 1.2 The elliptical incision for mastectomy. Notice that it should include the biopsy site

- Using a laparotomy pad, countertraction is applied on the breast in the caudal direction.
- Superior flap is created by dividing the Cooper's ligament which extend between superficial fascia of the breast and subdermal adipose tissue. The correct plane is known by minimal or no bleeding (Fig. 1.3).
- Upper limit of dissection is at the level of the clavicle (Fig. 1.4).

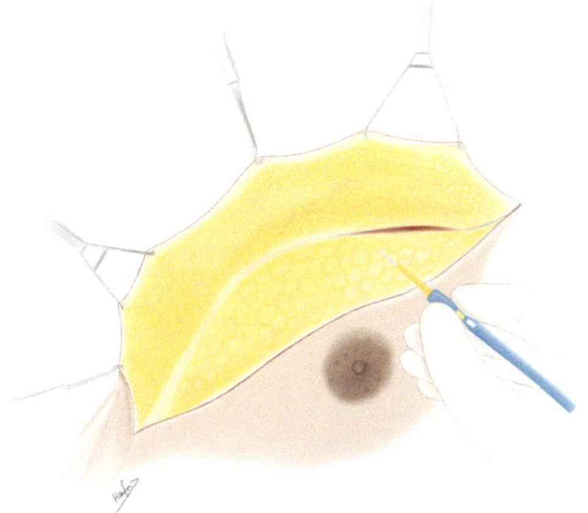

Fig. 1.3 Creation of the upper flap by dividing the Cooper's ligament

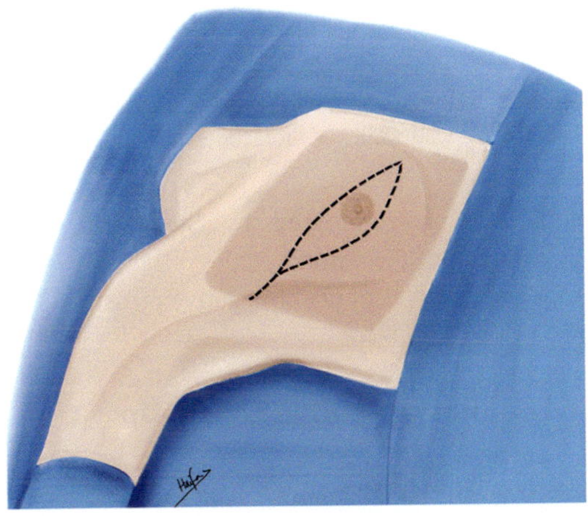

Fig. 1.4 The flaps should be dissected till the subclavicular area superiorly, to the inframammary fold inferiorly, and from the lateral edge of the sternum medially to the midaxillary line laterally

- The pectoralis major fascia is identified from medial margin to lateral edge of pectoralis major muscle.
- Once the upper flap is created, it should be covered with moist pad.
- Using the same technique, the inferior flap is created.
- The inferior flap extends down to the rectus sheath and from the edge of the fifth rib medially to the latissimus dorsi laterally.
- The breast tissue is dissected along with the pectoralis fascia from the underlying muscle (Fig. 1.5).
- Once the breast tissue is freed near the lateral sternal edge, the dissection is continued until lateral edge of the pectoralis major muscle.
- Further dissection from this point depends on whether total or modified radical mastectomy is to be performed.
- If modified radical mastectomy is being performed, attention is now directed toward performing the axillary dissection [14].

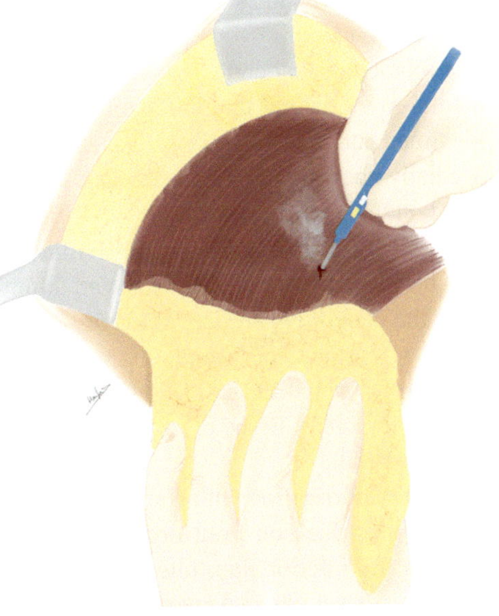

Fig. 1.5 The breast tissue is dissected along with the pectoralis fascia from the underlying muscle

Axillary Lymph Node Dissection:

- Once lateral edge of the pectoralis major muscle is dissected free, retract it upward with two right angle retractors.
- This exposes the interpectoral fat and Rotter lymph node.
- The interpectoral fat sharply dissected with Metz to be included in the specimen and skeletonized the underlying pectoralis minor muscle.
- Lateral pectoral nerve and vessels lying along the medial border of pectoralis minor are carefully identified and preserved.
- To gain access to the axilla, the clavipectoral fascia along the lateral border of pectoralis minor muscle is incised.
- Pectoralis minor muscle is retracted to expose level II lymph node.
- The axillary vein is identified, small tributaries are ligated and divided using 3-0 silk as they are encountered.
- Fascia over the length of the vein is incised (Fig. 1.6).
- Dissection above the vein should be avoided.
- Proceed with dissection by releasing the axillary tissue from lateral chest wall and laterally until axillary tissue is freed from latissimus dorsi tendon.
- The thoracodorsal bundle, which lies posteromedial to the lateral thoracic vein, should be identified and preserved (Fig. 1.7).
- Medially, the long thoracic nerve can be identified on the lateral chest wall.
- After identifying both nerves, the axillary tissue between them can be dissected bluntly from the underlying subscapularis muscle.
- The intercostobrachial nerve if possible, to preserve it once identified or just divide it.
- Finally, the breast tissue is freed from the lateral chest wall.
- Hemostasis, irrigation with warm saline.
- Two 10-mm Jackson Pratt drains are passed through the inferior flap, one under the flap and one in the axilla, making sure the tip of the drain does not lie against the vein to prevent its damage by the suction.
- The dermis is approximated with 3-0 absorbable suture followed by subcuticular 4-0 sutures.

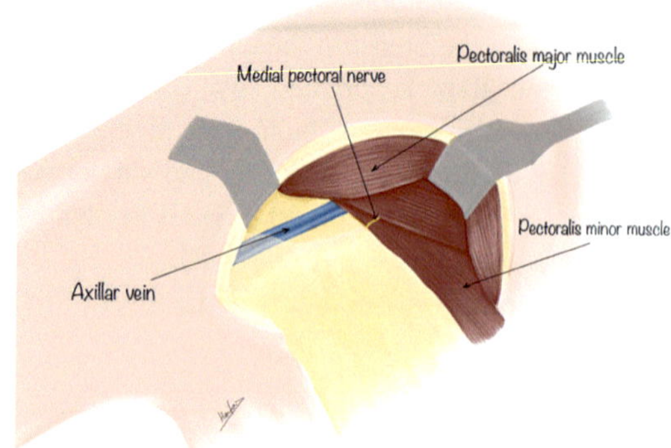

Fig. 1.6 The upper limit of the axillary dissection is the axillary vein

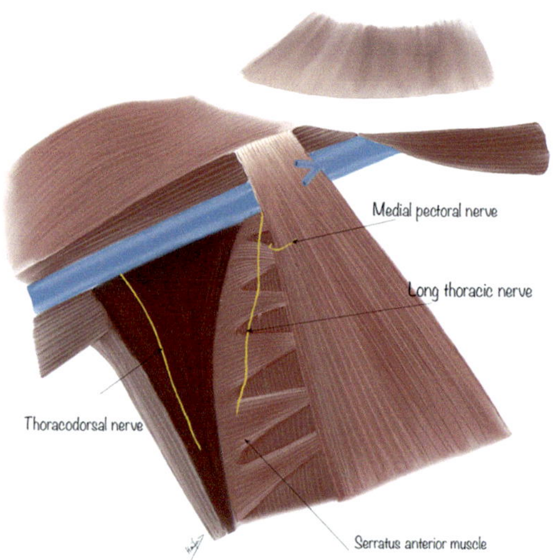

Fig. 1.7 The long thoracic nerve lies medially over the lateral chest wall while the thoracodorsal bundle laterally

- Closure is reinforced by Steri-Strip, then dressing of the wound.
- The drain is kept under negative pressure [14].

1.1.6 Postoperative Follow-Up

Early postoperative care:

- Resume diet once fully awake.
- Medication to be given:
  - Analgesia
  - Antibiotic if indicated
  - DVT prophylaxis and ulcer prophylaxis if indicated

- Encourage early mobilization.
- Monitor the drain output for the amount and color.
- Monitor the patient vital signs.
- If the drain output is <20 ml, remove it and discharge the patient.
- If the output is still high, patient can be discharged with the drain with instruction.

First outpatient visit:

- Check if the patient has any complaint.
- Examine the wound.
- Remove the sutures or clips if there is any.
- Check the final pathology result.
- Arrange for multidisciplinary team discussion.
- Refer to medical oncology or radiation therapy as indicated.

Long-term follow-up [2]**:**

- History and physical exam 1–4 times per year as clinically appropriate for 5 years, then annually
- **Genetic screening:**
  - Periodic screening for changes in family history and genetic testing indications and referral to genetic counseling as indicated
- **Post-surgical management:**
  - Educate, monitor, and refer for lymphedema management.
  - Mammography every 12 months.
  - Routine imaging of reconstructed breast is not indicated.
- **Screening for metastases:**
  - In the absence of clinical signs and symptoms suggestive of recurrent disease, there is no indication for laboratory or imaging studies for metastases screening.
- **Endocrine therapy:**
  - Assess and encourage adherence to adjuvant endocrine therapy.
  - Patients on tamoxifen: gynecologic assessment every 12 months if uterus present. Routine annual pelvic ultrasound is not recommended.
  - Patients on an aromatase inhibitor or who experience ovarian failure secondary to treatment should have monitoring of bone health with a bone mineral density determination at baseline and periodically thereafter [2].

1.2 Part II: Practice

Practice is the hardest part of learning, and training is the essence of transformation.
—Ann Voskamp

1.2.1 Case Scenarios for Practice

Tips:

- Practice with a friend and try to mimic the real exam!
- Don't forget to set the timer!
- Some twist points are suggested after each case and can be used to change the scenario to more difficult one.

Case No. 1:
A 25-year-old female patient presented to surgery clinic complaining of breast lump for 1-month duration.

Questions for discussion:

1. How will you approach the patient?
2. What is your next step (after clinical history and physical examination)?
3. Based on the result of the radiological investigation, what should be your plan of management?
4. What are the indications of surgical excision of her lump?
5. The patient came to you after 6 months with increase in the size of her breast lump to the double. What will be your decision?
6. Further assessment confirms the diagnosis (Fibroadenoma), size now is 30 × 29 mm. How will you prepare her for the operation?
7. What are the possible complications?
8. What is your long-term follow-up plan?

Possible twist points:

- The final pathology is cancer or DCIS. What will you do?

- The patient presents later on with seroma collection. How will you manage it?

Case No. 2:

A 42-year-old female patient referred to you from primary health care with abnormal finding in her screening mammogram.

Questions for discussion:

1. How will you approach the patient?
2. What is your next step (after clinical history and physical examination)?
3. Based on the result of the radiological investigation, what should be your plan of management?
4. The histopathology result is normal breast tissue. What will be your decision?
5. How will you prepare her for the operation?
6. What are the possible complications?
7. The final pathology result is ductal carcinoma in situ, tumor size is 2 cm, low grade, no comedo necrosis, triple negative receptors, margins are free except the posterior margin was positive. What will be your decision?
8. What are the indications of SLNB in DCIS?
9. What is your long-term follow-up plan?

Possible twist point:

- The diagnosis is upgraded to invasive carcinoma on the final pathology!
- Patient has a contraindication to radiation therapy; for example, she has been diagnosed to have scleroderma!

Case No. 3:

A 56-year-old female patient presented to you with 6-weeks history of breast pain and swelling.

Questions for Discussion:

1. How will you approach the patient?
2. What is your next step (after clinical history and physical examination)?
3. Based on the result of the radiological investigation, what should be your next step of management?
4. The histopathology result is invasive ductal carcinoma, grade 3, triple negative, Ki67 is 60%, FNA is positive for malignant cells. What is your plan of management?
5. The staging CT and bone scan are negative. What is her clinical stage?
6. Patient received eight cycles of chemotherapy as neoadjuvant and came to you. What will be your plan of management?
7. She is asking, since she has a good response to chemotherapy, is there any role for breast-conserving surgery in her condition?
8. What will you do with the axilla?
9. How will you prepare her for the operation?
10. What are the possible complications?
11. What is your long-term follow-up plan?

Possible Twist Points:

- Patient has metastasis on staging work up on L4. What will you do?
- Patient presents later on with inability to raise her arm to comb her hair. What is the cause and how you will manage it?

Case No. 4:

A 43-year-old male patient presented to you complaining of breast lump for 3 months.

Questions for Discussion:

1. How will you approach the patient?
2. What is your next step (after clinical history and physical examination)?
3. Based on the result of the radiological investigation, what should be your plan of management?
4. The histopathology result is invasive ductal carcinoma, grade 2, ER positive, PR positive, HER2Neu negative, Ki67 is 30%. What is your plan of management?
5. The staging CT and bone scan are negative. What is his clinical stage?
6. How will you prepare him for the operation?
7. What is your long-term follow-up plan?

Possible Twist Points:

The patient has matted lymph nodes on physical examination. How you will manage him?

Case No. 5:

A 39-year-old pregnant female patient presented to surgery clinic complaining of breast lump for 1 month.

Questions for Discussion:

1. How will you approach the patient?
2. What is your next step (after clinical history and physical examination)?
3. Based on the result of the radiological investigation, what should be your plan of management?
4. The histopathology of her biopsy is invasive ductal carcinoma, grade2, triple negative receptors, ki67 is 40%. What will be your management plan?
5. Is there any other option for management?
6. What is your long-term follow-up plan?

Possible Twist Points:

- The patient is in her first trimester!
- The patient is in her third trimester!
- The histopathology of her biopsy is invasive ductal carcinoma, grade2, ER, PR positive HER2 negative, ki67 is 40%. What will be your management plan?

Checklist

History	Items	Done	Not done	Not applicable
General	Introduce herself/himself to the patient			
	Patient personal data (name, age, gender, nationality)			
	Chief complaint			
	Duration			
Pain	Onset			
	Site			
	Character			
	Radiation/shifting			
	Aggravating/reliving			
	Severity			
	Relation to menstruation			
Lump	How did she notice it?			
	Any change since that time?			
	Any other lumps in the body?			
Nipple discharge	Unilateral or bilateral			
	Spontaneous or induced?			
	Nature (milk, blood, serous, greenish)			
	Lactating or not?			
Associated symptoms	Fever			
	Arm swelling			
Constitutional symptoms	Weight loss			
	Decrease appetite			
	Night sweating			
Risk factors	Menarche/menopause			
	Number of pregnancies			
	History of radiation			
	Age at first childbirth			
	Hormonal replacement therapy/hormonal contraceptives			
	Family history of breast, colon, ovarian, and prostate cancers			
	Personal history of any cancers			
Differential diagnosis	History of trauma (fat necrosis)			

(continued)

History	Items	Done	Not done	Not applicable
Symptoms of metastasis	Bone pain			
	Headache			
	Abdominal pain/jaundice			
	Cough/shortness of breath			
PMH	Previous similar complaint			
	Previous mammogram/ultrasound			
	Previous biopsy			
	Chronic illness			
PSH				
Social history				
Medication				
Allergy				
Systemic review				
Physical Examination				
General principle	Position			
	Permission			
	Privacy			
	Exposure			
	Wash hands			
General examination	Appearance			
	Body built			
	Color			
	Distress/decubitus			
	Environment			
Vital signs	Bp, HR, temp., RR, Spo_2			
Inspection	Inspection while arms raised behind the head and while pressing over her hips			
	Breast size			
	Asymmetry			
	Skin changes			
	Nipple inversion			
	Tethering			
	Visible masses			
Palpation	Start with the normal side			
	Systemic palpation of all areas including axillary tail			
Lump	Site			
	Number			
	Size			
	Shape			
	Consistency			
	Tenderness			
	Temperature			
	Mobility			
	Nipple discharge			
Lymph node	Palpable node (axillary, supraclavicular)			
	Which group			
	Single or multiple			
	Matted or mobile			
	Arm lymphedema			

History	Items		Done	Not done	Not applicable
Other system for metastasis	Palpate the lower back				
	Palpate the abdomen for hepatomegaly				
	Examine the lungs				
Differential diagnosis					
Investigation					
Blood	CBC				
	Coagulation				
	ALP				
	LFT				
	RFT				
Imaging	Ultrasound				
	Mammogram				
	MRI				
	Others: for example, ductogram				
Biopsy	Trucut				
	Stereotactic				
	MRI guided				
	Put a clip post biopsy				
Management (Depends on the Diagnosis)					
Breast cancer	Staging				
	MRI breast (if she will go for neoadjuvant)				
	Discuss in tumor board				
	Inform the patient and explain the plan				
	If neoadjuvant is indicated	Neoadjuvant chemotherapy			
		Re-evaluation			
		Re-staging			
		Discuss the response in tumor board			
		Inform the patient about the decision			
	Admission				
	Consent				
	Preoperative preparation (anesthesia evaluation, NPO, IV fluid, prophylaxis)				
	Preoperative medication (DVT prophylaxis, prophylactic antibiotic, stress ulcer prophylaxis if needed)				
	Surgical site marking				
	Surgery (lumpectomy/mastectomy/MRM/wire localization and excision, SLNB/ALND)				
DCIS/pleomorphic LCIS	Inform the patient and explain the plan				
	Admission				
	Consent				
	Preoperative preparation (anesthesia evaluation, NPO, IV fluid, prophylaxis)				
	Preoperative medication (DVT prophylaxis, prophylactic antibiotic, stress ulcer prophylaxis if needed)				
	Surgical site marking				
	Surgery (lumpectomy/mastectomy/wire localization and excision, ± SLNB)				

(continued)

History	Items	Done	Not done	Not applicable
Phyllodes	Discuss in tumor board			
	Chest imaging			
	Preoperative preparation			
	Surgical site marking			
	Admission			
	Consent			
	Excision with 1 cm margin/mastectomy			
LCIS classic	Reassure the patient that this is not cancer or premalignant It is a marker for high risk			
	Explain the options: 1. Close follow-up 2. Chemoprevention 3. Prophylactic bilateral mastectomy			
Fibroadenoma	Reassure the patient			
	Interval follow-up			
Abscess	Antibiotics			
	Aspiration/drainage			
Cyst	Aspirate ± cytology			
Postop Care				
Follow up	Clinical evaluation (history and physical examination)			
	Remove suture if applicable			
	Check the final pathology, margins			
	Discuss in a tumor board if cancer or DCIS			
	Refer to oncologist or radiotherapist if needed			
	Genetic counselling			
	Explain the long-term follow-up			

1.2.2 Answer Key

Case No. 1:

A 25-year-old female patient presented to surgery clinic complaining of breast lump for 1-month duration.

Questions for Discussion:

1. **How will you approach the patient?**

- Using triple assessment approach. The patient is a 25-year-old female who complains of right breast lump for 1 month. She felt the mass while she was taking shower. There is no change in the size since she first noticed it, and not associated with pain or any nipple discharge. She is single, her menarche at age of 15 years and her menstrual cycle is regular. She has no history of trauma, weight loss, decreased appetite, fever, or sweating. She has no history of radiation exposure, nor personal history of family history of cancers. She has no relevant past medical or surgical history, not on any regular medication. She is a smoker and allergic to egg; other systemic review is unremarkable.

- On physical examination, she looks well, obese lady, lying comfortable on the bed, not pale or jaundiced.

- Her both breasts are symmetrical, no obvious mass, tethering, skin erythema. Nipple and areola complex look normal. There is palpable well-defined right breast mass, at 3 O'clock position, 2 × 2 cm, round shape, smooth surface, and freely mobile.
- Other breast and both axillae are free from masses.

2. **What is your next step (after clinical history and physical examination)?**

- Ultrasound showed well-defined, hypoechoic solid mass, has a diameter of 20 × 18 mm.

3. **Based on the result of the radiological investigation, what should be your plan of management?**

- This patient most likely has fibroadenoma which requires no treatment at this point. The plan is to reassure her and to give her appointment for follow-up.

4. **What are the indications of surgical excision of her lump?**

- Continuous increase in size
- Cosmetic or the patient wants surgery
- >2 cm in size

5. **The patient came to you after 6 months with increase in the size of her breast lump to the double. What will be your decision?**

- Repeat the clinical assessment and ultrasound ± biopsy, and most likely she will need surgical excision.

6. **Further assessment confirms the diagnosis (Fibroadenoma), size now is 30 × 29 mm. How you will prepare her for the operation?**

- Operation can be done as day surgery.
- CBC, coagulation, and blood grouping as baseline investigation.
- Patient has to quit smoking before the operation by at least 1 month.
- Patient will be instructed to be fasting from midnight and to take a shower that night.
- No need for antibiotic prophylaxis.
- Surgical site to be marked.
- Informed consent to be taken.

7. **What are the possible complications?**

- Specific: infection, bleeding, and fluid collection
- General: DVT, PE, atelectasis, and pneumonia

8. **What is your long-term follow-up plan?**

- Patient will be instructed upon discharge to ambulate, eat and drink normally.
- Analgesia to be given to her.
- Appoint for follow up in the clinic.
- Patient will be assessed in the clinic for any complaint.
- Wound will be examined.
- To review the histopathology result, if the result is fibroadenoma no further treatment needed.
- Patient will be discharged from the clinic.

Possible Twist Points:

- The final pathology is cancer or DCIS!
- The patient presents later on with seroma collection. How you will manage it?

Case No. 2:

A 42-year-old female patient referred to you from primary health care with abnormal finding in her screening mammogram.

Questions for Discussion:

1. **How will you approach the patient?**

- Starting by clinical assessment (history and physical examination). She is a 42-year-old female with no active breast complaint. She started on screening program when she was 40 years. Currently she was referred due to a suspicious feature on her mammogram (a cluster of microcalcification at the upper outer quadrant of her right breast). Her menarche at age of 12 years and her menstrual cycle is regular. She is a mother of four kids, she delivered the first baby when she was 29 and the youngest is 4 years old. She used hormonal contraceptive pills between her pregnancies with a cumulative time of 5 years. Her mother died of breast cancer when she was 51 years old. She has no history of breast trauma and her last screening mammogram was normal.
- Her PMH, PSH, and FH otherwise unremarkable. She is not known allergic, and currently

she is on OCP. Systemic review is unremarkable.

- Physical examination:
- Obese otherwise healthy-looking lady. Normal vital signs.
- Both breast and axillary examinations are normal.

2. **What is your next step (after clinical history and physical examination)?**

- Repeat her mammogram (diagnostic) with complementary ultrasound.
- It showed a cluster of microcalcification at 10 O'clock position. No mass could be identified. No radiological detected abnormal lymph nodes (BIRAD IV).

3. **Based on the result of the radiological investigation, what should be your plan of management?**

- Stereotactic core needle biopsy and making sure to leave a clip.

4. **The histopathology result is normal breast tissue. What will be your decision?**

- The result is discordant to the radiological finding. Wire localization and excisional biopsy is the best option in this case.

5. **How will you prepare her for the operation?**

- Preoperative preparation:
- Anesthesia evaluation, CXR, ECG.
- NPO, IV fluid, consent. (Explain to the patient that this is a diagnostic step, and she might need further operation according to the final pathology.)
- Instruct the patient to take a shower the night before the operation.
- Surgical site marking.
- Arrange with the radiologist for insertion of wire localization and to image the excised breast tissue to confirm complete excision of the target lesion.

6. **What are the possible complications?**

- Bleeding, wound infection, seroma
- General complication like DVT, PE, MI

7. **The final pathology result is ductal carcinoma in situ, tumor size is 2 cm, low grade, no comedo necrosis, ER, PR negative, and margins are free except the posterior margin was positive. What will be your decision?**

- Break the bad news to the patient.
- Discuss the case in a multidisciplinary team meeting.
- She needs re-excision of the posterior margin.
- Postoperative radiation therapy (van Nuys score is 8).
- No need for adjuvant endocrine therapy since receptor status is negative.
- SLNB is not indicated in her condition.

8. **What are the indications of SLNB in DCIS?**

- Presence of palpable mass
- Nipple discharge
- High grade/comedo necrosis
- Large size >4 cm

9. **What is your long-term follow-up plan?**

- History and physical examination every 6–12 months for 5 years
- Mammogram every 12 months (first mammogram 6–12 months after BCS)

Possible Twist Point:

- The diagnosis is upgraded to invasive carcinoma on the final pathology!

- Patient has a contraindication to radiation therapy; for example, she has been diagnosed to have scleroderma!

Case No. 3:

A 56-year-old female patient presented to you with 6-weeks history of breast pain and swelling.

Questions for Discussion:

1. **How will you approach the patient?**

- Starting by clinical assessment. She is a 56-year-old female. She is complaining of left breast pain for the last 6 weeks. The pain started gradually and is dull aching in nature, not radiated or shifted, no specific aggravating or relieving factors, mild to moderated in severity, associated with swelling of the ipsilateral breast and erythema, not associated with fever or nipple discharge. She sought medical advice before 3 weeks and received a course of antibiotics, but she felt no improvement. No history of trauma to the breast. She is postmenopause. She has no kids. During the last 20 years, she was receiving hormonal therapy to treat her infertility, no significant family history of breast cancer. She is diabetic on insulin, and in her past surgical history, she underwent cholecystectomy long time ago.
- Other systemic review is of no clinical significance

- On physical examination, she looks ill, average body built, not jaundice or pale. Her vital sign within the normal limits. Her breast examination revealed asymmetry, left breast is swollen, skin is erythematous, and has peau d'orange appearance. The left breast is hard, tender with a palpable mass at 2 O'clock position. The mass is about 4 cm, ill defined, hard, fixed to skin. Nipple areola complex is free. The right breast is normal. Freely mobile left axillary lymph nodes are palpable. Right axilla is free.
- No tenderness over the spine and no hepatomegaly.

2. **What is your next step (after clinical history and physical examination)?**

- Bilateral mammogram with ultrasound.
- Imaging revealed a BI-RADs V breast lesion with suspicious multiple left axillary lymph nodes.
- Right breast is classified as B-IRADs I.

3. **Based on the result of the radiological investigation what should be your next step of management?**

- Core needle biopsy of her breast and FNA of the axillary lymph node

4. **The histopathology result is invasive ductal carcinoma, grade 3, triple negative, Ki67 is 60%, FNA is positive for malignant cells. What is your plan of management?**

- She meets the criteria of inflammatory breast cancer (rapid onset of breast edema, erythema that involve at least one third of the breast, biopsy confirms invasive cancer).
- Management plan should be:
  - Break the bad news to the patient.
  - Staging CT CAP, bone scan.
  - Discuss the case in a multidisciplinary team meeting.
  - The decision most likely will be neoadjuvant chemotherapy.

- (N.B. No need for breast MRI because it will not change the management of the affected breast.)

5. **The staging CT and bone scan are negative. What is her clinical stage?**

- T4d, N1, M0, stage III B.

6. **Patient received eight cycles of chemotherapy as neoadjuvant and came to you. What will be your plan of management?**
   - Repeat clinical assessment.
   - Assess the tumor response.
   - Repeat staging imaging.
   - Rediscuss her condition in tumor board meeting.
   - Prepare her for surgery MRM after 3–4 weeks from her last dose of chemotherapy.

- Her tumor markedly regresses after chemotherapy, no palpable axillary lymph node is palpable, and her staging imaging is free.

7. **She is asking, since she has a good response to chemotherapy, is there any role for breast conserving surgery in her condition?**

- No role for BCS in her condition even if there is good response as her diagnosis is inflammatory breast cancer.

8. **What will you do with the axilla?**

- Axillary lymph node dissection.

9. **How will you prepare her for the operation?**
   - Anesthesia evaluation
   - Make sure her DM is controlled
   - ECG ± echocardiography
   - Admission
   - Explain the procedure to the patient and take her consent
   - Instruct the patient to take shower the night before the surgery and to shave the axilla if needed
   - Surgical site marking
   - DVT prophylaxis if indicated
   - Stress ulcer prophylaxis
   - Antibiotic prophylaxis (as indicated)
   - Check her base line CBC, coagulation profile, LFT, RFT, blood group

10. **What are the possible complications?**

- General: DVT, PE, MI, atelectasis, and pneumonia
- Specific: wound infection, bleeding, seroma, flap necrosis, nerve injury, lymphedema of the arm

11. **What is your long-term follow-up plan?**
    - Every 6 months history and physical examination
    - Mammogram annually
    - In the absence of symptoms or signs of metastatic disease, no need for routine metastatic work up

Possible Twist Points:

- Patient has metastasis on staging work up on L4. What will you do?
- Patient presents later on with inability to raise her arm to comb her hair. What is the cause and how you will manage it?

Case No. 4:

A 43-year-old male patient presented to you complaining of breast lump for 3 months.

Questions for Discussion:

1. **How will you approach the patient?**

- Starting by clinical assessment. He is a 43-year-old male patient who noticed a right breast lump 3 months ago. It was small, then starts to increase in size with time. No other lumps on the body. No pain or nipple discharge. His sister diagnosed with breast cancer when she was 45 years old. He has no history of breast trauma. He has no significant PMH or PSH. He is a smoker and allergic to penicillin.
- On physical examination, he looks well, with average body built. His vital signs are normal. His right breast has obvious swelling at 6 O'clock, no skin erythema, edema, or ulceration. Both nipples are normal. There is a non-tender, palpable mass at right breast, about 3 cm with irregular margin that felt hard and is not attached to skin or underlying muscle. The left breast and both axillae are normal.
- No tenderness over the spine, and there is no hepatomegaly.

2. **What is your next step (after clinical history and physical examination)?**

- Bilateral breast mammogram and ultrasound for both breasts and axillae.
- Image showed a right breast speculated mass at 6 O'clock position consistent with BI-RADs V.

3. **Based on the result of the radiological investigation, what should be your plan of management?**

- Core needle biopsy of the breast mass.

4. **The histopathology result is invasive ductal carcinoma, grade 2, ER positive, PR positive, HER2Neu negative, Ki67 is 30%. What is your plan of management?**
   - Break the bad news to the patient.
   - No need for staging imaging (according to his clinical stage).
   - Discuss in a tumor board.
   - Prepare for surgery mastectomy +SLNB if positive ALND.

5. **What is his clinical stage?**

- T2, N0, M0, stage IIA.

6. **How will you prepare him for the operation?**
   - Anesthesia evaluation.
   - ECG, CXR.
   - Admission.
   - Explain the procedure to the patient and take his consent.
   - Instruct the patient to take shower the night before the surgery and to shave the axilla.
   - Surgical site marking.
   - DVT prophylaxis if indicated.
   - Stress ulcer prophylaxis.
   - Antibiotic prophylaxis (as indicated).
   - Check his base line CBC, coagulation profile, LFT, RFT, blood group.

7. **What is your long-term follow-up plan?**
   - Refer for genetic counselling
   - Adjuvant chemotherapy and endocrine therapy (tamoxifen); every 6 months history and physical examination.
   - No need for contralateral mammogram.
   - In the absence of symptoms or signs of metastatic disease, no need for metastatic work up.

Possible twist point:

- The patient has matted lymph node on physical examination. How you will manage him?

Case No. 5:
A 39-year-old pregnant female patient presented to surgery clinic complaining of breast lump for 1-month.

Questions for Discussion:

1. **How will you approach the patient?**

- The patient is a 39-year-old pregnant lady in her second trimester (24 weeks). She noticed a left breast lump before 1 month that is getting bigger with time, not associated with pain or nipple discharge. She did not notice any other lumps in her body. Her menarche at age of 13 years old and she has two other kids, she delivered the first one when she was 27 years old. She has no significant family history of breast cancer. She was on OCP for 5 years.
- No other significant PMH, PSH, or social history.
- On physical examination, she looks well, stable vital signs.
- Her left breast was larger than the right, her left nipple is retracted, no skin changes. There is a palpable hard mass at her left breast in the retro-areolar area, about 4 cm, irregular shape, and is not tender.
- Left axilla was positive for matted lymph nodes, right side is normal.

2. **What is your next step (after clinical history and physical examination)?**

- Bilateral mammogram and ultrasound showed BI-RADs V lesion on her left breast multiple suspicious left axillary lymph node. Right breast and axilla are unremarkable.

3. **Based on the result of the radiological investigation, what should be your next step of management?**

- Core needle biopsy of her breast mass.

4. **The histopathology of her biopsy is invasive ductal carcinoma, grade2, triple negative receptors, ki67 is 40%. What will be your management plan?**
   - Break the bad news to the patient.
   - Staging work up for T1 and T2 are CXR with shielding, LFT; for T3 or clinically positive axilla, add liver ultrasound and consider MRI of thoracic and lumbar spine without contrast.
   - Discuss the case in a tumor board meeting.
   - The decision most likely will be neoadjuvant chemotherapy followed by surgery postpartum.

5. **Is there any other option for management?**

- Upfront surgery followed by adjuvant chemotherapy postpartum.

6. **What is your long-term follow-up plan?**
   - Every 6 months history and physical examination.
   - Mammogram annually.
   - In absence of symptoms or signs of metastatic disease, no need for routine metastatic work up.

Possible Twist Points:

- The patient is in her first trimester!
- The patient is in her third trimester!
- The histopathology of her biopsy is invasive ductal carcinoma, grade2, ER, PR positive HER2 negative, ki67 is 40%. What will be your management plan?

References

1. Khouri N. Breast imaging. In: Cameron J, Cameron A, editors. Current surgical therapy. 12th ed. Canada: Elsevier; 2016.
2. ["Referenced with permission from the NCCN Clinical Practice Guidelines in Oncology (NCCN Guidelines®) for Breast Screening V.1.2020. © National Comprehensive Cancer Network, Inc. 1. All rights reserved. Accessed [February 18, 1]. To view the most recent and complete version of the guideline, go online to NCCN.org. NCCN makes no warranties of any kind whatsoever regarding their content, use or application and disclaims any responsibility for their application or use in any way."].
3. Jieqiong L, Jacobs L. The management of benign breast disease. In: Cameron J, Cameron A, editors. Current surgical therapy. 12th ed. Canada: Elsevier; 2016.
4. Parker C, Damodaran S, Bland K, Hunt K. The breast. In: Brunicardi F, editor. Schwartz's principles of surgery. 11th ed. United States: McGraw-Hill Education; 2019.
5. Camp M. Ductal and lobular carcinoma in situ of the breast. In: Cameron J, Cameron A, editors. Current surgical therapy. 12th ed. Canada: Elsevier; 2016.
6. Gray R. Margins: how to and how big? In: Cameron J, Cameron A, editors. Current surgical therapy. 12th ed. Canada: Elsevier; 2016.
7. Euhus D. Breast cancer: surgical therapy. In: Cameron J, Cameron A, editors. Current surgical therapy. 12th ed. Canada: Elsevier; 2016.
8. Rosso K, Newman L. Advances in neoadjuvant and adjuvant therapy for breast cancer. In: Cameron J, Cameron A, editors. Current surgical therapy. 12th ed. Canada: Elsevier; 2016.
9. McCartan D, Gemignani M. The management of the axilla in breast cancer. In: Cameron J, Cameron A, editors. Current surgical therapy. 12th ed. Canada; Elsevier; 2016.
10. Gangi A, Giuliano A. Lymphatic mapping and sentinel lymphadenectomy. In: Cameron J, Cameron A, editors. Current surgical therapy. 12th ed. Canada: Elsevier; 2016.
11. Puig C, Boughey J. The management of recurrent and metastatic breast cancer. In: Cameron J, Cameron A, editors. Current surgical therapy. 12th ed. Canada: Elsevier; 2016.
12. Plichta J, Smith B. Inflammatory breast cancer. In: Cameron J, Cameron A, editors. Current surgical therapy. 12th ed. Canada: Elsevier; 2016.
13. Cody H. Male breast cancer. In: Cameron J, Cameron A, editors. Current surgical therapy. 12th ed. Canada: Elsevier; 2016.
14. Zollinger R, Ellison E. Breast cancer: surgical therapy. Zollinger's atlas of surgical operation. 9th ed. United States: McGraw-Hill Education; 2011.

2 Surgical Aspects of Thyroid Diseases for Clinical Board Exams

2.1 Part I: Knowledge

> Knowledge is power? No. Knowledge on its own is nothing, but the application of useful knowledge, now that is powerful.
> —Rob Liano

2.1.1 History of Thyroid Complaint

Possible Chief Complaint:

- Lump
- Symptoms of hypothyroidism or hyperthyroidism
- Compression symptoms
- Invasion (hoarseness)

Differential Diagnosis of Neck Mass:

- Benign thyroid nodule
- Multinodular goiter
- Toxic thyroid nodule
- Toxic goiter
- Thyroid cancer
- Thyroglossal cyst
- Enlarged lymph nodes
- Parathyroid adenoma
- Metastatic nodule
- Cystic hygroma
- Aneurysm
- Bronchocele
- Laryngocele
- Carotid body tumor

History:

- Introduce yourself to the patient.
- Personal data: name, age, occupation, sex, nationality.
- Chief complaint, duration.
- History of presenting illness.
  - **Analysis of chief complaint**

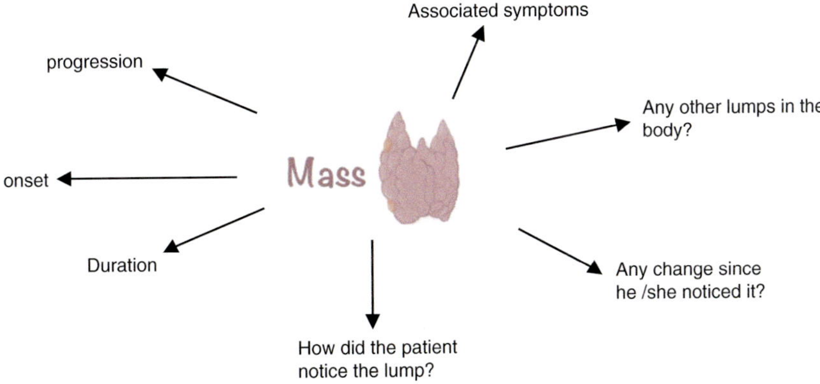

H. Alotaibi, *Study Surgery*, https://doi.org/10.1007/978-981-16-2305-9_2

- **Associated symptoms:**
  Symptoms of hypothyroidism (weight gain, decreased appetite, fatigue, constipation, cold intolerance, amenorrhea, depression, or loss of hair)
  Symptoms of hyperthyroidism [weight loss, increased appetite, diarrhea, heat intolerance, agitation, palpitation, sweating, menorrhagia, or eyes symptoms (pain/dryness)]
- **Constitutional symptoms:** weight loss, fever, night sweating, decreased appetite
- **Compression symptoms:** dysphagia, shortness of breath, cough, wheezes, hoarseness
- **Risk factors:**
  History of radiation, family history of thyroid, adrenal, and colon cancers (If yes, what is the degree of relationship and age at the diagnosis?)
- **Differential diagnosis:**
  Recent infection (lymph node)
  Symptoms of primary hyperparathyroidism (abdominal pain, renal stone, bone pain, psychological problem)
- **Previous similar attack**, previous investigation (ultrasound, CT, FNA)
- **Systemic review of the related system:**
  Endocrine system (headache, palpitation, hypertension, DM, weakness)

- Past medical history
- Past surgical history
- Family history
- Medication (current and previous), allergy, blood transfusion
- Social history (smoking, alcohol, drug abuse)
- Systemic review
  - **CNS:** (headache, blurred vision, hearing symptoms, numbness, paralysis)
  - **CVS:** (chest pain, palpitation, paroxysmal nocturnal dyspnea, orthopnea)
  - **RS:** (shortness of breath, cough, sputum)
  - **GIT:** (nausea, vomiting, diarrhea, constipation, distention)
  - **Renal:** (dysuria, hematuria, flank pain)
  - **MSK:** (arthritis, bone pain, weakness)

Physical Examination

- Introduce yourself to the patient.
- Ask permission for examination.
- Assure privacy.
- Position: sitting.
- Exposure: neck and upper chest.
- Handwashing.

General examination:

- Appearance (ill, well, underclothes or wearing layered heavy clothes)
- Body built (underweight, overweight, normal weight)
- Color (jaundice, pale)
- Distress/decubitus
- Environment

Vital signs: BP, PR, temperature, Spo_2, RR
Hands:

- Feel the pulse (tachycardia, bradycardia, atrial fibrillation).
- Is there tremor? Extend the patient arms, elbow, and wrist straight, fingers apart, look for fine tremor.
- Look for muscle wasting, nails (thyroid acropathy, onycholysis).
- Palm (warm and moist/sweaty, dry/cold).
- Water hammer pulse.

Eyes:

- Eyebrow: loss of hair in lateral one third.
- Lid retraction: upper eyelid is higher than normal and lower eyelid is normal.
- Lid lag: delay in moving the eyelid as the eyes move downwards.
- Exophthalmos: Eyeball is pushed forward by an increase in retro-orbital fat, edema, and cellular infiltration. Sclera becomes visible below the lower edge of the iris. Patient can look up without wrinkling the forehead.
- Corneal ulceration.
- Ophthalmoplegia: patient cannot look upward and outward due to paralysis of the superior and lateral recti muscle.
- Chemosis: edema of the conjunctiva.

Neck:
Inspection:

- Look for any visible swelling.
- Ask the patient to swallow.
  Thyroid swelling ascends during swallowing.
- Ask the patient to protrude the tongue.
  If the lump moves up: it is thyroglossal cyst.
- Look for any distended neck veins or scars.
- Ask the patient to raise the hands above the head (Pemberton's sign); indicate thoracic outlet obstruction.

Palpation:

- From the front:
  – Confirm your visual impression
  – (size, shape, surface, tenderness, and temperature)
  – Position of the trachea and carotid artery pulsation
  – Position of the thyroid cartilage
- From behind (the most important part)
  – Stand behind the patient.
  – Tilt patient head slightly forward to relax the anterior neck muscles.
  – Press on one side and palpate the opposite lobe each time.
  – Ask the patient to swallow and confirm that any swelling moving with swallowing.
  – Assess (site, size, shape, surface, consistency, tenderness, fixation to skin or muscle).
  – Check for the lower border; determine whether you can or cannot go below it which may indicate retrosternal extension.
  – Palpate the whole neck for any cervical and supraclavicular lymph nodes.
  – Noticed that normal thyroid gland is not palpable.

Percussion:

- Over manubrium sterni: to define the lower extent of the swelling
- Auscultation
- Systolic bruit over the swelling (thyrotoxic gland)

CVS:

- Heartrate
- Any sign of heart failure

CNS:

- Tremor
- Agitation
- Reflexes (sluggish in myxedema)
- Proximate myopathy

Skin: Pretibial myxedema (deposit of myxoid tissue within the skin)

2.1.2 Approach to Patient with Thyroid Nodule

- History and physical examination as described earlier
- Serum TSH
- Serum calcitonin (not routinely, if suggested MTC by history)
- Ultrasound of thyroid and neck:
  – **High suspicion:** solid hypoechoic or partially cystic with solid hypoechoic component with one or more of features like irregular margins, microcalcification, taller than wider, extrathyroidal extension
  – **Intermediate suspicion:** hypoechoic solid nodule without microcalcification, extrathyroidal extension
  – **Low suspicion:** isoechoic or hyperechoic nodule
  – **Very low suspicion:** spongiform without suspicious sonographic features
  – **Benign:** pure cystic
- Radioisotope scanning:
  – If suppressed TSH (hyperthyroidism)
  – Can use:
    Technetium 99 (disadvantage: taken up by salivary gland and major vasculature
    ^{123}I: low dose of radiation (30 mCi), shorter half-life (12–13 h), and mainly use for diagnostic purposes
    ^{131}I: optimal in case of cancer, high radiation, long half-life (8 days), and mainly used for therapeutic, for example, post-

operative ablation in high-risk thyroid cancer
- PET scan
- CT/MRI:
  - To evaluate local and retrosternal extension in more advanced stage of thyroid cancer
  - Concerns in CT (Iodide contrast):
    If patient is hyperthyroid: may trigger thyroid storm.
    Patient must be iodine depleted before therapeutic RAI treatment of thyroid cancer (4 weeks is the adequate time for clearance of iodine after CT).
  - Staging in MTC
- FNA:
  - Small gauge needle (23-27 gauge) with capillary or suction technique.
  - Can be done with ultrasound guided or without.
  - Use ultrasound if heterogenous, nonpalpable, posterior located, cystic nodule.
  - Indication of FNA:
    High suspicion nodule on ultrasound: FNA at ≥1 cm
    Intermediate suspicion: FNA at ≥1 cm
    Low suspicion: FNA at ≥1.5 cm
    Very low suspicion: FNA at ≥2 cm or observe without FNA
    Benign: no indication for FNA
  - Result of FNA: according to Bethesda classification
  - Notes:
    Cellular features can diagnose PTC, but for FTC, capsular and vascular invasion are needed for the diagnosis.
    Pure cystic lesion does not require FNA, but aspiration of cystic fluid to relieve mass effect may be done.
    Cyst that has residual mass, or benign cytology that recur should be considered for thyroid lobectomy.
  - If multiple nodules in ultrasound >1 cm:
    FNA the nodule with suspicious features.
    If RAI scan was done: FNA the cold nodule.
  - Bethesda classification:
    Bethesda I (Non diagnostic):
    - Repeat FNA after 3 months. If it is Bethesda I again, either continue close follow up or do thyroid lobectomy.

    Bethesda II (Benign):
    - Repeat ultrasound after 3–6 months if there are suspicious features in ultrasound.
    - Repeat ultrasound after 12–24 months if there are low or intermediate suspicious features in ultrasound.
    - Repeat ultrasound after 2 years if features are benign in both ultrasound and FNA.
    - If the repeated ultrasound performed for the nodule with benign biopsy shows either increase in the volume by 50% or increase in dimensions by 20%, repeat the FNA under ultrasound guidance.

    Bethesda III (atypia or follicular lesion of undetermined significance): Repeat FNA or molecular testing.
    Bethesda IV (follicular neoplasm or suspicious of follicular neoplasm): Perform diagnostic lobectomy, or upfront total thyroidectomy, if the lesion is more than 4 cm, presence of contralateral nodule, history of radiation, or family history is significant for thyroid cancer.
    Bethesda V (suspicious for malignancy): refer to Tables 2.1, 2.2, and 2.3.
    Bethesda VI (malignant): refer to Tables 2.1, 2.2, and 2.3 [1].

2.1.3 Management of Common Benign Thyroid Disease

2.1.3.1 Thyroiditis

- Symptoms: neck pain, tenderness, enlargement of the thyroid, and rarely fever
- **Hashimoto's thyroiditis:**
  - Progressive autoimmune disorder.
  - Characterized by lymphocytic infiltration, follicular cell atrophy, Hürthle cell metaplasia, Hürthle cell nodule, and fibrosis.
  - Increase the risk of thyroid lymphoma "B cell non-Hodgkin's": rapid enlarging goiter with Hashimoto's thyroiditis.

Table 2.1 Management of differentiated thyroid cancer [4, 5]

Type	Pathology	Prognostic indicators	Surgical management		
			Thyroid	Central lymph node	Lateral lymph node
Papillary thyroid cancer (PTC): • Most common 80% • Female: male ratio 2:1 • Patient usually is euthyroid • Slow growing • Symptoms mean advanced disease • Lymph node involvement is common, "lateral aberrant thyroid," i.e., metastasis to lateral lymph nodes • Most common sites of metastasis are lung, bone, liver, brain	FNAB of thyroid mass or lymph node show • Cells are cuboidal • Crowded nuclei "orphan Annie" • Psammoma bodies • Follicular variant classified as PTC • Multifocal 80% • Another variant: Tall cells, insular, columnar, diffuse sclerosing, clear cell, trabecular cells • Prognosis with these variants is poor	General: good prognosis **AGES:** Age, grade, extrathyroidal metastasis, size **MACIS:** Metastasis, age at presentation >40, completeness of resection, invasion, size **AMES:** Age at presentation (male <40, female <50, metastasis, extrathyroidal disease, size < or >5 cm	**>4 cm:** total thyroidectomy **>1 cm and <4 cm + low risk features:** (unifocal, absence of history of radiation, clinical and radiological negative lymph nodes): thyroid lobectomy (if low risk) or total thyroidectomy (if high risk) **<1 cm (microcarcinoma):** 1. Observation without immediate surgery for very low-risk tumors without extrathyroidal extension or lymph node metastases, if progress during observation treat it by surgery. OR 2. Thyroid lobectomy	• Enlarged lymph node "therapeutic" • T3 or T4 "Prophylactic central node dissection"	• Positive lateral lymph node "do central and lateral dissection" • Prophylactic lateral neck dissection is not necessary for PTC
Follicular thyroid cancer (FTC): • Account for 10% of all thyroid cancers • Male to female ratio 3:1 • Mean age: 50 years • Cervical lymph node metastases are uncommon • <1% of patient has hyperfunctioning thyroid	FNAB: unable to distinguish benign from cancer Considered malignant if there is capsular or vascular invasion		If FNA: follicular lesion • Do thyroid lobectomy (80% will be benign) • No frozen section • If positive for cancer in final pathology, total thyroidectomy If FNA showed atypia, size >4 cm, or the patient has history of radiation exposure or positive family history of thyroid cancer, up front total thyroidectomy	• Enlarged lymph node "therapeutic" • T3 or T4 "prophylactic central node dissection"	• Positive lateral lymph node "do central and lateral dissection" • Prophylactic lateral neck dissection is not necessary for PTC
Hürthle cell carcinoma: • Account for 3% of all thyroid cancer • It is a subtype of FTC • Cannot be diagnose by FNA • Differ from FTC in: usually bilateral, multifocal and do not take RAI • Metastasize to lymph node	Contain sheet of eosinophilic cells Considered malignant if there is capsular or vascular invasion		Do diagnostic lobectomy and isthmectomy: if adenoma, no further treatment is needed if carcinoma, total thyroidectomy is indicated	Should undergo routine central node dissection	Modified radical lateral neck dissection for palpable or image detected cervical lymph node

(continued)

Table 2.1 (continued)

Postoperative treatment	Follow-up
1. Radioiodine therapy: Indications: • Known metastasis • Extrathyroidal extension • Size >4 cm • High risk feature: (tall cell, columnar, insular, poor differentiated, intrathyroid vascular invasion, multifocal disease) • 1–4 cm with high-risk feature or lymph node metastasis Not indicated for: • Unifocal <1 cm without high-risk feature • Multifocal all <1 cm without high-risk feature Remnant ablation: Either by hormone withdrawal or recombinant TSH Hormonal withdrawal: 1. T4 therapy to be discontinued 6 weeks before ablation 2. Start T3 during this time and discontinue it 2 weeks before ablation 3. Target TSH: 30 4. Low-iodine diet during these 2 weeks Protocol of RAI ablation: • Screening dose 1–3 mCi and measure the uptake 24 h later • Therapeutic dose after 72 h (dose: for low-risk patient: 30–100 mCi, high-risk patient: 100–200 mCi), (maximum dose: at one time 200 mCi, cumulative: 1000–1500 mci) If the patient has elevated Tg but negative RAI scan: treat with mci of 131 I and repeat image 1–2 weeks after **2. Radiotherapy and chemotherapy:** No role of routine chemotherapy Radiation: for unresctable, locally invasive, bone metastases **3. Novel therapy**: kinase inhibitors **4. Thyroid hormone**: give T4 to suppress TSH. Target TSH: <0.1: persistent disease 0.3–2.0: clinical and biochemical free from disease, low risk patient 0.1–0.5: high risk patient	**Tg and anti Tg antibodies:** Every 6 months • Low-risk patients who have low suppressed Tg in the first year: measure Tg after T4 withdrawal or rTSH 12 months after ablation • Undetectable Tg: followed annually with clinical exam and Tg level on T4 treatment • Single rTSH-stimulated Tg <0.5 with absence of antibodies indicate 99.5% probability of complete free of disease on follow-up • Tg > 2 following rTSH indicate recurrence **Imaging:** after first post treatment scan • Low-risk patient, negative rTSH stimulated Tg, and negative ultrasound: do not require whole body scan • High-risk or intermediate-risk patient: scan 6–12 months, then annually for 3–5 years Note: if ultrasound showed suspicious nodule, manage according to size *>5–8 mm: biopsy and measure Tg in the aspiration *small nodule: follow-up and biopsy it if increase in size Note: if the patient has positive Tg and negative RAI scan: do PET scan

Table 2.2 Other types of thyroid cancers [4, 5]

			Surgical management			Postoperative treatment and follow-up
Type	Diagnosis	Pathology	Thyroid	Central lymph node	Lateral lymph node	
Medullary thyroid cancer (MTC): • Account for 5% of all thyroid cancer • Arise from parafollicular C cells • Concentrated superolateral in the thyroid • Most are sporadic • 25% are familiar (familial MTC, MEN2A, MEN2B), due to mutation in RET protooncogene • Sporadic: unilateral 80% • Familial: bilateral, multifocal • Female to male ratio 1.5:1 • Patients with hypercalcemia and elevated parathyroid hormone at time of thyroidectomy; only obviously enlarged gland should be removed while other parathyroid glands are marked and preserved Note: if you will auto transplant parathyroid gland in MEN2A, transplant it in forearm but in MEN2B transplant it in sternocleidomastoid	• Neck mass with or without lymph node • Pain is common • Local invasion (dysphagia, dyspnea, dysphonia) • Metastases: liver, bone (osteoblast), lung • MTC secrete: calcitonin, CEA, histaminadase, PGE2, PGF2 alpha, serotonin • Diarrhea occurs with distant metastases • Cushing syndrome from ectopic ACTH • All new patient with MTC should be screened for RET mutation, pheochromocytoma, and hyperparathyroidism • Calcitonin and CEA used to identify patient with recurrence or persistent MTC • Calcitonin is sensitive for screening • CEA is better predictor of prognosis Palpable lymph node or calcitonin >400: do CT triphasic for the liver + CT chest	C cell hyperplasia is premalignant Microscopically: sheet of infiltrating neoplastic cells separated collagen and amyloid Presence of amyloid is diagnostic	• Total thyroidectomy • Locally recurrent or widely metastatic: tumor debulking is advised not only to control symptoms of flushing, diarrhea but decrease the death from recurrent or metastatic disease • Liver metastases tend to be multiple and unresectable	Routine Note: central neck dissection should be avoided in children with RET positive, calcitonin negative	• If no distant metastasis: ipsilateral or bilateral lateral neck dissection is advised • Role for prophylactic lateral neck dissection is controversial; some favor this if the patient has positive central lymph node or the primary is >1.5 cm	Vanidetanib is used for treatment of advanced and progressive MTC Prophylactic thyroidectomy is indicated in RET mutation once mutation is confirmed (mutation in codon 634, i.e., MEN2A before age of 5, MEN2B before first year of age) **Follow-up:** • Annual calcitonin, CEA, and ultrasound + history and examination • Ultrasound, CT, MRI, FDGPET/CT to assess local recurrent Prognosis is related to disease stage. Survival is influenced by the disease type. It is the best in a non-MEN familial MTC followed by MEN2A, sporadic and MEN2B is the worst

Table 2.3 Further types of thyroid cancer [4, 5]

Type	Diagnosis and pathology	Management
Anaplastic thyroid cancer: • Less than 1% of all thyroid cancers • Most aggressive thyroid cancers • Women are more commonly affected than men • Mean age at diagnosis 70–80 • Typically, the patient has longstanding neck mass that rapidly enlarged and may be painful • Dysphagia, dyspnea, and dysphonia are common • Tumor may be fixed or ulcerated • Lymph nodes are usually palpable	• FNAB: giant and multinucleated cells • Core biopsy occasionally is needed to confirm the diagnosis when FNAB is necrotic material • Three histological growth patterns: spindle cells, squamoid, and pleomorphic • Ultrasound, CT, MRI, PET/CT should be obtained to assess respectability • Preoperative laryngoscopy to assess the status of the vocal cord	• Total or near total thyroidectomy with therapeutic lymph node dissection • If extrathyroidal extension is present, enbloc resection should be considered if all gross disease can be removed (R1 resection) • Tracheostomy should be avoided as possible unless impending airway loss • Cytotoxic chemotherapy is typically given currently and has been associated with prolong survival
Lymphoma: • Less than 1% of all thyroid cancer • Non-Hodgkin's B cell • Most develop in chronic thyroiditis • Painless rapidly enlarging mass	• Ultrasound: well-defined hypoechoic mass • FNAB may be diagnostic	• CHOP + radiotherapy • Thyroidectomy for airway obstruction or if not responding to treatment • Prognosis depends on histological grade and whether lymphoma confined or disseminated
Metastatic cancers to thyroid: From kidney, breast, lung, melanoma	FNAB is diagnostic	Resection of the thyroid, usually lobectomy may be helpful depending on the status of the primary

- Diagnosis:
  Antimicrosomal antibodies.
  Antithyroglobulin antibodies.
  FNA: lymphocytes with histocytes.
  Thyroidectomy is indicated for patient with large goiter and compressive symptoms or if there is a nodule with suspicion of cancer.

- **De Quervian's thyroiditis:**
  - Subacute granulomatous thyroiditis.
  - After viral upper respiratory tract infection.
  - It can last for 1–3 months.
  - Self-limited condition.
- **Acute suppurative thyroiditis:**
  - Life threatening
  - Mortality about 10%
  - Most common organisms: *Staphylococcus aureus*, *Streptococcus pyrogenous*
  - Treatment: empiric antibiotics and drainage of the abscess
- **Riedel's thyroiditis:**
  - Chronic idiopathic.
  - Characterized by fibrosis of the gland.
  - Multisystem involvement.
  - Definitive diagnosis requires open biopsy.
  - If there are compressive symptoms, isthmectomy to relieve the obstruction.
  - Extensive surgery is risky.
  - Mainstay treatment is with high dose corticosteroids.
- **Radioiodine-induced thyroiditis:**
  - Happens in patient receiving radioactive iodine, for example, ablation for Graves' disease.
  - Occurs in 1% of patients.
  - Symptoms usually resolve after a week, but sometimes anti-inflammatory is indicated [2].

2.1.3.2 Hyperthyroidism

- Overt thyrotoxicosis: low TSH (<0.1 mU/L), high level of serum free T3 and free T4
- Subclinical hyperthyroidism: low TSH but normal T3 and T4
- **Graves' disease:**
  - Most common cause of hyperthyroidism.
  - It is an autoimmune systemic disorder.
  - Caused by thyrotropin receptor antibodies binding to and stimulating TSH receptors.
  - The gland is enlarged diffusely and symmetrically.
  - Should be evaluated in usual fashion.
  - Eye signs are common.
  - Management:

    Antithyroid drugs:
    - Thioamides (propylthiouracil PTU): three times a day
    - Methimazole: once daily
    - Decrease thyroid hormone synthesis and control hyperthyroidism in 90% of patients
    - Side effect includes agranulocytosis (0.5%), hepatotoxicity with PTU
    - FDA recommend limiting use of PTU in patients in their first trimester of pregnancy or to those allergic or intolerant to methimazole

    Radioactive iodine (^{131}I):
    - Highly effective in Graves' disease.
    - Relieves hyperthyroidism in 90% of patients with a single dose.
    - Side effect: neck pain, radiation thyroiditis, sialadenitis and dry mouth, and worsens Graves' ophthalmopathy.
    - Contraindications: pregnancy and lactation.

    Surgery:
    - Effective 100% in curing hyperthyroidism.
    - The patient will need replacement T4 treatment.
    - Can be done in the second trimester.
    - Preoperative preparation is absolutely required with B blockers, antithyroid medication for 3–6 weeks to nearly normalize the T3 and T4 and potassium iodide (Lugol's solution).
    - Complications: recurrent laryngeal nerve damage either permanent or transient neuropraxia, hypoparathyroidism [3].
- **Toxic single adenoma:**
  - The nodule usually 3 cm or larger
  - Virtually never malignant
  - Management:

    Antithyroid drug:
    - Can control the hyperthyroidism but remission does not occur, and lifelong treatment is unacceptable.

    Radioactive iodine:
    - Euthyroidism is reestablished in 80% of patients with a single dose.
    - The nodule may shrink but rarely disappear with little risk to the surrounding structures from radiation.
    - Contraindicated in pregnancy and lactation.

    Surgery:
    - Lobectomy is 100% effective in controlling hyperthyroidism.
    - The risk of injury to the recurrent laryngeal nerve is 1% or less, hypoparathyroidism is not a concern, and other complications are rare [3].
- **Toxic multinodular goiter (Plummer's disease):**
  - Unremitting condition and often developed slowly.
  - Symptoms are more subtle than Graves' disease and without eye signs.
  - Cardiac symptoms such as tachycardia, atrial fibrillation, or arrythmia are most frequent.
  - Compressive symptoms are common.
  - Management:

    Antithyroid drugs:
    - Never used as definitive treatment but rather as preoperative preparation

Radioactive iodine:

- As an alternative to surgery in patients who have high operative risk.
- Resolution of hyperthyroidism with ^{131}I takes 5–6 months on average.
- The goiter size is reduced by about 40%.

Surgery:

- Prompt resolution of hyperthyroidism.
- Removal of goiter, resolving any associated compressive symptoms.
- The surgical risk is higher because of the size of multinodular goiter.
- The RLN may be more difficult to identify due to anatomic displacement [3].

2.1.4 Operation for Thyroid Gland

Preoperative Preparation:

- Tumor board
- Full staging
- Vocal cord assessment if indicated
- Review investigation, imaging
- Blood group and save serum
- Consent
- DVT prophylaxis, stress ulcer prophylaxis if indicated
- Surgical site marking if indicated
- NPO
- IV fluid

Consent for Thyroidectomy:

- Explain the procedure itself (total vs lobectomy): If lobectomy is decided for diagnostic purpose, inform the patient about the possibility of completion thyroidectomy as indicated.
- Explain the reason for the procedure.
- Explain if there is any alternative.
- Explain the risks and complications:
  - *Specific complications*

    Voice change (temporary or permanent)

    Unilateral injury to recurrent laryngeal nerve

    Bilateral injury to recurrent laryngeal nerve that may require permanent tracheostomy

    Injury to superior laryngeal nerve

    Low calcium level

    Bleeding: if significant may need return to OR

    Hypothyroidism and need for thyroxine lifelong

    Other complications like swallowing difficulty, scar, wound infection
  - *General complications:*

    DVT, PE, MI, wound infection

Total Thyroidectomy:

- Position: supine with the neck hyperextended.
- Anesthesia: general with endotracheal intubation.
- Time out: to confirm correct patient, correct procedure, correct side, and if any specific instruments are need.
- Prepping and draping in usual sterile fashion.
- Incision: curvilinear (collar or Kocher) incision is placed within skin crease two finger breadth above the sternal notch and between the medial borders of sternocleidomastoid muscle (Fig. 2.1).
- Divide the platysma, create the sub platysmal flaps. The landmarks are the thyroid cartilage superiorly and down to the sternal notch (Fig. 2.2).

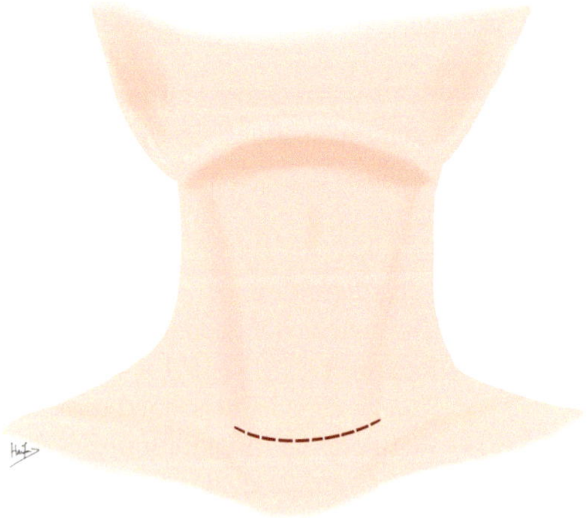

Fig. 2.1 Thyroid gland can be accessed through open cervical incision; 2 cm above the sternal notch

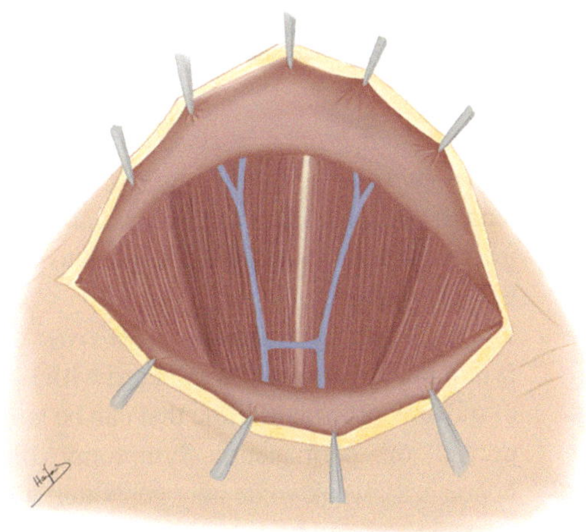

Fig. 2.2 Raise the subplatysmal flap from the sternal notch downwards to the thyroid cartilage upward

- Apply the self-retaining retractors.
- Expose the anterior surface of the thyroid by separating the strap muscles at the midline.
- Starting with the diseased lobe, retract the thyroid medially and divide the middle thyroid vein (Fig. 2.3).
- Retract the thyroid downward and expose the superior pole of the gland and divide the superior thyroidal artery by hooking it medial to lateral, taking care not to injure the external branch of the superior laryngeal nerve and superior parathyroid gland which is usually located at the level of the upper two third of the gland and in a posterior position.
- Moving with blunt dissection laterally and downward till reaching the inferior pole of the gland and divide the inferior thyroidal artery taking care not to injure the recurrent laryngeal nerve and inferior parathyroid gland which is usually located anterior and medially to the recurrent laryngeal nerve.
- Divide the Berry's ligament and take care not to injure the recurrent laryngeal nerve which is usually in close to the ligament and avoid using cautery in this area.
- Do the same thing in the opposite side if the operation is total thyroidectomy.
- Irrigation and hemostasis of any bleeding point.
- If indicated insert a drain in thyroid bed.

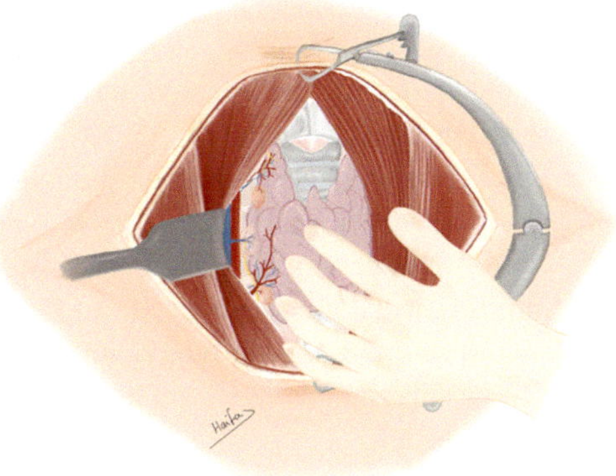

Fig. 2.3 Retract the thyroid lobe anteromedially to expose the middle thyroid vein

- Approximate the strap muscles.
- Close the platysma using interrupted absorbable sutures.
- Close the skin using subcuticular stitch and apply dressing [6].

Important Points Related to Thyroidectomy Operation

- *Boundaries of central lymph node compartment:*
  - Superior: hyoid bone
  - Laterally: carotid artery on both sides
  - Inferiorly: the innominate artery
- *Level VI lymph node dissection should include:*
  - Prelaryngeal Delphian node
  - Pretracheal lymph nodes inferiorly
  - Paratracheal lymph nodes laterally and in the tracheoesophageal groove
- *Lateral neck dissection:*
  - Indicated if the lymph node involved, prophylactic dissection is not typically indicated.
  - Berry picking of lateral compartment should be avoided.
  - Incision: extension of thyroidectomy incision superior and lateral along the border of sternocleidomastoid muscle.
  - Raise the subplatysmal flaps.
  - Divide the omohyoid muscle.
  - Nodes over the carotid artery and internal jugular vein should be removed.

- Nodes over the vagus nerve should be dissected.
- Thoracic duct on the left side may be protected or ligated specially if injured.
- Spinal accessory nerve passes superior and oblique across level II, and injury to it will cause shoulder syndrome. Lymph node inferior medial to the nerve is level IIa and should be dissected, but lymph node group that lie superior and medial is level IIb and should be left.
- Leave a drain after lymph node dissection [6].

- *Substernal goiter:*
  - Usually amenable for resection through the cervical incision
  - It may need partial sternotomy if it is:
    In reoperative field
    Retrosternal thyroid malignancy
    Extend below the margin of the aortic arch
    Reach the carina
    Extended to posterior mediastinum [5]
- *The gold standard way to identify the recurrent laryngeal nerve is:*
  direct anatomic identification
- *Landmarks for the recurrent laryngeal nerve location:*
  - Tracheoesophageal groove.
  - It crosses the inferior thyroid artery medial, lateral, and between its branches.
  - Superior parathyroid gland located posterior and lateral to the nerve.
  - Inferior parathyroid gland located anterior and medial to the nerve.
  - The nerve passes immediately medial to the tubercle of Zuckerkandl.
  - It enters the cricothyroid about 2 cm posterior to the anterior border of the trachea at the level of the cricoid ring [7] (Fig. 2.4).

Complications:

- Hypocalcemia
- Nerve injury
  - *The external branch of superior laryngeal nerve (motor):*
    lead to voice change, poor volume and projection, voice fatigue, and inability to sing at higher range
  - *The recurrent laryngeal nerve (mixed):*
    If unilateral, paralyzed vocal cord with loss of movement from midline that can be temporary or permanent. Symptoms like hoarseness, weak voice may get better with time 3–6 months, if the voice did not improve, the patient need voice therapy.
    If bilateral, need tracheostomy.
- Bleeding once recognized check
  - If the patient not in stridor or distress, shift him/her immediately to the OR.
  - If there are symptoms of airway compromise, open the wound immediately [7].

Follow-Up:

Early postoperative:

- NPO till full recovery and resume the diet gradually once possible.
- Monitor the vital signs.
- Check calcium and albumin level Q6h.
- Monitor the drain output.
- Keep the intubation set to be standby if needed.
- Monitor the patient for any respiratory symptoms or neck swelling.
- Encourage mobilization.
- Encourage use of incentive spirometry.
- Analgesia, antibiotic as indicated, for example, immunocompromised patient, stress ulcer, and DVT prophylaxis

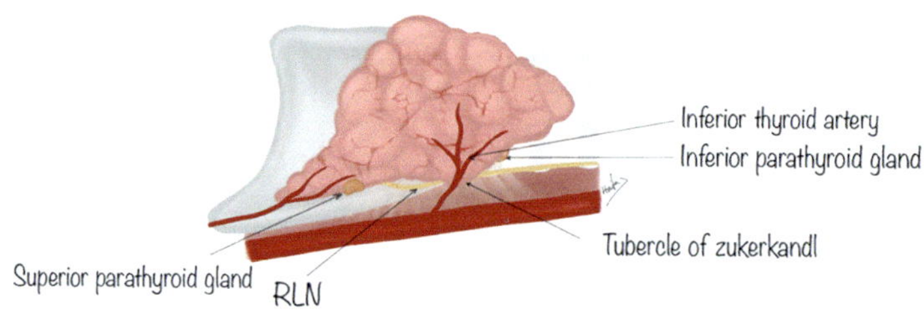

Fig. 2.4 Landmarks for recurrent laryngeal nerves

Before discharge, make sure that:

- The patient has no significant complaint.
- Tolerating oral diet.
- Check the wound status.
- Calcium and vitamin D to be started if needed.
- Thyroid hormone replacement (the dose 1.6 mcg/kg/day) and check TSH 6 weeks later.

First outpatient visit:

- Clinical assessment.
- Examine the wound and remove the sutures.
- Review the final pathology result.
- Discuss in multidisciplinary team when the pathology is cancer.

Long-term follow-up (in case of malignancy)

- Refer to the table of thyroid cancer management.

2.2 Part II: Practice

Practice makes the master.
—Patrick Rothfuss

2.2.1 Case Scenarios for Practice

Tips:

- Practice with a friend and try to mimic the real exam!
  Do not forget to set the timer!
- The clinical data are provided in the answer key section.
- Some twist points are suggested after some cases and can be used to change the scenario to a more difficult one.

Case No. 1:
A 32-year-old female patient pregnant in her 17 weeks gestational age after multiple attempts of IVF complaining of neck mass for 2 months.

Questions for Discussion:

1. How will you approach this patient?
2. What will be your next step?
3. How will you investigate this patient?
4. What will be your next step?
5. What will you do?
6. What will you do?
7. How will you follow up this patient (short-term follow-up)?
8. How will you follow up this patient (long-term follow-up)?

Case No. 2:
A 57-year-old male patient who presented to the surgery clinic complaining of neck swelling for 6 months.

Questions for Discussion:

1. How will you approach the patient?
2. What is your differential diagnosis?
3. How will you confirm the most likely diagnosis?
4. What will you do next?
5. How will you manage the patient?
6. Intraoperative finding as described. What will you do?
7. On early postoperative period, the patient is complaining of spasm in his hands. What will you do?
8. What further management may you offer the patient?

Case No. 3:
A 44-year-old female patient presented to the clinic complaining of left neck mass for 3 months.

Questions for Discussion:

1. How will you approach the patient?
2. What will you do next?
3. What will be your next step?
4. How will you manage that?
5. The intraoperative finding as described. What will you do?
6. How will follow up the patient (short-term follow-up)?

7. What will you do?
8. How will you follow up the patient (long-term follow-up)?

Case No. 4:

A 27-year-old female patient presented to the clinic complains of left neck mass for 3 months.

Questions for Discussion:

1. How will you approach the patient?
2. What is your differential diagnosis?
3. How will you confirm the most likely diagnosis?
4. How will you manage the patient?
5. On day 0 postoperative, the patient is complaining of difficulty in breathing. What will you do?
6. How will you follow up the patient postoperatively?

Checklist

History	Items	Done	Not done	Not applicable
General	Introduce herself/himself to the patient			
	Patient personal data (name, age, sex, etc.)			
	Chief complaint			
	Duration			
Lump	How did she notice it?			
	Any change since that time?			
	Any other lumps in the body?			
Associated symptoms	Symptoms of hyperthyroidism (weight loss, increase appetite, sweating, diarrhea)			
	Symptoms of hypothyroidism (weight gain, constipation, hair loss)			
	Pain			
	Discharge			
	Symptoms of other MEN syndrome (gastritis, PUD, uncontrol BP, palpitation, sweating)			
Pressure/invasion symptoms	Hoarseness			
	Dysphagia			
	SOB			
Constitutional symptoms	Fever			
	Weight loss			
	Decrease appetite			
	Night sweating			
Risk factors	Radiation therapy			
	Family history of thyroid cancer			
	Family history of MEN or personal history of MEN			
Differential diagnosis	Recent oral/ear infection			
	Symptoms of parathyroid adenoma			
	Family or personal history of hematological malignancy			

History	Items	Done	Not done	Not applicable
Symptoms of metastasis	Bone pain			
	Headache			
	Abdominal pain/jaundice			
	Cough/shortness of breath			
PMH	Previous similar complaint			
	Previous ultrasound			
	Previous FNA			
	Chronic illness			
PSH				
Social history				
Medication				
Allergy				
Systemic review				
Physical examination				
General principle	Position			
	Permission			
	Privacy			
	Exposure			
	Wash hands			
General examination	Appearance			
	Body built			
	Color			
	Distress/decubitus			
	Environment			
Vital signs	Bp, HR, temp., RR, Spo_2			
Hand	Pulse			
	Moist/dry			
	Tremor			
Eye	Exophthalmos			
	Lid lag			
	Lid retraction			
	Eyebrow			
Neck inspection	Ask the patient to swallow?			
	Ask the patient to protrude the tongue?			
	Look for any distended neck veins			
Palpation from the front	Confirm your visual impression			
	Position of the trachea			
	Position of the thyroid cartilage			

(continued)

History	Items	Done	Not done	Not applicable
Palpation from behind	Stand behind the patient			
	Tilt patient head slightly forward to relax the anterior neck muscle			
	Press on one side and palpate the opposite lobe each time			
	Ask the patient to swallow and confirm that any swelling moving with swallowing			
	Palpate the whole neck for any cervical and supraclavicular lymph nodes			
If there is any lump	Site			
	Number			
	Size			
	Shape			
	Consistency			
	Tenderness			
	Temperature			
Percussion	Over manubrium sterni: to define the lower extent of the swelling			
Auscultation	Systolic bruit over the swelling (thyrotoxic gland)			
Other system for metastasis	Palpate the lower back			
	Palpate the abdomen for hepatomegaly			
	Examine the lungs			
Investigation				
Blood	CBC			
	Coagulation profile			
	ALP			
	LFT			
	RFT			
	TFT			
	Thyroglobulin (Tg) with thyroglobulin antibodies			
	Calcitonin			
	Screening for MEN syndrome when indicated (gastrin level, parathyroid hormone, calcium, catecholamine level)			
Imaging	Ultrasound			
	CT neck			
	Thyroid scan			
Biopsy	FNA from the thyroid nodule			
	FNA from clinically positive lymph node			

History	Items	Done	Not done	Not applicable
Management				
Hyperthyroidism	Inform the patient			
	Antithyroid medication			
	Radioactive ablation			
	Surgery:			
	• Preoperative preparation			
	• Vocal cord assessment			
	• Surgical site marking			
	• Consent			
	• Type of surgery (lobectomy, total, subtotal thyroidectomy)			
Thyroid cancer	Staging if indicated			
	Multidisciplinary team discussion			
	• Admission			
	• NPO			
	• IV fluid			
	• Prophylaxis			
	• Anesthesia consultation			
	• Vocal cord assessment			
	• Consent			
	• Surgical site marking			
	Type of surgery (lobectomy vs. total thyroidectomy)			
	Lymph node dissection (central, modified lateral, both)			
Early follow-up	Clinical assessment			
	Check the final pathology report			
	Multidisciplinary team discussion			
	Thyroid replacement to reach the target TSH			
	Tg and Tg antibodies every 6 months			
	Ultrasound neck every 6 months			
	Radioactive iodine ablation if indicated			

2.2.2 Answer Key

Case No. 1:
A 32-year-old female patient pregnant in her 17 weeks gestational age after multiple attempts of IVF complaining of neck mass for 2 months.

Questions for Discussion:

1. **How will you approach this patient?**
   A 32-year-old female patient was referred from an obstetric clinic due to a central neck mass. She noticed the mass accidentally. It has

been growing since that time, painless, no discharge, no symptoms of hyper or hypothyroidism, no pressure symptoms. Constitutional symptoms are negative. She has no family history of thyroid or endocrine malignancy, and she has never been exposed to radiation therapy. She has no previous similar complain. PMH, PSH are unremarkable. She is on folic acid and multivitamins. She is not known to have allergy.

Physical examination:

No signs of hyper or hypothyroidism.

There is lump at the anterior surface of the neck that moves with swallowing but not with the protrusion of the tongue. The mass is on the left thyroid lobe, about 2 × 2 cm, round shape, hard, not tender.

No palpable cervical lymphadenopathy.

2. **How will you investigate this patient?**

   TSH: 3.1 mU/L.

   T3 and T4 are normal.

   Ultrasound neck: left thyroid lobe cystic mass with large solid component measuring 2.1 × 1.7 cm in its greatest dimensions. It shows significant internal vascularity. No extrathyroidal extension or cervical lymphadenopathy.

3. **What will be your next step?**

   FNA result: (papillary thyroid cancer).

4. **What will you do?**

   Discuss in multidisciplinary team.

   Break the bad news.

   Follow up with ultrasound after 4–6 weeks.

   Thyroid hormone (target TSH < 2).

   During the sonographic follow-up, you noticed significant growth of the tumor.

   At 23 gestational age (after 6 weeks), ultrasound was performed, and the size of the thyroid nodule increased to 4.1 cm with no abnormal cervical lymph node.

5. **What will you do?**
   - Explain to the patient that she needs surgery.
   - Vocal cord assessment.
   - Prepare for total thyroidectomy.
   - Admission.
   - NPO.
   - IV fluid.
   - Prophylaxis (stress ulcer and DVT prophylaxis).
   - Anesthesia consultation.
   - Obstetric consultation.
   - Consent

   The patient underwent uneventful total thyroidectomy with no obstetric complication, and she was discharged after few days.

6. **How will you follow up this patient (short-term follow-up)?**
   - Clinical assessment.
   - Check the final pathology report.
   - Tumor board.
   - Thyroid hormone replacement

   The final pathology report showed unifocal PTC measuring 3.5 × 3.8 cm. No extracapsular invasion. No lymphovascular invasion.

7. **How will you follow up this patient (long-term follow-up)?**
   - Tg and Tg antibodies every 6 months
   - Ultrasound neck every 6 months
   - Target TSH 0.3–2.0 mU/L

Case No. 2:

A 57-year-old male patient who presented to the surgery clinic complaining of neck swelling for 6 months.

Questions for Discussion:

1. **How will you approach the patient?**

   A 57-year-old male patient presented to the surgical clinic due to neck swelling for 6 months. He noticed the mass accidentally. It has been growing since that time, painless, no discharge, no symptoms of hyper or hypothyroidism. He has hoarseness of voice but no dysphagia or dyspnea. Constitutional symptoms are negative. He has no family history of thyroid or endocrine malignancy, and he was never being exposed to radiation therapy. He has no previous similar complain. He is diabetic on insulin, otherwise healthy man.

   Physical examination:

   No signs of hyper or hypothyroidism.

   There is a huge neck swelling that moves with swallowing but not with the protrusion of the tongue. The thyroid gland contains multiple large nodules bilaterally but the most prominent one on the right side, measuring 6 × 5 cm, hard, ill defined.

He has multiple enlarged right anterior cervical lymph nodes.

2. **What is your differential diagnosis?**
   - Thyroid cancer
   - Multinodular goiter
   - Parathyroid cancer
   - Lymphoma
3. **How will you confirm the most likely diagnosis?**

   TFT: normal.

   Ultrasound neck: multiple thyroid nodules bilaterally. The largest and the most suspicious one is on the right side, hypoechoic 6.4 × 5.2 cm with area of macrocalcification and prominent internal vascularity. Multiple enlarge right lateral cervical lymph nodes.

   FNA (thyroid): papillary thyroid cancer.

   FNA (lymph nodes): positive for metastasis.
4. **What will you do next?**

   CT neck: huge enlarged soft tissue mass, measuring 6.4 × 5.2 cm. the thyroid gland is enlarged with multiple nodules bilaterally. Multiple right-side enlarged lymph node. Mild deviation of the trachea to the left side.

   CT chest: no signs of metastasis.

   Vocal cord assessment: right vocal cord is immobile.
5. **How will you manage the patient?**
   - Discuss the case in multidisciplinary team meeting.
   - Break the bad news to the patient.
   - Admission.
   - NPO.
   - IV fluid.
   - Prophylaxis (antibiotic, DVT, stress ulcer).
   - Consent for total thyroidectomy, central neck dissection and right modified lateral neck dissection.
   - Inform the patient that one of the vocal cords is already paralyzed and mention the risk of injury to other nerve and possibility of tracheostomy.

   Intraoperatively, the right recurrent laryngeal nerve is invaded by the tumor. The tumor was involving the right internal jugular vein.
6. **Intraoperative finding as described. What will you do?**

   The internal jugular vein can be ligated and resect the thyroid in addition to central and right modified lateral neck dissection.
7. **In the early postoperative period, the patient is complaining of spasm in his hands. What will you do?**

   Measure the serum calcium and albumin level.

   Start the patient on IV calcium gluconate.
8. **What further management may you offer the patient?**

   Radioactive iodine ablation

   Thyroid hormone replacement to suppress the TSH to reach the target (0.1–0.5)

   Follow-up with Tg and anti-Tg antibodies to check for recurrence or metastasis

Case No. 3:

A 44-year-old female patient presented to the clinic complaining of left neck mass for 3 months.

Questions for Discussion:

1. **How will you approach the patient?**

   The patient is 44-year-old female patient who presented to surgery clinic due to neck mass for 3 months. Her husband noticed the mass, and it has been growing since that time. It is not associated with pain, discharge, and symptoms of hyper or hypothyroidism. She has no hoarseness of voice. Her mother was diagnosed with thyroid cancer when she was 50 years old. She has no history of radiation exposure. She is not known to have chronic illness and has no previous surgical history

   On examination:

   No signs of hyper or hypothyroidism.

   Neck: there is a palpable nodule at the left thyroid lobe 3 × 2 cm, round shape, smooth surface, firm, moving up and down with swallowing. No other palpable nodule or lymph nodes.

2. **What will you do next?**

   TFT: normal.

   Ultrasound neck: there is heterogenous left thyroid nodule measuring 3.2 cm (length) × 2.5 cm (width).
3. **What will be your next step?**

   FNA: follicular lesion of undetermined significance (Bethesda III).
4. **How will you manage that?**
   - Inform the patient.
   - Vocal cord assessment: both cords are mobile.
   - Prepare for total thyroidectomy (because she has high risk of thyroid cancer).
   - Admission.
   - NPO.
   - IV fluid.
   - Prophylaxis (DVT and stress ulcer).
   - Consent.

     Intraoperatively, you started with the left (diseased) side. The left recurrent laryngeal nerve was difficult to identify. Later you recognized that you cut the nerve accidentally.
5. **The intraoperative finding as described. What will you do?**

   Remove the left lobe. Terminate the procedure and wait for the final pathology result.

   You did that, and the patient had smooth post-op recovery apart from hoarseness of voice.

   And discharge home.
6. **How will follow up the patient (short-term follow-up)?**
   - Clinical assessment.
   - Examine the wound and remove the sutures.
   - Review the final pathology result: single focus of follicular variant of papillary thyroid cancer measuring 3 × 2 cm
   - Discuss in multidisciplinary team.
7. **What will you do?**

   Inform the patient that she has cancer and she needs to undergo completion thyroidectomy with higher risk of tracheostomy giving the complication that happened in her previous surgery.

   The patient underwent an uneventful completion thyroidectomy and discharged home.
8. **How will you follow up the patient (long-term follow-up)?**
   - Refer to the endocrine team for adjuvant radioactive ablation.
   - Tg and Tg antibodies every 6 months.
   - Ultrasound neck every 6 months.
   - Thyroid replacement to reach the target TSH (0.1–0.5 mU/L).

Case No. 4:

A 27-year-old female patient presented to the clinic complains of left neck mass for 3 months.

Questions for Discussion:

1. **How will you approach the patient?**

   The patient is 27-year-old female patient presented to the clinic due to a left neck mass for 3 months. She noticed the mass herself, and it looks the same with no change in the size since she noticed it. She has history of weight loss, diarrhea, increase in appetite, inability to tolerate the hot weather. She has no family history of thyroid or endocrine malignancy. No history of radiation exposure

   Recently, she delivered her first child, and she is currently lactating

   On examination:

   She looks restless, underweight.

   Eye: no abnormality.

   Vital signs: BP: 121/82 mmHg, PR: 121 bpm temperature: 37.3 °C.

   Neck: there is palpable left neck swelling which moves with swallowing. It is about 3 × 2 cm, firm, round shape, smooth surface, well defined edges.

   No palpable lymph nodes.
2. **What is your differential diagnosis?**

   Toxic solitary nodule

   Toxic multinodular goiter

   Graves' disease

   Thyroid cancer
3. **How will you confirm the most likely diagnosis?**

   TFT: suppressed TSH, high T4 and T3.

Ultrasound; single hyperechoic thyroid nodule on the left side measuring 3.1 × 2.3 cm. No abnormal lymph node is detected.

Thyroid scan: hot nodule at the left thyroid lobe.

4. **How will you manage the patient?**
   - Antithyroid medication to normalize her TFT
   - Beta blocker
   - Left thyroid lobectomy

   The patient was started on antithyroid medication and B blocker then she was taken for left thyroid lobectomy
5. **On day 0 postoperative, the patient is complaining of difficulty in breathing. What will you do?**

   Examine the neck.

   Immediate opening of the sutures to decompress the hematoma followed by exploration in OR to ensure hemostasis.
6. **How will you follow up the patient postoperative?**
   - **Early postoperative:**
     - NPO till full recovery and resume the diet gradually once possible.
     - Monitor the vital signs.
     - Monitor the drain output.
     - Keep the intubation set to be standby if needed.
     - Monitor the patient for any respiratory symptoms or neck swelling.
     - Encourage mobilization.
   - **First outpatient visit:**
     - Clinical assessment.
     - Examine the wound and remove the sutures.
     - Review the final pathology result.
   - Check TFT after 3 months and give thyroid hormone replacement if needed.

References

1. Pasternak JD. The management of thyroid nodule. In: Cameron J, Cameron A, editors. Current surgical therapy. 12th ed. Canada: Elsevier; 2016.
2. McHenry CR. The management of thyroiditis. In: Cameron J, Cameron A, editors. Current surgical therapy. 12th ed. Canada: Elsevier; 2016.
3. Grant CS. Hyperthyroidism. In: Cameron J, Cameron A, editors. Current surgical therapy. 12th ed. Canada: Elsevier; 2016.
4. Haugen BR, Alexander EK, Bible KC, Doherty GM, Mandel SJ, Nikiforov YE, et al. 2015 American Thyroid Association Management Guidelines for Adult patients with thyroid nodules and differentiated thyroid cancer: The American Thyroid Association Guidelines Task Force on Thyroid Nodules and Differentiated Thyroid Cancer. Thyroid. 2016;26(1):1–133.
5. Glenda G, Callender RU. In: Cameron J, Cameron A, editors. Current surgical therapy. 12th ed. Canada: Elsevier; 2016.
6. Zollinger R. Thyroid: surgical therapy. Zollinger's atlas of surgical operation. 9th ed. United States: McGraw-Hill Education; 2011.
7. Clark GLOH. Thyroid, parathyroid and adrenal. In: Brunicardi F, editor. Schwartz's principles of surgery. United States: McGraw-Hill Education; 2019.

3 Surgical Aspects of Parathyroid Diseases for Clinical Board Exams

3.1 Part I: Knowledge

The difference between a successful person and others is not a lack of strength, not a lack of knowledge, but rather a lack of will.
—Vince Lombardi

The patient could present with one of the following:

- Symptoms of hypercalcemia
- Abnormal elevation in serum calcium

History:

- Introduce yourself to the patient.
- Personal data: name, age, gender, nationality, occupation.
- Chief complaint and duration (most of the time, the scenario will be a referral from a family physician due to high calcium level).
- History of presenting illness:
  - Symptoms of hyperparathyroidism (Table 3.1).
  - Symptoms of hyperthyroidism: heat intolerance, weight loss, diarrhea, sweating, and agitation.
  - History of neck swelling if positive, clarify more.
  - Personal history of malignancy: breast, lung, kidney, ovary, multiple myeloma.
  - History of tuberculosis (TB) or contact with patient having TB.
  - Family history of hypercalcemia, pancreatic, adrenal, and pituitary problems.

Table 3.1 Symptoms of hyperparathyroidism [1]

Renal	Bone	GIT	Neuropsychiatry	Others
Polyurea Nocturia Flank pain Hematuria History of renal stone Polydipsia History of HTN	Bone pain Joint pain Fractures	Abdominal pain Heartburn Decrease appetite Nausea Vomiting Hematemesis Constipation Diarrhea Melena History of PUD History of pancreatitis Pruritis Jaundice	Anxiety Depression Fatigue Memory loss Decrease level of consciousness	Fatigue Muscle weakness (proximal group) Gout/pseudogout Cardiac symptoms MI Heart failure

H. Alotaibi, *Study Surgery*, https://doi.org/10.1007/978-981-16-2305-9_3

- Personal history of pituitary, pancreatic, and adrenal disease (MEN1, MEN2A).
- Drugs: lithium, thiazide, vitamin D.
- History of immobilization.
- History of watery diarrhea (VIPoma).
- Constitutional symptoms.
- Compressive or invasion symptoms: hoarseness, dysphagia, SOB.
- Previous related investigation (ultrasound, calcium level, PTH level).

- Past medical history: HTN, previous admission
- Past surgical history
- Social history: alcohol, smoking
- Family history
- Medication (past and current)
- Allergy and blood transfusion history
- Systemic review:
  - **CNS:** headache, visual disturbance, numbness, paralysis.
  - **CVS:** chest pain, orthopnea, paroxysmal nocturnal dyspnea, palpitation, lower limb edema.
  - **Respiratory system:** cough, wheezes, hemoptysis.
  - **GIT, renal, and musculoskeletal systems** are covered in the presenting illness.

Physical Examination:
General Examination:

- Appearance: ill, well, agitated, dehydrated
- Body built
- Color: pallor or jaundice
- Distress or not
- Environment

Vital signs: BP, PR, temperature, RR, SPO_2.

Eye: jaundice, keratopathy, signs of hyperthyroidism, for example, exophthalmos, lid lag, lid retraction.

Neck: similar to the thyroid examination.

Look mainly for masses, lymph nodes, or jaw tumor.

Chest: examine the CVS, respiratory system.

Breast examination looking for signs of breast cancer.

Abdomen: look for tenderness, organomegaly, ascites.

Musculoskeletal: arthritis, weakness (power).

Differential Diagnosis of Hypercalcemia:

1. Hyperparathyroidism
2. Malignancy: hematologic (e.g., multiple myeloma) or solid tumor due to release of parathyroid hormone releasing peptide (PTHrP) (e.g., lung, breast, kidney, and ovarian cancers) even if there is no bone metastasis
3. Endocrine disease: hyperthyroidism, Addison crisis, VIPoma
4. Granulomatous disease: sarcoidosis, TB
5. Milk alkali syndrome
6. Drugs: thiazide, lithium, vitamin A or D intoxication
7. Familial hypercalcemic hypocalciuric
8. Paget's disease
9. Immobilization

3.1.1 Approach to Patient with Hypercalcemia

- **History and physical examination as described earlier**
- **Diagnostic Investigation:**
  - CBC, electrolytes (mainly calcium, phosphorus, chloride, magnesium).
  - Liver function test (LFT): mainly albumin, ALP, bilirubin.
  - Renal function test (RFT).
  - Blood group and cross match.
  - Coagulation profile.
  - Parathyroid hormone level.
  - Thyroid-stimulating hormone (TSH).
  - Uric acid.
  - Vitamin D.
  - Chloride: phosphorus ratio.
  - Calcium: Creatinine clearance ratio.
  - 24-h urine test for calcium.
  - Hand and skull X-ray.
  - Bone mineral density.
  - Abdominal ultrasound (looking for renal stone).

- If suspecting MEN from the clinical assessment, do biochemical markers accordingly.
  Gastrin level
  Prolactin level
  Calcitonin
  Serum catecholamine level

Primary Hyperparathyroidism:

- If PTH level, calcium level, and urine calcium are high, the diagnosis is primary hyperparathyroidism.
- If the diagnosis is confirmed, it is time to do neck ultrasound and sestamibi scan for localization.
- Other options for localization:
  - Noninvasive preoperative tests like:
    4D CT
    MRI
    Single photon emission CT
  - Invasive preoperative tests like:
    FNA
    Venous sampling
- **Indications of Parathyroidectomy:**
  - Symptomatic
  - Asymptomatic if:
    Age <50 years.
    Serum calcium >1 mg/dL above the upper limit.
    Glomerular filtration rate (GFR) <60 mL/min.
    24-h urine calcium >400.
    Decrease in BMD at lumbar spine, total hip, femoral neck, or distal radius >2.5 SD, T score < −2.5, vertebral fracture by X ray/CT/or MRI.
    Increase stone risk by biochemical stone risk analysis or presence of nephrolithiasis by ultrasound/CT/or MRI.
    Long-term medical surveillance is not desired (annual calcium and creatinine level, BMD at three sites every 1–2 years).
- **Medical Treatment of Primary Hyperparathyroidism:**
  - Bisphosphonate
  - Hormone replacement therapy
  - Selective estrogen receptor modulator, for example, Raloxifene
- **A Successful Parathyroidectomy will Result in:**
  - Resolution of osteitis fibrosa cystica.
  - Decrease the formation of the stone.
  - Improve BMD.
  - Decrease fracture risk by 50%.
  - Improve fatigue, polydipsia, polyurea, and nocturia.
  - HTN is the least likely to improve after parathyroidectomy.
- **Surgical Options:**
  - Unilateral neck exploration
    If the patient has primary HPT and the neck ultrasound and the sestamibi scan independently identify same gland + intraoperative parathyroid hormone assay decrease by 50% after 10 minutes, terminate the procedure.
  - Bilateral neck exploration If:
    Parathyroid localization or IOPTH is not available
    Localization study failed to identify abnormal gland
    Patient has history of familial hyperparathyroidism, MEN1, or MEN2A regardless the result of localization
    Concomitant thyroid disorder requires bilateral exploration
    Secondary or tertiary hyperparathyroidism
  - Radio-guided parathyroidectomy
  - Endoscopic parathyroidectomy
  - Robotic parathyroidectomy [1, 2]

Recurrent or Persistent Hyperparathyroidism:

- Patients who do not achieve or maintain eucalcemia in 6 months postoperatively have persistent disease.
- If the patient has an apparently successful operation (with temporary normalization of serum calcium and parathyroid hormone [PTH] levels) but then develops hypercalcemia with inappropriately elevated PTH levels after having cure for 6 months, the patient is diagnosed with recurrent disease.

- The most common cause of persistent hyperparathyroidism is a missed diseased parathyroid gland.
- Anatomic locations that can harbor missed glands are commonly the deep tracheaesophageal groove, the thyroid gland, the thymus, the posterior mediastinum, the base of the skull, and the carotid sheath.
- Diagnostic evaluation:
  - Review the medical history mainly family history.
  - Physical examination of the patient placement of the incision, body habitus, voice changes.
  - Confirm diagnosis of hyperparathyroidism (assess vitamin D levels).
  - Vocal cord assessment.
  - Review prior imaging studies, records from the initial operation, and pathology reports from initial operation.
  - Localization:
    - Perform a combination of cervical US, sestamibi, and 4D CT.
    - Consider FNA to obtain PTH levels and cytology.
    - Utilize venous sampling selectively.
  - If the location of a single missed gland is confirmed, proceed to reoperation.
  - If multifocal disease is suspected, review location of glands removed, plan completion, subtotal parathyroidectomy.
  - If abnormal gland(s) are not identified, continue monitoring, reevaluate the patient's status with new imaging studies in 1–2 years [3].

Secondary Hyperparathyroidism:

- Increased PTH production in response to external stimuli, most commonly chronic kidney disease.
- It can occur in the setting of vitamin D deficiency in patients with normal renal function.
- Characterized by low to normal serum calcium levels and significant elevation of PTH levels.
- **Medical Management:**
  - When it is due to vitamin D deficiency and renal function is normal, aggressive vitamin D supplementation is recommended.
  - In patients with secondary hyperparathyroidism due to chronic kidney disease, medical management is dependent on the severity of renal disease:
    - Early-stage renal disease: dietary restriction of phosphorus (eating foods that are low in protein).
    - Advanced disease: phosphate-binding medications may be required like aluminum salts, calcium-containing phosphate binders, such as calcium carbonate and calcium acetate, and cinacalcet [4].
- **Indications of Parathyroidectomy in Secondary Hyperparathyroidism:**
  Bone pain & pruritis in addition to any of the following:
  - Ca/Ph product ≥70
  - Ca >11 mg/dL
  - PTH >800 pg/mL
  - Calciphylaxis (a limb and life-threatening condition)
  - Progressive renal osteodystrophy
  - Soft tissue calcification despite maximum medical treatment
  - Osteoporosis and pathological fracture [4]

Tertiary Hyperparathyroidism:

- Autonomous hypersecretion of PTH even after causes of SHPT have been corrected
- Characterized by elevated serum calcium levels and elevated PTH levels
- **Indications of Parathyroidectomy in Tertiary Hyperparathyroidism:**
  - Autonomous parathyroid hormone secretion persistent over 1 year after successful transplant in patient with hypophosphatemia
  - Low BMD, severe osteopenia
  - Fatigue, pruritis, peptic ulcer disease, nephrocalcinosis [4]

Important Surgical Considerations:

- Secondary and often tertiary hyperparathyroidism are associated with parathyroid hyperplasia.
- Bilateral exploration is always indicated, and preoperative imaging studies for localization of abnormal glands are usually unnecessary.
- Subtotal parathyroidectomy is the resection of three (or more, if supernumerary glands are present) glands and 50–75% removal of the last gland, with preservation of a viable, histologically confirmed remnant.
- Disadvantages include the potential need for re-operative cervical surgery if HPT recurs and the possibility of inadvertently devascularizing the in situ parathyroid remnant.
- Total parathyroidectomy removes all identified parathyroid glands, including supernumerary glands. In patients who develop recurrent HPT, reimplantation into the forearm allows for easier debulking, avoiding the need for re-operative surgery in the neck, and easier confirmation of graft-related recurrence.
- Disadvantages of total parathyroidectomy include the need for much more aggressive postoperative management of hypocalcemia to avoid complications, especially because autograft failure can lead to persistent, potentially profound hypoparathyroidism.
- Patients should start taking oral calcium supplementation immediately after surgery [4].

Standard Bilateral Neck Exploration:

- General anesthesia and endotracheal intubation.
- Supine position with the neck extended.
- Time out: confirm the correct patient, procedure, site, surgeon, and the need for any specific instrument, or tests like frozen section or IOPTH assay.
- Prepping and draping in usual sterile fashion.
- Curvilinear transverse (collar) incision two fingerbreadths above the sternal notch.
- Divide the platysma and raise the subplatysmal flaps (being carefully to stay above the anterior jugular vein).
- Apply the retractor.
- Divide the strap muscle in the midline.
- Sternohyoid and sternothyroid muscle are elevated off the anterior surface of the thyroid gland.
- It is important to address one side at a time.
- Gently mobilize the thyroid lobe anteriorly and medially.
- Ligate and divide the middle thyroid vein, continue mobilization of the thyroid lobe medially using blunt dissection with peanut.
- Identify and preserve the recurrent laryngeal nerve.
- Systematically search for the parathyroid gland (it is typically 4–6 mm length, mustard brown color) considering the following:
  - Bloodless field is important to allow identification of the parathyroid gland.
  - Parathyroid is partially surrounded by fat, fat at the typical location should be explored, and the thin facia over the fat sharply incised. If there is a parathyroid gland, it will "pop" out.
  - Parathyroid gland needs to be distinguished from normal fat, lymph node, and thyroid nodule. (Lymph node will be light beige to whitish and glassy. Thyroid nodule will be more vascular, firm, dark or reddish brown.)
  - If you are not sure, FNA and check the parathyroid hormone level.
  - Superior gland is above the inferior thyroid artery entrance and dorsal to the nerve.
  - Inferior gland is below the entrance of the inferior thyroid artery entrance and ventral to the nerve (Fig. 3.1).
- If the inferior gland not found in its typical location:
  - Mobilize the thyro-thymic ligament and the thymus.
  - If still not found, open the carotid sheath from the bifurcation to the base of the neck.
  - If still not found, check for intrathyroidal gland by intraoperative ultrasound, incise the thyroid capsule on its posterolateral side, or perform thyroid lobectomy (Fig. 3.2).

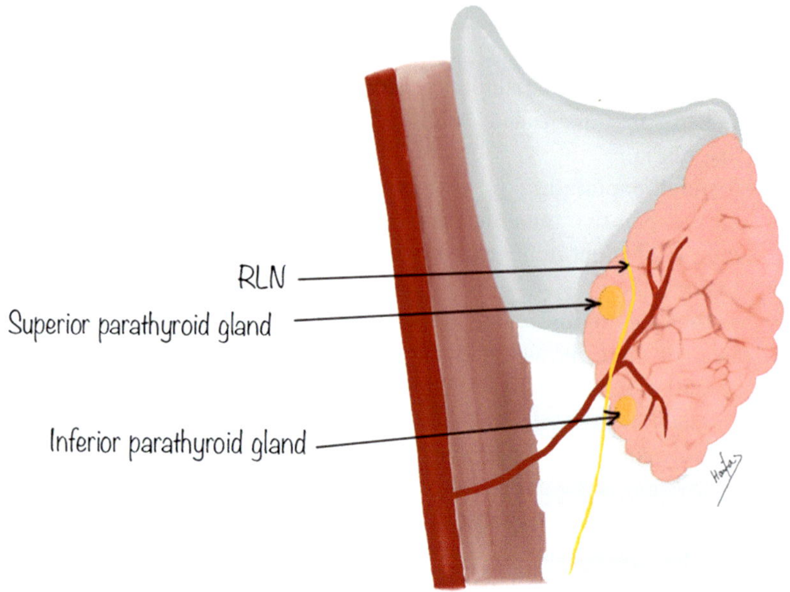

Fig. 3.1 Normal position of superior parathyroid gland is dorsal and lateral to the RLN, while the inferior parathyroid gland usually lies ventral and medial to the nerve

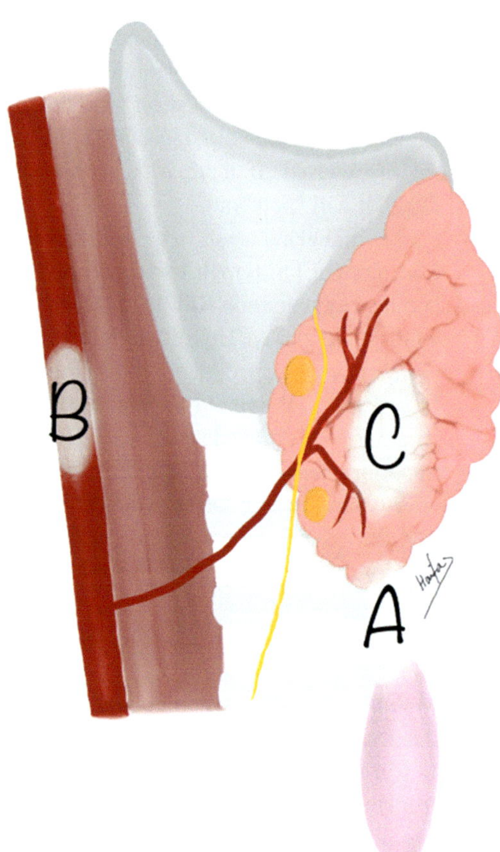

Fig. 3.2 The ectopic inferior parathyroid gland is commonly found in the thyro-thymic ligament and thymus (A), in the carotid sheath (B), or intrathyroidal (C)

- Upper gland is more consistent in position, ectopic gland may be found in:
  - Carotid sheath
  - Tracheoesophageal groove
  - Retroesophageal
  - Posterior mediastinum (Fig. 3.3)
- Every attempt should be made to identify all the four glands.
- Treatment depends on the number of the abnormal gland.
  - Single adenoma, the others are normal: remove the abnormal, clip the pedicle, check intraoperative parathyroid hormone level.
  - Two adenomas and two normal glands or triple adenomas: if the remaining is/are normal (confirmed), excise the abnormal and clip the pedicle.
  - All are abnormal: do subtotal parathyroidectomy (leave 50 mg of the most normal and apply clip, or total parathyroidectomy with auto transplantation).
  - Important considerations:

    If possible, subtotal the inferior gland (easier to be identified if re-excision is required).

    Autotransplantation in a nondominant forearm by making horizontal incision over the brachioradialis, 1–2 pieces of

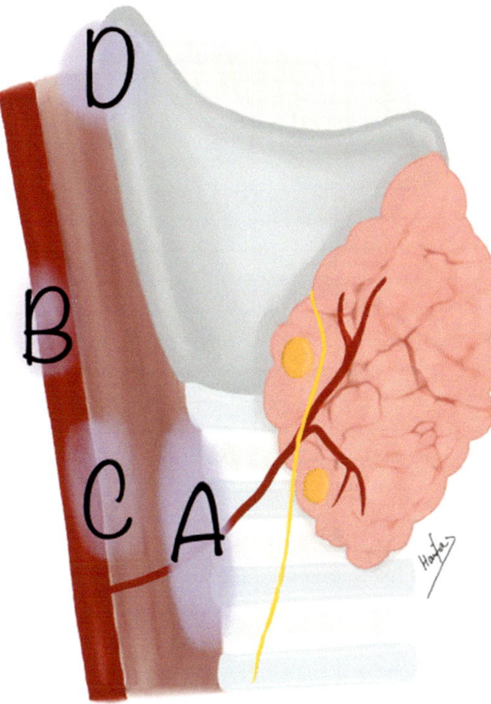

Fig. 3.3 The ectopic superior thyroid gland is commonly found in the tracheoesophageal groove (**A**), in the carotid sheath (**B**), retroesophageal (**C**), or high near the upper part of the thyroid cartilage (**D**)

1 mm size place in each pocket, 12–14 pieces is transplanted.
Other sites for autotransplantation include sternocleidomastoid muscle, brachioradialis, intercostal muscle, or pretibial area.

- **Indications for Sternotomy:**
  - Not recommended as initial unless calcium >13 mg/dL.
  - Only 5% of patient may need sternotomy.
  - If needed, partial sternotomy is enough.
- **Post-Parathyroidectomy Complications:**
  - Operative failure
  - Hematoma
  - Postoperative hypocalcemia
  - Recurrent laryngeal nerve injury
  - Wound infection
  - Bone hunger syndrome [1]

3.2 Part II: Practice

It's not necessarily the amount of time you spend at practice that counts; it's what you put into the practice.
—Eric Lindros

3.2.1 Case Scenarios for Practice

Tips:

- Practice with a friend and try to mimic the real exam!
  Do not forget to set the timer!
- The clinical data is provided in the answer key section.

Case No. 1:
A 43-year-old female patient referred from PHC due to hypercalcemia.
Questions for Discussion:

1. How will you approach this patient?
2. What is your differential diagnosis?
3. How will you investigate this patient?
4. What is your diagnosis?
5. What will you do next?
6. What will you do?
7. How will you differentiate between a parathyroid gland, a thyroid nodule, and a lymph node?
8. Where will you look for the inferior parathyroid gland?
9. What will you do?
10. You found a single inferior parathyroid adenoma. What will you do?
11. What will you do?
12. What are the post-parathyroidectomy complications?

Checklist

History	Items	Done	Not done	Not applicable
General	Introduce herself/himself to the patient			
	Patient's personal data (name, age, sex, nationality, occupation)			
	Ask for any complaint			
	Duration			
Renal	Dysuria			
	Hematuria			
	Flank pain			
	Nocturia			
	History of renal stones			
GIT	Epigastric pain			
	History of pancreatitis			
	History of gastritis/PUD			
	Nausea			
	Vomiting			
	Jaundice			
	Pruritis			
Bone/MSK	Bone pain			
	Fractures			
	Arthritis			
	Fatigue			
	Muscle weakness			
Psychology	Depression			
	Anxiety			
Other symptoms	MI			
	Heart failure			
Associated symptoms	Neck swelling			
	Symptoms of hyperthyroidism (weight loss, increase appetite, sweating, diarrhea)			
	Symptoms of other MEN syndrome (gastritis, PUD, amenorrhea, palpitation, HTN)			
Pressure/invasion symptoms	Hoarseness			
	Dysphagia			
	SOB			
Constitutional symptoms	Fever			
	Weight loss			
	Decrease appetite			
	Night sweating			
Risk factors	Radiation therapy			
	Family history of parathyroid disease			
	Family history of MEN or personal history of MEN			
Differential diagnosis	History of tuberculosis (TB) or contact with patients having TB			
	Personal history of malignancy (metastasis)			
	History of immobilization			
	Drugs: lithium, thiazide			
	Diarrhea			

History	Items	Done	Not done	Not applicable
Symptoms of metastasis	Bone pain			
	Headache			
	Abdominal pain/jaundice			
	Cough/shortness of breath			
PMH	Previous similar complaint			
	Previous ultrasound			
	Previous FNA			
	Chronic illness			
PSH				
Social history				
Medication				
Allergy				
Systemic review				
Physical examination				
General principle	Position			
	Permission			
	Privacy			
	Exposure			
	Wash hands			
General examination	Appearance			
	Body built			
	Color			
	Distress/decubitus			
	Environment			
Vital signs	Bp, PR, temp., RR, Spo_2			
Hand	Pulse			
	Moist/dry			
	Tremor			
Eye	Signs of hyperthyroidism			
Neck inspection	Ask the patient to swallow			
	Ask the patient to protrude the tongue			
	Look for any distended neck veins			
	Any jaw swelling			
Palpation from the front	Confirm your visual impression			
	Position of the trachea and carotid pulse			
	Position of the thyroid cartilage			
Palpation from behind	Stand behind the patient			
	Tilt patient head slightly forward to relax the anterior neck muscle			
	Press on one side and palpate the opposite lobe each time			
	Ask the patient to swallow and confirm that any swelling moving with swallowing			
	Palpate the whole neck for any cervical and supraclavicular lymph nodes			

(continued)

History	Items	Done	Not done	Not applicable
If there is any lump	Site			
	Number			
	Size			
	Shape			
	Consistency			
	Tenderness			
	Temperature			
Percussion	Over manubrium sterni: to define the lower extent of the swelling			
Auscultation	Systolic bruit over the swelling (thyrotoxic gland)			
Other systems for metastasis	Palpate the lower back			
	Palpate the abdomen for hepatomegaly			
	Examine the lungs			
MSK	Muscle power			
Differential diagnosis	Parathyroid adenoma			
	VIPoma			
	Milk alkali syndrome			
	Granulomatous disease (TB, sarcoidosis)			
	FHH			
	Immobilization			
	Malignancy (primary or secondary)			
Investigation				
Blood and urine	CBC			
	Coagulation			
	Electrolytes (mainly calcium, phosphorus, chloride, magnesium)			
	ALP			
	LFT (albumin)			
	RFT			
	TFT			
	PTH			
	Urine calcium			
	Vitamin D			
Imaging (localization)	Ultrasound			
	Sestamibi scan			
	4D CT			
	Venous sampling			
Management Primary hyper parathyroidism	Explain to the patient the need for surgery			
	Focused exploration or bilateral exploration			
	Vocal cord assessment			
	Prepare for surgery (focused neck exploration or bilateral exploration + parathyroidectomy + IOPTH essay)			
	Admission			
	NPO			
	IV fluid			
	Prophylaxis			
	Anesthesia consultation			
	Consent			

History	Items	Done	Not done	Not applicable
Intraoperative	Lymph node will be light beige to whitish and glassy			
	Thyroid nodule will be more vascular, firm, dark, or reddish brown			
	Parathyroid gland is golden brown and surrounded by fat; once the fat is incised, it will pop out			
	Inferior gland is below the entrance of the inferior thyroid artery entrance and ventral to the nerve			
	Superior gland is above the entrance of the inferior thyroid artery entrance and dorsal to the nerve			
If the inferior gland is not found	Mobilize the thyro-thymic ligament and the thymus			
	If still not found, open the carotid sheath from the bifurcation to the base of the neck			
	If still not found, check for intrathyroidal gland by intraoperative ultrasound, incise the thyroid capsule on its posterolateral side, or perform thyroid lobectomy			
If the superior gland is not found	Carotid sheath			
	Tracheoesophageal groove			
	Retroesophageal			
	Posterior mediastinum			
If one abnormal adenoma is found	Remove the abnormal, check intraoperative parathyroid hormone level			
	Clip the pedicle			
	Check intraoperative parathyroid hormone level			
If two adenomas and two normal glands or triple adenomas	If the remaining is/are normal (confirmed), excise the abnormal			
	Clip the pedicle			
All are abnormal	Subtotal parathyroidectomy (leave 50 mg of the most normal and apply clip)			
	Total parathyroidectomy with autotransplantation			
Complications	Bleeding			
	Nerve injury			
	Hypocalcemia			
	Bone hunger syndrome			
	Infection			

3.2.2 Answer Key

Case No. 1:
A 43-year-old female patient referred from PHC due to hypercalcemia.

Questions for Discussion:

1. **How will you approach this patient?**
   The patient is 43 years old, medically free. She has no active complaint and was following with the family physician for routine checkup.

   No personal or family history of endocrine malignancy.

   She has no contact with patients having TB.

   PSH: laparotomy and graham patch for perforated duodenal ulcer 6 months ago for which she is on proton pump inhibitors occasionally.

   Physical examination:
   No signs of hyper or hypothyroidism
   No palpable cervical lump
   No palpable cervical lymphadenopathy

2. **What is your differential diagnosis?**
   - Hyperparathyroidism
   - Malignancy
   - Endocrine disease
   - Granulomatous disease: sarcoidosis, TB
   - Milk alkali syndrome
   - Drugs: thiazide, lithium, vitamin A or D intoxication
   - Familial hypercalcemic hypocalciuric
   - Paget's disease
   - Immobilization

3. **How will you investigate this patient?**
   PTH and Ca (serum and urine) are high.
   ALP is 199.
   Vitamin D, RFT, and 24-h urine calcium are normal.
   Ultrasound shows small? Left inferior parathyroid adenoma.
   The thyroid gland is normal.
4. **What is your diagnosis?**
   Primary hyperparathyroidism.
5. **What will you do next?**
   Sestamibi scan shows left inferior parathyroid adenoma.
6. **What will you do?**
   - Explain to the patient that she needs surgery.
   - Vocal cord assessment.
   - Prepare for focused left neck exploration + parathyroidectomy + IOPTH essay.
   - Admission.
   - NPO.
   - IV fluid.
   - Prophylaxis (DVT, stress ulcer, antibiotic as indicated).
   - Anesthesia consultation.
   - Consent.

7. **How will you differentiate between a parathyroid gland, a thyroid nodule, and a lymph node?**
   Lymph node will be light beige to whitish and glassy.
   Thyroid nodule will be more vascular, firm, dark, or reddish brown.
   Parathyroid gland is golden brown and surrounded by fat; once the fat is incised, it will pop out.
8. **Where will you look for the inferior parathyroid gland?**
   Inferior gland is below the entrance of the inferior thyroid artery entrance and ventral to the nerve.
9. **You could not identify it in its usual position. What will you do?**
   - Mobilize the thyro-thymic ligament and the thymus.
   - If still not found, open the carotid sheath from the bifurcation to the base of the neck.
   - If still not found, check for intrathyroidal gland by intraoperative ultrasound, incise the thyroid capsule on its posterolateral side, or perform thyroid lobectomy.
10. **You found a single inferior parathyroid adenoma. What will you do?**
    - Remove the abnormal and check intraoperative parathyroid hormone level.
    - Clip the pedicle.
    - Check intraoperative parathyroid hormone level.

The intraoperative parathyroid hormone dropped by 60% from her baseline.

11. **What will you do?**
    Terminate the procedure.
12. **What are the post-parathyroidectomy complication?**
    - Bleeding
    - Nerve injury
    - Hypocalcemia
    - Bone hunger syndrome
    - Infection

References

1. Azar FK. Primary hyperparathyroidism. In: Cameron J, Cameron A, editors. Current surgical therapy. 12th ed. Canada: Elsevier; 2016.
2. Clark GLOH. Thyroid, parathyroid and adrenal. In: Brunicardi F, editor. Schwartz's principles of surgery. 11th ed. United States: McGraw-Hill Education; 2019.
3. Christakis IA. Management of recurrent and persistent hyperparathyroidism. In: Cameron J, Cameron A, editors. Current surgical therapy. 12th ed. Canada: Elsevier; 2016.
4. Wang TS. Management of secondary and tertiary hyperparathyroidism. In: Cameron J, Cameron A, editors. Current surgical therapy. 12th ed. Canada: Elsevier; 2016.

4 Surgical Aspects of Adrenal Diseases for Clinical Board Exams

4.1 Part I: Knowledge

> The best advice I ever got was that knowledge is power and to keep reading.
> —David Bailey

The patient may present with one of the following:

1. Symptoms of hyper-functionality
2. Abdominal mass/pain
3. Incidental finding

History:

- Personal data: name age, sex, nationality
- Chief complaint and duration
- History of presenting illness
  - **Analysis of the Chief Complaint**
    Symptoms of functionality (Table 4.1)
    Mass: onset, how did the patient noticed the mass?, any changes since it was first noticed?
    Pain: onset, site, radiation/shifting, aggravating/reliving factors, progression, severity, course
  - **Associated symptoms:** abdominal pain, vomiting, nausea, diarrhea, symptoms of hypercalcemia (i.e., MEN2A), pigmentation (i.e., neurofibromatosis)
  - **Constitutional symptoms:** weight loss, decrease appetite, fever, sweating
  - **Risk Factors:**
    Personal history of endocrine syndromes
    Family history of endocrine syndromes
  - **Differential Diagnosis (Table 4.2):**
    History of trauma
    History of TB or contact with patient has TB
    History of other cancer especially renal
    Personal history of pancreatic cyst, renal cyst, that is, Von Hippel-Lindau syndrome
  - **Symptoms of metastases:** abdominal pain, ascites, SOB, cough, or bone pain
- PMH
- PSH
- Social history
- Family history of thyroid, adrenal, parathyroid diseases
- Allergy, transfusion, medication
- Systemic review:
  - **CNS:** headache, blurred vision, hearing symptoms, epilepsy, numbness
  - **CVS:** dyspnea, paroxysmal nocturnal dyspnea, orthopnea, chest pain, lower limb edema
  - **Respiratory:** cough, hemoptysis, SOB, wheezes
  - **GIT:** change in appetite, dysphagia, heartburn, nausea, vomiting, change bowel habit
  - **Urological symptoms:** flank pain, dysuria, hematuria
  - **MSK:** weakness, arthritis, bone pain, back pain

H. Alotaibi, *Study Surgery*, https://doi.org/10.1007/978-981-16-2305-9_4

Table 4.1 Symptoms of functional tumors [1, 2]

Cushing syndrome	Pheochromocytoma	Hyperaldosteronism
• Weight gain • Hirsutism • Plethora • Striae • Acne • Ecchymosis • HTN • DM • Hyperlipidemia • Generalized weakness • Osteopenia • Emotional lability, depression, psychosis • Polyurea, renal stone • Impotence, decrease libido, menstrual irregularities • Sleep disturbance	• Headache • Palpitation • Diaphoresis • Anxiety • Paresthesia • Flushing • Shortness of breath • Chest pain • Cardiac complication, for example, MI • CVA • Tremor	• HTN • Muscle weakness • Polydipsia • Polyurea • Nocturia • Headache • Fatigue

Table 4.2 Differential diagnosis of adrenal mass

Functional tumor	Nonfunctional tumor	Malignant
Pheochromocytoma Cortisol-secreting adenoma Aldosterone-secreting adenoma Primary adrenal hyperplasia	Nonfunctional adenoma Myelolipoma Adrenal hematoma Adrenal cyst Ganglioneuroma Lymphoma Tuberculosis	Adrenocortical cancer Metastasis to adrenal gland

Physical Examination:

- Introduce yourself to the patient.
- Obtain permission.
- Assure privacy.
- Wash hands.
- Position: supine.
- Exposure.

General Examination:

- Appearance: ill, well, agitated, restless, hirsutism, acne
- Body built, for example, cachexia, obesity, buffalo hump, moon face
- Color: facial plethora, ecchymosis
- Distress
- Environment

Vital signs: BP, PR, temperature, RR, SPO_2
CVS: look for signs of heart failure
Respiratory: air entry, crackles
Neck: look for any neck mass, lymph nodes

Abdomen:

- Inspection: distention, striae, scars, ecchymosis, obvious swelling, hernial orifices
- Palpation: tenderness, organomegaly, ascites
- Percussion: ascites, dullness
- Auscultation: bowel sound, for example, ileus with hypokalemia
- DRE and groin

Extremities: edema, power
Differential diagnosis: Table 4.2
Adrenal Anatomy:
Refer to Fig. 4.1.

4.1.1 Approach to Patient with Adrenal Incidentaloma

Three Important Steps:

1. Verify that the lesion is in the adrenal gland: review the images, repeat it if needed to con-

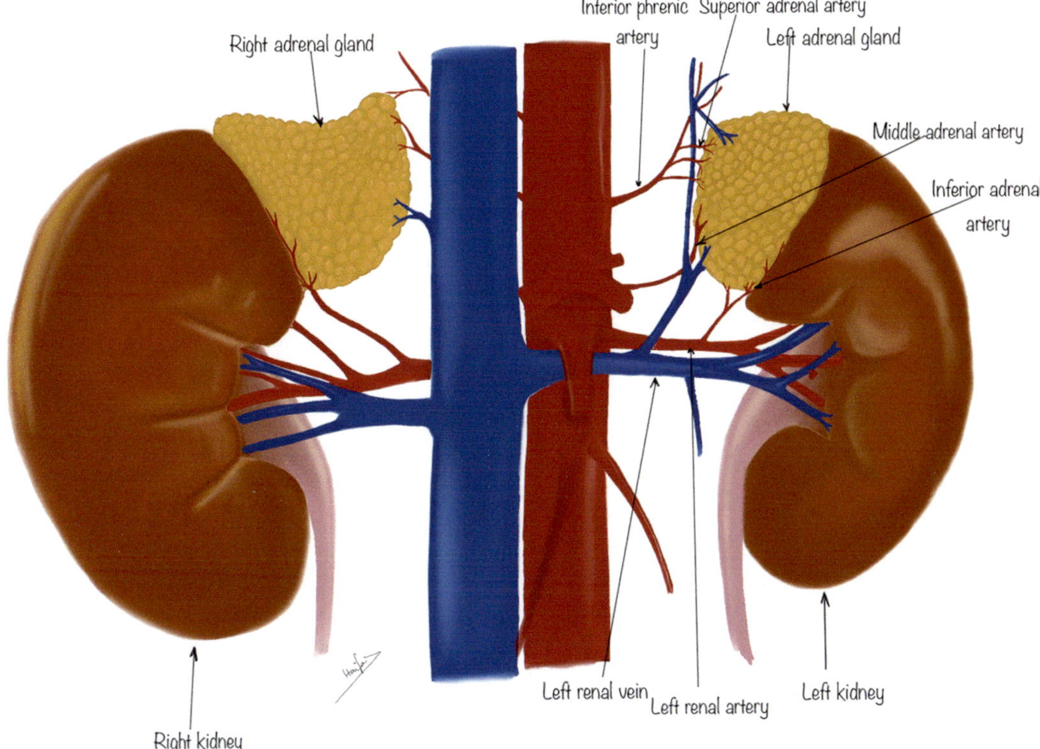

Fig. 4.1 Adrenal glands anatomy

firm it is from the adrenal, and see the characteristic features.

2. Determine if the lesion is hypersecreting hormones: clinical and biochemical.
3. Assess whether it is potentially malignant.

A. ***Clinical assessment:*** as described earlier

B. ***Biochemical Assessment:***

- CBC, electrolytes, liver function test (LFT), renal function test (RFT), blood group, coagulation profile.
- Do screening test to check for functionality. If any screening test is positive, do the confirmatory test related to that condition (Table 4.3).

C. ***Management:***

- If you confirm that the lesion is functional: do adrenalectomy.
- If the lesion is not functional:
  - <4 cm adenoma: repeat images after 3–6 months then annual for 2 years and repeat biochemical assessment at 12–24 months for 5 years.
  - >4 cm or has suspicious features: adrenalectomy.
  - Myelolipoma: observe [1, 2].

4.1.2 Pheochromocytoma

- **Classic Triad:**
  - Headache
  - Palpitation
  - Diaphoresis
- Most common clinical sign is paroxysmal hypertension.
- **Diagnostic Test:**
  - Initial biochemical testing: Screening tests:

    24-h urine metanephrine and normetanephrine (98% sensitive, 98% specific)

    Plasma metanephrine and normetanephrine:

Table 4.3 Screening and confirmatory tests for functionality assessment [1, 2]

	Hyperaldosteronism (Conn's)	Cushing	Pheochromocytoma
Screening tests	Plasma aldosterone and renin level (only if the patient is HTN± hypokalemic) N.B. Make sure the patient is off ACE inhibitors and spironolactone	Overnight 1 mg of dexamethasone at 11:00 pm Measure the plasma cortisol at 8:00 am	Measure plasma catecholamine level
Confirmatory tests	If the aldosterone level >15 or the ratio >20–25 Confirm the result by: Saline test: Keep the patient on high salt diet or give 2 L of saline and measure 24-h urine or aldosterone, Na, and K N.B. If aldosterone is >12, adrenalectomy if only unilateral adenoma	If not suppressed (plasma level >3 mcg), measure 24-h urine for cortisol level and measure plasma ACTH	If high, measure 24-h urine catecholamines and metanephrine

- Should be drawn in supine position after overnight fasting.
- Cut value for diagnosing is >200 pg/mL for norepinephrine and 200 pg/mL for epinephrine.

– Chromogranin A: adjunct to urinary metanephrine (help to decrease false positive result)

– Clonidine:

Can suppress neurologically mediated catecholamine but not secretion from pheochromocytoma.

Normal clonidine suppression test defined by decrease basal catecholamines to <500 pg/mL within 2–3 h after an oral dose of 0.3 mg of clonidine.

If not suppressed, diagnosis is pheochromocytoma.

– Imaging:

To localize the tumor once the diagnosis has been made.

CT scan of the abdomen (including diaphragm): pheochromocytoma appears homogeneous or heterogenous (Hounsfield >10), may have necrotic part with calcification, and can be solid or cystic.

CT neck and chest if needed to exclude extra-adrenal pheochromocytoma.

MRI abdomen: pheochromocytoma has high signal intensity in T2.

Functional Imaging:

- F^{18}—FDG PET/CT and ^{68}Ga—Dota peptide PET/CT: helps to localize pheochromocytoma or rule out metastasis.
- ^{123}I-MIBG scan should be used when planning radiotherapy with ^{131}I-MIBG for patient with metastatic disease.

- **Preoperative Preparation:**

1. **Alpha-Adrenoreceptor Antagonist**
   - Decrease blood pressure.
   - Reverse volume depletion.
   - Decrease peripheral vascular resistance.
   - Should be started 7–14 days preoperatively to normalize blood pressure and heart rate.
   - Warrant the patient of orthostatic hypotension.
   - Agent and Doses:

     Phenoxybenzamine 10 mg BID, dose can be increased by 10–20 mg every 2–3 days

     Goal blood pressure 130/80 mmHg while setting and 100/80 mmHg while standing

     Other options:

     - Doxazosin 2 mg OD
     - Prazosin 2 mg BID
     - Terzosin 2 mg OD
2. **Beta Blockers:**
   - Should be added to control heart rate

  - Typically, 2–3 days after alpha blocker and hydration
  - Agents:

    Selective drugs such as atenolol or metoprolol to reach the target heart rate 60–70 bpm.

    Do not use nonselective drugs, for example, Labetalol.
3. **Hydration:**
  - To avoid postoperative hypotension with loss of vasoconstriction after tumor removal
4. **Calcium Channel Blockers:**
  - Nicardipine can be used preoperative and intraoperative to control high blood pressure.

- **Intraoperative Measures:**
  - Use invasive and noninvasive monitoring.
  - Avoid stress during anesthesia induction.
  - Use inhaled agents like Isoflurane and Euflurane; they have minimal cardiac depressant effect.
  - Avoid fentanyl, ketamine, and morphine; it can stimulate catecholamine release from the tumor.
  - The goal is to resect the tumor completely with minimal tumor manipulation and avoid rupture of the tumor capsule.
  - Ligate the vein first.
  - To control intraoperative high blood pressure, use nitroprusside, nitroglycerin, phentolamine, and nicardipine.
  - To control intraoperative arrhythmia, use short-acting beta blocker, for example, esmolol.
  - To control intraoperative hypotension, use fluids and noradrenaline.
  - Open anterior approach is better for bilateral tumor, extra-adrenal, and metastatic lesions.
  - Tumors <5 cm can be safely removed laparoscopically.
  - If blood pressure did not drop post resection, either metastatic tumor or lesions in ectopic location [1, 3].

4.1.3 Cushing Syndrome

- **Cushing disease:** pituitary tumor
- **Cushing syndrome:** complex of symptoms and signs resulting from hypersecretion of cortisol regardless the etiology
- Mostly sporadic
- Female to male ratio is 8:1
- May be found in MEN1, result from ACTH secreting pituitary tumor (Table 4.4)

- **Signs and Symptoms:**
  - Progressive truncal obesity (most common occurring symptom ~95%).
  - Other features, see Table 4.1.
  - Most common symptoms in children are obesity and stunted growth.

Table 4.4 Cushing syndrome [1, 4]

ACTH dependent 70%	ACTH independent 20–30%	Others
• Pituitary adenoma (Cushing disease) ~70% • Ectopic ACTH production ~10% • Ectopic CRH production <1% (from bronchial carcinoid, pheochromocytoma, and other tumors)	• Adrenal adenoma ~10–15% • Adrenal hyperplasia 5% • Micronodular • Macronodular • Massive macronodular • Primary pigmented nodular adrenocortical disease: • Small <5 mm • Black nodule • May be associated with Carney complex (Atrial myxoma, Schwannoma, and pigment nevi) • Adrenal carcinoma 10–15%	Pseudo-Cushing: • Major depression • Alcoholism • Pregnancy • Chronic renal failure • Stress • Iatrogenic

Table 4.5 Diagnostic tests for Cushing syndrome [1, 4]

Confirm the diagnosis	Determine the etiology
1. Low dose dexamethasone test (screening test): Give 1 mg of dexamethasone at 11 pm and measure plasma cortisol level at 8 am (a) Suppressed to <3 mcg: normalFalse negative seen in mild disease (b) Not suppressed: Cushing syndromeFalse positive seen in CRF, depression, and in patient on phenytoin N.B: If negative test but high clinical suspicion: Perform classic low dexamethasone test (0.5 mg Q6h for eight doses or 2 mg over 48 h) **2. 24-h urine cortisol level:** (a) Very sensitive 95–100%, specific 98%. (b) Can identify patient with pseudo-Cushing (c) Level <100 mcg/dL exclude hypercortisolism **3. Salivary cortisol measurement has superior sensitivity** N.B: 24-h urine free cortisol + overnight dexamethasone test at 5 mcg/dL cut off has highest specificity for the diagnosis of Cushing syndrome	**1. Plasma ACTH level (normal 10–100 pg/mL):** (a) <5 pg/mL: primary cortisol secreting adrenal tumor (b) 15–500 pg/mL: adrenal hyperplasia due to Cushing disease (pituitary) or CRH secreting tumor (c) >1000 pg/mL: ectopic ACTH **2. High dose dexamethasone test:** (a) Used to differentiate between the cause of ACTH dependent Cushing (pituitary vs. ectopic) (b) Give 2 mg dexamethasone Q6h for 2 days or 8 mg dexamethasone overnight, then measure 24-h urine for cortisol and 17 hydroxysteroid: Failed to suppress by 50%: ectopic ACTH producing tumors (patient should undergo testing for medullary thyroid cancer and pheochromocytoma) Suppressed: pituitary cause **3. Bilateral petrosal vein sampling:** differentiate between Cushing disease (pituitary) and ectopic Cushing syndrome **4. CRH test:** Give 1 mg/kg of CRH intravenous then take serial measurement for ACTH every 15 min for 1 h (a) >30 pg/mL: ACTH dependent (b) <10 pg/mL: Adrenal

  - Skin hyperpigmentation if present suggest ectopic ACTH producing tumor.
- **Diagnostic Tests:**
  - Refer to Table 4.5.

- **Radiological Studies:**
  - CT and MRI abdomen:

    Can identify adrenal tumors with 95% sensitivity

    Can help to distinguish adenoma from carcinoma

    Adrenal adenoma darker than the liver on T2
  - NP-59:

    Can distinguish adenoma from hyperplasia
  - Inferior petrosal sinus sampling for ACTH before and after CRH injection has been helpful in identifying pituitary tumors.

    Sensitivity 100%

    Ratio of petrosal to peripheral vein ACTH > 2 in basal state and >3 after CRH stimulation is diagnostic.
  - CT and MRI (chest and anterior mediastinum first then neck abdomen and pelvis second if the first is negative) for patient with suspected ectopic ACTH production.
- **Treatment:**
  - Laparoscopic adrenalectomy is the treatment of choice for adrenal adenoma.
  - Open adrenalectomy is reserved for large tumor ≥6 cm or suspected cancer.
  - Bilateral adrenalectomy is curative for primary adrenal hyperplasia.
  - For Cushing disease (pituitary):

    Trans-sphenoidal excision of pituitary adenoma.

Radiation for persistent or recurrent tumor.

Stereotactic adrenalectomy.

Medical adrenalectomy (ketoconazole, metyrapone, and aminoglutethimide)

- Ectopic ACTH production:

  Treatment of the primary including the recurrence.

  Medical or bilateral adrenalectomy has been used to palliate patient with unresectable disease or those whose ectopic ACTH secreting tumor cannot be localized.

- Give pre- and postoperative steroid (the contralateral gland is suppressed).
- Give anticoagulant (those patients at increased risk of thromboembolic complication from increased clotting factors including factor VIII, VW factor, and impaired fibrinolysis) [1, 4].

4.1.4 Approach to Patient with Suspected Hyperaldosteronism

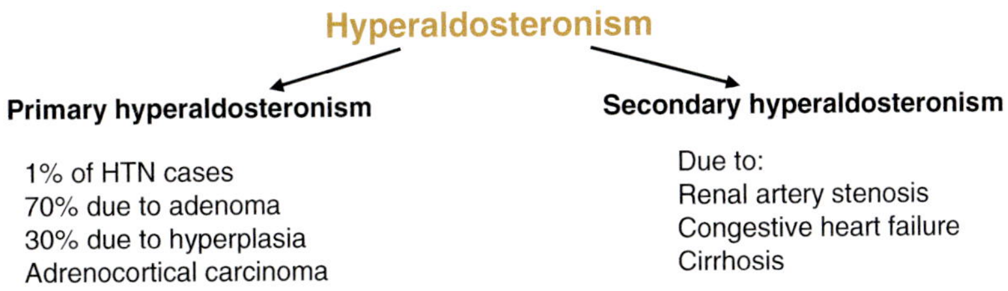

I. **Suspect the Diagnosis**
- Any hypertensive patient with coexisting spontaneous hypokalemia <3.2 mmol/L or hypokalemia <3 mmol/L while on diuretics and despite potassium (K) replacement.
- Before testing, the patient must receive adequate K and Na and the antihypertensive medication should be held.

II. **Confirm the Diagnosis**
- Elevated plasma aldosterone level:
  - Suppressed renin activity
  - Ratio 1:25 to 1:30
  - False positive may be seen in patient with congestive heart failure
- Na loading test:
  - 5 days of high Na diet, then measure 24-h urine for Na, cortisol and aldosterone.
  - Or 2–3 days of low Na diet, then give 2 L of saline while patient in supine position, and then measure 24-h urine for Na, cortisol, and aldosterone.
- Plasma level of aldosterone <5 or 24-h urine aldosterone <14 exclude hyperaldosteronism.

III. **Determine Whether Bilateral or Unilateral Disease:**
- CT abdomen (0.5 cm cuts) localizes adenoma with sensitivity of 90%.
- MRI is less sensitive but more specific.
- Selective venous catheterization and adrenal vein sampling:
  - Sensitivity 95%, specificity 90%.
  - Procedure: cannulate the adrenal veins, then draw blood for aldosterone and cortisol levels from both adrenal veins and IVC after administration of ACTH.
  - Measurement of cortisol confirms a proper placement of the catheter in the adrenal vein.
  - Aldosterone to cortisol ratio >4-folds difference indicates unilateral tumor.
  - Indications of adrenal vein sampling:

    Tumor cannot be localized.

    Bilateral adrenal enlargement.

    Suspected adrenocortical carcinoma.

    Familial hyperaldosteronism type I and type III.

- Scintigraphy with ^{131}I-6B-iodomethyl-noriodocholestrol (NP-59)
  - This compound is taken up by the cortex and remain in the gland without metabolism.
  - Adenoma appear as hot nodule and hyperplasia will show bilateral increase uptake.
- 11-C-metomidate with PET-CT.

IV. **Treatment of Hyperaldosteronism**

A. Preoperative:
- Control HTN
- Correct hypokalemia to >3.5 mmol/L
- Medications that can be used: spironolactone, amiloride, nifedipine or captopril

B. Operative:
- Unilateral tumor: adrenalectomy.
- Laparoscopic resection is the preferred approach or posterior open approach.
- If carcinoma is suspected, the best approach is anterior abdominal approach.
- Only 20–30% of patients with hyperaldosteronism secondary to bilateral hyperplasia benefit from surgery.
- Adrenal vein sampling (AVS) is useful to predict which patient will respond.

C. Post-operative:
- Transient hypoaldosteronism require mineralocorticoid for up to 3 months.
- High risk for post resection hypokalemia:
  - Old patient
  - Long duration of hypertension
  - Impaired kidney function
  - High preoperative aldosterone level
- Patient who responds to spironolactone therapy and those with short duration of HTN achieve more improvement in HTN.
- Male patients, older than 50 years, are least likely to benefit from adrenalectomy.
- Acute Addison disease may happen 2–3 days after adrenalectomy.
- Post adrenalectomy >90% of hypokalemia and >70% of HTN will improve [1, 4].

4.1.5 Adrenocortical Cancer

- Bimodal age: children and adult in fourth to fifth decades of life
- Majority sporadic
- Familial:
  - P53: Li Fraumeni syndrome
  - MENIN: MEN1
  - Loci on P11: Beckwith Wiedemann syndrome
  - 2p: carney complex
- **Symptoms and Signs:**
  - 50% are nonfunctioning:
    Presented with enlarging abdominal mass, abdominal or back pain, and rarely with weight loss and nausea
  - 50% functioning:
    Cortisol 30%, androgen 20%, estrogen 10%, and aldosterone 2%
    Multiple hormones in 35%
- **Diagnostic Tests:**
  - Serum electrolytes (to rule out hypokalemia).
  - Urinary catecholamines (to rule out pheochromocytoma).
  - Overnight 1 mg dexamethasone suppression test, 24-h urine cortisol, and 17 keto-steroid (to rule out Cushing).
  - CT and MRI: the size of the adrenal mass on the imaging is the single most important criterion to help diagnose malignancy. More than 92% of adrenal cancers are >6 cm. Other characteristic features include tumor heterogenicity, irregular margin, presence of hemorrhage, lymph node, and metastasis.
  - In T2:
    Has moderately enhancing signal
    Shows significant lesion enhancement
    Slow washout after injection of gadolinium
    Evidence of local invasion to adjacent tissue, liver, IVC, distant metastases
  - PET or PET/CT has some utility in distinguishing benign from malignant lesion.
  - Once adrenal cancer diagnosed, do CT CAP or PET for staging.

- Capsular or vascular invasion is the most reliable sign for cancer because it is difficult to distinguish adenoma from carcinoma by histology.
- **Treatment**:
  - Most important predictor of survival is adequacy of resection.
  - Enbloc resection of the tumor and the involved lymph node or organs (diaphragm, kidney, pancreas, liver, IVC) is the treatment of choice.
  - Best approach is open adrenalectomy via subcostal incision or thoracoabdominal (on the right side).
  - Wide exposure is needed to minimize chance of capsular rupture, tumor spillage, and allow vascular control of aorta, IVC, and renal vessels.
  - Adjuvant treatment: Mitotane, o,p-DDD,1,1 dichoro-2-(o-chlorophenyl)-2-(p-chlorophenyl) ethane can be used in the adjuvant setting and for the treatment of unresectable or metastatic disease due to their adrenolytic activity.
  - Common site for metastases is liver, lung, and bone.
  - Management of isolated, recurrent disease is debulking.
  - Adrenocortical cancer is relatively insensitive for radiation, but radiation therapy can be used for bone metastases or palliation [1, 4].

4.1.6 Adrenalectomy

Preoperative Preparation:

- Special preparation: depends on the pathology as described earlier
- General:
  - Admission
  - Nothing per oral (NPO)
  - IV fluid
  - Prophylaxis: antibiotics, DVT, and stress ulcer prophylaxis
  - Anesthesia consultation
  - ICU consultation for possible postoperative admission
  - Surgical site marking
  - Consent

Informed Consent:

- *Describe the procedure to the patient:* under general anesthesia, the surgeon will perform (left/right) adrenalectomy using (open/laparoscopic) approach. Mention if there is any need for Enbloc resection of nearby organs in case of malignancy.
- *Mention if there are any alternatives* like medical adrenalectomy or follow-up.
- *Mention the possible complications:* bleeding, infection, collection, atelectasis, pneumonia, injury to nearby organs, intraoperative hyper/hypotension, arrythmias, and post-operative adrenal crisis.

4.1.7 Laparoscopic Adrenalectomy

Procedure:

- The operating room is set up with the monitors just off the patient's shoulders.
- General anesthesia and endotracheal intubation.
- Position: lateral decubitus position with the side of the tumor up.
- Time out: confirm correct patient, procedure, side, surgeon, and availability of any required instruments.
- The surgeon stands facing the patient's abdomen.
- The patient's entire side extending down the abdomen and the back is prepped and draped in normal sterile fashion.
- The lower chest and entire abdomen are draped into the field to allow maximal access.
- The positions for port sites are marked approximately 1–2 fingerbreadths below the costal margin extending from the posterior axillary line to the midclavicular line with at least 6 cm between them.

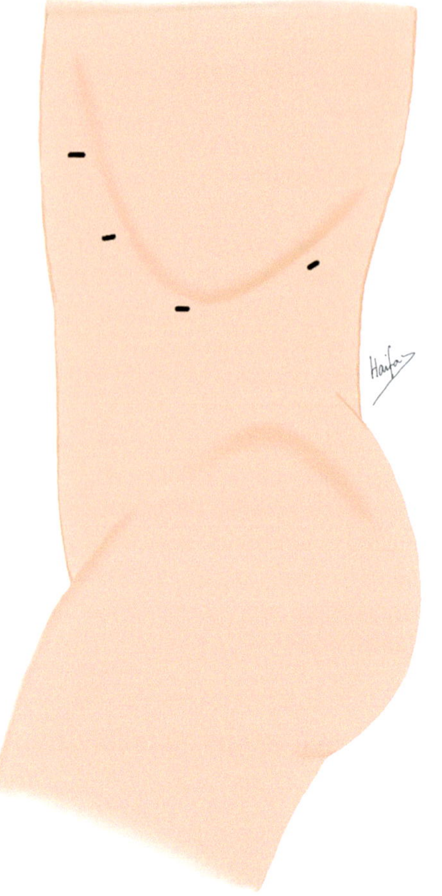

Fig. 4.2 The positions for port sites are marked approximately 1–2 fingerbreadths below the costal margin extending from the posterior axillary line to the midclavicular line with at least 6 cm between them

- A pneumoperitoneum is then created with a Veress needle inserted through a small nick in the skin.
- After creating the pneumoperitoneum, a 10-mm port is placed into the peritoneal cavity.
- The 30° laparoscope is then inserted, and the additional three ports are placed in the positions identified (Fig. 4.2). It may be necessary to take down the lateral attachments of the left colon to place the last port on the left side or mobilize a portion of the right lobe of the liver on the right side.
- For left-sided adrenalectomy, the lateral attachments of the spleen are divided with a harmonic scalpel. This allows the spleen to fall medially, taking the tail of the pancreas with it and opening up the retroperitoneal space.

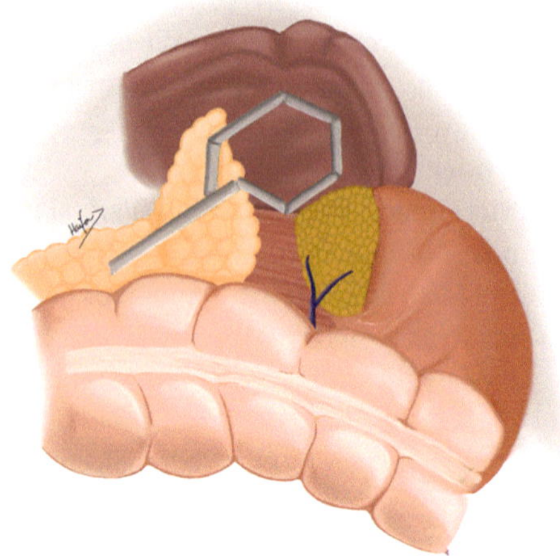

Fig. 4.3 Laparoscopic left adrenalectomy, try to avoid injury to the nearby structure mainly pancreas

- On the right side, it is necessary to enter the retroperitoneum at the posterior aspect of the right lobe of the liver so that the liver can be retracted anteriorly. The harmonic scalpel is used to separate the tissue to allow identification of the inferior vena cava.
- On the left side, the kidney is identified and the tissue superior and medial to it is inspected to allow identification of the left adrenal gland (Fig. 4.3). If there is difficulty identifying the gland, a laparoscopic ultrasound probe can be used to identify an adrenal mass in the retroperitoneal fat.
- On the right side, the dissection involves also identifying the kidney and then identifying the adrenal gland in the tissue medial and superior to the kidney. No matter which side is being dissected, the harmonic scalpel should be used at this point to carefully dissect the tissue lateral and inferior to the adrenal gland in order to better define the extent of the gland.
- If a pheochromocytoma is present, the adrenal vein should be controlled first, by identifying the vessel, doubly clipping it, and then dividing it. The right adrenal vein is quite short and can cause significant problems with hemorrhage if not carefully dissected and divided.

- The posterior and superior attachments of the adrenal gland are divided with the harmonic scalpel, allowing the gland to be carefully separated from all of the surrounding tissues.
- Once the gland is completely separated from the surrounding tissues, it is placed within a bag inside the patient. It is then removed through one of the port sites, extending the port as necessary to allow the gland to be removed intact in the bag.
- The port is then reinserted into the patient for further examination of the bed of the adrenal gland. This space is inspected, irrigated, and drained of fluid to allow adequate hemostasis to be confirmed.
- The ports are then removed, and the fascia closed on each with interrupted O Vicryl sutures.
- The skin is closed with monofilament absorbable subcuticular stitches [5].

Postoperative Complications:

- Acute adrenal crisis
- Postoperative hypotension
- Hemorrhage
- Peritonitis due to injury of any of the organs in proximity to the adrenal gland, such as the colon, spleen, or liver [1, 5]

4.2 Part II: Practice

> You need to put what you learn into practice and do it over and over again until it's a habit
> —Brett Hoebel

4.2.1 Case Scenarios for Practice

Tips:

- Practice with a friend and try to mimic the real exam!
- Do not forget to set the timer!
- The clinical data is provided in the answer key section.

Case No. 1:

A 55-year-old male patient referred to your clinic due to accidental finding of left adrenal mass that is found on abdominal ultrasound done for another reason.

Questions for Discussion:

1. How will you approach this patient?
2. What is your differential diagnosis?
3. How will you investigate this patient?
4. What will you do next?
5. How will you manage this patient?
6. How will you prepare this patient for operation?
7. What are the intraoperative precautions?
8. How will you control intraoperative high BP and arrythmias?
9. After resection of left adrenal gland, the patient is severely hypotensive. How will you manage that?

Case No. 2:

A 46-year-old female patient referred from endocrinologist due to the presence of right adrenal mass.

Questions for Discussion:

1. How will approach the patient?
2. What is the most likely diagnosis?
3. How will investigate the patient?
4. How will you manage the patient?
5. Second day, the patient is febrile and hypotensive. What could be the cause and how will you manage that?

Checklist

History	Items	Done	Not done	Not applicable
General	Introduce herself/himself to the patient			
	Patient personal data (name, age, sex, etc.)			
	Chief complaint			
	Duration			
General	Abdominal pain			
	Abdominal distention			
	Vomiting			
	Nausea			
Cushing	Weight gain			
	Hirsutism			
	Plethora			
	Striae			
	Acne			
	Ecchymosis			
	HTN			
	DM			
	Hyperlipidemia			
	Generalized weakness			
	Osteopenia			
	Emotional lability, depression, psychosis			
	Polyurea, renal stone			
	Impotence, decrease libido			
	Sleep disturbance			
Pheochromocytoma	Headache			
	Palpitation			
	Diaphoresis			
	Anxiety			
	Paresthesia			
	Flushing			
	Shortness of breath			
	Chest pain			
	Cardiac complication, for example, MI			
	CVA			
	Tremor			
Aldosterone secreting adenoma	HTN			
	Muscle weakness			
	Polydipsia			
	Polyurea			
	Nocturia			
	Headache			
	Fatigue			
Associated symptoms	Symptoms of other MEN syndromes (gastritis, PUD, palpitation, HTN), neck swelling			

History	Items	Done	Not done	Not applicable
Constitutional symptoms	Fever			
	Weight loss			
	Decrease appetite			
	Night sweating			
Risk factors	Family history of MEN or personal history of MEN syndromes			
Differential diagnosis	History of tuberculosis (TB) or contact with TB patient			
	History of trauma			
	History renal cancer			
	History of pancreatic cyst, renal cyst			
Symptoms of metastasis	Bone pain			
	Headache			
	Abdominal pain/jaundice			
	Cough/shortness of breath			
PMH	Chronic illness			
	Previous abdominal imaging			
PSH				
Social history				
Medication				
Allergy				
Systemic review				
Physical examination				
General principle	Position			
	Permission			
	Privacy			
	Exposure			
	Wash hands			
General examination	Appearance			
	Body built			
	Color			
	Distress/decubitus			
	Environment			
Vital signs	Bp, HR, temp., RR, Spo_2			
Hand	Pulse			
	Moist/dry			
	Tremor			
CVS	Signs of heart failure			
RS	Pulmonary edema or crackles			
Neck	Look for any masses			
	Look for any distended neck veins			
Abdomen inspection	Distention			
	Ecchymosis			
	Striae and scars			
	Obvious swelling			
	Hernial orifices			
Palpation	Tenderness			
	Palpable masses			
	Organomegaly			

(continued)

History	Items	Done	Not done	Not applicable
Percussion	Ascites			
	Over the mass if present			
Auscultation	Bowel sound			
DRE	DRE			
MSK and extremities	Muscle power			
	Peripheral edema			
Differential diagnosis	Pheochromocytoma			
	Cortisol-secreting adenoma			
	Aldosternoma			
	Primary adrenal hyperplasia			
	Nonfunctional adenoma			
	Myelolipoma			
	Adrenal hematoma			
	Adrenal cyst			
	Ganglioneuroma			
	Lymphoma			
	Adrenal tuberculosis			
	Adrenocortical cancer			
	Metastasis to adrenal gland			
Investigation				
Blood tests	CBC			
	Coagulation			
	Electrolytes			
	LFT			
	RFT			
	Chromogranin A			
Screening for functionality	Plasma aldosterone and renin level			
	Overnight 1 mg of dexamethasone at 11:00 pm Measure the plasma cortisol at 8:00 am			
	Measure plasma catecholamine level			
Confirmatory test (depends on which of the screening tests is positive)	Measure 24-h urine catecholamines and metanephrine			
	Saline test			
	If cortisol is not suppressed (plasma level >3 mcg), measure 24-h urine for cortisol level and measure plasma ACTH			
Imaging	CT abdomen/MRI			
	NP-59			
	Dota scan/PET scan			

History	Items	Done	Not done	Not applicable
Management				
Pheochromocytoma:				
Preoperative alpha blocker	Phenoxybenzamine 10 mg BID, dose can be increased by 10–20 mg every 2–3 days			
	Goal blood pressure 130/80 mmHg while setting and 100/80 while standing.			
Preoperative Beta blocker	2–3 days after alpha blocker			
	Selective drugs such as atenolol or metoprolol to reach the target heart rate 60–70 bpm			
Fluid	Hydration			
CCB	For example, Nicardipine			
General preparation	Admission			
	NPO			
	IV fluid			
	Prophylaxis			
	ECG			
	CXR			
	Anesthesia consultation			
	ICU consultation			
	Surgical site marking			
	Consent			
	Adrenalectomy			
Intraoperative precautions	Use invasive and noninvasive monitoring			
	Avoid stress during anesthesia induction			
	Use inhaled agents like Isoflurane and Euflurane; they have minimal cardiac depressant effect			
	Avoid fentanyl, ketamine, and morphine; it can stimulate catecholamine release from the tumor			
	The goal is to resect the tumor completely with minimal tumor manipulation or rupture of the tumor capsule			
	Ligate the vein first			
Intraoperative control of hypertension and arrhythmia	To control intraoperative high blood pressure, use nitroprusside, nitroglycerin, phentolamine, and nicardipine			
	To control intraoperative arrhythmia, use short-acting beta blocker, for example, esmolol			
Control of intraoperative hypotension	To control intraoperative hypotension, use fluids and noradrenaline			

(continued)

History	Items	Done	Not done	Not applicable
Cushing syndrome:	Admission			
	NPO			
	IV fluid			
	Prophylaxis			
	ECG			
	CXR			
	Anesthesia consultation			
	ICU consultation			
	Surgical site marking			
	Consent			
	Preoperative cortisone			
	Adrenalectomy			
	Postoperative cortisone			
Hyper-aldosterone secreting adenoma:				
Preoperative	Control HTN			
	Correct hypokalemia to >3.5			
	Medications that can be used: spironolactone, amiloride, nifedipine, or captopril			
	Admission			
	NPO			
	IV fluid			
	Prophylaxis			
	ECG			
	CXR			
	Anesthesia consultation			
	ICU consultation			
	Surgical site marking			
	Consent			
Operative	Adrenalectomy			
Postoperative	Manage the transient hypoaldosteronism with mineralocorticoid			
	Manage the hypokalemia			
	Manage acute Addison crises if happens			
Adrenocortical cancer	Staging			
	Multidisciplinary team			
	Break the bad news			
	Preoperative preparation			
	Adrenalectomy			
	Refer for adjuvant treatment if indicated			

4.2.2 Answer Key

Case No. 1:

A 55-year-old male patient referred to your clinic due to accidental finding of left adrenal mass that is found on abdominal ultrasound done for another reason.

Questions for Discussion:

1. **How will you approach this patient?**
   The patient is 55 years old, hypertensive on two antihypertensive medications; however, his BP is uncontrolled.
   He was following with gastroenterologist for hepatitis, and ultrasound was requested to assess his liver and they discovered this adrenal mass.
   He has history of chronic headache, occasional chest pain, and palpitation.
   He has no personal or family history of endocrine diseases or malignancy.
   And no other significant symptoms.
   PSH: free.
   PMH: HTN and hepatitis.
   Medication: anti-hypertensive.
   Not known allergic.
   Physical examination: unremarkable.
2. **What is your differential diagnosis?**
   - Pheochromocytoma
   - Cortisol secreting adenoma
   - Aldosternoma
   - Primary adrenal hyperplasia
   - Nonfunctional adenoma
   - Myelolipoma
   - Adrenal hematoma
   - Adrenal cyst
   - Ganglioneuroma
   - Lymphoma
   - Tuberculosis
   - Adrenocortical cancer
   - Metastasis to adrenal gland
3. **How will you investigate this patient?**
   - CBC, coagulation profile, electrolytes, LFT, RFT, Chromogranin A, Plasma aldosterone, and renin level.
   - Overnight 1 mg of dexamethasone at 11:00 pm. Measure the plasma cortisol at 8:00 am. Measure plasma catecholamine level CT abdomen.
   - Basic labs within normal. The screening test reveals high plasma catecholamine levels (four times the normal).
   - CT abdomen: left adrenal mass 5 × 6 cm.

4. **What will you do next?**
   Measure 24-h urine catecholamines and metanephrine (confirmatory test).
   Three times the normal level.
5. **How will you manage this patient?**
   Left adrenalectomy after proper preoperative preparation.
6. **How will you prepare this patient for operation?**
   - Alpha blocker:
     - Phenoxybenzamine 10 mg BID, dose can be increased by 10–20 mg every 2–3 days.
     - Goal blood pressure 130/80 mmHg while setting and 100/80 while standing.
   - Beta blocker:
     - 2–3 days after alpha blocker:
     - Selective drugs such as atenolol or metoprolol to reach the target heart rate 60–70 bpm

- Hydration
- Calcium channel blocker, for example, Nicardipine
- Admission
- NPO
- IV fluid
- Prophylaxis
- ECG
- CXR
- Anesthesia consultation
- ICU consultation
- Surgical site marking
- Consent

7. **What are the intraoperative precautions?**
   - Use invasive and noninvasive monitoring.
   - Avoid stress during anesthesia induction.
   - Use inhaled agents like Isoflurane and Euflurane; they have minimal cardiac depressant effect.

- Avoid fentanyl, Ketamine, and Morphine; it can stimulate catecholamine release from the tumor.
- The goal is to resect the tumor completely with minimal tumor manipulation or rupture of the tumor capsule.
- Ligate the vein first.

8. **How will you control intraoperative high BP and arrythmias?**
   - To control intraoperative high blood pressure, use nitroprusside, nitroglycerin, phentolamine, and nicardipine.
   - To control intraoperative arrhythmia, use short-acting beta blocker, for example, esmolol.
9. **After resection of left adrenal gland, the patient is severely hypotensive, how will you manage that?**
   By fluid administration and noradrenaline.

Case No. 2:

A 46-year-old female patient referred from endocrinologist due to the presence of right adrenal mass.

Questions for Discussion:

1. **How will approach the patient?**
   The patient is a 46-year-old female patient. She is following with endocrinologist due to progressive symptoms of weight gain, easily bruises, hirsutism, menstrual irregularity for 1 year. CT was requested and it showed right adrenal mass. She has no history of abdominal pain or mass. She has no family or personal history of endocrine disease and no history of trauma. She is recently diagnosed with diabetes mellites on oral hypoglycemic medications and has no previous surgical history.
   On examination:
   The patient looks obese.
   Vital signs: normal.
   Face: has the classic picture of moon face and hirsutism.
   Abdomen: redundant abdomen with stretch marks. No palpable masses, ascites, or organomegaly.
   Extremities: multiple bruises marks.
2. **What is the most likely diagnosis?**
   Cushing syndrome.
3. **How will investigate the patient?**
   - Low dose dexamethasone test (screening test):
     1 mg of dexamethasone at 11 pm and measure plasma cortisol level at 8 am (not suppressed).
   - 24-h urine cortisol: elevated.
   - Plasma ACTH: 3 pg/mL.
   - Review the CT: there is right adrenal mass 4 × 3 cm.
4. **How will you manage the patient?**
   Right adrenalectomy.
5. **Second day, the patient is febrile and hypotensive. What could be the cause and how will you manage that?**
   Acute adrenal insufficiency due to suppressed contralateral gland.
   Give 100 mg IV hydrocortisone.

References

1. Clark GLOH. Thyroid, parathyroid and adrenal. In: Brunicardi F, editor. Schwartz's Principles of surgery. 11th ed. United States: McGraw-Hill Education; 2019.
2. Brunt LM. Adrenal incidentaloma. In: Cameron J, Cameron A, editors. Current surgical therapy. 12th ed. Canada: Elsevier; 2016.
3. Dhaval Patel NN, Kebebew E. The management of pheochromocytoma. In: Cameron J, Cameron A, editors. Current surgical therapy. 12th ed. Canada: Elsevier; 2016.
4. Konstantinos Makris APBD. The management of adrenal cortical tumor. In: Cameron J, Cameron A, editors. Current surgical therapy. 12th ed. Canada: Elsevier; 2016.
5. Angelos P. Adrenalectomy. In: Bell DBK RH, editor. Northwestern handbook of surgical procedures. 11th ed. United States: LANDES BIOSCIENCE; 2005.

5 Surgical Aspects of Liver Diseases for Clinical Board Exams

5.1 Part I: Knowledge

I would encourage you be informed—knowledge is power.
—Matt Bevin

5.1.1 History of Right Upper Abdominal Pain or Mass

The differential diagnosis of the possible hepatic-related complaints (Table 5.1)

History:

- Introduce yourself to the patient
- Name, Age, Occupation, Sex, Nationality
- History of the presenting illness:
  - Analysis of the chief complaint

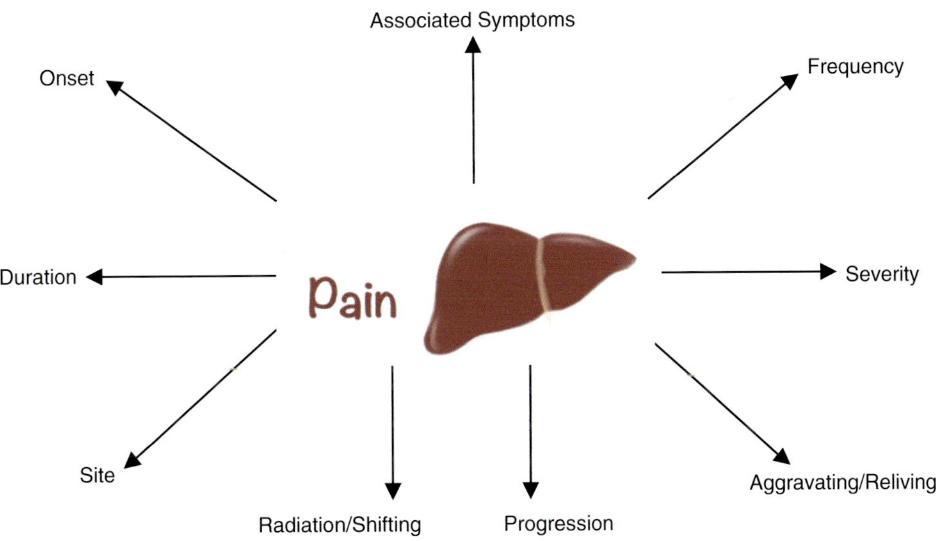

H. Alotaibi, *Study Surgery*, https://doi.org/10.1007/978-981-16-2305-9_5

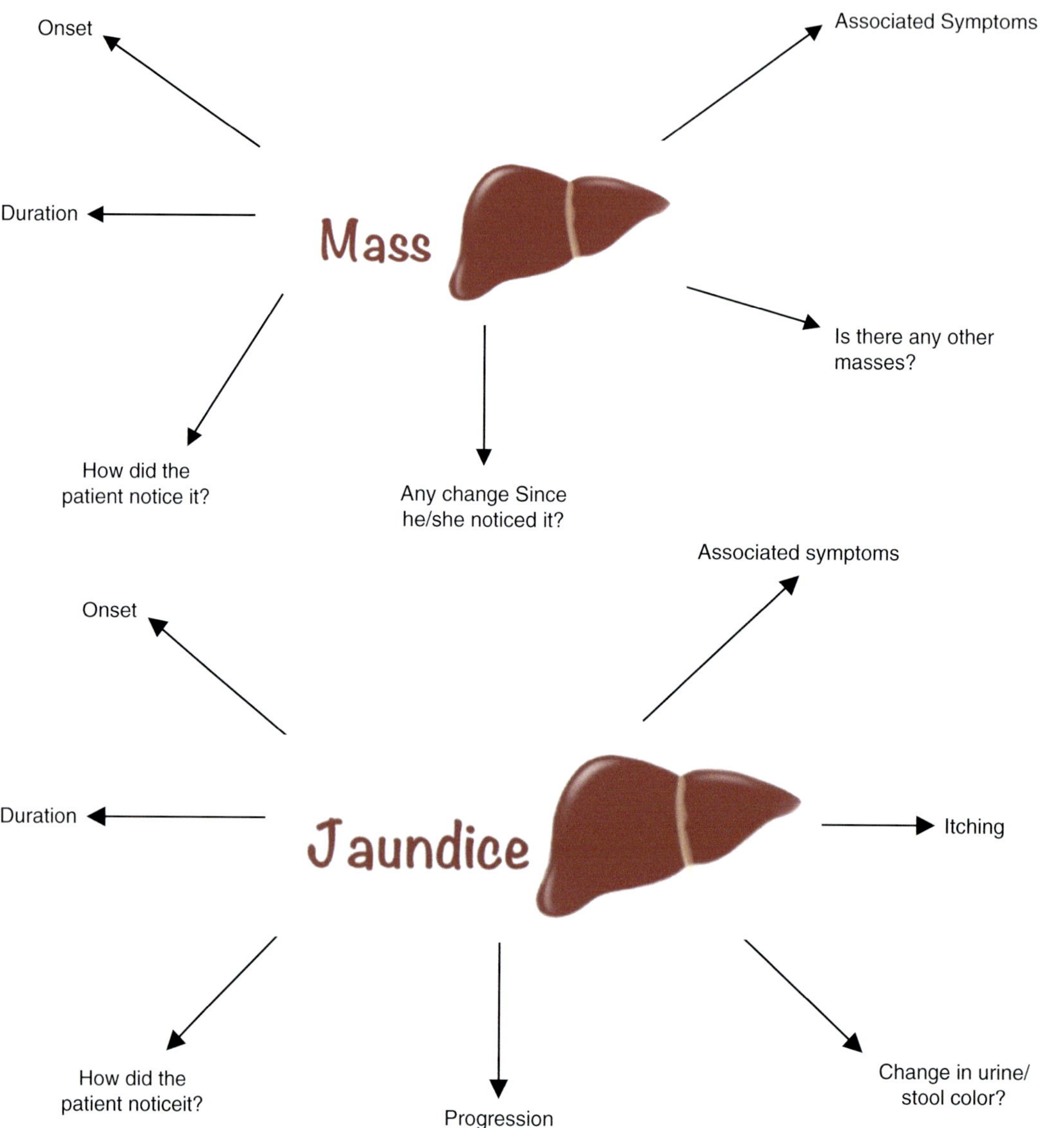

Table 5.1 Differential diagnosis

Right upper quadrant pain	Right upper quadrant mass	Jaundice
Gallstone disease	Distended gallbladder	**Prehepatic:**
Liver abscess	Liver mass (benign or malignant)	Hemolytic anemia
Hepatitis	Choledochal cyst	Hemolysis
Symptomatic hemangioma or adenoma	Liver cyst	**Hepatic:**
Hydatid cyst	Hernia, e.g., incisional	Cirrhosis
Amebic abscess	Lipoma	Gilbert's syndrome
Hepatocellular carcinoma (HCC)		Hepatitis
Gallbladder cancer		**Posthepatic:**
Lower lobe pneumonia		Choledocholithiasis
Myocardial infarction		Cholangiocarcinoma
Musculoskeletal pain		Stricture
Trauma		Mirrizi syndrome
		Periampullary cancer

- Associated symptoms
- Pain, fever, jaundice, nausea, vomiting, diarrhea, constipation, change in urine or stool color, itching, or abdominal distention
- Constitutional symptoms:
- Weight loss, decrease in appetite, night sweating, or fever
- Symptoms of metastasis
- Back pain, abdominal distention, cough, or shortness of breath (SOB)
- Risk factors:
  Rapid weight loss
  History of cirrhosis
  Oral contraceptive pills (OCPs)
  Alcohol
  Family history of a similar complaint or malignancy
  Personal history of cancer
  Medication history (anabolic steroid, acetaminophen)
  History of blood transfusion
  Vaccination
  Contact with sick patients
  Contact with animals
  Previous hepatobiliary surgery
  History of traveling
  Smoking
  History of inflammatory bowel disease (IBD)
- **Differential diagnosis**
  Chest pain (myocardial infarction (MI))
  Cough, fever, SOB (pneumonia)
  Recent history of trauma
- **Previous similar attack**, previous admission, previous investigation
- **Systemic review of a related system** (gastrointestinal tract (GIT) system):
  Dysphagia, heartburn, hematemesis, melena, history of bleeding, or ecchymosis.

- Progessive macular hypomelanosis (PMH)
- Paroxysmal sympathetic hyperactivity (PSH)
- Family history
- Social history
- Medication, transfusion, allergy
- Systemic review

  - Central nervous system (CNS): headache, eye and hearing symptoms, epilepsy, numbness, paralysis
  - Cardiovascular (CVS): chest pain, orthopnea, paroxysmal nocturnal dyspnea (PND), lower limb edema, palpitation
  - Respiratory: cough, fever, chest pain, hemoptysis
  - Renal: dysuria, flank pain, hematuria
  - Musculoskeletal (MSK): weakness, arthritis, skin erythema

Physical examination:

- Introduce yourself to the patient
- Ask permission for examination
- Assure patient's privacy
- Position: supine
- Exposure: nipple to mid-thigh
- Handwashing

General examination:

- **A**ppearance: ill, well, dehydrated
- **B**ody built: cachectic, obese
- **C**olor: pale, jaundice
- **D**istress
- **E**nvironment and connection to monitor or intravenous (IV) fluids

Vital signs: blood pressure (BP), heart rate (HR), temperature, respiratory rate (RR), oxygen saturation (SPO_2)

Hands:

- Muscle wasting
- Palmar erythema
- Clubbing
- Koilonychia (iron deficiency anemia)
- Leukonychia (hypoalbuminemia)
- Flapping tremor
- Pulse rate and its characteristics (rhythm, volume, etc.)

Eye:

- Jaundice
- Pallor

Mouth:

- Jaundice in mucus membrane, below the tongue
- Fetor hepaticus

Neck:

- Lymphadenopathy
- Thyroid swelling

Chest:

- Spider nevi
- Gynecomastia
- Respiratory and CVS examination

Abdomen:

- Inspection:
  - Distention
  - Asymmetry
  - Visible veins
  - Scars/Striae
  - Dilated veins (caput medusae)
  - Hernial orifices
  - Stretch marks
  - Visible peristalsis
  - Signs of retroperitoneal hemorrhage (Grey turner, Cullen, and Fox signs)
- Palpations:
  - Superficial then deep palpation
  - Look for any tenderness
  - Palpable masses
  - Ascites
  - Cough impulse at hernial orifices
  - Organomegaly
- Percussion:
  - Shifting dullness
  - Fluid thrill
  - Organomegaly
- Auscultation:
  - Bowel sounds
  - Bruit, venous hum

Groin, digital rectal examination (DRE), proctoscopy

Lower limbs: edema, swelling, skin rash, weakness

Back: for tenderness

5.1.2 Approach to Patient with Liver Mass

- History and physical examination, as described earlier in this chapter
- Management plan:
  - Investigations:

    Complete blood count (CBC) with differential

    Electrolytes

    Coagulation profile

    Blood grouping

    Liver function test (LFT): alanine transaminase (ALT), aspartate transaminase (AST), γ-glutamyl transpeptidase (GGT), alkaline phosphatase (ALP), total bilirubin, direct bilirubin, and albumin

    Amylase/lipase

    Renal function test (RFT)

    C-reactive protein (CRP)/erythrocyte sedimentation rate (ESR)

    Hepatitis profile

    Serology: Fluorescent antibodies test for Entamoeba histolytica, enzyme-linked immunosorbent assay (ELISA) for Echinococcus antigens

    Blood culture

    Ultrasound abdomen

    Triphasic computed tomography (CT) scan for the abdomen

    Tumor markers (alpha-fetoprotein (AFP), carcinoembryonic antigen (CEA), carbohydrate-associated antigen 19-9 (Ca19-9))

    Magnetic resonance imaging/magnetic resonance cholangiopancreatography (MRI/MRCP)
  - Admission, if indicated
  - Nothing per oral (NPO)/Diet
  - IV fluid when NPO
  - Antibiotics, if indicated (e.g., if the clinical picture is going with abscess)
  - Analgesia, antipyretic as needed
  - Prophylaxis (deep vein thrombosis (DVT), stress ulcer prophylaxis)
  - Differential diagnosis of liver mass (Table 5.2)

Pyogenic Liver Abscess

- More on the right side
- May be single or multiples
- **Most common organisms:**
  - *E. coli*(2/3 of cases)
  - *Streptococcus faecalis, Klebsiella, Proteus*
  - *Bacteroid*
  - *Staphylococcus & streptococcus* (in patient with infective endocarditis or infected catheter)
- **Causes:**
  - Portal
  - Hepatobiliary
  - Arterial
  - Traumatic
  - Cryptogenic
- **Presentation:**
  - RUQ pain & fever
  - Jaundice (1/3 of patients)
  - Increased WBC, ALP, and ESR
  - Blood culture (positive in 50% of cases)
- **Imaging:**

Chest x-ray:
elevated right dome of diaphragm: subdiaphragmatic air fluid level, pneumonitis extending toconsolidation, or presence of air in liver, biliary tree, or air fluid levels in the liver.

Ultrasound:
Round or oval hypoechoic lesion with well-defined edges with variable internal echo and air fluid level (2, 5)

Amebic Liver Abscess

- Most common type of liver abscess worldwide
- Presentation:
  - History of antecedent diarrhea.
  - Tender hepatomegaly
  - Leukocytosis 70%
  - Hyperbilirubinemia (1/3 of cases)
  - Enzyme Linked Immunoassay (ELISA) positive in 95% of patients
- Caused by Entamoeba histolytica, an anaerobic parasite
- Reach the liver through the portal vein
- Common site: superior and anterior surface of the right hemi-liver
- It contains proteolytic enzymes that destroy the hepatocytes and lead to the special characteristic of amebic abscess (anchovy Sause appearance)
- CT & ultrasound are sensitive but not specific
- Diagnosis is made by positive fluorescent antibodies test
- **Treatment:**
- Metronidazole 750 mg TID for 7 days
  - chloroquine is administered in combination with low dose emetine for metronidazole resistant strains.
  - Metronidazole used to treat both intestinal and extraintestinal disease. (2, 5)

Therapeutic aspiration
Aspiration has been indicated in the following circumstances:

- Lack of clinical improvement for more than 5 to 7 days after druginitiation
- Large left hemi-liver abscess
- Large abscess > 10 cm
- Thin rim of liver tissue around the abscess (< 10 mm)
- Seronegative abscess
- Metronidazole therapy is contraindicated e.g., pregnancy.(1)

Hydatid Liver cyst

- Caused by tape worm Echinococcus
- The human is the intermediate host
- 70% of the hydatid cyst is in the liver, commonly in the right hemi-liver

Diagnosis:
ELISA
Eosinophilia is present in 30%
Ultrasound and CT ± MRI
MRCP to rule out communication with biliary tree

- Know the World Health Organization Informal Working Group on Echinococcosis (WHO-IWGE) Ultrasonographic Classification

1. **Medical management:**

Indication: Cyst < 5cm
CE1 –CE3
Inoperable disease
Multiorgan involvement
Peritoneal cyst
Albendazole 10-15 mg/kg/day

2. **Puncture, Aspiration, Injection and Re-aspiration (PAIR)**:

Indications:

- Cyst <5cm
- Unilocular CE1-CE3
- Accessible
- Inoperable patient
- Pregnant or children not fit for surgery
- Relapse after surgery
- Refuse surgery
- Failure to respond to Pharmacological treatment.

Contraindication:
Complicated (infection, rupture, communicated with biliary system)

- Albendazole should be started at least 4 hours before the procedure and for 1 month after.

Leave a drain if the cyst > 10 cm (2, 6)

Pyogenic Liver Abscess

CT: (highly sensitive in localization)
Well defined hypodense round lesion with wall enhancement & peripheral zone of edema may contain air fluid level.

- **Management:**

Correct underlying cause
IV antibiotics at least 6-8 weeks

- Two weeks course of IV antibiotics followed by 4 weeks of oral antibiotic therapy
- To switch to oral patient should be afebrile, with a white cell count trend toward normal and adequate oral intake and GI absorption.
- The duration of the treatment should be guided by clinical and radiographic improvement in the patient.(1)
- IV antibiotics according to the presumed source and culture result later
  - **Biliary:**piperacillin + tazobactam
  - **GIT:**Third generation cephalosporine or fluroquinolone + Metronidazole
  - **Severe, recurrent:**Meropenem
  - **Liver transplant:**Cover candida

Percutaneous drainage
Surgical drainage is indicated if:

- Coexistence of intra-abdominal disease (biliary or bowel) that requires operative management.
- Patients with loculated or multiple abscesses that are not amenable to percutaneous drainage because of location.
- Failure/contraindication of percutaneous aspiration or drainage.
- Signs of peritonitis resulting from intraperitoneal rupture of pyogenic liver abscess.

Important point:keep in mind necrotic hepatic malignancy. (2, 5)

Amebic Liver Abscess

The common indications for surgery are:
1. Free perforation into the peritoneal cavity with frank generalizedperitonitis.
2. Erosion into surrounding organs (partial resection andclosure of the involved organis necessary)
3. Septicemia from amoebic abscesses secondarily infected,especially when percutaneous drainage fails.
4. Failed conservative management of abscesses(1)

Hydatid Liver cyst

3. Surgical Management:
The gold standard for large, complex cyst
Indications:

- Large
- Complicated
- Risk of rupture (superficial)
- Multiple daughter cyst CE2
- Causing pressure on adjacent structure

Surgical Options:

A. Conservative:
Endocystectomy (removal of endocyst and keep the pericyst)

B. Radical:
Pericystectomy
Segmental Resection
Liver transplantation

Important point: start perioperative treatment with Albendazole at least 1 monthbefore the operation and continue it for 1 month after.

Laparoscopic vs open approach

Laparoscopic	Open
• Easily accessible e.g. (segments III, IVb, V, VI) • High risk of spillage (2, 3)	• Large, multiloculated • Complicated • Deep • Suspected cyst-Biliary fistula (2, 3)

Table 5.2 Differential diagnosis of liver mass

Infectious	Benign	Neoplastic	
		Primary	Secondary
Liver abscess Amebic abscess Hydatid cyst	Liver cyst Adenoma Hemangioma FNH Regenerative nodule Biliary hamartoma	Hepatocellular carcinoma (HCC) Fibrolamellar HCC Intrahepatic cholangiocarcinoma Lymphoma	Colorectal cancers Cholangiocarcinoma Pancreatic cancer Renal cell carcinoma Neuroendocrine tumors Breast cancer

5.1.3 Benign Liver Lesions

A. **Benign Liver Cyst:**

- Majority is asymptomatic.
- Neoplasia should be suspected, in case of:
  - Nodularity of the wall
  - Loculations/septations
  - Papillary projections.
- Ultrasound: well-defined, anechoic lesion.
- CT: avascular, water dense lesion.
- MRI: in T1 it is hypointense or hyperintense if there is hemorrhage, while in T2 it is hyperintense.
- MRCP, if there is concern about biliary communication.
- Treatment:
  - Not needed, unless symptomatic
  - Ultrasound-guided aspiration (contraindicated, if a hydatid cyst is suspected), if it recurs, to do sclerotherapy (agents: ethanol 95%, minocycline, or tetracycline)
  - Maximum dose of ethanol is 120 ml, to avoid severe ethanol intoxication
  - Contraindication of sclerotherapy: suspected biliary fistula, recent hemorrhage
  - Surgical treatment: fenestration, unroofing (do not forget to send the wall for pathological assessment) [1, 6, 7]

B. **Hemangioma:**

- The most common solid benign mass that occurs in the liver.
- Four times more common in women.
- Hemangioma >10 cm is considered giant.
- Estrogen receptor found on the surface (that is why it is more common in female and its growth gets increased in response to steroids, OCP, and during pregnancy).
- Blood supply to the hemangioma is from the hepatic artery.
- Symptoms:
  - 50–90% are asymptomatic.
  - Symptoms develop with larger lesions and depend on where the lesion is located within the liver.
  - Large lesions can cause early satiety, abdominal pain due to it stretching of Glisson's capsule, biliary obstruction secondary to biliary compression, and/or ascites secondary to portal compression.
  - Large hemangioma causes arteriovenous (AV) shunting and congestive heart failure (CHF).
  - Life-threatening complications include rupture, hemorrhage, and Kasabach-Merritt syndrome.
  - Kasabach-Merritt syndrome: consumptive thrombocytopenia triggered by a simple dental procedure. The mortality reaches 30%.
- Imaging:
  - Ultrasound: well-defined hyperechoic mass
  - CT:
    Noncontrast CT: isodense to the liver tissue
    Contrast CT: Arterial phase: asymmetric peripheral nodular enhancement
    Portovenous phase: progressive centripetal enhancement
    Delayed phase: retention of the contrast
  - MRI: in T1; hypointense, in T2; hyperintense with delayed relaxation time "light bulb sign"
- Biopsy: is contraindicated
- Tagged red blood cell (RBC) scan: limited to lesion deep in the liver
- Laboratory investigation:
  - Generally normal
  - Thrombocytopenia in Kasabach-Merritt syndrome

  - Obstructive jaundice pattern, if it is causing external compression
- Treatment:
  - Asymptomatic: observation, even if pregnant or on OCP
  - Indications of intervention:
    - Severe symptoms (extreme pain, mass effect, hemorrhage, rupture)
    - Ruptured hemangioma: embolization after resuscitation followed by resection
    - Kasabach-Merritt syndrome
    - Diagnostic uncertainty
  - Surgical options: enucleation, anatomical and nonanatomical resection
  - Transarterial embolization (TAE): as a bridge to surgery or in the case of intraperitoneal hemorrhage
    - Thermal ablation
- Follow-up: it is not typically required [1, 7, 8]

C. **FNH:**

- The second most common benign tumor after hemangioma.
- It has no malignant potential.
- Presentation:
  - More common in female.
  - Majority discovered accidentally.
- Imaging:
  - CT: well-circumscribed hypodense on the arterial phase, isodense on the venous phase, and hyperdense central scar on the venous phase.
  - MRI:
    - T1: Hypointense without attenuation of the central scar
    - T2: Hyperintense with hyperintense central scar with early enhancement, if gadolinium is administered.
- Biopsy: is not recommended
- Treatment:
  - Conservative.
  - Resection: only if symptomatic (pain or weight loss) or inability to rule out malignancy [1, 7].

D. **Hepatic Adenoma:**

- Rare, benign tumor of the liver.
- Perfused only by large peripheral artery.
- Histology: sheet of hepatocytes containing glycogen and lipid with the absence of Kupffer cells and bile ductile.
- Hemorrhage is common.
- Can be found anywhere in the liver but it is more common in the right hemi-liver.
- The main concern is transition from benign to malignant in about 4.2%, with majority occurring in adenoma >5 cm,
- The main risk factors:
  - OCP (when taking the history, ask about the dose and duration)
  - Anabolic androgenic steroid use
  - Long-term steroid therapy
  - Glycogen storage disease types 1 and 3
- Presentation:
  - More common in female.
  - Age 20–40 years.
  - Rarely found in males.
  - Most commonly asymptomatic.
  - If symptomatic, the patient can present with right upper quadrant (RUQ) pain or epigastric pain.
- Imaging:
  - Ultrasound: well-demarcated heterogeneous mass
  - CT: round, well-encapsulated lesion, iso- to hypodense on a noncontrast CT, and hyperdense on the arterial phase, when there is active or recent hemorrhage.
  - MRI: isointense to hyperintense on T1 and T2, especially if here is hemorrhage.
- Management:
  - Asymptomatic and <5 cm: discontinue OCP or steroid
  - If regress: follow-up
  - If there is an increase in growth while off OCP, symptomatic, or the size is >5 cm: resection to achieve negative margin as in malignant lesion.
  - Radiofrequency ablation: if small, multiple, and not amenable for resection.
  - Life-threatening hemorrhage:
    - Stable: embolization then elective resection
    - Unstable: Laparotomy, Pringle's maneuver, and packing
    - Formal resection is not necessary in this operation [1, 7].

5.1.4 Malignant Liver Lesions

HCC

- Most common primary malignant liver tumor
- Risk factors: cirrhosis of any cause, in absence of cirrhosis it can be associated with HBV or it is fibrolamellar type
- Screening ultrasound every 6 months for patient at high risk:
  HCV, HBV, Primary biliary cirrhosis, Hemochromatosis, and alpha-1- antitrypsin.
- AFP may be used for screening in addition to ultrasound.
- Diagnostic imaging:
  CT & MRI: Homogenous enhancement in arterial phase, wash out in porto-venous phase.
- Biopsy is not needed if the clinical and radiological pictures are typical for HCC.
- HCC tend to spread via portal venous tributaries
- If the diagnosis is HCC:
  1. Assess the degree of liver disease using CHILD (table 5.3) & MELD scores
  2. Staging
  3. Measure the amount of future liver remnant
  4. Determine resectability and transplantability (table 5.4)
- **Management options:**

A.Resection

- Standard of care for patient with HCC and no underlying liver disease
- Resection should be anatomical with free margin = 1cm
- If no enough liver remnant: do portal vein embolization (contraindicated in CHILD B &C) (2, 3)

Intrahepatic Cholangiocarcinoma

- Second most common primary liver malignancy
- Risk factors:
  - ➢ Sclerosing cholangitis (8-20% lifetime risk)
  - ➢ Choledochal cyst (3-28% lifetime risk)
  - ➢ Cirrhosis
- Three subtypes:
  - ➢ Mass forming
  - ➢ Periductal infiltration (most common & the worst prognosis)
  - ➢ Intraductal
- Jaundice as presentation most likely indicates advanced stage!
- **Investigations:**
  - ➢ Role out other primary tumors (upper & lower endoscopy, chest CT and mammogram)
  - ➢ LFT, Serology test, CEA, CA19-9, chromogranin A
- CT:
  - ➢ Low attenuation
  - ➢ Minor peripheral enhancement
  - ➢ Upstream biliary dilatation
  - ➢ Capsule retraction
- **Diagnosis**:
  Biopsy: adenocarcinoma & no other primary (negative endoscopy, mammogram, and CT chest)
- **Treatment:**
  The only curative option is resection with negative margin + hilar lymphadenectomy
- Goal of resection: negative margins
- Positive margins or positive lymph nodes are associated with worst prognosis (2, 3)

Metastatic colorectal cancer

- 50% of patient with colorectal cancer have synchronous or metachronous liver metastasis
- CT: hypovascular & hypodense in portal phase
- **Treatment:**
- ➢ The surgical resection is the best curative option
- ➢ The goal of resection is to remove all metastasis with negative margins (microscopically)
- ➢ **Synchronous lesion: liver & colon**
  - One stage or multistage procedure
  - Use concomitant approach (both primary and secondary) when:
    - o Minor liver resection is required
    - o When colon surgery is straight forward
  - Use the "liver 1stapproach" when:
    1. Extensive liver disease that may progress to unresectable
    2. Patient with rectal cancer that will require time between radiation and resection of the primary
- ➢ **Hepatic & Extrahepatic metastasis**
  - o Surgery can be done as long as other extrahepaticis resectable & limited
  - o If preoperative chemotherapy used should be limited to few months because side effect of the chemotherapy on the liver and small lesion (< 2cm) may disappear and recur later (2, 3)

HCC

- **Tumor is resected when:**

Negative margins can be obtained (1 cm) while:
  - Adequate liver remnant
  - Intact inflow (hepatic artery & portal vein)
  - Intact outflow (Hepatic veins)
  - Biliary drainage
- **Resection is limited to patient with:**
  - No cirrhosis
  - Child A without portal HTN
  - Single tumor

B. Transplantation

- It is the gold standard for patient with child B & C and in patient with limited liver reserved.
- Transplantation criteria: Follow Barcelona Clinic Liver Cancer (BCLC) System.

C. Ablation:

- Thermal ablation for lesions < 3cm equivalent to surgical resection
- Ablation of tumor > 4cm or near major vessels should be avoided because it is associated with high rate of incomplete tumor destruction and recurrence

D. Embolization:

- Embolization for lesion in patient not candidate for curative treatment by resection, ablation, transplantation.
- Embolization can be used as bridge to liver transplantation or before ablation for tumor between 3-5 cm.
- Total bilirubin > 3mg/dl is relative contraindication for TACE, RFA
- Portal vein thrombosis is relative contraindication for TACE, TAE (these patients can be treated with radiation) (4)

Intrahepatic Cholangiocarcinoma

- **Multiple liver lesions (intrahepatic metastasis):**
  - Poor prognosis
  - Resection only in highly selected patient
- **Contraindications for resection:**
  - Extrahepatic disease
  - Lymph nodes outside porta hepatis
  - Portal hypertension
  - Locally advanced tumor involving either inflow or outflow bilaterally
  - Multiple bilateral intrahepatic tumors
  - Small localized satellite lesions
- **Adjuvant treatment (can be considered in high-risk patient after R0 resection):**
  - Fluoropyrimidine based regimen
  - Gemcitabine based regimen
- **Treatment of locally advance disease:**
  - Trans-arterial embolization (TAE)
  - Trans-arterial chemoembolization (TACE)
  - Trans-arterial radioembolization (TARE)
  - External beam radiation
  - Ablation (RFA, microwave, PDT) (2, 3)

Metastatic colorectal cancer

- **Poor Prognostic signs:**
  1. Disease free interval < 12 months between the primary and secondary
  2. Size of the liver tumor > 5cm
  3. Extrahepatic disease
  4. Nodal status of the primary
  5. CEA > 200 ng/mL
  6. More than one tumor (2, 3)

Table 5.3 Child-Pugh score [9]

Parameter	1 point	2 points	3 points
Albumin, g/dl	>3.5	3.0–3.5	<3.0
Bilirubin mg/dl	<2	2–3	>3
International normalized ratio (INR)	<1.7	1.7–2.2	>2.2
Ascites	None	Controlled	Refractory
Encephalopathy	0 (none)	I–II (minimal)	III–IV (advanced)
Class A = 5–6 points			
Class B = 7–9 points			
Class C = 10–15 points			

Table 5.4 Transplantability criteria [9]

Milan criteria
Three tumors maximum with a maximum size of 3 cm for each
Single tumor ≤5 cm
The University of California, San Francisco (USCF) criteria
Maximum three tumors, the largest ≤4.5 cm
Single tumor ≤6.5 cm
Total tumor diameter ≤8 cm

5.1.5 Portal Hypertension

- Definition: portal venous pressure >5–7 mmHg.
- The most accurate method to determine the portal pressure is hepatic venography.
- Causes:
  - Prehepatic.
  - Hepatic.
  - Posthepatic.
- The most common cause in the USA is cirrhosis from alcohol or hepatitis C virus (HCV).
- The most clinically relevant variceal network is between coronary and short gastric veins to the azygous vein forming esophageal varices.
- Other sites: retroperitoneal, hemorrhoidal, and caput medusae.
- Larger size varices and worsening hepatic function Child B or C are the risk factors for hemorrhage.
- Fifty percent of patients with cirrhosis have esophageal varices and one third of them will develop hemorrhage.
- Each episode of bleeding has 20–30% risk of mortality [10, 11].
- **Prevention of Variceal Bleeding:**
  - Nonselective B blocker (propranolol, nadolol): prevents up to 45%.
- **Management of Portal Hypertensive Esophageal Varices Bleeding:**

1. **Medical:**
   - Acute bleeding needs intensive care unit (ICU) admission, resuscitation followed by definitive management.
   - Target hemoglobin (Hb) is 7–8 mg/dl. Overresuscitation worsens portal hypertension and increases bleeding.
   - Nonselective B blocker: decreases the cardiac output, while splanchnic vasoconstriction leads to a decrease in portal venous pressure.
   - Prophylactic antibiotic should be started.
   - Infection, in addition to bleeding, results in failure to control bleeding, early rebleeding, increased days of hospitalization, and death.
   - Ceftriaxone and ciprofloxacin are the recommended regimen.
   - Vasoactive medication such as vasopressin decreases splanchnic blood flow ± nitroglycerin (to avoid extreme hypertension, MI, and arrythmias).
   - Octreotide (long-acting somatostatin analog) is a splanchnic vasoconstrictor, which is used in addition to endoscopy to control acute bleeding.
   - Proton pump inhibitor (PPI) should be initiated at the time of acute variceal bleeding and should be continued for short course after definitive therapy [10, 11].
2. **Luminal tamponade:**
   - Sengstaken-Blackmore tube or self-expanding metallic stent control bleeding in 90% of cases.
   - Balloon tamponade should not be kept for more than 36 h.
   - Disadvantages:

     Fifty percent of the recurrence hemorrhage rate, once the tamponade is released.

Esophageal rupture, necrosis, and aspiration are noticed in 30%.

It must be removed within 24–36 h.

Stents carry the risk of migration and tracheal compression.

- Due to a high risk of recurrence, it is a temporary measure, until there is a definitive plan to control bleeding [10, 11].

3. **Endoscopic**:
   - Primary diagnostic and therapeutic modalities in acute variceal bleeding in conjugation with aggressive resuscitative measures.
   - Esophagogastroduodenoscopy (EGD) should be performed on an emergency basis.
   - Variceal banding and sclerotherapy are the primary interventions performed (control 90% of bleeding).
   - Sclerotherapy (by cyanoacrylate): injecting a sclerosing agent directly into the varix or the surrounding tissue.
   - Possible complications of sclerotherapy: ulceration, perforation, stricture, fibrosis, and renal or pulmonary complications.
   - Banding: placing a tight band around the varix that stops bleeding and causes thrombosis of the vessels. It has a favorable safety profile and has become the standard for endoscopic intervention over sclerotherapy for acute variceal bleeding.
   - Injection sclerotherapy should not be used routinely, if band ligation is available.
   - Injecting sclerotherapy should be used in case where bleeding is refractory to endoscopic band ligation.
   - Isolating gastric varices from splenic vein thrombosis is best treated by splenectomy and should not be treated endoscopically [10, 11].
4. **Transjugular intrahepatic portosystemic shunt (TIPS):**
   - May be considered as a rescue therapy for initially uncontrolled variceal bleeding after failure of endoscopic management (10–20% of patient) or re-bleeding.
   - TIPS is more definitive management because it corrects the underlying problem of portal hypertension, at least temporarily.
   - Decrease in portal pressure will lead to decrease in gastropathy, decrease in ascites, and decrease in hydrothorax [10, 11].
   - Indications:

     Standard of care:

     I. Portal variceal bleeding refractory to medical and endoscopic management

     II. Ascites refractory to medical management

     III. Budd-Chiari syndrome not responsive to anticoagulation

     IV. Hepatic hydrothorax refractory to diuretics

     Emergency:

     Child B or Child C with acute variceal bleeding, in addition to endoscopic and medical treatment
   - Absolute contraindications:

     Severe increased right-side pressure

     Severe tricuspid regurgitation

     Severe pulmonary hypertension

     Severe congestive heart failure (CHF)

     Severe encephalopathy

     Uncorrectable bleeding diathesis

     Active systemic or hepatic bacterial infection

     Unrelieved biliary obstruction [10, 11]
   - Procedure:

     Percutaneous guidance of wire from the right internal jugular vein into the right hepatic vein, then through hepatic parenchyma into portal branches (right portal vein).

     The parenchymal tract is dilated by a balloon dilator and then portography is performed and an expandable stent is inserted [10, 11].
   - Most frequent complications: stent stenosis or thrombosis
   - Other complications: encephalopathy, bleeding, sepsis, liver infarction, and liver failure.

- Mortality: 5–40%, higher mortality in poorly compensated cirrhotic shunts placed or on an emergent basis [10, 11].

5. **Surgical shunts:**
   To be considered, only if:
   - Model for end-stage liver disease (MELD) < 15 and the patients are not candidates for transplantation.
   - Limited access to TIPS.
     Selective shunts:
     Provide selective decompression of portal-azygous system while preserving portal inflow into the liver, for example, distal splenorenal (decrease in encephalopathy but it is contraindicated in the patient with intractable ascites)
     Nonselective shunts:
     Divert all the portal flow away from the liver
     - End-to-side portocaval shunt (Eck fistula): historical, associated with a high rate of encephalopathy.
     - Side-to-side portocaval shunt.
     - Splenorenal (Warren's) shunt: most currently used and most difficult to perform. It has the advantage of low rate of encephalopathy and does not interfere with future transplantation.
     - Mesocaval shunt (H-graft between superior mesenteric vein (SMV) and IVC): can be used as a bridge to transplantation and can be ligated at the time of transplantation.
   - All portosystemic shunts decrease gastroesophageal varices and reduce the risk of hemorrhage [10, 11].
6. **Nonshunt surgical management of refractory variceal bleeding:**
   - Sugiura procedure:
     Extensive devascularization of stomach and distal esophagus
     Transection of esophagus
     Splenectomy
     Truncal vagotomy and pyloroplasty
   - Hassab procedure:
     Splenectomy
     Devascularization of the esophagus and proximal stomach
     Vagotomy and pyloroplasty [10, 11]
7. **Liver transplantation** [10, 11]

Budd-Chiari Syndrome

- Primary: intraluminal hepatic vein thrombosis.
- Secondary: veins are compressed or invaded.
- Obstruction of two or more veins: hepatomegaly, liver congestion, and RUQ pain. If not treated, it will lead to portal hypertension and ascites.
- Caudate lobe hypertrophy found in 50% of cases because it drains directly to inferior vena cava (IVC), but if enlarged it will cause more obstruction to the IVC.
- Initial investigation is ultrasound that will show:
  - Absence of hepatic venous flow
  - Spider web hepatic veins
  - Collateral hepatic veins
- Definitive diagnostic method: hepatic venography
- Treatment:
  - Initial medical treatment (treat the underlying disease and start anticoagulation)
  - If not responding, radiological or surgical shunt (TIPS and thrombolytics are preferred or side-to-side portocaval shunt)
  - Progressive or end-stage liver disease: liver transplantation [12]

5.1.6 Hepatic Operations

Preoperative Preparation:

- Admission
- Diet (NPO, regular or fat-free diet)
- IV fluid
- Medication: analgesia, antibiotic (prophylactic or therapeutic), stress ulcer prophylaxis, and DVT prophylaxis, as indicated
- If the procedure is for hydatid liver disease, make sure the patient is on albendazole and prepare hypertonic saline (20%) to be used intraoperatively

- Review the relevant clinical information
- Review the laboratory investigations (CBC, LFT, electrolytes, RFT, blood group, coagulation profile, tumor marker, inflammatory marker, hepatitis profile, and biopsy result)
- Review the preoperative images: ultrasound, MRCP/MRI, triphasic CT abdomen, endoscopic ultrasound (EUS), or endoscopic retrograde cholangiopancreatography (ERCP))
- Evaluate the cardiopulmonary system
- Chest x-ray (CXR), electrocardiogram (ECG)
- Instruct the patient to take shower the night before surgery
- Explain the procedure to the patient and obtain informed consent

Consent for major hepatectomy:

- *Mention the procedure:* removal of right/left hemi-liver through abdominal incision and under general anesthesia ± lymphadenectomy ± removal of the gallbladder and closure of the abdomen after placement of suction drain
- *Mention any alternative:* locoregional therapy like radiofrequency ablation (RFA), transcatheter arterial chemoembolization (TACE), transarterial radioembolization (TARE)
- *Mention the possible complications*:
  Specific complications: bleeding, hematoma, bile leak, biloma, liver failure, injury to the bile ducts or the surrounding structure

  General complications: wound infection, atelectasis, pneumonia, DVT, pulmonary embolism (PE), adhesion, or incisional hernia

Surgical Anatomy of the Liver:

- Arterial anatomy (Fig. 5.1)
- Venous anatomy (Fig. 5.2)
- Sections and segments (Fig. 5.3)

Preoperative Assessments:

A. **Evaluating Tumor Extent:**

- CT with liver protocol (triphasic and slice thickness of 2.5–5 mm) to evaluate the tumor extent and its relationship with biliary tree and vascular structures.
- CT volumetry.
- CT chest to identify lung metastases.
- Routine use of MRI is not recommended. However, MRI should be performed for further characterization of presumably benign or atypical liver tumor, when the CT is not conclusive.

B. **Evaluating Determinants of Postoperative Liver Function:**

- Liver function after liver resection depends on the quality of the liver parenchyma, the volume of future liver remnant (FLR), and regenerative liver capacity of the liver.

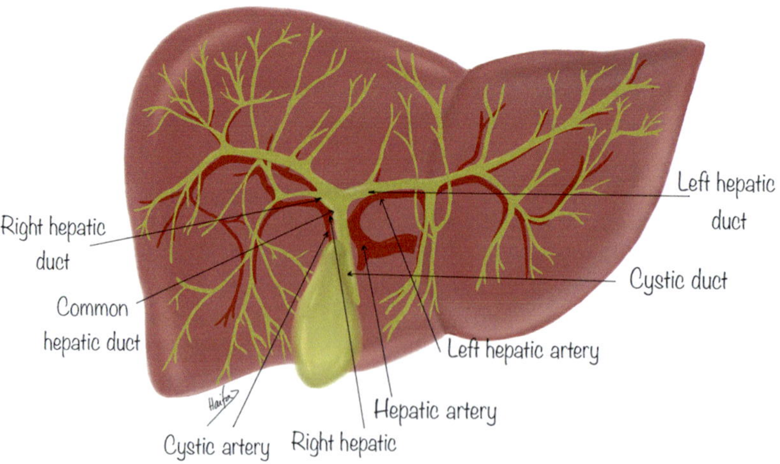

Fig. 5.1 Arterial supply and bile ducts of the liver

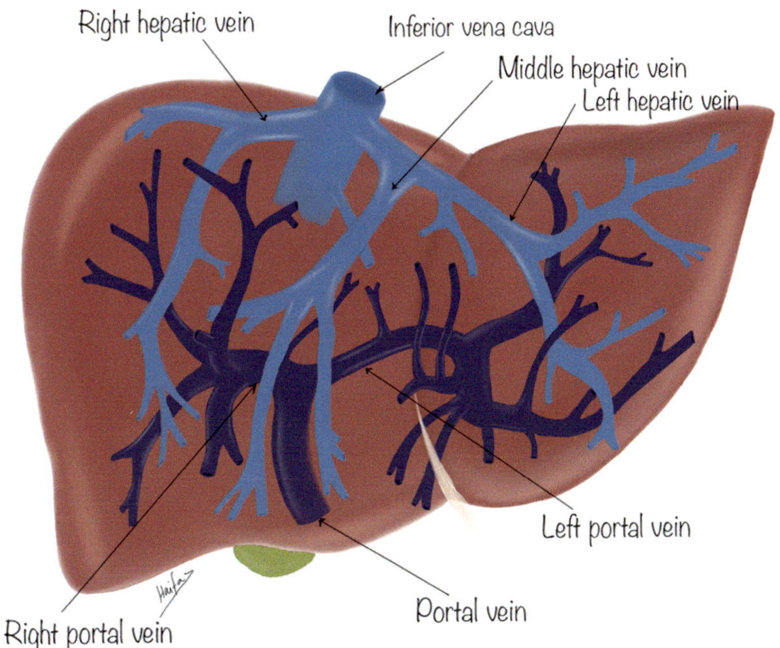

Fig. 5.2 Hepatic and portal veins

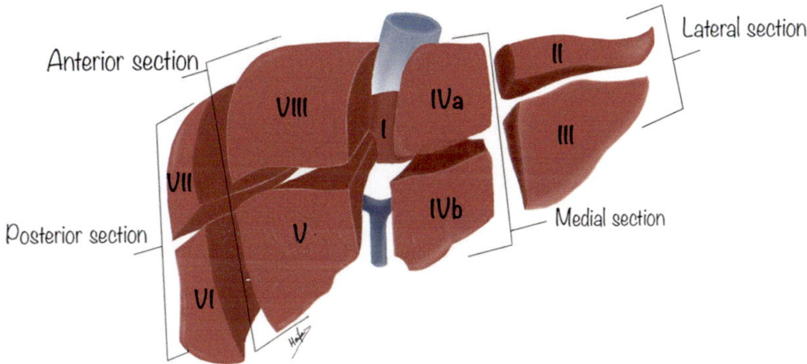

Fig. 5.3 Liver segments and sections

- The risk of postoperative liver failure should be estimated preoperatively to determine whether resection is safe and to optimize the postoperative outcome.
- Screen for clinical signs of undiagnosed portal hypertension (ascites, collateral veins), biological assessment (platelet count), and imaging (evidence of venous collaterals or splenomegaly).
- Assess the liver function and presence of an underlying liver disease (by biopsy of nontumorous liver parenchyma or indocyanine green (ICG) clearance).
- Evaluate the future liver remnant.
- In patient with small FLRs, portal vein embolization (PVE) can be used to promote hypertrophy of FLR, making curative resection possible.

C. **Type of Resection:**

- Depends on the type of lesion (benign tumor, primary malignant liver tumor, or metastases) and the extent of the disease
- Liver resection can be classified as anatomical (removal of one or more liver segments) or nonanatomical (wedge) resection.
- Terminology:

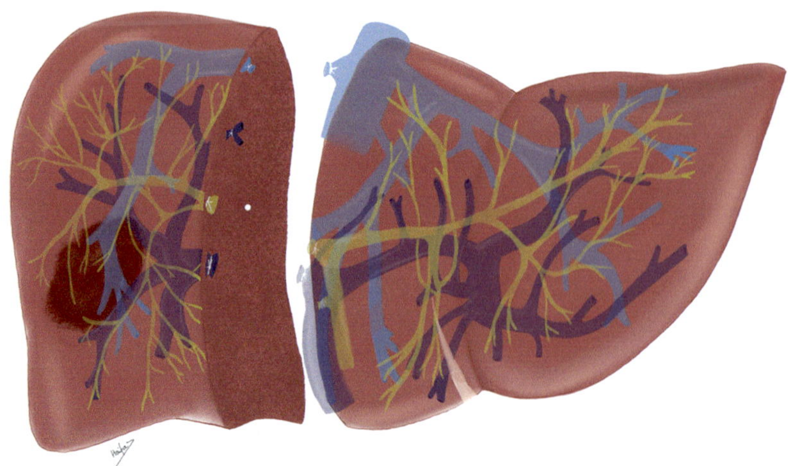

Fig. 5.4 Right hepatectomy

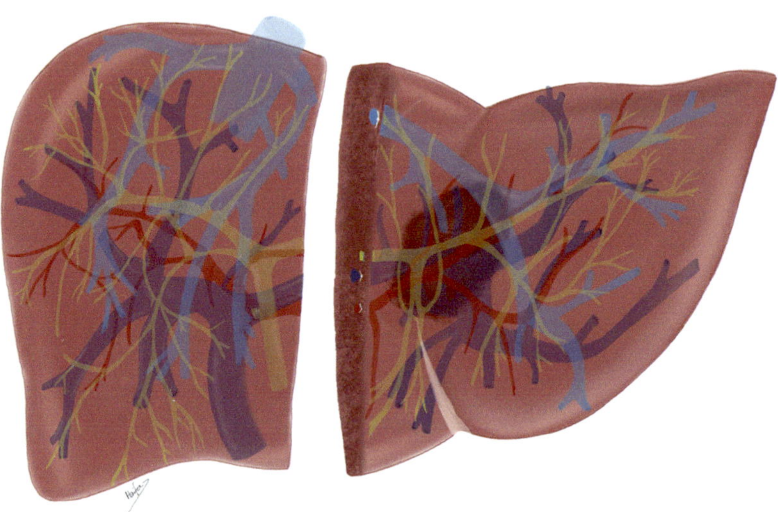

Fig. 5.5 Left hepatectomy

- Right hepatectomy or right hemi-hepatectomy (segments V, VI, VII, and VIII) (see Fig. 5.4)
- Left hepatectomy or left hemi-hepatectomy (segments II, III, and IV) (see Fig. 5.5)
- Right tri-sectionectomy or extended right hepatectomy (segments IV, V, VI, VII, and VIII)
- Left tri-sectionectomy or extended left hepatectomy (segments II, III, IV, V, and VIII)
- Left lateral sectionectomy (segments II and III) (Fig. 5.6)
- Right posterior sectionectomy (segments VI and VII)

• Regardless of the approach used for resection, tumor-free resection margins should be achieved [13–15].

D. **Exposure:**

Skin incisions: inverted T (Mercedes) incision, the bilateral subcostal (chevron) incision, right/left subcostal (Kocher/Kehr) incisions, Makuuchi incision (J incision), or inverted L (hockey-stick) incision are used to achieve a good exposure.

E. **Principle of Parenchymal Transection:**

Intraoperative ultrasonography has contributed to major improvements in liver resection techniques. It confirms the preoperative imag-

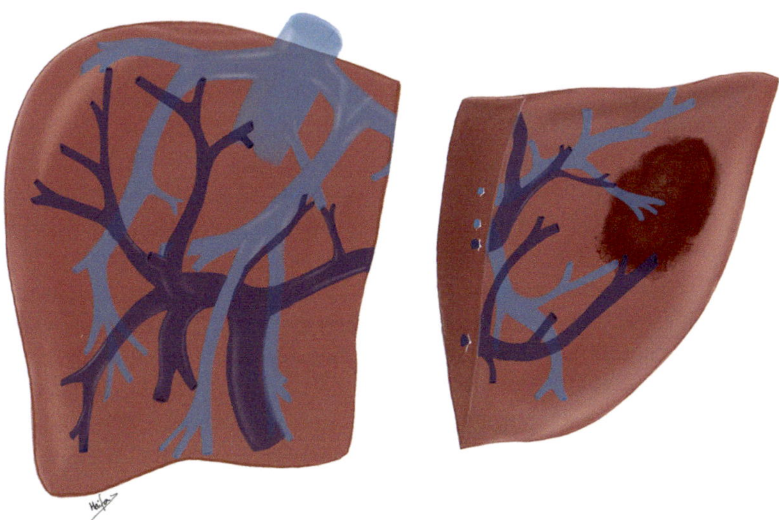

Fig. 5.6 Left lateral sectionectomy

ing finding and helps define the extent of the tumor and its relationship with major vascular and biliary structures. Intraoperative ultrasound (IOUS) is used to define the plane of transection while indicating the location and direction of the hepatic veins.

Tools available for transection: clamps, staplers, jet cutters, ultrasonic surgical aspirators (cavitron ultrasonic surgical aspirator (CUSA)), saline-linked cautery (TissueLink), bipolar electrocoagulation devices, radiofrequency transection devices, harmonic scalpels, and microwave coagulators [13–15].

Operative Procedures:

1. **Right hepatectomy:**
   - Under general anesthesia and endotracheal intubation.
   - Position: supine with table in slightly reverse Trendelenburg position.
   - The abdomen is prepped from nipple to the symphysis pubis.
   - Patient is draped in sterile fashion.
   - Incision: extended right or bilateral subcostal incision with midline extension to the xiphoid can provide an excellent exposure.
   - Details of the procedure:
     - Extent of the tumor involvement in the right hemi-liver is verified by inspection of a bimanual palpation.
     - Inspect the peritoneal surface.
     - Using intraoperative ultrasound, the extent and the exact location of the tumor is noted.
     - Understanding the relationship of the lesion in question with major vascular structures is essential to minimize blood loss.
     - The liver is mobilized by dividing the falciform ligament and right triangular ligament as well as freeing the liver posteriorly from the diaphragm.
     - Cystic artery and cystic duct are ligated, and the gallbladder removed, since the gallbladder bed is the dividing line between the left and right hemi-liver.
     - The right hepatic duct is easier to visualize after removal of the gallbladder. A clear exposure of the right hepatic duct is essential to avoid interference with the area of bifurcation supplying the left hepatic duct.
     - The right hepatic duct is divided under clear vision and double-sutured with one or more transfixing sutures.
     - After the right duct is divided, the variable arterial supply is exposed. The surgeon

should at this time review imaging, alert to the possibility that the right hepatic artery may arise from the superior mesenteric artery. The right hepatic artery is ligated and divided.

- The left hepatic artery must be visualized to be certain it has not been obstructed or compromised in anyway.
- The right and left branches of the portal vein are clearly exposed, before the right branch of the portal vein is doubly clamped with straight Cooley vascular clamps.
- Both ends of the portal vein are oversewn with a continuous 4-0 nonabsorbable suture. Alternatively, the right portal vein may be divided using a vascular stapler.
- After the vessels and other structures are gently dissected away from the liver, a logical area is exposed for the division between the right liver and the medial segment of the left hemi-liver.
- The right hepatic liver is freed up from the diaphragm and rotated medially away from the diaphragm, exposing the small hepatic veins communicating with the inferior vena cava. These small vessels are carefully and securely ligated.
- The caval ligament must be divided to expose the inferior border of the right hepatic vein. Caution must be executed, as an accessory right hepatic vein may traverse this ligament and drain into the inferior vena cava (IVC). The major right hepatic vein is exposed.
- A loop is passed around the large right hepatic vein, and the liver tissue gently pushed away to permit the application of two curved Cooley vascular clamps to the vein. Sufficient vein must extend beyond the vascular clamps in order to secure the open ends. After the vein has been divided, two rows of nonabsorbable vascular sutures are used to secure the ends of the right hepatic vein. Alternatively, a vascular stapler may be used.
- The concave line of demarcation following the color change subsequent to ligation of the blood supply may be superficially outlined with a cautery.
- The liver tissue is divided with an ultrasound dissector, laser, or electrocautery unit.
- Larger vessels and branches from the middle hepatic vein may require double ligation.
- After all bleeding and bile leakage have been controlled, the omentum may be brought up to cover the raw surface of the left hemi-liver. Sufficient sutures are taken to secure the omentum in place.
- The falciform ligament is reapproximated to ensure stability of the left liver. Closed system Silastic suction drainage may be used.
- A routine closure of the abdominal wall is performed [13–15].

2. **Left hepatectomy:**
   - Under general anesthesia and endotracheal intubation.
   - Position: supine position with table in slightly reverse Trendelenburg position.
   - The abdomen is prepped from nipple to the symphysis pubis.
   - Patient is draped in sterile fashion.
   - Incision: bilateral subcostal incision with midline extension to the xiphoid can provide excellent exposure or midline laparotomy as an alternative.
   - Details of the procedure:
   - Extent of the tumor involvement in the left hemi-liver is verified by inspection of a bimanual palpation.
   - Inspect the peritoneal surface.
   - Using intraoperative ultrasound, the extent and the exact location of the tumor is noted.
   - Understanding the relationship of the lesion in question with major vascular structures is essential to minimize blood loss.
   - The left hemi-liver is mobilized by division of the falciform and coronary ligaments.
   - Since the median margin of the left hemi-liver extends into the gallbladder bed, a cholecystectomy is performed after liga-

tion and division of the cystic artery and cystic duct.
- Removal of the gallbladder improves the exposure for the identification of the major hepatic ducts and vessels to be divided and ligated.
- The left hepatic duct is freed up for the sufficient distance to allow passage of a right-angle clamp. The duct is doubly ligated and then divided.
- The division of the left hepatic duct exposes the underlying left hepatic artery, which usually arises from the common hepatic artery. Notice, if there is any aberrant anatomy.
- The left hepatic artery is gently freed up a short distance from its point of origin and doubly tied with 2-0 nonabsorbable sutures proximally.
- The area of the arterial bifurcation is inspected to ascertain that the blood supply to the right hemi-liver is intact and that the artery is divided between the ligatures.
- The left branch of the portal vein is now exposed. The area of the bifurcation of the portal vein is carefully freed up and the left branch mobilized and divided.
- If the caudate (Segment 1) is to be preserved, the surgeon must take care to divide the left portal vein distal to the caudate branch at the base of the umbilical fissure.
- The left lateral segment (Segments 2 and 3) can be lifted to expose the ligamentum venosum. When this is divided at its most cranial extent, a window is opened along the inferior border of the left hepatic vein as well as the middle hepatic vein depending upon their point of convergence.
- The path of the middle hepatic vein must be visualized as separate from the left hepatic vein.
- The left hepatic vein is freed of liver substance, until a sufficient distance is gained to permit the application of a pair of long curved Cooley vascular clamps and then divided. A vascular stapler may be utilized to control the left hepatic vein.
- A line of demarcation between the right and left hemi-livers develops after the left hepatic vein has been ligated.
- This line tends to curve in a concave manner to the left, until the dome of the liver is reached.
- Ultrasonic dissecting instruments are available for dividing and aspirating the liver tissue with easier exposure for ligation of the larger ducts and vessels, especially the venous branches of the middle hepatic vein.
- Alternatively, an electrocautery or laser device may be used to divide the liver parenchyma, or an endoscopic GIA stapler can be used.
- The raw surface of the right hemi-liver is carefully inspected for bleeding points as well as for bile leakage, which may require a suture ligature.
- The omentum can be mobilized and anchored over the divided surface of the right hemi-liver. Closed system Silastic suction drain can be used.
- A routine closure of the abdominal wall is performed [13–15].

3. **Pericystectomy for hydatid liver cyst:**
   - The main principle of the surgery is to eradicate the parasite and prevent intraoperative spillage of the cyst content avoiding peritoneal spread and anaphylactic reaction.
   - Pericystectomy provides a radical treatment removing the whole cyst "en bloc" including the adventitia without resection of healthy liver tissue.
   - Indication: peripheral hydatid cyst of the liver.
   - Contraindication:
     - Deep cyst within the liver parenchyma.
     - Invasion of main right or left hepatic ducts.
   - Preoperative treatment of albendazole 10–14 mg/kg/day in two doses administered 2 weeks preoperatively and to be continued for 1 month postoperatively.

- Under general anesthesia and endotracheal intubation.
- Position: supine position with table in slightly reverse Trendelenburg position.
- The abdomen is prepped from nipple to the symphysis pubis.
- Patient is draped in sterile fashion.
- Incision: extended right or bilateral subcostal incision with midline extension to the xiphoid can provide excellent exposure.
- Details of the procedure:
  - Careful exploration of the abdominal cavity is done to exclude extrahepatic disease.
  - Cover the surrounding organs with gauzes soaked in hypertonic saline.
  - Intraoperative ultrasound can be used to confirm the location and number of the cysts and the relation with important vascular structures.
  - Vessel loop is placed around the porta hepatis to control the inflow in case of bleeding.
  - Mobilize the liver.
  - Pack the whole space around the liver with gauze soaked in hypertonic saline.
  - Two suctions should be available in case of rupture of the cyst.
  - Stay sutures with 2-0 silk sutures are placed in the liver parenchyma around the emerging part of the cyst to enable traction and better exposure during resection.
  - The liver capsule is incised with diathermy.
  - Identification of correct plane is crucial to avoid bleeding and spillage of the cyst content.
  - Dissect through the liver parenchyma using bipolar forceps or any of the transection methods described earlier.
  - Small vessels and bile duct are carefully identified and tied.
  - Hemostasis of the exposed raw surface of the liver.
  - Insert suction drain and close the abdomen [13–15].

Postoperative care:

- Admission to a high dependency ward or ICU.
- Early mobilization and DVT prophylaxis, whenever possible.
- Introduction of enteral nutrition as early as possible.
- Analgesia, gastric acid suppressors.
- Daily blood and liver function.
- Prothrombin time (PT) seems to be most predictive of hepatic functional recovery.
- Electrolyte assessments and replacement of K, Mg, and phosphate, as needed.
- Significant blood loss from drains may require replacement.
- Meticulous attention must be paid to minimizing infectious risks.
- Leakage of fluid from the wound should not be tolerated and aggressively corrected.
- If there is a bile leak of greater than 100 ml/day, then an endoscopic biliary stent should be considered.
- If there is an ascites leak, the wound should be revised.
- Long-term follow-up should include frequent examinations with periodic liver function tests [13–15].

Prevention and Treatment of Common Postoperative Complications:

- **Postoperative Bleeding:**
  Severe postoperative bleeding after liver resection is uncommon, except in the context of severe liver failure. Blood transfusion may be avoided in an otherwise stable patient, when there is no evidence of active bleeding or hemodynamic instability.
- **Postoperative Liver Dysfunction:**
  The risk of postoperative hepatic insufficiency is closely related to volume and function of FLR. It is manifested by nonobstructive jaundice, fluid retention, coagulopathy, and increase in susceptibility to septic complications. It is best managed by prevention rather than treatment.

Predictive factors of postoperative insufficiency include:
- patient factors (age, body mass index (BMI))
- Liver factors (FLR < 20% in a normal liver)
- Surgeon factors (blood loss and requirements of intraoperative transfusions)

- Some factors like age and BMI are nonmodifiable, but it is possible to decrease the risk of hepatic insufficiency by increasing the volume of the FLR with PVE and limiting intraoperative blood loss to reduce the risk of transfusions. The occurrence of postoperative liver dysfunction should be detected early in the postoperative period, and associated complication such as fluid collections and infections should be treated aggressively in order to prevent progression to liver failure.
- **Perioperative Fluid Collections and Bile Leaks:**
  Fluid collection may be related to infections or bile leaks. In most cases, postoperative fluid collections are asymptomatic; however, in some cases, they are associated with fever, abdominal pain, upper gastrointestinal (GI) symptoms, or pleural effusion. Fluid collections are diagnosed with CT or ultrasonography and may be treated with percutaneous drainage. Bile leak is another major complication and most of the time it appears to arise from an injured major ductal branch or biliary enteric anastomosis in case of combined liver and biliary tract resections [13–15].

5.2 Part II: Practice

Knowledge is of no value unless you put it into practice.
—Anton Chekhov

5.2.1 Case Scenarios for Practice

Tips:

- Practice with a friend and try to mimic the real exam!
  Don't forget to set the timer!
- The clinical data are provided in the Answer Key section.
- Some twist points are suggested after some cases and can be used to change the scenario to a more difficult one.

Case No. 1:
A 38-year-old female patient presented to the surgery clinic complaining of epigastric pain for 1 month.

Questions for Discussion:

1. How will you approach this patient?
2. What is your differential and provisional diagnosis based on the given clinical data?
3. What will you do to confirm the most likely diagnosis?
4. How will you manage this patient? Why?
5. How will you prepare the patient for surgery?
6. What are the possible complications?
7. How will you follow this patient?

Suggested Twist Points:

- The patient wants to delay the surgery, then she presented to the emergency department few weeks later with shock and severe abdominal pain. What could be the cause and how will you manage that?
- The final pathology result shows that the excised lesion is malignant, what will you do?

Case No. 2:
A 51-year-old alcoholic male patient was referred from the hepatology clinic due to RUQ mass for 6 weeks.

Questions for Discussion:

1. How will you approach this patient?
2. What is your differential diagnosis based on the given clinical data?
3. What will you do next?
4. Do you need to confirm the diagnosis by tissue biopsy? Why?
5. How will you manage this patient?
6. How will you prepare this patient for OR?
7. What are the possible complications?
8. How will you follow this patient?

Suggested Twist Points:

- The future liver remnant is less than the required, what will be your plan of management?
- On day 4 postoperative, the patient has bile in the drainage tube, what are the possible causes and how will you manage it?

Case No. 3:
A 42-year-old male patient presented to the emergency department complaining of right upper abdominal pain for 3 days.

Questions for Discussion:

1. How will you approach this patient?
2. Based on the given clinical information, what is your differential diagnosis?
3. What is your next step?
4. Based on the radiological image, how would you classify the patient's condition?
5. How will you manage such patients?
6. What are the pre- and intraoperative precautions you should take?
7. The patient underwent endocystectomy with suture ligation of few small bile ducts that were communicating with the cyst. On the third postoperative day, the drain output is bile, what should you do?
8. What are the other options to treat such a condition?

Suggested Twist Point:

- The cystic lesion is communicating with one of the major biliary ducts. What will be your surgical option?

Case No. 4:
A 33-year-old female patient presented to the clinic complaining of right upper quadrant pain and she noticed a slight yellow discoloration of her eyes for 2 weeks.

Questions for Discussion:

1. How will you approach the patient?
2. What is your differential diagnosis?
3. How will you confirm the most likely diagnosis?
4. Based on the given information, what is your diagnosis?
5. How will you manage the patient?
6. How will you prepare the patient for operation?
7. How will you follow the patient?

Suggested Twist Point:

- The patient refused surgery, then later she presented to the emergency department with severe abdominal pain and hemodynamic instability. How will you manage her?

Case No. 5:
A 46-year-old female was referred to the surgery clinic complaining of right upper abdominal pain for 1 month.

Questions for Discussion:

1. How will you approach the patient?
2. What investigations you would like to ask for?
3. Based on clinical information, what is your differential diagnosis?
4. What do you want to do to confirm the most likely diagnosis?
5. What is your diagnosis?
6. What is your plan of management?
7. How will you follow the patient postoperatively?

Checklist

History	Items	Done	Not done	Not applicable
General	Introduce himself/herself to the patient			
	Patient personal data (name, age, sex, nationality)			
	Chief complaint			
	Duration			
Pain	Onset			
	Site			
	Character			
	Radiation/shifting			
	Aggravating/relieving			
	Severity			
	Progression			
	Frequency			
Mass	Onset			
	Site			
	How did the patient notice it?			
	Any change since it was first noticed?			
	Other masses			
Jaundice	Onset			
	Itching			
	Change in stool or urine color			
	Progression			
Associated symptoms	Pain			
	Fever			
	Nausea			
	Vomiting			
	Diarrhea			
	Constipation			
	Abdominal distention			
Constitutional symptoms	Weight loss			
	Decrease in appetite			
	Night sweating			
Symptoms of metastases	Back pain			
	Cough			
	Shortness of breath			
	Abdominal distention			
Risk factors	Rapid weight loss			
	History of cirrhosis			
	Medication: OCP, anabolic steroid, acetaminophen			
	Alcohol, drug abuse			
	Smoking			
	History of IBD			
	Contact with animal			
	Previous hepatobiliary surgery			
	History of traveling			
	History of contact with sick people			
	Personal history of malignancy			
	Family history of a similar complaint			

(continued)

History	Items	Done	Not done	Not applicable
Differential diagnosis	Chest pain (MI)			
	Cough, SOB (pneumonia)			
	Recent history of trauma			
PMH	Previous similar attack			
	Previous investigation			
	Previous admission			
	Chronic illnesses			
PSH	Previous surgery			
Family history	Of cancers or hepatic problem			
Social history	Occupation			
	Habits (smoking, alcohol, drugs)			
Other	Medication			
	Allergy			
	Transfusion			
Systemic review				
Physical examination				
General principle	Patient position			
	Exposure			
	Privacy			
	Wash hands			
General examination	Appearance			
	Body built			
	Color			
	Distress/decubitus			
	Environment			
Vital signs	BP, HR, temperature, RR, SPO_2			
Hand signs	Muscle wasting, palmar erythema, clubbing, flapping tremor, leukonychia, koilonychia			
Eyes	Jaundice, pallor			
Mouth	Jaundice, fetor hepaticus			
Neck	Lymphadenopathy			
Chest	Spider nevi, gynecomastia, respiratory and CVS examination			
Abdomen: Inspection	Distention			
	Asymmetry			
	Dilated veins			
	Striae			
	Visible peristalsis			
	Scars			
	Signs of retroperitoneal hemorrhage			
Palpation	Superficial then deep palpation			
	Tenderness			
	Palpable masses			
	Organomegaly			
	Cough impulse at hernial orifices			
Percussion	Shifting dullness			
	Fluid thrill			
	Organomegaly			

History	Items	Done	Not done	Not applicable
Auscultation	Bowel sounds			
	Bruit, venous hum			
Groin				
DRE and proctoscopy				
Back tenderness				
Differential diagnosis	According to the given scenario			
Investigations				
General laboratory test	CBC with differential			
	Electrolytes			
	Liver function test (ALT, AST, GGT, albumin, total bilirubin, and direct bilirubin)			
	Amylase and lipase			
	Coagulation profile (PT, INR, aPTT)			
	Blood grouping			
	RFT			
	CPR/ESR			
	Blood culture			
Specific tests	Tumor marker (AFP, CEA, Ca19-9)			
	Hepatitis profile			
	ELISA for *Echinococcus*			
	Fluorescent antibody test of *Entamoeba histolytica*			
Imaging	Ultrasound abdomen			
	Triphasic CT abdomen			
	MRI/MRCP			
Biopsy	When indicated			
Provisional diagnosis	According to the given scenario			
Management (depending on the diagnosis)				
Liver abscess	Admission			
	Diet (NPO if for procedure)			
	IV fluid			
	Empirical antibiotic then de-escalates according to the culture (duration 6–8 weeks)			
	Antipyretic			
	Prophylaxis (DVT and stress ulcer)			
	Search for the underlying cause (biliary, GIT, hematogenous)			
	Percutaneous drainage			
	Surgical drainage, if drainage failed			
Amebic liver abscess	Admission			
	Diet			
	IV fluid, if NPO			
	Medication: antipyretic, antiemetic, DVT prophylaxis, and stress ulcer prophylaxis, as needed			
	Metronidazole 750 mg TID for 7 days			
	Drainage, only if there is a large abscess or the patient is not responding to medical treatment			

(continued)

History	Items	Done	Not done	Not applicable
Hydatid cyst	Admission			
	NPO, if required			
	IV fluid			
	Analgesia			
	Antiemetic			
	Albendazole			
	DVT and stress ulcer prophylaxis			
	Intervention as indicated (percutaneous aspiration, injection, and reaspiration (PAIR) vs surgical)			
	Prepare hypertonic saline			
	Prepare standby epinephrine and hydrocortisone			
	Consent, if surgery is indicated			
	Surgery (PAIR, nonradical resection, radical resection)			
Liver cyst	If asymptomatic: no intervention			
	Symptomatic: ultrasound-guided aspiration			
	Sclerotherapy			
	Surgical treatment, if aspiration failed (fenestration or unroofing)			
	If treated surgically, send the wall for pathological assessments			
Hemangioma	Asymptomatic: follow-up			
	Symptomatic: surgical interventions (enucleation, anatomic vs nonanatomic resection)			
	If ruptured: resuscitation			
	embolization			
	resection			
FNH	Conservative treatment Surgery, only if symptomatic or inability to rule out malignancy			
Adenoma	If asymptomatic, discontinue OCP or steroid			
	If symptomatic or increase in size >5 cm, carry out resection to achieve negative margins			
	If there is life-threatening hemorrhage and the patient is stable, embolization is followed by elective resection			
	If there is life-threatening hemorrhage and the patient is unstable, laparotomy, Pringle's maneuver, and packing are carried out			

History	Items	Done	Not done	Not applicable
HCC	Admission			
	Assess the degree of liver disease using CHILD and MELD scores			
	Measure the amount of future liver remnant			
	Staging			
	Multidisciplinary team discussion			
	Determine the resectability and transplantability			
	Decide the management plan (resection, transplantation, ablation, or embolization)			
	If the treatment is resection:			
	o Prepare the patient for OR			
	o Anesthesia consultation			
	o ICU consultation			
	o Prepare the standby blood			
	o Consent			
	o NPO			
	o IV fluid			
	o Prophylactic antibiotic			
Intrahepatic cholangiocarcinoma	Rule out other primary (colonoscopy, upper and lower endoscopy, CT chest, and mammogram)			
	Multidisciplinary team discussion			
	Assess resectability and resect, if possible			
	If the treatment is resection:			
	o Prepare the patient for OR			
	o Anesthesia consultation			
	o ICU consultation			
	o Prepare standby blood			
	o Consent			
	o NPO			
	o IV fluid			
	o Prophylactic antibiotic			
Metastatic colorectal tumor	Multidisciplinary team approach			
	One-stage procedure, if the colon surgery is straightforward and the liver resection is minor, otherwise multistage procedure			
Postoperative care				
Early postoperative	Admission to high dependency unit (HDU) or ICU			
	Early mobilization and DVT prophylaxis			
	Enteral nutrition as early as possible			
	Analgesia			
	Stress ulcer prophylaxis			
	CBC and LFT daily			
	Coagulation profile, especially PT			
	Electrolyte assessment			
	Monitor drain output and the nature of the fluid (blood, bile, serous)			

(continued)

History	Items	Done	Not done	Not applicable
First outpatient visit	Clinical assessment			
	Remove sutures			
	Review the final pathology report			
	Arrange for multidisciplinary discussion, if the case is cancer			
	Refer to oncology, if adjuvant treatment is required			
Long-term follow-up	For HCC: Imaging and AFP every 3–6 months for 2 years then annually			
	For intrahepatic cholangiocarcinoma: Computed tomography chest abdomen pelvis (CT CAP) every 3–6 months for 2 years then annually for up to 5 years			

5.2.2 Answer Key

Case No. 1:

A 38-year-old female patient presented to the surgery clinic complaining of epigastric pain for 1 month.

Questions for Discussion:

1. **How will you approach this patient?**

- The patient is a 38-year-old female. She was doing well till last month when she gradually started to have epigastric pain, which was dull aching pain. It was not radiated or shifted to another place. She describes her pain to be continuous. Her pain was not associated with nausea, heartburn, or other significant symptoms. She has no history of weight loss or recent history of traveling or contact with sick patients. She has no chronic medical problem, and her past surgical history was positive for appendectomy 10 years ago. She has been on oral contraceptive pills for 5 years. She has no family or personal history of malignancy.
- On examination, she was lying comfortably on the bed and did not look jaundiced or pale. Her vital signs were within normal limits. She had no stigmata of chronic liver disease. Her abdomen was not distended, soft with mild tenderness over the epigastric area. There was well-defined, 5 × 5 cm, mildly tender, nonpulsatile mass over the epigastric area.

2. **What is your differential and provisional diagnosis based on the given clinical data?**
   - Benign liver mass (adenoma, hemangioma, FNH)
   - Malignant liver lesion (primary, secondary)
   - Benign liver cyst
   - Hydatid cyst
   - Liver abscess
   - Choledochal cyst
   - Lipoma
   - Gastric mass
   - Hernia (diversion recti)

provisional diagnosis: hepatic adenoma

3. **What will you do to confirm the most likely diagnosis?**

- CBC, LFT, coagulation profile, amylase, lipase, and inflammatory marker are normal. Ultrasound abdomen showed a well-demarcated left side heterogeneous mass of about 5.3 × 5.1 cm in its greatest dimensions.
- Triphasic CT abdomen revealed a solitary well-encapsulated lesion on segments II and III. It is isodense on a noncontrast phase and shows a homogeneous enhancement in the arterial phase which returns to isodense on portal and delayed phases. No other lesions or abnormal lymph nodes.

4. **How will you manage this patient? Why?**

- This patient has symptomatic hepatic adenoma which has a size >5 cm, and the appropriate management should be surgical resection to achieve negative margins (left lateral hepatectomy), due to increased risk of both malignancy and rupture.

5. **How will you prepare the patient for surgery?**
   - Explain the diagnosis and the plan of management to the patient
   - Admission
   - NPO before surgery
   - IV fluid
   - Medication: analgesia, prophylactic antibiotic and stress ulcer prophylaxis, and DVT prophylaxis, as indicated
   - Review the laboratory investigations, prepare standby blood
   - Review the preoperative images: ultrasound, CT
   - Evaluate the cardiopulmonary system
   - CXR, ECG
   - Anesthesia consultation
   - Instruct the patient to take shower the night before surgery
   - Explain the procedure to the patient and obtain informed consent
6. **What are the possible complications?**

- Complications related to the procedures like bleeding, bile leak, hematoma, and injury to the nearby structures
- General complications like atelectasis, pneumonia, DVT, PE, wound infection, adhesions, and incisional hernia

7. **How will you follow this patient?**

- Early postoperative:
  - NPO till full recovery then start feeding gradually
  - Early mobilization whenever possible and DVT prophylaxis
  - Analgesia, gastric acid suppressor
  - Daily blood tests and liver function test
  - Coagulation profile assessment
  - Electrolyte assessment and replacement of K, Mg, and phosphate, as needed
  - Monitor the amount and the color of the drain output.
- First outpatient visit:
  - Clinical assessment of the patient's general condition and the wound.
  - Remove sutures/clips.
  - Check the final pathology report.
  - If the diagnosis is adenoma, no further management is required, and the patient can be discharged.

Suggested twist points:

- *The patient wants to delay the surgery, then she presented to the emergency department few weeks later with shock and severe abdominal pain.*

  The management of ruptured adenoma depends on stability:
  - Stable: embolization then elective resection.
  - Unstable: Laparotomy, Pringle's maneuver, and packing

    Formal resection is not necessary in this operation.
- *The final pathology result shows that the excised lesion is malignant (HCC), what will you do?*
  - Multidisciplinary discussion
  - Assess the degree of liver disease if it presents using CHILD or MELC scores (this patient has normal liver)
  - Staging: CT chest, abdomen, and pelvis, consider bone scan if there is any symptom
  - Measure the amount of future liver remnant (should be more than 25%)
  - Determine resectability. if possible, re-resect to achieve negative margin
  - Refer to oncologist or radiotherapist, if further treatment is recommended by the multidisciplinary team

Case No. 2:

A 51-year-old alcoholic male patient was referred from the hepatology clinic due to liver mass found on ultrasound 6 weeks ago.

Questions for discussion:

1. **How will you approach this patient?**

- The patient is a 51-year-old male who is known to be alcoholic for the last 30 years. He is following in the hepatology clinic due to liver cirrhosis and has been referred to the surgery clinic, due to a liver mass that was discovered during an ultrasound examination. He did not notice any new abdominal swelling and does not have abdominal pain. He is jaundiced ever since he was diagnosed with cirrhosis. His weight has decreased over the past 3 months by 7 kg (from 75 to 68 kg). He has no significant family history. He is not known to have any other chronic illness and has no history of previous surgery.
- On examination:
- The patient looks ill, jaundiced. With obvious stigmata of chronic liver disease in the form of palmar erythema, flapping tremor, and spider nevi. His vital signs are normal. His abdomen is slightly distended but soft with no localized area of tenderness. There is an ill-defined mass palpable at the RUQ area, approximately 2 × 2 cm, hard, and its surface is irregular. He does not have ascites. The other examination is normal.

2. **What is your differential diagnosis based on the given clinical data?**
   - Malignant liver lesion (HCC mainly)
   - Secondary liver tumors
   - Regenerative liver nodule
   - Benign liver lesion
   - Hydatid cyst
   - Liver abscess
   - Choledochal cyst
   - Lipoma
   - gastric mass

Table 5.5 Blood test for Case No. 2

Test	Result	Normal value
WBC (white blood cells) (k/ul)	7	4.8–10.8
Hb (g/dl)	13	12.6–16.5
PLT (K/ul)	150	130–400
ALT (U/l)	120	10–130
AST (U/l)	31	10–34
Total bilirubin (mg/dl)	1.9	0–0.8
Direct bilirubin (mg/dl)	1	0–0.3
Albumin (g/dl)	3.6	2.4–4
Creatinine (mg/dl)	1	0.7–1.2
PT (seconds)	12	10–13
INR	1	1
AFP	350	<7
CEA (ng/ml)	4	<5
Ca19-9 (u/ml)	26	0–27
Hepatitis profile	Negative	Negative

3. **What will you do next?**

- Blood tests: Table 5.5.
- Triphasic CT abdomen shows cirrhotic liver with a hypervascular lesion on arterial phase with a rapid washout during the portal phase. The lesion is about 2.2 × 3.1 cm and is located in the area between segments V and VIII. No other lesions or abnormal lymph node are noticed and there are no signs of portal hypertension.

4. **Do you need to confirm the diagnosis by tissue biopsy? Why?**

- The diagnosis is HCC, and no further testing is necessary.
- Biopsy is not indicated because the radiological picture of the lesion is typical for HCC and the clinical evidence of cirrhosis is enough to confirm the diagnosis.

5. **How will you manage this patient?**
   - Multidisciplinary discussion
   - Assess the degree of liver disease using CHILD or MELC scores (this patient is Child A)

- Staging: CT chest, abdomen, and pelvis, consider bone scan if there is any symptom
- Measure the amount of future liver remnant (more than 40%)
- Determine resectability and transplantability:
- This patient is candidate for curative liver resection in the form of right anterior sectionectomy or right hepatectomy to achieve 2-cm negative margins.

6. **How will you prepare this patient for OR?**
   - Explain the diagnosis and the plan of management to the patient
   - Admission
   - NPO before surgery
   - IV fluid
   - Medication: prophylactic antibiotic and stress ulcer prophylaxis, and DVT prophylaxis, as indicated
   - Review the laboratory investigations, prepare standby blood
   - Review the preoperative images: ultrasound, CT.
   - Evaluate the cardiopulmonary system
   - CXR, ECG
   - Anesthesia consultation
   - Instruct the patient to take shower the night before surgery
   - Explain the procedure to the patient and obtain informed consent
7. **What are the possible complications?**

- General complications:
- Bleeding, wound infection, atelectasis, pneumonia, MI, DVT, PE, adhesion, incisional hernia
- Specific complications:
- Bile leak, biloma, hematoma, liver failure

8. **How will you follow this patient?**

- Early postoperative:
  - Admission to ICU or HDU
  - NPO till full recovery then start feeding gradually
  - Early mobilization whenever possible and DVT prophylaxis
  - Analgesia, gastric acid suppressors
  - Daily CBC, renal function, liver function
  - Coagulation profile assessment
  - Electrolyte assessments and replacement of K, Mg, and phosphate, as needed
  - Monitor the amount and the color of the drain output.
- First outpatient visit:
  - Clinical assessment of the patient general's condition and the wound
  - Remove sutures/clips
  - Check the final pathology report
  - Multidisciplinary team discussion
  - Refer to a medical oncologist or radiotherapist, if further treatment is indicated
- Long term follow-up:
  - CT chest, abdomen, and pelvis every 3–6 months for 2 years, then 6–12 months for up to 5 years.

Suggested twist points:

- **The future liver remnant is less than required, what will be your plan of management?**
  Portal vein embolization to induce hypertrophy of the liver remnant
- **On day 4 postoperative, the patient has bile in the drainage tube, what is the possible cause and how will you manage it?**
  Bile leak from the row surface of the liver or bile duct injury could explain the patient's symptoms. The cause can be determined by cholangiography (MRCP or ERCP).

  MRCP was done and the leak came from the row surface. It can be managed by ERCP and sphincterotomy.

Case No. 3:

A 42-year-old male patient presented to the emergency department complaining of right upper abdominal pain for 3 days.

Questions for discussion:

1. **How will you approach this patient?**

- The patient is a 42-year-old male who works as a shepherd presented to the emergency department complaining of upper abdominal pain. His pain started gradually, stabbing in nature, and radiated to the right shoulder sometimes. The pain is associated with nausea and fever (38°C). His wife noticed that his eyes were yellow. He confirmed that his urine turned to be darker and his stool was pale. There was no history of diarrhea or vomiting.

- No history of contact with a sick patient or any recent history of traveling. The patient is diabetic on insulin, otherwise healthy.
- On examination:
- He looks ill and jaundiced. His vital signs are as follows: BP: 125/87 mmHg, temperature: 37.8 °C, and pulse: 92 bpm.
- The abdomen is soft with mild fullness at the RUQ and tenderness on palpation and negative Murphy's sign. No signs of chronic liver disease.

2. **Based on the given clinical information, what is your differential diagnosis?**

- Hydatid liver disease
- Pyogenic liver abscess
- Choledocholithiasis
- Cholangitis
- Amebic liver abscess
- Hepatitis

3. **What is your next step?**

- Blood tests: Table 5.6.
- Ultrasound abdomen shows a well-defined cystic lesion measuring 8.0 cm × 7.4 cm in the right hemi-liver of the liver (segments VII and VIII) with low level of internal echoes. The cyst shows a detached membrane inside it, which appears to float within the content. There is dilatation of both intra- and extrahepatic bile ducts. The gallbladder looks normal with no stones.

4. **Based on the radiological image, how would you classify the patient's condition?**

- Based on the World Health Organization's (WHO's) classification, it is CE3a (water lily sign).

Table 5.6 Blood test for Case No. 3

Test	Result	Normal value
WBC (k/ul)	12	4.8–10.8
Hb (g/dl)	13	12.6–16.5
PLT (K/ul)	230	130–400
ALT (U/l)	140	10–130
AST (U/l)	39	10–34
Total bilirubin (mg/dl)	2	0–0.8
Direct bilirubin (mg/dl)	1.5	0–0.3
Albumin (g/dl)	3.6	2.4–4
Creatinine (mg/dl)	1	0.7–1.2
PT (seconds)	12	10–13
INR	1	1
CRP (mg/l)	20	<3
ESR (mm/h)	36	0–29
Blood culture	Negative	Negative
ELISA for *Echinococcus*	Positive	Negative
Antibodies for ameba	Negative	Negative

5. **How will you manage such patients?**

- *First: confirm or rule out communication with biliary tree by MRCP/ERCP.*
- ERCP was done and there was a gelatinous material inside the CBD, which was cleared, and the cholangiogram revealed communication between intrahepatic bile ducts and the cyst.
- *Second: start the patient on medication*
- Albendazole 10–15 mg/kg/day, analgesia, antiemetic, antibiotics
- Prophylaxis against DVT and stress ulcer, as indicated
- *Third: prepare the patient for operation*

6. **What are the pre- and intraoperative precautions you should take?**

- Preoperative:
  - rule out communication with the biliary tree
  - start the patient on albendazole
  - prepare 20% of hypertonic saline to be used intraoperatively, when needed
- Intraoperative:
  - prepare epinephrine and hydrocortisone in the case of cyst rupture and anaphylaxis
  - prepare two large suctions to control any possible spillage

7. **The patient underwent endocystectomy with suture ligation of few small bile ducts that were communicating with the cyst. On the third postoperative day, the drain output is bile, what should you do?**

- Most likely, there is bile leak from the site of the cyst or unrecognized injury to the bile ducts.
- Cholangiography is needed to confirm the diagnosis (either MRCP or ERCP) and to be managed according to the finding.
- MRCP shows small bile leak from the site of endocystectomy.
- The management is endoscopic sphincterotomy to decrease the intrabiliary pressure and promote healing of the leaking duct.

8. **What are the other options to treat such a condition?**

- Medical treatment alone is enough, if the cyst is indicated in
  - Cyst <5 cm
  - CE1–CE3
  - Inoperable disease
  - Multiorgan involvement
  - Peritoneal cyst
- Albendazole 10–15 mg/kg/day
- PAIR is indicated in:
  - Cyst <5 cm
  - Unilocular CE1–CE3
  - Accessible
  - Inoperable patient
  - Pregnant women and children not fit for surgery

Suggested twist point:

- **The cystic lesion is communicating with one of the major biliary ducts. What will be your surgical option?**
  Radical surgery like resection will be indicated, if the cyst is communicating with one of the major hepatic ducts.

Case No. 4:

A 33-year-old female patient presented to the clinic complaining of right upper quadrant pain and she noticed a slight yellow discoloration of her eyes for 2 weeks.

Questions for discussion:

1. **How will you approach the patient?**

- The patient is a 33-year-old female who presented to the surgery clinic complaining of right upper quadrant pain for 2 weeks. Her pain started gradually, dull aching pain, not radiated or shifted anywhere else. Associated with yellowish discoloration of her eyes, itching, dark urine, and pale stool. No history of fever, weight loss, or night sweating. No recent history of traveling or contact with sick patients. She has no chronic medical problem; no previous surgery and she is not on any regular medications.
- On examination:
- She looks jaundiced, in mild pain. Her vital signs are normal.
- Her abdomen is soft with mild tenderness at right upper quadrant area, but Murphy's sign is negative. No palpable mass, ascites, or organomegaly.

2. **What is your differential diagnosis?**
   - Choledocholithiasis
   - Benign liver lesion
   - Cholangiocarcinoma
   - Biliary stricture
   - Mirizzi's syndrome
   - Periampullary cancer
3. **How will you confirm the most likely diagnosis?**

- Blood tests: Table 5.7
- Ultrasound abdomen shows a hyperechoic well-defined liver lesion at segment VII measuring 4.5 cm × 5.1 cm causing mass effect and the proximal intrahepatic biliary tree is

Table 5.7 Blood test for Case No. 4

Test	Result	Normal value
WBC (k/ul)	8	4.8–10.8
Hb (g/dl)	13	12.6–16.5
PLT (K/ul)	165	130–400
ALT (U/l)	135	10–130
AST (U/l)	35	10–34
Total bilirubin (mg/dl)	3	0–0.8
Direct bilirubin (mg/dl)	2.2	0–0.3
Albumin (g/dl)	4	2.4–4
Creatinine (mg/dl)	1.1	0.7–1.2
PT (seconds)	13	10–13
INR	1	1
CRP (mg/l)	1	<3
ESR (mm/h)	25	0–29
Blood culture	Negative	Negative
ELISA for *Echinococcus*	Negative	Negative
Antibodies for ameba	Negative	Negative

dilated. The gallbladder is normal with no stones.

- Triphasic CT abdomen shows hypoattenuating lesion on a noncontrast study that shows nodular peripheral enhancement in the arterial phase that progresses in portal phase with more centripetal fill-in.

4. **Based on the given information, what is your diagnosis?**

- Symptomatic liver hemangioma

5. **How will you manage the patient?**

- Surgical management is indicated, since the patient has symptoms (mass effect) and enucleation is the appropriate option.

6. **How will you prepare the patient for operation?**
   - Explain the diagnosis and the plan of management to the patient
   - Admission
   - NPO before surgery
   - IV fluid
   - Medication: prophylactic antibiotic and stress ulcer prophylaxis, and DVT prophylaxis, as indicated
   - Review the laboratory investigations and prepare standby blood
   - Review the preoperative images: ultrasound, CT.
   - Evaluate the cardiopulmonary system
   - CXR, ECG
   - Anesthesia consultation
   - Instruct the patient to take shower the night before surgery
   - Explain the procedure to the patient and obtain informed consent

7. **How will you follow the patient?**

- Early postoperative:
  - NPO till full recovery then start feeding gradually
  - Early mobilization whenever possible and DVT prophylaxis
  - Analgesia, gastric acid suppressors
  - Daily blood tests and liver function
  - Coagulation profile assessment
  - Electrolyte assessments and replacement of K, Mg, and phosphate, as needed
  - Monitor the amount and the color of the drain output
- First outpatient visit:
  - Clinical assessment of the patient's general condition and the wound.
  - Remove sutures/clips.
  - Check the final pathology report.
  - If no further management is required, the patient can be discharged.

Suggested twist point:

- **The patient refused surgery then presented to the emergency department with severe abdominal pain and hemodynamic instability. How will you manage her?**
  Resuscitation, embolization followed by resection

Case No. 5:
A 46-year-old female is referred to the surgery clinic complaining of right upper abdominal pain for 1 month.

Questions for discussion:

1. **How will you approach the patient?**

- The patient is a 46-year-old female patient who presented to the surgery clinic complaining of a gradual onset of right upper quadrant pain that is not radiated or shifted anywhere else. The pain is associated with nausea, anorexia, and weight loss (more than 8 kg in 1 month). No history of GI bleeding, no change in the bowel habit. No jaundice or change in urine or stool color. No history of traveling or contact with sick patients. No personal history or family history of malignancy.
- The patient is known to have hypertension controlled with medication. She underwent laparoscopic cholecystectomy when she was 30 years old.
- On physical examination:
- She looks ill, underweight. Not pale or jaundiced.
- Vital signs are normal.
- No abnormal lymphadenopathy.
- The abdomen is not distended, soft, nontender, no ascites or organomegaly.

2. **What investigation would you like to ask for?**

- Blood tests: Table 5.8.
- Ultrasound: homogeneous mass at the left hemi-liver that shows intermediate echogenicity with a peripheral hypoechoic halo of compressed liver parenchyma. It is well delineated but irregular in outline and is associated with capsular retraction.

Table 5.8 Blood test for Case No. 5

Test	Result	Normal value
WBC (k/ul)	10	4.8–10.8
Hb (g/dl)	12.1	12.6–16.5
PLT (K/ul)	200	130–400
ALT (U/l)	120	10–130
AST (U/l)	23	10–34
Total bilirubin (mg/dl)	0.8	0–0.8
Direct bilirubin (mg/dl)	0.2	0–0.3
Albumin (g/dl)	4	2.4–4
Creatinine (mg/dl)	0.9	0.7–1.2
PT (seconds)	10	10–13
INR	1	1
CRP (mg/l)	2	<3
ESR (mm/h)	25	0–29

- Triphasic CT: there is a mass measuring 5.2 × 3.4 cm occupying the segments II and III and shows homogeneous attenuation on noncontrast scan and demonstrates heterogeneous minor peripheral enhancement. The mass does not seem to invade the nearby organs. Capsular retraction is noted and the bile ducts distal to the mass are dilated. No abnormal lymph nodes are seen.

3. **Based on clinical information, what is your differential diagnosis?**

- Malignant liver lesion could be primary (intrahepatic cholangiocarcinoma, HCC) or metastatic tumors form GIT, lung, or breast.

4. **What do you want to do to confirm the diagnosis?**

- Tumor marker: Table 5.9
- Biopsy: adenocarcinoma
- CT chest: normal
- Upper and lower endoscopy: normal
- Mammogram: normal

5. **What is your diagnosis?**

- Intrahepatic cholangiocarcinoma

6. **How will you manage the patient?**

- Staging CT CAP, if not done before.
- Multidisciplinary team approach.
- Staging laparoscopy can be done before surgery or in conjunction with surgery.
- The tumor is resectable, the only curative treatment is resection to achieve negative margin (left hepatectomy) with lymphadenectomy.

Table 5.9 Tumor marker for Case No. 5

Test	Result	Normal value
CEA (ng/ml)	4	<5
Ca19-9 (u/ml)	150	0–27
AFP	4	<7

7. **How will you follow the patient postoperatively?**

- Early postoperative:
  - Admission to ICU or HDU
  - NPO till full recovery then start feeding gradually
  - Early mobilization whenever possible and DVT prophylaxis
  - Analgesia, gastric acid suppressors
  - Daily blood tests and liver function
  - Coagulation profile assessment
  - Electrolyte assessments and replacement of K, Mg, and phosphate, as needed
  - Monitor the amount and the color of the drain output.
- First outpatient visit:
  - Clinical assessment of the patient's general condition and the wound.
  - Remove sutures/clips
  - Check the final pathology report
  - Multidisciplinary team
  - Referral to oncology, if adjuvant systematic chemotherapy is indicated
- Long-term follow-up:
  - CT chest, abdomen, and pelvis every 3–6 months for 2 years, then 6–12 months for up to 5 years.

References

1. Geller DA, Goss JA, Busuttil RW, Tsung A. The liver. In: Brunicardi F, editor. Schwartz's principles of surgery. 11th ed. United States: McGraw-Hill Education; 2019.
2. Durand CM. The management of hepatic abscess. In: Cameron J, Cameron A, editors. Current surgical therapy. 12th ed. Canada: Elsevier; 2016.
3. Thapar ANSVB. In: Chu QD, editor. Hepato-pancreato-biliary and transplant surgery. 12th ed. Canada: Beaux Books Publishing, LLC; 2018.
4. Calvin Eriksen VGA. The management of echinococcal cyst disease of the liver. In: Cameron J, Cameron A, editors. Current surgical therapy. 12th ed. Canada: Elsevier; 2016.
5. Richard D, Schulick ALG. The management of liver tumors. In: Cameron J, Cameron A, editors. Current surgical therapy. 12th ed. Canada: Elsevier; 2016.
6. Keri E, Lunsford FMK. The management of cystic disease of the liver. In: Cameron J, Cameron A, editors. Current surgical therapy. 12th ed. Canada: Elsevier; 2016.
7. Katherine E, Poruk MJW. The management of benign liver lesions. In: Cameron J, Cameron A, editors. Current surgical therapy. 12th ed. Canada: Elsevier; 2016.
8. Kevin C, Soares TMP. The management of liver hemangioma. In: Cameron J, Cameron A, editors. Current surgical therapy. 12th ed. Canada: Elsevier; 2016.
9. Adam Bodzin RWB. Hepatic malignancy: resection versus transplantation. In: Cameron J, Cameron A, editors. Current surgical therapy. 12th ed. Canada: Elsevier; 2016.
10. Arun Chockalingam BPH, Hong K. Transjugular intrahepatic portosystemic shunt. In: Cameron J, Cameron A, editors. Current surgical therapy. 12th ed. Canada: Elsevier; 2016.
11. Christine E, Haugen AMC. Portal hypertension and the role of shunting procedures. In: Cameron J, Cameron A, editors. Current surgical therapy. 12th ed. Canada: Elsevier; 2016.
12. Hamilton JP. The management of Budd Chiari syndrome. In: Cameron J, Cameron A, editors. Current surgical therapy. 12th ed. Canada: Elsevier; 2016.
13. Jean Nicolas Vauthey JS. Liver. In: Fischer JE, editor. Master techniques in general surgery. Hepatobiliary and pancreatic surgery. 9th ed. United States: Lippincott Williams and Wilkins; 2013.
14. Zollinger R, Ellison EC. liver. Zollinger's atlas of surgical operation. 9th ed. United States: McGraw-Hill Education; 2011.
15. Clavien P-A. Liver. In: MGS P-AC, Fong Y, editors. Atlas of upper gastrointestinal and hepato-pancreatic-biliary surgery. 9th ed. Germany: Springer; 2007.

6 Surgical Aspects of Biliary Diseases for Clinical Board Exams

6.1 Part I: Knowledge

Knowledge has to be improved, challenged, and increased constantly, or it vanishes.
—Peter Drucker

History:

- Introduce yourself to the patient
- Name, age, occupation, sex, nationality
- History of presenting illness:
  - **Analysis of the chief complaint**

H. Alotaibi, *Study Surgery*, https://doi.org/10.1007/978-981-16-2305-9_6

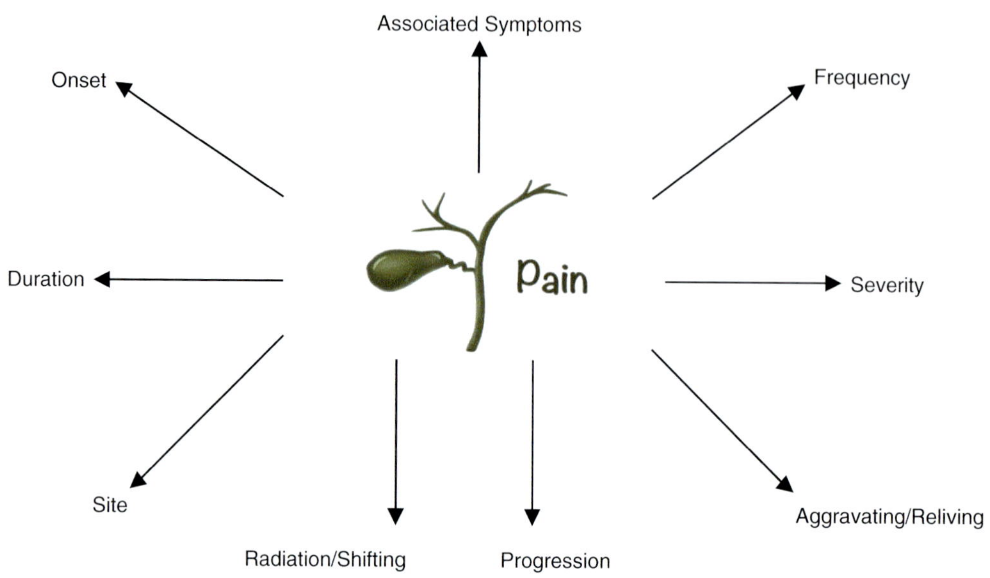
Associated Symptoms
Onset
Frequency
Pain
Duration
Severity
Site
Radiation/Shifting
Progression
Aggravating/Reliving

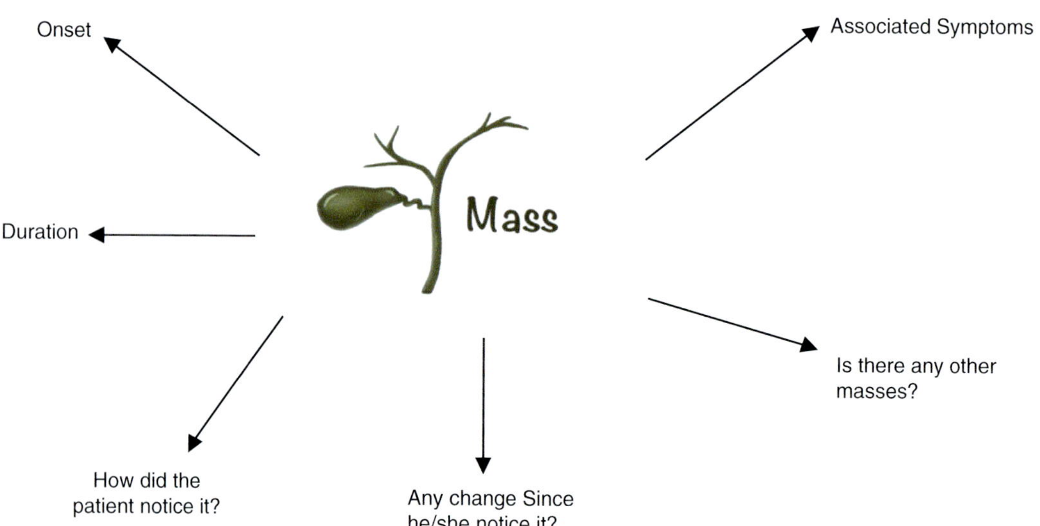
Onset
Associated Symptoms
Mass
Duration
How did the patient notice it?
Any change Since he/she notice it?
Is there any other masses?

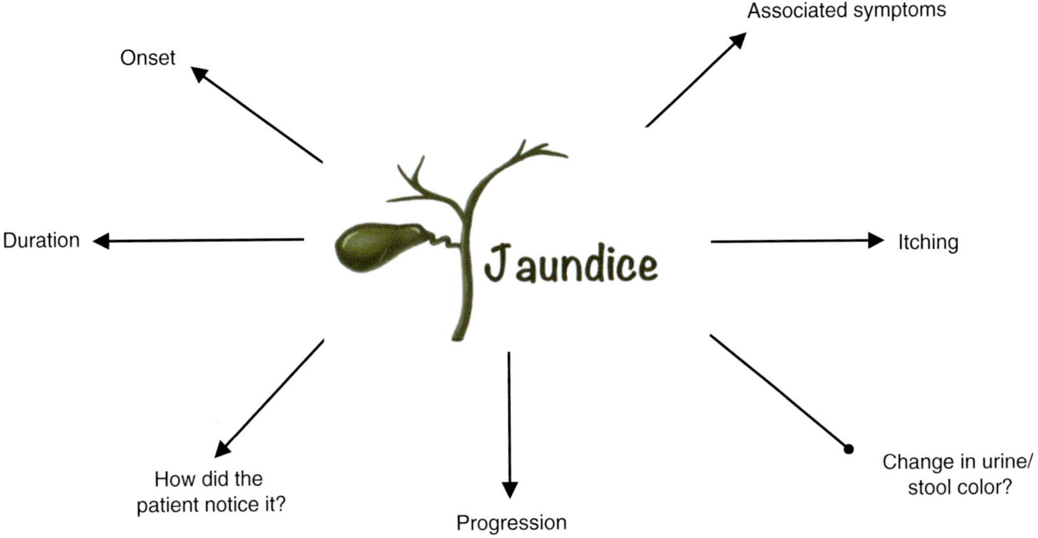

- **Associated symptoms:**
  Pain, fever, jaundice, nausea, vomiting, diarrhea, constipation, change in urine or stool color, itching, abdominal distention
- **Constitutional symptoms:**
  Weight loss, decreased appetite, night sweating, fever
- **Symptoms of metastasis:**
  Back pain, abdominal distention, cough, shortness of breath
- **Risk factors:**
  Rapid weight loss
  History of cirrhosis
  Oral contraceptive pills (OCP)
  Alcohol
  Family history of similar complaint or malignancy
  Personal history of cancer
  History of blood transfusion
  Vaccination
  Contact with sick patient
  Contact with animal
  Previous hepatobiliary surgery
  History of traveling
  Smoking
  History of IBD
- **Differential diagnosis**
  Chest pain (MI)
  Cough, fever, SOB (pneumonia)
  Recent history of trauma
- Previous similar attack, previous admission, previous investigation
- Systemic review of related system (GIT):
  Dysphagia, heart burn, hematemesis, melena, history of bleeding, ecchymosis

- PMH
- PSH
- Family history
- Social history
- Medication, transfusion, allergy
- Systemic review
  - CNS: headache, vision and hearing problems, epilepsy, numbness, paralysis
  - CVS: chest pain, orthopnea, paroxysmal nocturnal dyspnea, lower limb edema, palpitation
  - Respiratory: cough, fever, chest pain, hemoptysis
  - Renal: dysuria, flank pain, hematuria
  - MSK: weakness, arthritis, skin erythema

Physical examination:

- Introduce yourself to the patient
- Ask permission for examination
- Assure privacy

- Position: supine
- Exposure: nipple to mid-thigh
- Handwashing

General examination:

- **A**ppearance: ill, well, dehydrated
- **B**ody built: cachectic, obese
- **C**olor: pale, jaundice
- **D**istress
- **E**nvironment and connection to monitors, IV fluids, drains

Vital signs: BP, HR, temperature, RR, SpO_2
Hands:

- Muscle wasting
- Palmer erythema
- Clubbing
- Koilonychia (iron deficiency anemia)
- Leukonychia (hypoalbuminemia)
- Flapping tremor
- Pulse rate and its characteristics (rhythm, volume, etc.)

Eye:

- Jaundice
- Pallor

Mouth:

- Jaundice in mucus membrane, below the tongue
- Fetor hepaticus

Neck:

- Lymphadenopathy

Chest:

- Spider nevi
- Gynecomastia
- Respiratory and CVS examination

Abdomen:

- Inspection:
  - Distention
  - Asymmetry
  - Visible veins
  - Scars/striae
  - Dilated veins (caput medusa)
  - Hernial orifices
  - Stretch marks
  - Visible peristalsis
  - Signs of retroperitoneal hemorrhage (Grey Turner, Cullen, and Fox signs)
- Palpations:
  - Superficial then deep palpation
  - Look for any tenderness
  - Palpable masses
  - Ascites
  - Cough impulse at hernial orifices
  - Organomegaly
- Percussion:
  - Shifting dullness
  - Fluid thrill
  - Organomegaly
- Auscultation:
  - Bowel sounds
  - Bruit, venous hum

Groin, DRE, proctoscopy
Lower limbs: edema, swelling, skin rash, weakness
Back: for tenderness

6.1.1 Management of Asymptomatic Gallstones

- Incidentally discovered gallstones are those found on imaging performed for another purpose and the patient has no subjective symptoms related to gallstones.
- Only 20% of patients with asymptomatic cholelithiasis develop biliary symptoms.
- Prophylactic cholecystectomy:
  It is not indicated for asymptomatic cholelithiasis, with very few exceptions.

- **Polyps and gallstones:**
  The greatest concern with their presence is progression to adenocarcinoma.
  Patient with polyps >1 cm and those with radiographic evidence of vascular stalks should undergo cholecystectomy
- **Gallbladder wall calcifications:**
  There are two pathological calcifications in the gallbladder: selective focal and diffuse (porcelain gallbladder)
  The incidence of gallbladder cancer with selective calcification is higher than with the diffuse type
  The decision to proceed with prophylactic cholecystectomy in an asymptomatic patient with gallbladder wall calcification should be individualized to the patient
- **Small bowel resection:**
  Prophylactic cholecystectomy can be considered at the time of small bowel resection for carcinoid tumor if somatostatin therapy is to be used [1]

6.1.2 Management of Acute Cholecystitis

- Diagnostic criteria for acute cholecystitis:
  A. Local signs of inflammation:
    - Murphy's sign
    - RUQ mass/pain/tenderness
  B. Systemic signs of inflammation:
    - Fever
    - Elevated CRP
    - Elevated WBC count
  C. Imaging finding:
    - Imaging finding characteristic of acute cholecystitis
  Suspected diagnosis: one item in A + one item in B
  Definite diagnosis: one item in A+ one item in B + C
- Ultrasound abdomen is the recommended first-choice imaging modality for the morphological diagnosis of cholecystitis
  Diagnostic features in ultrasound:
  - Pericholecystic fluid
  - Distended gallbladder
  - Edematous wall
  - Posterior acoustic shadow of stones
  - Sonographic Murphy's sign
- Severity grading and management of acute cholecystitis (Table 6.1)
- What is the optimal timing of cholecystectomy for acute cholecystitis?
  The Tokyo Guidelines 2013 recommend early surgery regardless how much time passed since the onset of symptoms [3]
- Management: Table 6.1

6.1.3 Approach to Patient with Jaundice

- History and physical examination as described earlier
- Blood investigations:
  - CBC with differential
  - Electrolytes
  - Coagulation profile
  - LFT: ALT, AST, GGT, ALP, total bilirubin, direct bilirubin, albumin
  - Lipase, amylase
  - Renal function test
  - CRP, ESR
  - Hepatitis profile
  - Blood grouping
  - Tumor markers (CA 19-9, AFP, CEA)
- Imaging (according to the possible diagnosis):
  - Ultrasound abdomen (initial imaging modality)
  - CT abdomen (triphasic CT or pancreatic protocol)
  - MRCP/MRI
  - ERCP
  - EUS
  - Chest X-ray
- Management plan:
  - Admission (regular ward/ICU)
  - Diet (NPO/fat-free diet)
  - IV fluid
  - Analgesia
  - Antibiotic
  - Anti-emetic

Table 6.1 Classification and management of acute cholecystitis [2]

Severity classification	Criteria	Medical management	Surgical management
III (severe)	Associated with dysfunction of one of the following organs/systems: o Cardiovascular dysfunction: hypotension requiring treatment with dopamine ≥5 μg/kg/min, or any dose of epinephrine o Neurological dysfunction: decreased level of consciousness o Respiratory dysfunction: PaO_2/FiO_2 ratio <300 o Renal dysfunction: oliguria, creatinine >2.0 mg/dl o Hepatic dysfunction: PT-INR >1.5 o Hematological dysfunction: platelet count <100,000/mm^3	• The degree of organ dysfunction should be determined, and attempts made to normalize function through organ support • Monitor respiration and hemodynamics • Intravenous fluid • Electrolyte correction • Analgesia • Antimicrobial: Group: Antibiotic Penicillin group: Piperacillin/tazobactam Cephalosporin: Cefepime or ceftazidime ± metronidazole Carbapenem: Imipenem, meropenem, or ertapenem Fluroquinolone: –	If the patient can withstand surgery, early laparoscopic cholecystectomy can be performed. If the patient cannot withstand surgery, conservative treatment with early biliary drainage should be performed
II (moderate)	Associated with any of the following: o Elevated WBC count >18,000/mm^3 o Palpable tender mass in the right upper abdominal quadrant o Duration of complaints >72 h o Marked local inflammation (gangrenous, pericholecystic abscess, biliary peritonitis, emphysematous cholecystitis)	• Monitor respiration and hemodynamics • Intravenous fluid • Electrolyte correction • Analgesia • Antimicrobial: Group: Antibiotic Penicillin group: Piperacillin/tazobactam Cephalosporin: Ceftriaxone, cefotaxime ± metronidazole Carbapenem: Ertapenem Fluroquinolone: Ciprofloxacin, levofloxacin, moxifloxacin ± metronidazole	Laparoscopic cholecystectomy should be ideally performed soon after the onset if the ASA-PS score suggests that the patient can withstand the surgery. If the patient cannot withstand the surgery, conservative management and biliary drainage should be considered

Table 6.1 (continued)

Severity classification	Criteria	Medical management		Surgical management
I (mild)	Does not meet the criteria of grade III and II acute cholecystitis. It can be defined as acute cholecystitis in a healthy patient with no organ dysfunction and mild inflammatory changes	• Monitor respiration and hemodynamics • Intravenous fluid • Electrolyte correction • Analgesia • Antimicrobial:		Laparoscopic cholecystectomy should ideally be performed soon after the onset of symptoms
		Group	Antibiotic	
		Penicillin group	–	
		Cephalosporin	Cefazolin or cefuroxime or ceftriaxone ± metronidazole	
		Carbapenem	Ertapenem	
		Fluroquinolone	Ciprofloxacin, levofloxacin, moxifloxacin ± metronidazole	

Table 6.2 Differential diagnosis of jaundice

Prehepatic	Hepatic	Posthepatic
Hemolytic anemia Hemolysis	Cirrhosis Hepatitis Liver failure Gilbert's syndrome	Choledocholithiasis Mirizzi syndrome Bile duct stricture/injury Cholangiocarcinoma Periampullary cancers

- DVT and stress ulcer prophylaxis
- Definitive management (ERCP, surgery, drainage)

Differential diagnosis: Table 6.2

6.1.4 Approach to Patient with Cholangitis

1. Assure stability:
   - Airway: assure airway patency
   - Breathing: oxygenation and ventilation
   - Circulation:
     - Insert two large cannulas
     - Start IV fluid (RL)
     - Start broad spectrum antibiotics
     - Draw blood for:

       CBC with differential
       Electrolytes
       Coagulation profile
       Blood grouping
       LFT
       RFT
       Inflammatory marker: ESR, CRP
       Pan culture
       Urine analysis
       Amylase, lipase
     - Chest X-ray
     - ECG
     - Ultrasound abdomen
     - ICU consultation
2. If the patient is stable or stabilized after initial resuscitation:
   Take a history and perform a physical examination and determine the severity classification
3. Management:
   - Admission (ICU, HDU, ward)
   - Monitor vital signs
   - NPO
   - IV fluid
   - Analgesia/antipyretic
   - DVT and stress ulcer prophylaxis
   - IV antibiotics
4. Definitive management:
   Decompression of the biliary system. According to the cause and level of obstruction:

A. **Distal obstruction due to choledocholithiasis, stricture:**
Urgent decompression by ERCP ± sphincterotomy ± stent

B. **Proximal obstruction or if ERCP is not available:**
Percutaneous transhepatic drainage (PTD)

C. **If ERCP and PTD are not available:**
CBD exploration

D. **External compression from, for example, Mirizzi syndrome:**
Cholecystectomy [4]

6.1.5 Management of Choledocholithiasis

- Majority of CBD stones are formed within the gallbladder and migrate down the cystic duct into the CBD (i.e., secondary CBD stones) and are usually cholesterol stone
- Primary CBD stone usually brown pigmented stones and associated with biliary infection and stasis
- **Clinical manifestations:**
  - May be silent and often discovered incidentally
  - May cause complete or incomplete obstruction or they may manifest with cholangitis or gallstone pancreatitis
  - The typical pain caused by stone in the bile duct are similar to the pain caused by impacted stone in the cystic duct
  - Physical examination may reveal mild tenderness in the epigastric or right upper quadrant as well as mild jaundice
  - The symptoms may be intermittent due to stone impact temporarily in the ampulla but moves subsequently known as "a ball valve"
  - Small stones may pass through ampulla spontaneously
  - Some stones may impact completely causing progressive jaundice
- **Diagnosis:**
  - Ultrasound is useful for documenting gallbladder stones as well as the size of the common bile duct
  - Dilated CBD (>8 mm in diameter) on ultrasound in a patient with gallstones, jaundice, and biliary pain is highly suggestive of common bile duct stones.
  - If the presence of bile duct stone is in question, MRCP provides excellent anatomic detail (sensitivity 95% and specificity 89%).
  - ERCP is highly effective at diagnosing choledocholithiasis. However, due to risk associated with the procedure, it is rarely used as a diagnostic modality, rather being reserved for cases in which therapeutic intervention is indicated.
  - EUS has good diagnostic ability but less therapeutic capabilities, making it less desirable tool for diagnosis.
  - Percutaneous transhepatic cholangiography (PTC) is rarely needed in patients with CBD stone but can be performed for diagnostic and therapeutic reasons in patient with contraindication to endoscopic or surgical approaches.
- **Treatment:**
  - For patient with symptomatic gallstones with suspected CBD stones, bile duct clearance and cholecystectomy are indicated, and this can be achieved by:
    Preoperative ERCP followed by surgery
    Upfront surgery with intraoperative cholangiogram and CBD exploration

Both approaches are safe and effective.

- If endoscopic or laparoscopic exploration failed or not feasible, open CBD exploration is indicated. Choledochotomy in large duct can be closed primarily, while smaller duct should be closed over a T-tube. T-tube cholangiogram should be obtained before its removal at least several weeks after its placement.
- Impacted stone which could not be cleared by endoscopic approach or CBD exploration, transduodenal sphincterotomy can be considered.
- If still could not be cleared, choledochoduodenostomy or Roux-en-Y choledochojejunostomy may be the available options to restore biliary continuity.
- Retained stone (left in place at the time of surgery or diagnosed shortly after cholecystectomy).
- Recurrent stones (diagnosed months or years later after).
- Retained or recurrent stones after cholecystectomy are best treated endoscopically. Repeat surgery should be a last resort if other interventions have failed [5].

6.1.6 Management of Mirizzi Syndrome

- It is caused by the obstruction of the CBD or CHD by external compression from impacted gallstone in the Hartman's pouch.
- Presenting symptoms: similar to symptoms of obstructive jaundice due to CBD stones.
- Classifications:
  - Type I: no fistula is present, just external compression, but the stone impacted in the infundibulum of the gallbladder or cystic duct.
  - Type II: cholecysto-choledochal fistula less than 1/3 of the bile duct diameter.
  - Type III: cholecysto-choledochal fistula up to 2/3 of the bile duct diameter.
  - Type IV: complete destruction of the bile duct wall.
  - Type V: presence of cholecystoenteric fistula along with Mirizzi syndrome.
- Diagnosis:
  - Ultrasound
  - MRCP: the preferred modality when Mirizzi syndrome is suspected
  - ERCP: the gold standard modality of choice
  - CT
- Treatment (is always surgical):
  - Type I: cholecystectomy (open is preferred than laparoscopic) without exploration of the bile ducts. Sometimes partial cholecystectomy is indicated.
  - Type II: subtotal cholecystectomy, stone extraction, and leaving remnant of the gallbladder wall over the fistula to aid closure of the destroyed bile duct.
  - Types III and IV: biliary enteric anastomosis (Roux-en-Y hepaticojejunostomy) [6].

6.1.7 Management of Gallstone Ileus

- Occur when a large gallstone erodes through the wall of the gallbladder directly into the intestine via choledochoenteric fistula.
- The stones can then pass through the intestinal tract until they reach an area of narrowing.
- Proximal fistula with the stomach can cause gastric outlet obstruction due to stones impacted in the pylorus or proximal duodenum "Bouveret syndrome."
- Some stones move travel distally until become lodged at surgical anastomoses or ileocecal valve where it causes small bowel obstruction.
- Gallstone ileus is responsible for <1% of all intestinal obstruction.
- These patients present with symptoms of obstipation, nausea, and abdominal pain.
- Plain abdominal X-ray may show an obstructive bowel gas pattern and gas delineating the biliary tree, but may fail to identify radiolucent stones.
- Ultrasound evaluation may be limited by extensive bowel gas.
- CT is highly sensitive and specific for gallstone ileus and the location of the obstruction.
- Management:
  - The aim is to relieve the obstruction and remove the stones.
  - In case of very proximal obstruction in the stomach or duodenum, endoscopic retrieval can be effective.
  - For more distal stones, enterolithotomy can be accomplished laparoscopically or open
  - Stones are removed through enterotomy (just proximal to the impacted stone), which are then repaired or resected depending on its size.
  - Cholecystectomy and closure of the fistula at the time of enterolithotomy or at a later time remain a topic of debate, but it should be considered in stable and young patients [7].

6.1.8 Management of Cystic Disorders of the Bile Duct

- Congenital cystic dilatation of the extrahepatic and/or intrahepatic biliary tree.

- Affect females 3–8 times more often than males.
- The exact cause is unknown, but it is believed that weakness of the bile duct wall and increased pressure secondary to partial biliary obstruction contribute to biliary cyst formation.
- 90% of patient have an anomalous pancreaticobiliary duct junction, with the pancreatic duct joining the common bile duct outside the duodenum, creating a long common channel >1.5 cm. This may allow reflux of pancreatic secretion into the biliary tract.
- The typical clinical triad of biliary cysts includes abdominal pain, jaundice, and a palpable mass.
- Adult patients may present with cholangitis.
- Diagnosis is made by ultrasound or CT scan.
- MRCP or ERCP are essential to assess the biliary anatomy and to plan the appropriate surgical treatment.
- The risk of cholangiocarcinoma is 20- to 30-fold higher than in the general population and varies with the patient's age and type of cyst [8].
- Classification: Table 6.3

6.1.9 Management of Bile Duct Injury

- Typically result from perceptional error in identifying the anatomy.
- Most common injury occur with excessive cephalad traction of the gallbladder or insufficient lateral traction of the infundibulum.
- Other causes include excessive thermal cautery medial to the gallbladder, aberrant biliary anatomy or excessive inflammation [9].
- **Safety strategies to minimize the risk of bile duct injury during cholecystectomy:**
  1. Use the critical view of safety method of identification of the cystic duct and cystic artery during laparoscopic cholecystectomy.
     - The hepatocystic triangle is cleared of fat and fibrous tissue.
     - The lower one third of the gallbladder is separated from the liver to expose the cystic plate.
     - Two and only two structures should be seen entering the gallbladder.
  2. Understand the potential aberrant anatomy in all cases.

Table 6.3 Classification of biliary cysts [8]

Type I	**Type II**	**Type III**
Fig. 6.1	Fig. 6.2	Fig. 6.3
Fusiform CBD dilatation ▪ Most common type (~50%) ▪ Hight risk of malignancy (>60%) ▪ Management: should be cyst resection and frozen section of the margins (gross margin should be nondilated duct) with Roux-en Y hepaticojejunostomy reconstruction	Saccular dilatation of the extrahepatic bile ducts Management: Simple diverticulectomy and closure of the CBD at the diverticulum neck	Intraduodenal Low risk of malignancy (~2%) Management: Endoscopic sphincterotomy Large cyst: transduodenal excision
Type IVa	**Type IVb**	**Type V**
Fig. 6.4	Fig. 6.5	Fig. 6.6
Both intrahepatic and extrahepatic cystic dilations	Only extrahepatic cystic dilatation, management like type I	Caroli disease ▪ Rare <1% ▪ It can affect the entire liver ▪ Managed by resection if unilobar and liver transplantation is required in the advanced stage

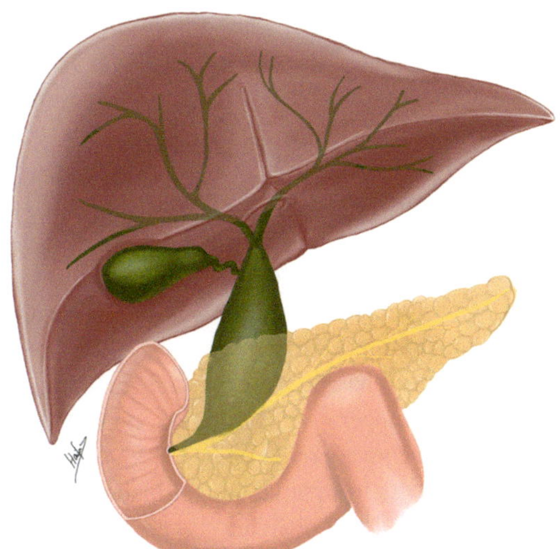

Fig. 6.1 Type I biliary cyst

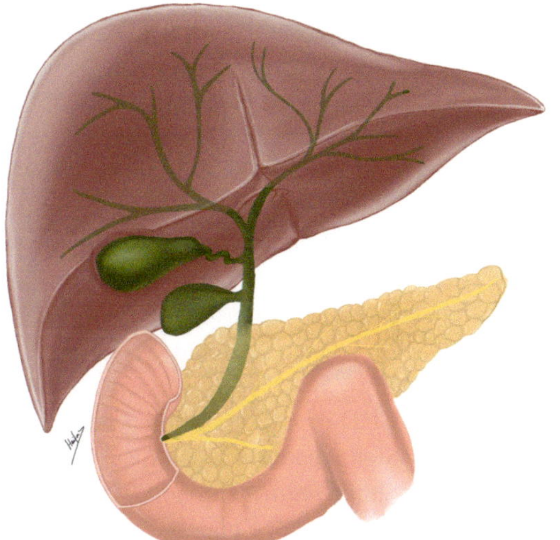

Fig. 6.2 Type II biliary cyst

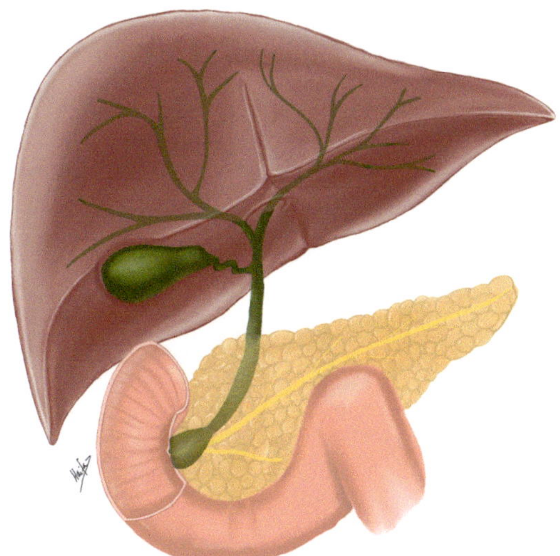

Fig. 6.3 Type III biliary cyst

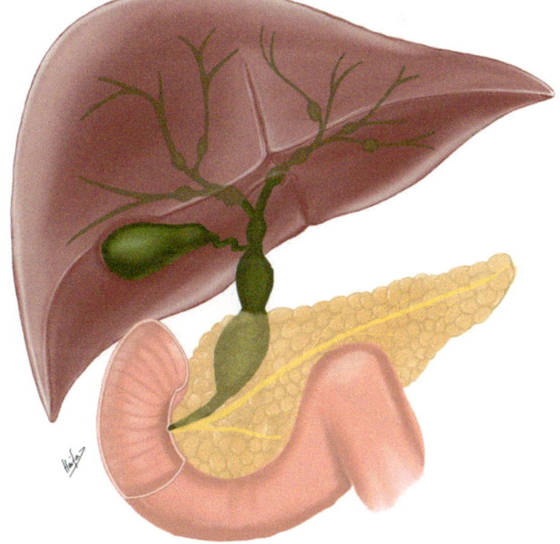

Fig. 6.4 Type IVa biliary cyst

3. Make liberal use of cholangiography or other methods to image the biliary tree intraoperatively.
4. Consider an intraoperative pause during laparoscopic cholecystectomy prior to clipping, cutting, or transecting any ductal structures.
5. Recognize when the dissection is approaching a zone of significant risk and halt dissection before entering the zone. Finish the operation by a safe method other than cholecystectomy if conditions around the gallbladder are too dangerous.
6. Get help from another surgeon when the dissection or condition are difficult [9, 10].

- **Clinical presentation:**
  - <40% discovered during the index of cholecystectomy

    <u>Off normal finding:</u>

    The standard 9-mm clip is insufficient to completely occlude the ductal structure

    Persistent leak of the bile from the liver

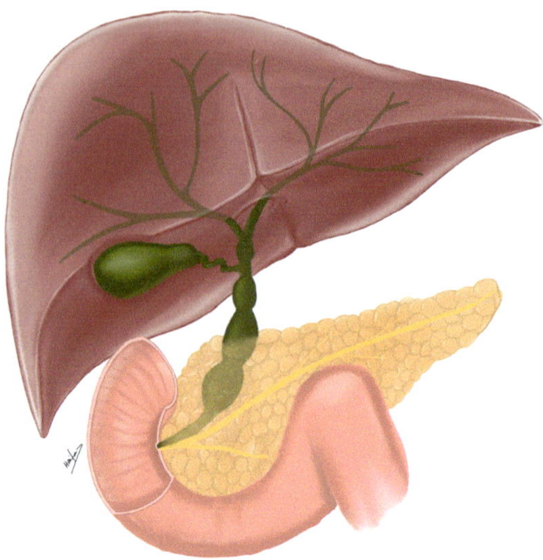

Fig. 6.5 Type IVb biliary cyst

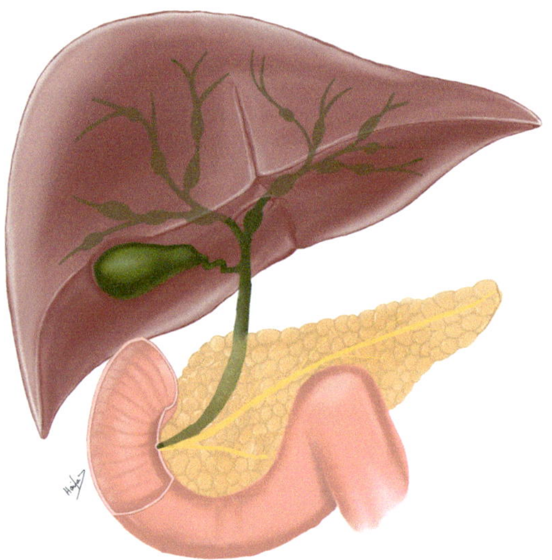

Fig. 6.6 Type V biliary cyst

Identification of second ductal structure
Extra soft tissue adjacent to the porta hepatis
Presence of large artery coursing behind the presumed cystic duct
Sustained bleeding from the area medial to the gallbladder
Excessive number of required clips
Inability to adequately identifying regional anatomic structure

– Because most of the biliary injury are unrecognized at the original operation, most common time is early postoperative period [9]

Management:

A. **Repair of immediately recognized injury:**
- Consult a second surgeon with significant hepatobiliary experience.
- Further characteristic of bile duct injury via intraoperative cholangiogram (IOC) or direct conversion to open.
- Attempts to remove the gallbladder if not already done, or ligate the proximal duct to allow dilatation should be avoided.
- Drainage of the gallbladder fossa or placing catheter in the proximal duct is advisable.
- If experienced surgeon available, repair in the original operation.
- If segmented or accessory duct <3 mm has been injured and IOC demonstrate segmental or subsegmental drainage: simple ligation.
- If the injured duct is ≥4 mm, more likely to drain multiple segments: operative repair (hepaticojejunostomy).
- All the repair should be drained externally.
- If the CHD or CBD is injured below the bifurcation: operative repair.
- If the injured segment is short (<1 cm) and the two ends can be opposed without tension: end-to-end anastomosis with T-tube through separate choledochotomy either above or below the anastomosis.
- End-to-end anastomosis should be avoided if the ductal injury near the bifurcation or if there is excessive loss of bile duct.
- If the injured segment is >1 cm: ligate the distal end and proximal end anastomosed in an end to side to Roux-en-Y jejunal limb.
- If no expert surgeon is available:
  – No repair should be attempt
  – No ligation of ducts
  – Drain via retrograde catheter

- Drain the subhepatic space
- Transfer to tertiary hepatobiliary center [9]

B. **Initial management after delayed recognition:**
- Immediate control of leak
- Evacuation of fluid collection
- Control of sepsis
- Empirical IV antibiotics and to be tailored according to the culture
- Complete cholangiography via PTC, MRCP, or ERCP
- CTA or MRA to rule out concurrent right hepatic artery injury (10–30%) [9]

C. **Definitive management of bile duct stricture:**
- Dilatation with angioplasty type balloon catheter
- Leave stent across the stricture to allow access to the biliary tree for repeat cholangiography, dilatation, and maintain the patency of the lumen
- Endoscopic balloon dilatation and reevaluation with cholangiography every 3–6 months [9]

Management according to the Strasberg-Bismuth classification: Table 6.4

6.1.10 Management of Gallbladder Cancer

- More in women than in men.
- The risk increased with age.
- **Risk factors:**
  - Cholelithiasis with the presence of chronic inflammation (the risk increases with the stone size)
  - Calcification of the gallbladder
  - Anomalous pancreaticobiliary duct junction
  - Gallbladder polyp >1 cm
  - Chronic typhoid infection
  - Primary sclerosing cholangitis
  - Inflammatory bowel disease
- It is often diagnosed at an advanced stage due to the aggressiveness and oftentimes asymptomatic in early stages, nature of the tumor, which can spread rapidly.

Table 6.4 Management of bile duct injury [9]

Type			Management
Type A	Fig. 6.7		ERCP and stent
Types B and C	Fig. 6.8	Fig. 6.9	Do not require operative intervention, but if the patient has repeated sepsis and cholangitis, right posterior sectionectomy may be performed
Type D	Fig. 6.10		Caused by cautery, require dilatation and stent. If operative approach is indicated, Roux-en-Y hepaticojejunostomy
Type E	Fig. 6.11	Fig. 6.12	Always require biliary enteric anastomoses Either single anastomosis or two anastomoses (right and left duct)
	Fig. 6.13	Fig. 6.14	
	Fig. 6.15		

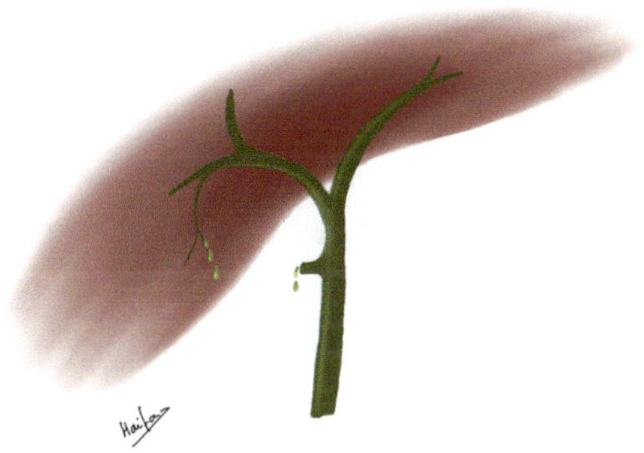

Fig. 6.7 Type A Strasberg bile duct injury

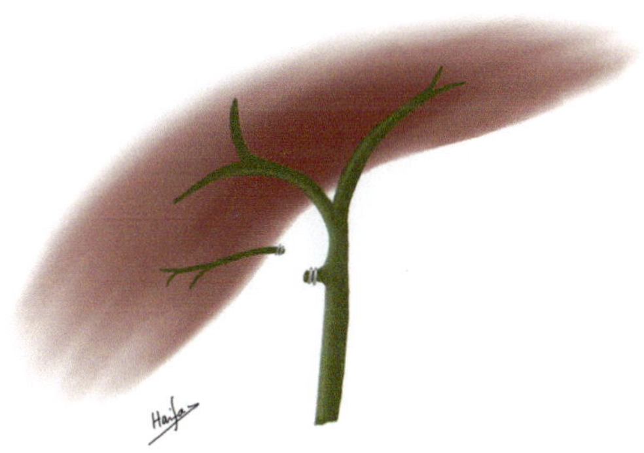

Fig. 6.8 Type B Strasberg bile duct injury

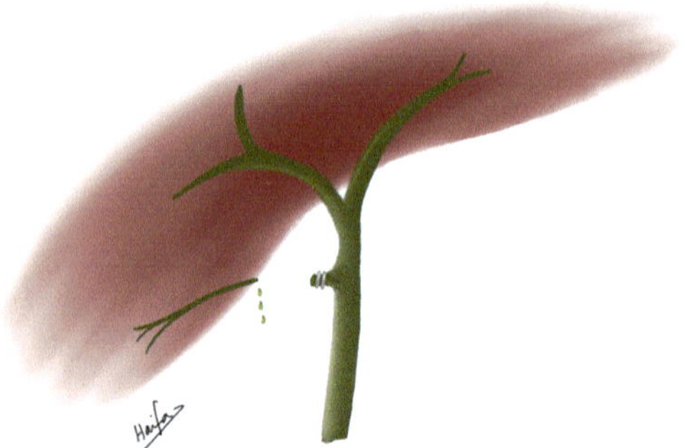

Fig. 6.9 Type C Strasberg bile duct injury

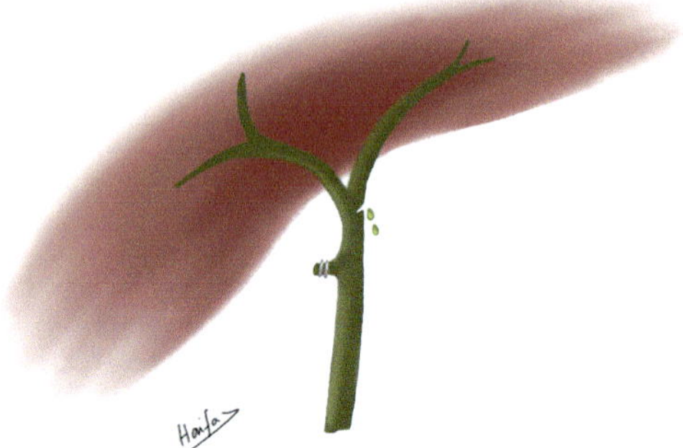

Fig. 6.10 Type D Strasberg bile duct injury

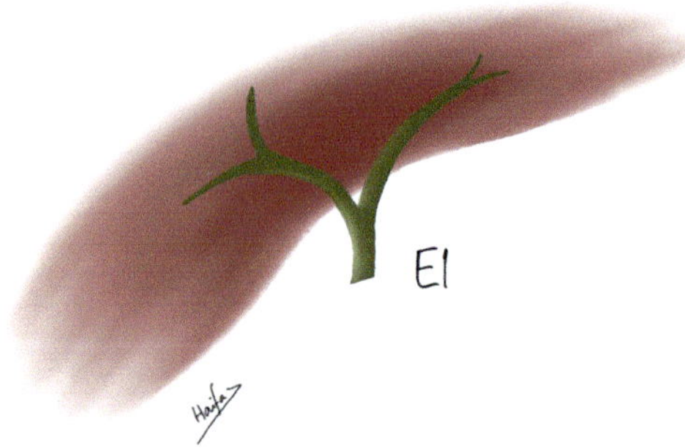

Fig. 6.11 Type E1 Strasberg bile duct injury

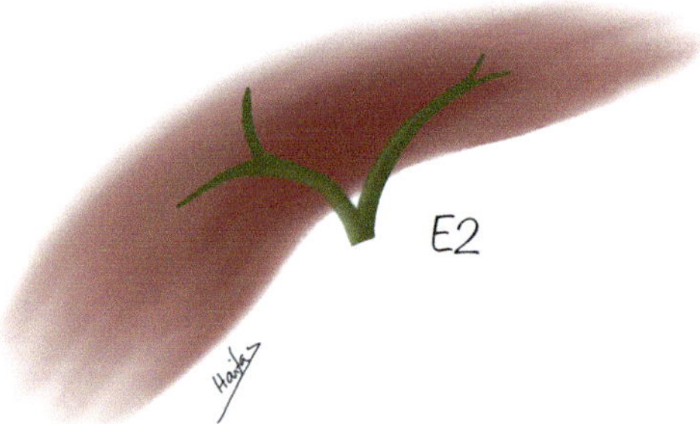

Fig. 6.12 Type E2 Strasberg bile duct injury

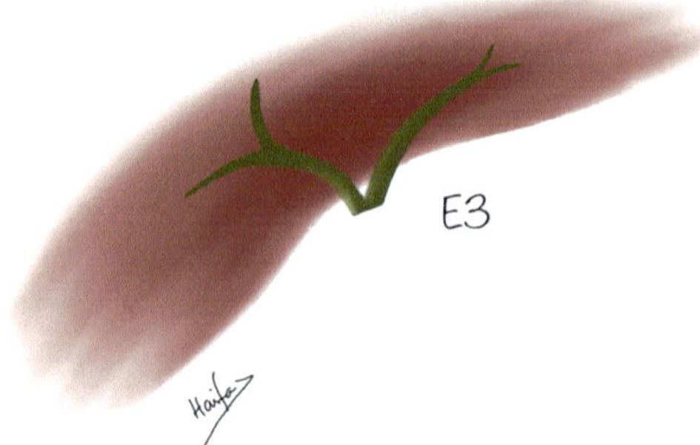

Fig. 6.13 Type E3 Strasberg bile duct injury

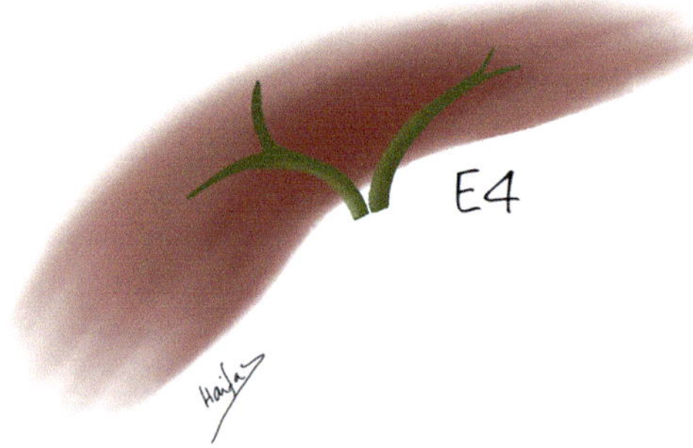

Fig. 6.14 Type E4 Strasberg bile duct injury

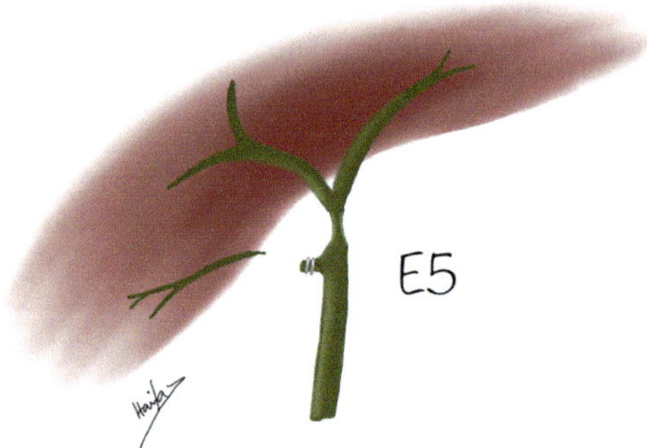

Fig. 6.15 Type E5 Strasberg bile duct injury

- It is common for the diagnosis of gallbladder cancer to be an incidental finding at cholecystectomy for presumed benign gallbladder disease or, more frequently, on pathologic review following cholecystectomy for symptomatic cholelithiasis.
- Other possible clinical presentation of gallbladder cancer is a suspicious mass detected on imaging.

- Any gallbladder mass, any gallbladder polyp >1 cm, or porcelain gallbladder should raise the suspicion of gallbladder cancer.
- The presence of jaundice with gallbladder cancer is associated with poor prognosis [11].
- **Workup:**
  - LFT
  - CT/MRI liver protocol
  - CT CAP
  - MRCP/ERCP/PTC for patient presenting with jaundice
  - CEA, CA 19-9
  - Biopsy is not recommended as it can result in peritoneal dissemination
- **Staging:** follow the AJCC TNM classification system
- **Surgical management:** depend on the stage
  1. **Tumor confined to lamina propria (T1a) (usually on the pathology report after cholecystectomy):**
     - Verify negative margin, including the cystic duct
     - Simple cholecystectomy
     - No lymphadenectomy is warranted
     - No further staging workup is recommended
     - If the cystic duct stump is involved, an excision of the common hepatic duct followed by Roux-en-Y hepaticojejunostomy
     - No routine postoperative treatment is required [11]
  2. **Tumor with muscular and perimuscular invasion (T1b and T2):**
     - Re-excision with radical or extended cholecystectomy (i.e., segments IVb/V hepatic resection) to achieve R0
     - Portal lymph node dissection (cystic, periportal, and hepatic artery lymph nodes. At least six lymph nodes must be removed)
     - Staging work up
     - Adjuvant treatment (fluoropyrimidine chemoradiation vs. gemcitabine-based or fluoropyrimidine-based chemotherapy)
     - Surveillance imaging (consider imaging every 3–6 months for 2 years then every 6–12 months for up to 5 years or as clinically indicated. Consider CEA and CA 19-9 as clinically indicated) [11]
  3. **Advanced tumor (T3 and T4):**
     - Staging work up
     - Consider diagnostic laparoscopy
     - Resection if no metastatic disease identified (M0)
     - Radical cholecystectomy (segments IVb/V resection, hepatic wedge resection, right hepatectomy, or trisectionectomy) to achieve R0
     - Portal lymphadenectomy
     - Adjuvant treatment (fluoropyrimidine chemoradiation vs. gemcitabine-based or fluoropyrimidine-based chemotherapy)
     - Surveillance imaging (consider imaging every 3–6 months for 2 years then every 6–12 months for up to 5 years or as clinically indicated. Consider CEA and CA 19-9 as clinically indicated) [11]
  4. **N2 and M1 disease:**
     - Contraindication to attempt at curative resection
     - Patients may require palliative operation for relieve of biliary obstruction (endoscopic/percutaneous drainage should be considered first-line treatment)
     - Palliative chemotherapy with gemcitabine/cisplatin therapy (fluoropyrimidine-based or gemcitabine-based chemotherapy regimens)
     - Resection of laparoscopic port site is not recommended [11]
- **Absolute contraindications for surgery:**
  - Medical comorbidities
  - M1 disease (including liver)
  - Involvement of N2 lymph nodes (peripancreatic, periduodenal, superior mesenteric)
  - Malignant ascites
  - Significant involvement of hepatoduodenal ligament
  - Encasement of major vasculature [11]

6.1.11 Management of Extrahepatic Cholangiocarcinoma

- More common than intrahepatic cholangiocarcinoma
- Occur anywhere within the extrahepatic bile duct from the junction of the right and left hepatic ducts to the common bile duct, including the intrapancreatic portion (and are further classified into hilar and distal tumor) [12]
- **Risk factors:**
  - Chronic inflammation
  - Primary sclerosing cholangitis
  - Choledochal cysts
  - Liver fluke infections
- **Hilar cholangiocarcinoma:**
  - It is the most common type of extrahepatic cholangiocarcinoma
  - Patients are likely to present with jaundice followed by evidence of a biliary obstruction or abnormality on subsequent imaging
  - Hilar stricture in the absence of previous biliary intervention is highly suspicious of cancer [12]
  - Work up:
    - LFT
    - CEA, Ca 19-9
    - Ultrasound
    - CT/MRI with IV contrast of the abdomen and pelvis (to assess lymph node status, presence of metastasis, extent of liver atrophy, presence of vascular involvement)
    - Assessment of the liver function and volume (many hilar resections include liver resection)
    - MRCP
    - ERCP/PTC is not recommended for the diagnosis of extrahepatic cholangiocarcinoma, since this is associated with complication and contamination of the biliary tree, but it helps to drain the biliary system (therapeutic)
    - Choledochoscopy
    - Brush cytology can be obtained for pathological evaluation [12]
- Right arterial invasion is more common than left arterial invasion because the right hepatic artery courses much closer to the confluence
- Staging: follow the AJCC guideline, TNM staging system
- Management:
  - Complete resection with negative margins is the only curative treatment for patient with resectable disease.
  - Patients suspected of having resectable disease should first undergo diagnostic laparoscopy.
  - Bismuth-Corlette type I and II (involving the bifurcation or proximal CHD) with no signs of vascular involvement are candidates for local tumor excision with portal lymphadenectomy, cholecystectomy, CBD excision, and bilateral Roux-en-Y hepaticojejunostomies.
  - If Bismuth-Corlette type IIIa or IIIb (tumors involve right or left hepatic duct), right or left hepatic lobectomy, respectively, should also be performed.
  - Resection of adjacent caudate lobe is required because of direct extension into caudate biliary radicals.
  - Normalize bilirubin by drainage is important, but the goal is <6–7 mg/dl prior to resection.
  - There is no proven role for adjuvant chemotherapy in the treatment of cholangiocarcinoma.
  - Type IV tumors, those with more extensive involvement of both hepatic ducts and intrahepatic spread, are often considered unresectable or only treatable with liver transplantation. However, there are very restrictive criteria for transplantation.
  - Nonoperative biliary decompression can be performed for patients with unresectable disease on initial presentation. Endoscopic placement of expandable metal stents is often the preferred approach.
  - Patients with unresectable disease can be offered palliative chemotherapy, typically with gemcitabine and cisplatin.
  - Criteria for unresectability:
    - Hepatic duct involvement up to secondary biliary radical bilaterally
    - Encasement or occlusion of the main portal vein proximal to its bifurcation

Atrophy of one hepatic lobe with contralateral encasement of portal vein branch
Atrophy of one hepatic lobe with contralateral involvement of secondary biliary radical
Unilateral tumor extension to secondary biliary radicals with contralateral vein branch encasement or occlusion [12]

- **Distal cholangiocarcinoma:**
  - The presentation is similar to that of other periampullary tumors
  - Painless jaundice, constitutional symptoms are the usual presenting symptoms
  - Work up:
    LFT
    Ultrasound
    CEA, CA 19-9
    CT pancreatic protocol
    MRCP/ERCP (routine ERCP and stenting are not recommended because it colonize the biliary tree with enteric organism and increase the postoperative complication)
    EUS
    Choledochoscopy
    Brush cytology
  - Unlike hilar cholangiocarcinoma, major hepatic resection is not required and no need to resolve the jaundice preoperatively
  - Staging: follow the AJCC TNM system
  - Management:
    Resection (i.e., pancreaticoduodenectomy)
    Criteria of resectability include the absence of both metastatic and locally advanced disease
    Frozen section biopsy of the bile duct and the pancreas should be obtained to confirm a negative margin
    Distal cholangiocarcinoma is not chemosensitive, but adjuvant treatment may be used in case of positive margin or lymph node
    Unresectable disease warrants either stenting or biliary bypass and consideration of chemotherapy and radiotherapy
- Long-term surveillance: consider imaging every 3–6 months for 2 years then every 6–12 months for up to 5 years or as clinically indicated [12]

6.1.12 Biliary Operations

Preoperative preparation:

- Admission
- NPO
- IV fluid
- Analgesia
- Prophylactic medications: antibiotic, DVT prophylaxis, stress ulcer prophylaxis
- Preoperative laboratory investigations: CBC, LFT, RFT, coagulation profile, blood group
- Review the preoperative imaging
- Explain the procedure to the patient and obtain informed consent
- Anesthesia consultation

Consent for Cholecystectomy ± IOC ± CBD Exploration:

1. *Explain the procedure:* Removal of the gallbladder under general anesthesia and through right subcostal incision/four small port incisions ± intraoperative cholangiogram through cystic duct or the CBD.
   Mention the possibility of conversion to open if the planned procedure is laparoscopic.
   If CBD exploration is to be done, mention that exploration of the biliary tree through the cystic duct/CBD to remove the stones and close the duct over a T-tube if it is via choledochotomy.
   The T-tube to be removed few weeks later after cholangiography.
2. *Explain if any alternative is available:* like conservative management or postoperative ERCP for stone removal.
3. *Explain the possible complications:*
   General: bleeding, wound infection, atelectasis, pneumonia, wound dehiscence, incisional hernia, DVT, PE, MI.

Specific: intra-abdominal fluid collection, bile leak, injury to bile ducts or other nearby organs, and bile duct stricture.

Open CBD Exploration:

- Under general anesthesia and endotracheal intubation.
- Time out: make sure correct patient, correct procedure, availability of special instruments like laparotomy set, Thompson retractor, Randall forceps, choledochoscopy, Fogarty catheter, glucagon, electrohydraulic lithotripsy, T-tube, Dormia basket, #15 blade, C-arm, set for cholangiogram.
- Position: supine.
- Prepping and draping in usual sterile fashion.
- Incision: upper midline, right subcostal.
- Open skin in layers, muscle cutting if Kocher incision till reaching the peritoneum.
- Kocher maneuver to expose the retro-duodenal CBD.
- Do cholangiography.
- Palpate the CBD to detect the location of any CBD stone.
- Aspirate to confirm CBD.
- Dissect out the CBD, remove areolar tissue anterior to CBD.
- Place two stay sutures, inferior to cystic duct takeoff, using fine monofilament absorbable suture, for example, PDS or Maxon.
- Putting gentle traction on the stay suture to elevate the anterior wall of CBD.
- Make small longitudinal incision (choledochotomy) between two stay sutures using #11 or #15 blade, then enlarge the opening to about 1.5 cm using Potts scissors.
- Be aware that the blood supply is running longitudinally at 3 O'clock position so, avoid the incision in these positions.
- Gently milk any stone into the choledochotomy using thumb and forefingers.
- Place a small red rubber Robinson catheter into cholechodotomy, pass it superiorly and inferiorly, irrigate with saline.
- Pass a biliary Fogarty catheter distal to any detected stone, inflate, and gently pull back on the catheter.
- If the above maneuvers are unsuccessful, Randal stone forceps can be gently passed to retrieve the stone, taking care not to make false passage during instrumentation.
- Perform choledochoscopy using a flexible choledochoscope (it should pass superiorly into hepatic ducts and inferiorly going through the ampulla into duodenum.
- Dormia basket should be passed through the working port of the scope to remove multiple stones.
- Fogarty balloon catheter can be passed under choledochoscopy to facilitate stone removal.
- Choledochoscopy should be continued until the entire extrahepatic ducts are clearly seen to be free.
- Cholechodotomy can be closed primarily or over a T-tube.
- Primary closure:
  - Use fine monofilament absorbable suture (PDS or Maxon), the size depends on the CBD size.
  - Large ductotomy can be closed in continuous fashion, while small duct should be closed by interrupted sutures (tie the sutures only after all of them have been placed).
  - Insert close suction drain near the choledochotomy.
- Closure over T-tube:
  - Use 16 fr T-tube (larger size for larger duct).
  - Cut off half of the circumference.
  - Insert the T-tube.
  - Close the cholechodotomy over the T-tube using running stitch of monofilament absorbable sutures to create watertight closure.
  - The tube should be moved down and cholechodotomy is sutures from above downward.
  - Irrigate the T-tube with saline to ensure that it is watertight.
  - Perform T-tube cholangiogram.
  - Bring the T-tube through separate stab skin incision.
  - Secure it with two sutures (2-0 Nylon).
  - Place close suction drain.

- Close the incision in layers.
- Close the skin by stapler [12].

Laparoscopic Cholecystectomy:

- Under general anesthesia and endotracheal intubation.
- Time out: make sure correct patient, correct procedure, availability of special instruments like two 5 mm trocars, two 10 mm trocars.
- If cholangiogram will be done, C-arm and cholangiography set to be available.
- Position: supine with slight reverse Trendelenburg position with the table slightly tilt to the left.
- Prepping and draping in usual sterile fashion.
- Access to intraperitoneal space:
  - Open (Hasson) technique: through supra/infra umbilical transverse incision, the base of the umbilicus is everted using clamp. Make a gap in the *Linea alba*. The trocar can be inserted directly into the peritoneal cavity. Use 30 degree telescope to confirm correct entry; insufflate CO_2 to reach pressure 14–15 mmHg. Placement of other trocars under direct vision as illustrated in Fig. 6.16.
- Exploration: start from the center (site of port entry) and explore all the quadrants, and report any positive finding.
- Retraction and dissection of the Calot's triangle:
  - Cephalad retraction of the fundus using the most lateral port and lateral retraction of the Hartman's pouch by the upper lateral port.
  - Incise the peritoneal attachment behind the Hartman's pouch to separate the pouch from the liver and further stretch out Calot's triangle.
  - Hook dissection can be used, staying close to the gallbladder to incise the anterior peritoneal attachments over the Calot's triangle.
  - Once the two ductal structures are seen, create a window between these two structures.

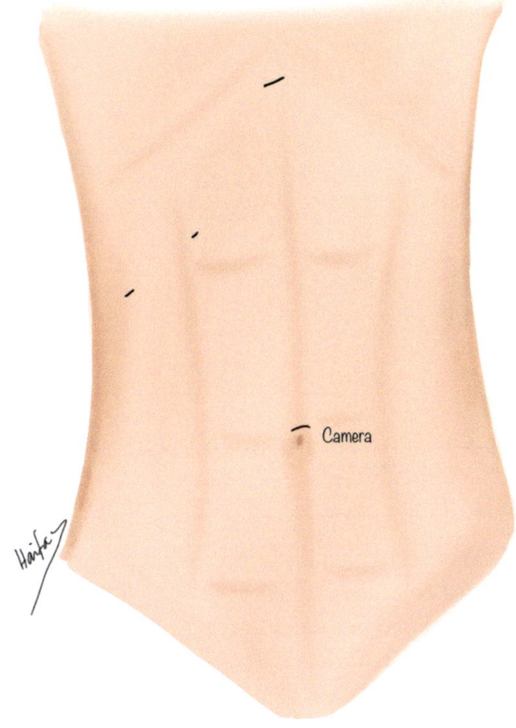

Fig. 6.16 Trocars positions in laparoscopic cholecystectomy

  - The lateral one third of the gallbladder is dissected from the underling liver surface to create the critical view of safety.
  - If two and only two structures are entering the gallbladder then the anatomy is determined, and the duct and the artery can be divided (Fig. 6.17).
- The cystic artery is divided between clips and a clip is placed below the Hartman's pouch on the proximal cystic duct and two clips are placed on the distal end (not too close to the CBD), then the duct is divided.
- Removal of the gallbladder from the liver using hook diathermy. This is done through a combination of elevation of the peritoneum, burning with the hook and pushing so that the gallbladder is removed toward the fundus and finally separated from the liver at the fundus.
- Then the gallbladder is removed by endo-bag through the epigastric port.

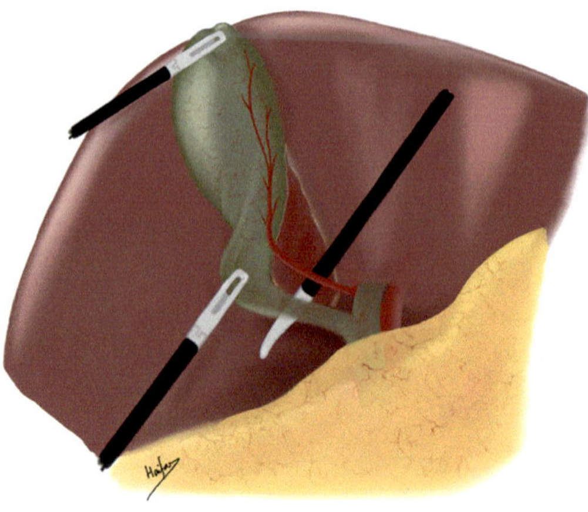

Fig. 6.17 Critical view of safety during dissection of the Calot's structures

- The insufflation is stopped, and the gas evacuated from the peritoneal cavity while removing the trocars under vision.
- The defect in the *Linea alba* is closed using absorbable braided sutures (vicryl 2-0).
- The skin is closed using sutures/clips [13–15].

Open Cholecystectomy:

- Under general anesthesia and endotracheal intubation.
- Time out: make sure correct patient, correct procedure, availability of special instruments like retractors, open cholecystectomy set ± cholangiography and C-arm to be available.
- Position: supine with slight reverse Trendelenburg position.
- Prepping and draping in usual sterile fashion.
- A right subcostal incision is made two finger's width below the costal margin. The rectus sheath is divided in the line of the incision and this is taken down to the peritoneal cavity using diathermy coagulation.
- Once the peritoneal cavity is entered, three packs are inserted, one behind the liver, one on the colon, and one over the gastroduodenal area and retractors are placed over the gastroduodenal area and over the liver to place the Calot's triangle on stretch.
- The key step of the open cholecystectomy is division of the cystic artery which allows the Hartman's pouch to swing out and allow clear definition of the biliary anatomy.
- The cystic duct is clipped and the gallbladder is retracted inferiorly and dissected free of the liver.
- Hemostasis and closure of the abdomen in layers [13–15].

Open Resection of Choledochal Cyst:

- Under general anesthesia and endotracheal intubation.
- Time out: make sure correct patient, correct procedure, availability of special instruments like Thompson retractor, open cholecystectomy set ± cholangiography and C-arm to be available.
- Position: supine position with the right arm tucked to the patient.
- Prepping and draping in usual sterile fashion.
- Incision: the choice is based on the surgeon preference and influenced by the body habitus of the patient, right subcostal incision or inverted L incision can be done.
- Cholecystectomy is started by incising the peritoneum overlying the gallbladder neck. The cystic duct typically arises from the lateral midportion of the fusiform cyst wall. The cystic artery is identified, isolated, clamped, and divided. A top-down dissection of the gallbladder from the liver bed.
- Kocher maneuver is done to mobilize the duodenum from the retroperitoneum.
- The peritoneum is incised on the superior border along the first part of the duodenum and it is reflected downward and medially to expose the anterior surface of the cyst wall.
- Continue dissection until the distal common bile duct is circumferentially isolated.
- The lower end of the cyst is encircled with a vessel loop and used for traction. This maneuver provides excellent exposure of the adjacent portal vascular structure.
- The dilation commonly extends behind the duodenum and into the substance of the pan-

creas. Therefore, care must be taken not to injure the underlying pancreatic duct.

- In order to achieve a complete cyst excision, it is essential to follow the distal extent of the cyst dissection until a normal sized duct is identified.
- Once identified, the normal size bile duct is divided and oversewn with 3-0 or 4-0 absorbable suture, the proximal end of the divided duct is also oversewn to avoid spillage of the bile.
- The choledochal cyst is then reflected upward to allow dissection away from the portal vein and hepatic artery. This tissue plan is usually areolar and flimsy and can be reflected by blunt dissection up to the hepatic bifurcation and the duct is divided at the point when transit to a normal caliber.
- Biliary-enteric reconstruction:
  - It is best done using a 70-cm retro colic Roux-en-Y hepaticojejunostomy.
  - The Roux enteric limb is prepared and the posterior raw of the hepaticojejunostomy is constructed with interrupted 4-0 or 5-0 absorbable monofilament suture that all tied after placement of all the sutures. The anastomosis is then completed as an end to side hepaticojejunostomy in the same way (Fig. 6.18).
  - Close suction drain is placed behind the anastomosis.
- Hemostasis and closure of the abdominal wall in layers [13–15].

Complications:

- Bleeding: The major intraoperative complication is bleeding. This is typically from a very short cystic artery or from right hepatic artery itself. Bleeding from the portal vein is rare.
- Bile duct injury.
- Postoperative bile leak.
- Subphrenic collection.
- Bile duct stricture.
- Pneumonia.
- Atelectasis.
- DVT.
- Pulmonary embolism (PE).

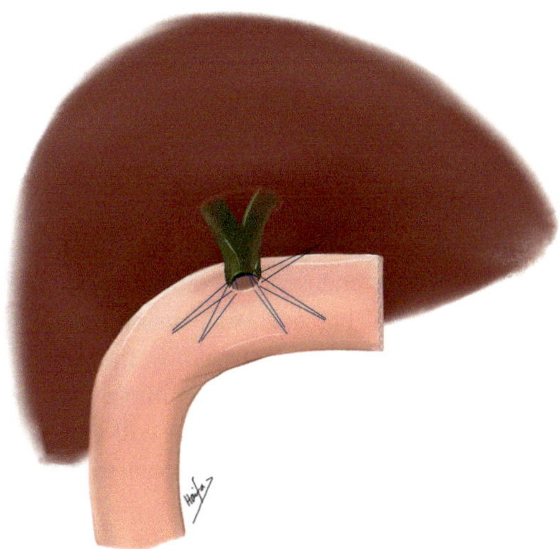

Fig. 6.18 Hepaticojejunostomy using interrupted sutures with knots tied to the inside of the posterior wall and to the outside of the anterior wall

- Myocardial infarction (MI).
- Wound infection or dehiscence.
- Incisional hernia.

6.2 Part II: Practice

Knowledge is of no value unless you put it into practice.
—Anton Chekhov

6.2.1 Case Scenarios for Practice

Tips:

- Practice with a friend and try to mimic the real exam!
  Do not forget to set the timer!
- The clinical data are provided in the answer key section.
- Some twist points are suggested after some cases and can be used to change the scenario to a more difficult one.

Case No. 1:

A 39-year-old male patient presented to the emergency department complaining of right upper abdominal pain, fever, and jaundice for 5 days.

Questions for Discussion:

1. How will you approach the patient?
2. What will you do next?
3. What will be your next step of the management?
4. ERCP shows multiple CBD stones (the largest is 9 mm), the endoscopist could remove most of the stones, but one stone was difficult to retrieve, so he did sphincterotomy, the patient's hemodynamics parameters are improving, but his bilirubin is still raising, what will you do?
5. What are the intraoperative options to remove the stone?
6. The patient was taken to operating room and laparoscopic cholecystectomy was done, a trial of laparoscopic CBD exploration was failed to remove the stone and the operation was converted to open exploration and the stone is removed. How will you close the CBD?
7. If you close over a T-tube, when will you remove it?
8. Six months later, the patient came with jaundice and abdominal pain and the MRCP revealed stricture at the closure site. How will you manage it?

Suggested Twist Point:

- You are in primary center and neither ERCP nor intervention radiologist are available. How will you manage the patient?

Case No. 2:
A 51-year-old male patient presented to the clinic complaining of upper abdominal pain for 6 months.

Questions for Discussion:

1. How will you approach the patient?
2. What will you do next?
3. What is your differential diagnosis?
4. How will you confirm the most likely diagnosis?
5. How will you manage him?
6. Intraoperative you sent a frozen section of the cystic duct and the result came as positive for malignant cells. How will you manage that?
7. What are the possible complications?

Suggested Twist Points:

- The patient presented with picture of acute cholecystitis and laparoscopic cholecystectomy was done. Later, the pathology revealed adenocarcinoma of the gallbladder that invades the muscularis layers. How you will manage?
- During exploration, you discovered distant metastasis to the liver. What will you do?

Case No. 3:
A 70-year-old male patient presented to the emergency department complaining of abdominal pain and vomiting for 3 days.

Questions for Discussion:

1. How will you approach this patient?
2. What is your differential diagnosis?
3. What are the investigations would you like to order for this patient?
4. What further investigations you want to do to confirm the diagnosis?
5. What is your final diagnosis?
6. How will you manage it?
7. What will you do with the biliary-enteric fistula?
8. You did the surgery and few days later the patient is complaining from foul smelling discharge from the wound. What will you do?
9. You opened the wound partially; the fluid looks like bowel content and you started the patient on IV antibiotic. What will you do after that?
10. The CT showed no intra-abdominal fluid collection, and the oral contrast is demonstrating a tract connecting the distal ileum to the wound. What is your diagnosis and how will you manage it?

Suggested Twist Points:

- The patient is young and healthy. How will you manage the biliary-enteric fistula?
- The stone was causing pressure necrosis on the small bowel wall. How will you deal with it?

Case No. 4:
A 29-year-old male patient presented to the clinic complaining of abdominal pain, jaundice for 2 months.

Questions for Discussion:

1. How will you approach this patient?
2. What is your differential diagnosis?
3. What are the investigations you would like to do?
4. What is your diagnosis?
5. How will you manage this patient? and why?
6. What will be your extent of resection?
7. How will you prepare the patient for operation?

Suggested Twist Points:

- Few days postoperation, the patient's drain brought greenish fluid. What will you do?
- Change the type of the biliary cyst.

Case No. 5:
A 37-year-old male patient presented to the emergency department complaining of right upper abdominal pain and vomiting for 3 days

Questions for Discussion:

1. How will you approach the patient?
2. What is your differential diagnosis?
3. What further investigation will you do?
4. How will you manage this patient?
5. The patient underwent a difficult laparoscopic cholecystectomy. On the third postoperative day, you removed the drain and discharged the patient. Three days later, the patient presented to the emergency department complaining of severe abdominal pain, fever, and jaundice. What is your differential diagnosis?
6. What will you do next?
7. The ultrasound showed dilated intrahepatic duct and no collection. The MRCP showed dilated intrahepatic biliary radicals and cutoff sign at the level of the CHD. What will you do next?
8. What is the type of this injury?
9. The patient underwent decompression of the biliary system via PTD and his symptoms improved. What will be the definitive management of his condition?

Suggested Twist Points:

- At the time of cholecystectomy, you noticed bile coming from the area of the porta hepatis, how will you manage it?
- During the perioperative period the drain output is bile. What will you do?

Checklist

History	Items	Done	Not done	Not applicable
General	Introduce himself/herself to the patient			
	Patient personal data (name, age, sex, nationality)			
	Chief complaint			
	Duration			
Pain	Onset			
	Site			
	Character			
	Radiation/shifting			
	Aggravating/relieving			
	Severity			
	Progression			
	Frequency			
Mass	Onset			
	Site			
	How did the patient notice it?			
	Any change since it was first noticed?			
	Other masses			
Jaundice	Onset			
	Itching			
	Change in stool or urine color			
	Progression			
Associated symptoms	Pain			
	Fever			
	Nausea			
	Vomiting			
	Diarrhea			
	Constipation			
	Abdominal distention			
Constitutional symptoms	Weight loss			
	Decrease appetite			
	Night sweating			
Symptoms of metastases	Back pain			
	Cough			
	Shortness of breath			
	Abdominal distention			
Risk factors	Rapid weight loss			
	History of cirrhosis			
	Alcohol, drug abuse			
	Smoking			
	History of IBD			
	Contact with animal			
	Contact with sick people			
	Previous hepatobiliary surgery			
	History of traveling			
	Personal history of malignancy			
	Family history of similar complain			
Differential diagnosis	Chest pain (MI)			
	Cough, SOB (pneumonia)			
	Recent history of trauma			

History	Items	Done	Not done	Not applicable
PMH	Previous similar attack			
	Previous investigation			
	Previous admission			
	Chronic illnesses			
PSH	Previous surgery			
Family history	Of cancers or hepatic problem			
Social history	Occupation			
	Habits (smoking, alcohol, drugs)			
Other	Medication			
	Allergy			
	Transfusion			
Systemic review				
Physical examination				
General principle	Patient position			
	Exposure			
	Privacy			
	Wash hands			
General examination	Appearance			
	Body built			
	Color			
	Distress/decubitus			
	Environment			
Vital signs	BP, HR, temperature, RR, SpO_2			
Hand signs	Muscle wasting, palmar erythema, clubbing, flapping tremor, leukonychia, koilonychia			
Eyes	Jaundice, pallor			
Mouth	Jaundice, fetor hepaticus			
Neck	Lymphadenopathy			
Chest	Spider nevi, gynecomastia, respiratory and CVS examination			
Abdomen: Inspection	Distention			
	Asymmetry			
	Dilated veins			
	Striae			
	Visible peristalsis			
	Scars			
	Signs of retroperitoneal hemorrhage			
Palpation	Superficial then deep palpation			
	Tenderness			
	Palpable masses			
	Organomegaly			
	Cough impulse at hernial orifices			
Percussion	Shifting dullness			
	Fluid thrill			
	Organomegaly			
Auscultation	Bowel sounds			
	Bruit, venous hum			
Groin				
DRE and proctoscopy				
Back tenderness				
Differential diagnosis	According to the given scenario			

(continued)

History	Items	Done	Not done	Not applicable
Investigations				
General laboratory test	CBC with differential			
	Electrolytes			
	Liver function test (ALT, AST, GGT, albumin, total bilirubin, direct bilirubin)			
	Amylase and lipase			
	Coagulation profile (PT, INR, aPTT)			
	Blood grouping			
	RFT			
	CPR/ESR			
	Blood culture			
Specific tests	Tumor marker (AFP, CEA, Ca19-9)			
Imaging	Ultrasound abdomen			
	Triphasic CT abdomen			
	MRI/MRCP			
	ERCP/choledochoscopy			
Biopsy	Brush cytology			
Provisional diagnosis	According to the given scenario			
Management (depends on the diagnosis)				
Acute cholecystitis	Admission			
	Fat-free diet/NPO			
	IV fluid			
	Antibiotics			
	Antipyretic			
	Prophylaxis (DVT and stress ulcer)			
	Cholecystectomy			
	Consent			
	Percutaneous drainage (cholecystostomy) if indicated			
Acute cholangitis	Assess stability (ABC)			
	Resuscitation			
	Admission to ICU/ward			
	Assess severity			
	Medication: antipyretic, antibiotics, antiemetic, DVT prophylaxis, and stress ulcer prophylaxis as needed			
	Decompression (ERCP, PTD, surgical)			
Biliary cyst	Admission			
	NPO if required			
	IV fluid			
	Analgesia			
	DVT and stress ulcer prophylaxis			
	Preoperative preparation			
	Consent			
	Surgical management			

History	Items	Done	Not done	Not applicable
Bile duct injury	Recognition			
	Further assessment of the injury (MRCP, ERCP, CTA)			
	Drainage if indicated (ERCP, PTD, percutaneous drainage for collection)			
	Referral to tertiary center or expert hepatobiliary surgeon			
	Preoperative preparation			
	Consent			
	Surgical management if indicated			
Gallbladder cancer	Staging if T1b and above			
	Multidisciplinary team discussion			
	Preoperative preparation if resectable			
	Admission			
	NPO			
	IV fluid			
	Consent			
	ICU consultation			
	Anesthesia consultation			
	Extended/simple cholecystectomy			
	Frozen section from the cystic duct margin			
	Resection of the extrahepatic duct if frozen result is positive			
Hilar cholangiocarcinoma	Staging			
	Multidisciplinary team discussion			
	Assess resectability			
	Preoperative management of jaundice (drainage)			
	Assess the future liver remnant			
	Admission			
	Consent			
	NPO			
	IV fluid			
	Prophylactic medication (DVT and stress ulcer and preoperative antibiotics)			
	Exploration			
	Resection			
	Frozen section of the margins			
	Reconstruction			
Distal cholangiocarcinoma	Staging			
	Multidisciplinary team discussion			
	Assess resectability			
	Admission			
	Consent			
	NPO			
	IV fluid			
	Prophylactic medication (DVT and stress ulcer and preoperative antibiotics)			
	Exploration			
	Resection			
	Frozen section of the margins			
	Reconstruction			
	Prophylactic antibiotic			

(continued)

History	Items	Done	Not done	Not applicable
Postoperative care				
Early postoperative	Admission to HDU or ICU			
	Early mobilization and DVT prophylaxis			
	Enteral nutrition as early as possible			
	Analgesia			
	Stress ulcer prophylaxis			
	CBC and LFT daily			
	Coagulation profile specially PT			
	Electrolyte assessment			
	Monitor drain output and the nature of the fluid (blood, bile, serous)			
First outpatient visit	Clinical assessment			
	Remove sutures			
	Review the final pathology report			
	Arrange for multidisciplinary discussion if the case is cancer			
	Refer to oncology if adjuvant treatment is required			

6.2.2 Answer Key

Case No. 1:

A 39-year-old male patient presented to the emergency department complaining of right upper abdominal pain, fever, and jaundice for 5 days.

Questions for Discussion:

1. **How will you approach the patient?**

- Before starting the history make sure the patient is hemodynamically stable. Otherwise start resuscitation.
- Confirm the patency of his airway and the adequacy of his breathing and start him on IV fluid and draw blood for investigation.
- The patient was hypotensive, he was started on IV fluid, and his pressure is slightly improving.
- The pain started gradually at the right upper quadrant, increasing in severity in over the last 2 days. It is stabbing pain that not radiated or shifted elsewhere. It is associated with yellowish discoloration of the sclera, dark urine, and pale stool. Since yesterday, he has documented fever at home reaching up to 39.5°C. He vomited twice after he ate. No history of weight loss or night sweating. He has no history of traveling or alcohol intake. He has no significant family history of malignancy. He is not on regular medication. He has no significant past surgical history.
- On physical examination:
  - He is ill, jaundice.
  - His vital signs: BP: 90/60 (was 85/42 mmHg), PR: 110 (was 123 bpm), temperature: 39°C
  - His abdomen is soft with localized tenderness at the RUQ area. Murphy's sign is negative
  - The rest of examination is not significant.

2. **What will you do next?**

- Blood investigation: Table 6.5
- CXR: normal
- Abdominal ultrasound: the gallbladder is contracted over multiple stones. There is extra- and intrahepatic biliary radical dilatation. CBD is measuring 9 mm with multiple stones seen inside it.

Table 6.5 Blood test for case 1

Test	Result	Normal value
WBC (k/μl)	22	4.8–10.8
HB (g/dl)	12	12.6–16.5
PLT (K/μl)	150	130–400
ALT (U/l)	135	10–130
AST (U/l)	38	10–34
Total bilirubin (mg/dl)	3	0–0.8
Direct bilirubin (mg/dl)	2.5	0–0.3
Albumin (g/dl)	3.6	2.4–4
Creatinine (mg/dl)	1	0.7–1.2
PT (seconds)	12	10–13
INR	1	1
Amylase (U/l)	100	60–180
Lipase (U/l)	35	0–160
Hepatitis profile	Negative	Negative

3. **What will be your next step of the management?**

- This patient is in cholangitis and he needs urgent decompression of the biliary system.
- So, he needs admission to the ICU, to keep him NPO and continue the administration of IV fluid, blood culture to be sent, and the antibiotic should be started as soon as possible along with other medications (antipyretic, antiemetic, and DVT and stress ulcer prophylaxis).
- Gastroenterology consultation for urgent ERCP.

4. **ERCP shows pus inside the CBD and cholangiogram revealed multiple stones (the largest is 9 mm), the endoscopist could remove most of the stones but one stone was difficult to retrieve, so he did sphincterotomy, the patient' hemodynamic parameters are improving, but his bilirubin is still raising, what will you do?**

- The patient has impacted stone at the CBD that could not be removed endoscopically. So he needs cholecystectomy with laparoscopic CBD exploration.

5. **What are the intraoperative options to remove the stone?**
   - Glucagon to relax the sphincter
   - Flushing with saline
   - Fogarty balloon catheter
   - Dormia basket
   - Flexible choledochoscopy
   - Laser lithotripsy or shockwave lithotripsy
6. **The patient was taken to operating room and laparoscopic cholecystectomy was done, a trial of laparoscopic CBD exploration was failed to remove the stone and the operation was converted to open exploration and the stone is removed. How will you close the CBD?**

- Depend on the size of the CBD.
- If the duct is dilated, it can be closed primarily using longitudinal running or interrupted stitches by 4-0 absorbable monofilament suture. Otherwise closure over a T-tube using 4-0 absorbable sutures.

7. **If you close over a T-tube, when you will remove it?**

- Two to three weeks later and after T-tube cholangiogram confirming no distal obstruction.

8. **Six months later the patient came with jaundice and abdominal pain and the MRCP revealed stricture at the closure site. How will you manage it?**

- It can be managed endoscopically with either balloon dilatation or stenting.

Suggested Twist Points:

- You are in primary center and neither ERCP nor intervention radiologist are available. How will you manage the patient?
- The stone was difficult to be removed even after converting to open CBD exploration. How will you manage that?

Case No. 2:

A 51-year-old male patient presented to the clinic complaining of upper abdominal pain for 6 months.

Questions for Discussion:

1. **How will you approach the patient?**

- The pain started gradually over the last 6 months and increased in severity over the last week. It is not radiated or shifted and aggravated by meal specially when is fatty. No history of jaundice, no vomiting, or change in bowel habit. He noticed a significant loss of his weight over the last 3 months (he lost 20 kg of his weight). He has no history of traveling or contact with sick patient. He has no significant family history. He is diabetic on insulin and has no previous surgical history.
- On examination:
  - He was conscious, cachectic with stable vital signs.
  - There are no stigmata of chronic liver disease.
  - His abdomen is not distended, soft with mild tenderness at the RUQ area. No guarding or rigidity. Murphy's sign is negative. No ascites or organomegaly.

2. **What will you do next?**

- Blood investigation: Table 6.6
- CXR: normal
- ECG: normal
- Ultrasound abdomen: showed asymmetrical wall thickening of the gallbladder wall at the level of the mid gallbladder measuring 2.1 cm at the thickest point. There are multiple gallstones. No signs of acute cholecystitis.

3. **What is your differential diagnosis?**

- Gallbladder cancer
- Gallbladder polyp
- Gallbladder stone
- Adenomyomatosis
- Chronic cholecystitis
- Primary hepatic tumor

Table 6.6 Blood test for case 2

Test	Result	Normal value
WBC (k/μl)	10	4.8–10.8
HB (g/dl)	11	12.6–16.5
PLT (K/μl)	200	130–400
ALT (U/l)	90	10–130
AST (U/l)	20	10–34
ALP (IU/l)	150	44–147
Total bilirubin (mg/dl)	0.7	0–0.8
Direct bilirubin (mg/dl)	0.1	0–0.3
Albumin (g/dl)	2.5	2.4–4
Creatinine (mg/dl)	1	0.7–1.2
PT (seconds)	12	10–13
INR	1	1
Amylase (U/l)	70	60–180
Lipase (U/l)	12	0–160
Hepatitis profile	Negative	Negative

4. **How will you confirm the most likely diagnosis?**

- Triphasic liver protocol CT scan and tumor markers
- Biopsy is not indicated if the radiological picture is clear (it showed heterogenous mass arising from posterior wall of the gallbladder at the level of middle of the gallbladder with patchy moderate enhancement. It is measuring 2.3 cm × 1.8 cm. There are suspicious lymph nodes at the porta hepatis. No other hepatic lesion)
- CEA: 4 ng/ml (normal)
- Ca19-9: 300 u/ml (high)
- AFP: 4 (normal)

5. **How will you manage him?**

- This patient has gallbladder cancer.
- Needs staging CT CAP.
- His case needs to be discussed in tumor board.
- If no distant metastasis, the decision most likely will be exploration and extended cholecystectomy (segment IVb and V) with lymphadenectomy and the cystic duct margin to be sent for frozen section and adjuvant chemotherapy postoperatively.

6. **Intraoperative you sent frozen section of the cystic duct and the result came back as positive for malignant cells. How will you manage that?**

- Resection of the extrahepatic bile duct and reconstruction as Roux-en-Y hepaticojejunostomy.

7. **What are the possible complications?**

- General complications: DVT, PE, MI, atelectasis, pneumonia, wound infection, adhesion, incisional hernia.
- Specific complications: bleeding, bile leak, bile duct injury, liver abscess, liver failure, stricture.

Suggested Twist Points:

- The patient presented with picture of acute cholecystitis and laparoscopic cholecystectomy was done. Later, the pathology revealed adenocarcinoma of the gallbladder that invades the muscularis layers. How you will manage?
- During exploration, you discovered distant metastasis to the liver. What will you do?

Case No. 3:
A 70-year-old male patient presented to the emergency department complaining of abdominal pain and vomiting for 3 days.

Questions for Discussion:

1. **How will you approach this patient?**

- The pain started gradually at the periumbilical area progressing with time, colicky in nature, associated with nausea and vomiting of whatever he eats or dinks. The last bowel motion was 3 days ago. And he did not pass flautas for 2 days. He has recurrent right upper abdominal pain due to gallstones, but his cholecystectomy was postponed due to his cardiac condition. He has no history of weight loss, fever, or other constitutional symptoms. He has no significant family history. He was admitted last year due to myocardial infarction for which he underwent PCI, but no stent was inserted. He is on aspirin and calcium channel blocker. He has previous surgical history of appendectomy when he was 20 years old.
- Physical examination:
  - Conscious, dehydrated old man.
  - No pallor or jaundice.
  - Vital signs: BP: 130/85, PR: 95 bpm, temperature: 37.7°C.
  - Abdomen is distended, with mild generalized tenderness. Tympanic on percussion. The hernial orifices are intact.
  - PR shows empty rectum with no local abnormalities.

2. **What is your differential diagnosis?**

- Picture of bowel obstruction: it could be secondary to colonic tumors, volvulus, gallstone ileus, intussusception, adhesion, or hernias.

3. **What are the investigations would you like to order for this patient?**

- Blood investigations: Table 6.7
- CXR: normal
- AXR: dilated small bowel with multiple air fluid levels

Table 6.7 Blood test for case 3

Test	Result	Normal value
WBC (k/μl)	13	4.8–10.8
HB (g/dl)	12	12.6–16.5
PLT (K/μl)	250	130–400
ALT (U/l)	90	10–130
AST (U/l)	20	10–34
ALP (IU/l)	154	44–147
Total bilirubin (mg/dl)	0.7	0–0.8
Direct bilirubin (mg/dl)	0.1	0–0.3
Albumin (g/dl)	3	2.4–4
Creatinine (mg/dl)	1	0.7–1.2
PT (seconds)	12	10–13
INR	1	1

4. **What further investigations you want to do to confirm the diagnosis?**

- CT abdomen with oral and IV contrast.
- It showed dilated small bowel up to the level of the terminal ileum and distal collapsed colon. The contrast did not reach the colon. At the area of the transition zone there is intraluminal radiopaque stone. The CT also showed a pneumobilia.

5. **What is your final diagnosis?**

- Small bowel obstruction due to gallstones

6. **How will you manage it?**

- By exploration and removal of the stone via longitudinal enterotomy proximal to the obstructing stone. The rest of the bowel should be examined for any other remaining stone. Closure of the enterotomy transversely.

7. **What will you do with the biliary-enteric fistula?**

- Since the patient condition is not suitable for major surgery. The fistula between the gallbladder and the bowel should not be addressed at this stage.

8. **You did the surgery and few days later the patient is complaining foul smelling discharge from the wound. What will you do?**

- Open the wound, drain the fluid, take swab for culture and sensitivity, and start the patient on antibiotics.

9. **You opened the wound partially; the fluid looks like bowel content and you started the patient on IV antibiotic. What will you do after that?**

- CT abdomen with oral and IV contrast to rule out any deep collection and clarify the source of this fluid.

10. **The CT showed no intra-abdominal fluid collection, and the oral contrast is demonstrating a tract connecting the distal ileum to the wound. What is your diagnosis and how you will manage it?**

- Enterocutaneous fistula.
- Initial medical management by controlling any sepsis, measuring the output of the fistula. If it is low output fistula, the patient can be fed orally otherwise NPO and start TPN. If there is no distal obstruction, foreign body, and the tract is short, most likely it will close spontaneously.
- If did not close, it may need surgical management in a form of take down the fistula resection of the affected bowel and anastomosis.

Suggested Twist Points:

- The patient is young and healthy. How will you manage the biliary-enteric fistula?
- The stone was causing pressure necrosis on the small bowel wall. How will you deal with it?

Case No. 4:
A 29-year-old male patient presented to the clinic complaining of abdominal pain, jaundice for 2 months.

Questions for Discussion:

1. **How will you approach this patient?**

- The pain started gradually at the right upper abdomen 2 months ago, dull aching, not radiated or shifted, with no specific aggravating or relieving factor. It is associated with yellowish discoloration of the sclera and his urine became darker and his stool is pale. No nausea or vomiting. No history of weight loss, fever, or night sweating. He has no history of traveling or contact with sick patient. Other systemic review is unremarkable.
- Physical examination:
  - Conscious, alert, looks jaundiced.
  - Vital signs: BP: 120/82 mmHg, PR: 89 bpm, temperature: 36.7°C.

– Abdomen: there is mild tenderness at the RUQ area. A mass is palpable at this area. It is about 3 cm × 5 cm, round shape, smooth surface. The percussion over the mass is dull. No ascites.

2. **What is your differential diagnosis?**
   - Distended gallbladder
   - Choledochal cyst
   - Liver mass (benign or malignant)
   - Liver cyst
   - Pancreatic cancer
   - Lipoma
3. **What are the investigations would you like to do?**

- Blood test: Table 6.8
- Ultrasound: there is cystic dilatation of the extrahepatic bile duct reach up to 2 cm in diameter. This dilatation is separated from the gallbladder. There is no intrahepatic biliary duct dilatation and there are no gallstones.
- MRCP showed fusiform dilatation of the common bile duct. The intrahepatic ducts and the hepatic ducts are of normal size. No lymph nodes or sign of malignant disease.

4. **What is your diagnosis?**

- Type I choledochal cyst

Table 6.8 Blood test for case 4

Test	Result	Normal value
WBC (k/μl)	9	4.8–10.8
HB (g/dl)	14	12.6–16.5
PLT (K/μl)	167	130–400
ALT (U/l)	90	10–130
AST (U/l)	20	10–34
ALP (IU/l)	160	44–147
Total bilirubin (mg/dl)	2	0–0.8
Direct bilirubin (mg/dl)	1.3	0–0.3
Albumin (g/dl)	4	2.4–4
Creatinine (mg/dl)	1	0.7–1.2
PT (seconds)	12	10–13
INR	1	1
AFP	5	<7
CEA (ng/ml)	4	<5
Ca19-9 (u/ml)	40	0–27

5. **How will you manage this patient? and why?**

- This patient needs to be managed by resection of the extrahepatic bile duct and reconstruction in the form of Roux-en-Y hepaticojejunostomy due to high risk of malignancy (up to 60%).

6. **What will be your extent of resection?**

- Normal diameter duct

7. **How will you prepare the patient for operation?**
   - Admission
   - NPO
   - IV fluid
   - Analgesia
   - Prophylactic medications: antibiotic, DVT prophylaxis, stress ulcer prophylaxis
   - Preoperative laboratory investigations: CBC, LFT, RFT, coagulation profile, blood group
   - Review the preoperative imaging
   - Explain the procedure to the patient and obtain informed consent
   - Anesthesia consultation

Suggested Twist Points:

- Few days postoperation, the patient's drain brought greenish fluid. What will you do?
- Change the type of the biliary cyst.

Case No. 5:

A 37-year-old male patient presented to the emergency department complaining of right upper abdominal pain and vomiting for 3 days.

Questions for Discussion:

1. **How will you approach the patient?**

- The pain started gradually after fatty meal at the RUQ, radiated to the right shoulder. It is associated with vomiting four times. He has history of undocumented fever at home. No history of jaundice, no change in bowel habit. No history of weight loss or night sweating. No significant family history. He is smoker, otherwise healthy man with no previous surgical history.

- On examination:
  - Conscious, alert, looks ill, not jaundiced.
  - Vital signs: BP: 110/80, PR: 110 bpm, temperature: 37°C.
  - Abdomen: not distended, soft, with localized tenderness at RUQ with positive Murphy's sign.

2. **What is your differential diagnosis?**
   - Acute cholecystitis
   - Liver abscess
   - Hepatitis
   - Symptomatic hemangioma or adenoma
   - Hydatid cyst
   - Amebic abscess
   - Hepatocellular carcinoma
   - Gallbladder cancer
   - Lower lobe pneumonia
   - Myocardial infarction
   - Musculoskeletal pain
   - Trauma
3. **What further investigation will you do?**

- Blood investigation: Table 6.9
- CXR: normal
- Abdominal ultrasound: distended gallbladder, thick wall >4 mm, with multiple gallstones, one of them impacted at the cystic duct. There is pericholecystic fluid.

4. **How will you manage this patient?**

- Admission
- NPO
- IV fluid
- IV antibiotic
- Prophylaxis: DVT and stress ulcer
- Analgesia
- Antiemetic
- Prepare the patient for urgent laparoscopic cholecystectomy
- Anesthesia consultation
- Cross match
- Consent for laparoscopic cholecystectomy ± open

5. **The patient underwent a difficult laparoscopic cholecystectomy. On third postoperative day, you removed the drain and discharged the patient. Three days later, the patient presented to the emergency department complaining of severe abdominal pain, fever, and jaundice. What is your differential diagnosis?**
   - Cholangitis due to retained stone
   - Bile duct injury
   - Infected collection or biloma
   - Liver abscess
6. **What will you do next?**

- Blood tests: Table 6.10
- Ultrasound and MRCP

Table 6.9 Blood test for case 5a

Test	Result	Normal value
WBC (k/μl)	14	4.8–10.8
HB (g/dl)	15	12.6–16.5
PLT (K/μl)	199	130–400
ALT (U/l)	140	10–130
AST (U/l)	20	10–34
ALP (IU/l)	170	44–147
Total bilirubin (mg/dl)	0.7	0–0.8
Direct bilirubin (mg/dl)	0.2	0–0.3
Albumin (g/dl)	4	2.4–4
Creatinine (mg/dl)	1	0.7–1.2
PT (seconds)	12	10–13
INR	1	1
Hepatitis profile	Negative	Negative

Table 6.10 Blood test for case 5b

Test	Result	Normal value
WBC (k/μl)	20	4.8–10.8
HB (g/dl)	15	12.6–16.5
PLT (K/μl)	300	130–400
ALT (U/l)	148	10–130
AST (U/l)	40	10–34
ALP (IU/l)	220	44–147
Total bilirubin (mg/dl)	2.7	0–0.8
Direct bilirubin (mg/dl)	2.0	0–0.3
Albumin (g/dl)	4	2.4–4
Creatinine (mg/dl)	1	0.7–1.2
PT (seconds)	12	10–13
INR	1	1

7. **The ultrasound showed dilated intrahepatic duct and no collection. The MRCP showed dilated intrahepatic biliary radicals and cutoff sign at the level of the CHD 3 cm distal to the confluence, what will you do next?**

- This patient in cholangitis and needs urgent decompression via PTD along with resuscitation and antibiotics.

8. **What is the type of this injury?** Type E1
9. **The patient underwent decompression of the biliary system via PTD and his symptoms improved. What will be the definitive management of his condition?**

- Biliary enteric anastomosis in a form of hepaticojejunostomy

Suggested Twist Points:

- At the time of cholecystectomy, you noticed bile coming from the area of the porta hepatis, how will you manage it?
- During the perioperative period the drain output is bile. What will you do?

References

1. Raigani S, Fiedler AG, Berger DL. The management of asymptomatic (silent) gallstones. In: Cameron J, Cameron A, editors. Current surgical therapy. 12th ed. Canada: Elsevier; 2016.
2. Gomi H, Solomkin JS, Schlossberg D, Okamoto K, Takada T, Strasberg SM, et al. Tokyo Guidelines 2018: antimicrobial therapy for acute cholangitis and cholecystitis. J Hepato-Biliary-Pancreatic Sci. 2018;25(1):3–16.
3. Fagenholz PJ, Velmahos G. The management of acute cholecystitis. In: Cameron J, Cameron A, editors. Current surgical therapy. 12th ed. Canada: Elsevier; 2016.
4. Theodore N, Pappas MLC. The management of acute cholangitis. In: Cameron J, Cameron A, editors. Current surgical therapy. 12th ed. Canada: Elsevier; 2016.
5. Santos BF, Strasberg MS. Management of common bile duct stones: laparoscopic common bile duct exploration. In: Cameron J, Cameron A, editors. Current surgical therapy. 12th ed. Canada: Elsevier; 2016.
6. Valderrama-Treviño AI, Granados-Romero JJ, Espejel-Deloiza M, Chernitzky-Camaño J, Barrera Mera B, Estrada-Mata AG, et al. Updates in Mirizzi syndrome. Hepatobiliary Surg Nutr. 2016;6(3):170–8.
7. Goldin SB, Mullinax J. The management of gallstone ileus. In: Cameron J, Cameron A, editors. Current surgical therapy. 12th ed. Canada: Elsevier; 2016.
8. Ahrendt SA. The management of cystic disorders of the bile ducts. In: Cameron J, Cameron A, editors. Current surgical therapy. 12th ed. Canada: Elsevier; 2016.
9. Ball CG, Lillemoe KD. The management of benign biliary strictures. In: Cameron J, Cameron A, editors. Current surgical therapy. 12th ed. Canada: Elsevier; 2016.
10. HE SAGES SAFE CHOLECYSTECTOMY PROGRAM. Strategies for minimizing bile duct injuries: adopting a universal culture of safety in cholecystectomy. https://www.sages.org/safe-cholecystectomy-program/.
11. Marmor RAJKS. The management of gallbladder cancer. In: Cameron J, Cameron A, editors. Current surgical therapy. 12th ed. Canada: Elsevier; 2016.
12. Naeem Goussous STP, Cunningham SC. The management of bile duct cancer. In: Cameron J, Cameron A, editors. Current surgical therapy. 12th ed. Canada: Elsevier; 2016.
13. Zollinger R, Ellison E. Bile duct: surgical therapy. Zollinger's atlas of surgical operation. 9th ed. United States: McGraw-Hill Education; 2011.
14. Jean Nicolas Vauthey JS. Liver. In: Fischer JE, editor. Master techniques in general surgery. Hepatobiliary and pancreatic surgery. 9th ed. United States: Lippincott Williams and Wilkins; 2013.
15. Clavien P-A. Liver. In: Pierre-Alain Clavien MGS, Fong Y, editors. Atlas of upper gastrointestinal and hepato-pancreatic-biliary surgery. 9th ed. Germany: Springer; 2007.

7 Surgical Aspects of Pancreatic and Splenic Diseases for Clinical Board Exams

7.1 Part I: Knowledge

> If four things are followed—having a great aim, acquiring knowledge, hard work, and perseverance—then anything can be achieved.
> —A. P. J. Abdul Kalam

History:

- Introduce yourself to the patient
- Name, age, occupation, gender, nationality
- History of presenting illness:
  - **Analysis of the chief complaint**

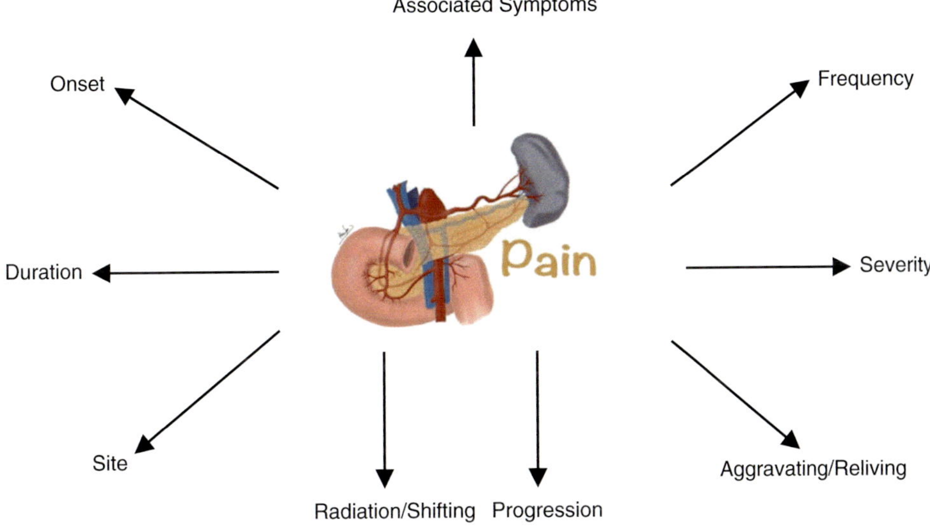

H. Alotaibi, *Study Surgery*, https://doi.org/10.1007/978-981-16-2305-9_7

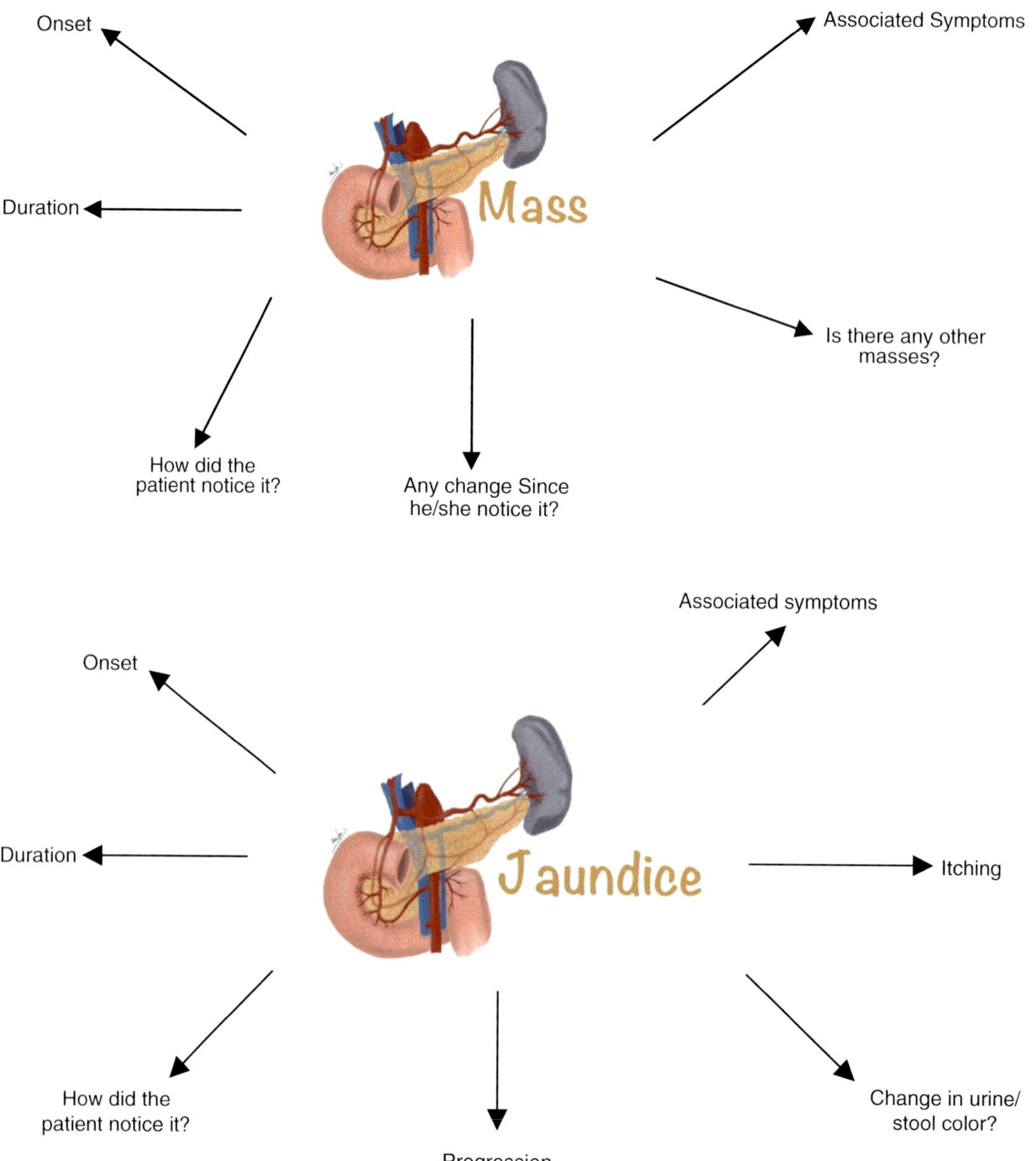

- **Associated symptoms**
  Pain, fever, jaundice, nausea, vomiting, diarrhea, constipation, change urine or stool color, itching, abdominal distention.
  Symptoms of functional neuroendocrine tumors (diarrhea, dermatitis, sweating, palpitation, DVT, epigastric pain, dizziness, fainting)
- **Constitutional symptoms:**
  Weight loss, decrease appetite, night sweating, fever.
- **Symptoms of metastasis**
  Back pain, abdominal distention, cough, shortness of breath.
- **Risk factors:**
  Gallstone
  Alcohol

Family history of similar complain or malignancy (pancreatic cancer, MEN syndrome, melanoma)
Personal history of cancer
Medication history (Thiazide, Steroids, Propofol, hormone replacement therapy
Contact with a sick patient
Previous hepatobiliary surgery
Previous attack of pancreatitis
Recent ERCP
Smoking
New-onset diabetes
Recent increase in insulin requirements
Diet (low fiber high fat diet increases the risk of pancreatic ca)

- **Symptoms or factors related to differential Diagnosis**
  Chest pain (MI)
  Cough, fever, SOB (pneumonia)
  Recent history of trauma
  Heartburn, gastric reflux (GERD, Peptic ulcer disease)
- Previous similar attack, previous admission, previous investigation.
- Systemic review of related system (GIT)
  Dysphagia, heart burn, hematemesis, melena, history of bleeding, ecchymosis.

- PMH
- PSH
- Family history
- Social history
- Medication, transfusion, allergy
- Systemic Review
  - **CNS:** headache, eye and hearing symptoms, epilepsy, numbness, paralysis.
  - **CVS:** chest pain, orthopnea, paroxysmal nocturnal dyspnea, lower limb edema, palpitation.
  - **Respiratory system:** cough, fever, chest pain, hemoptysis.
  - **Renal system:** dysuria, flank pain, hematuria.
  - **MSK:** weakness, arthritis, skin erythema.

Physical examination:

- Introduce yourself to the patient
- Ask permission for examination
- Ensure privacy and ask for chaperon
- Position: supine
- Exposure: from nipple to midthigh
- Handwashing

General Examination:

- **A**ppearance: ill, well, dehydrated
- **B**ody Built: Cachectic, obese
- **C**olor: Pale, Jaundice
- **D**istress/**D**ecubitus
- **E**nvironment and connection to monitors, IV fluids, or drain

Vital signs: BP, HR, Temperature, RR, SPO_2
Hands:

- Muscle wasting
- Palmer erythema
- Clubbing
- Koilonychia (Iron deficiency anemia)
- Leukonychia (Hypoalbuminemia)
- Pulse rate and its characteristics (Rhythm, Volume, etc.)

Eye:

- Jaundice
- Pallor

Mouth:

- Jaundice in mucus membrane, below the tongue
- Fetor Hepaticus

Neck:

- Lymphadenopathy

Chest:

- Respiratory and CVS examination

Abdomen:

- Inspection:
  - Distention
  - Asymmetry

- Visible veins
- Scars/Striae
- Dilated veins (Caput medusa)
- Hernial orifices
- Stretch marks
- Visible peristalsis
- Signs of retroperitoneal hemorrhage (Grey turner, Cullen, and Fox signs)

• Palpations:
- Superficial then deep palpation
- Look for any tenderness
- Palpable masses
- Organomegaly

• Percussion:
- Ascites:
  Shifting dullness
  Fluid thrill

• Auscultation:
- Bowel Sounds
- Bruit, venous hum

Groin: Examine the hernial orifices and if there is any hernia clarify its characteristic (site, reducibility, or presence of incarceration/strangulation)

DRE

Lower limbs: edema, swelling, skin rash, weakness

Back: for tenderness

7.1.1 Approach to Patient with Pancreatitis

• **History and physical examination as described earlier**

• **Investigations:**
- Blood test:
  CBC
  Electrolyte
  Coagulation profile
  Blood group
  LFT (AST, ALT, Bilirubin direct and total, ALP, GGT, albumin)
  Amylase and lipase
  LDH
  Blood glucose
  Lipid profile
  CRP, ESR
  ABG
- Imaging:
  CXR
  AXR
  Ultrasound abdomen
  CT abdomen pancreatic protocol
  MRCP/ERCP
  EUS

• **Diagnostic criteria of acute pancreatitis:**
If the patient has acute pancreatitis if he/she has two out of the three of the following:
- Abdominal pain consisting of acute pancreatitis (epigastric pain, radiated to the back, and relieved by leaning forward)
- Amylase and/or lipase three times the normal value
- Radiological evidence of acute pancreatitis [1–3]

• **Identify the cause of the pancreatitis**
- Ultrasound abdomen to confirm the presence or absence of gallstones as it is the most common cause of acute pancreatitis (45%)
- History of alcohol (a second most common cause of pancreatitis); the type of alcohol is less important than the amount and the pattern (100–150 g/day).
- Drugs: thiazide, estrogen replacement therapy, steroids, propofol
- Hyperlipidemia and hypercalcemia; In the absence of gallstones or significant history of alcohol use, serum triglyceride and calcium levels should be measured. Serum triglyceride levels over 11.3 mmol/l (1000 mg/dl) indicate it as the etiology.
- Post-ERCP pancreatitis: risk factors include younger age, female patient, absence of bile duct stone, multiple attempts of cannulation to the ampulla, sphincterotomy, sphincter of Oddi dysfunction, pancreaticogram [1–3].

• **Assessment of the severity of pancreatitis:**
- *BISAP (bedside index of severity of acute pancreatitis)*
  One point for each of the following:
  BUN > 25 mg/dl
  Abnormal mental status (GCS < 15)

Table 7.1 Ranson's criteria [1–3]

	Parameter	Gallstone pancreatitis	Non-gallstone pancreatitis
At admission	Age (years)	>70	>55
	WBC (×10³/mm³)	18	16
	Blood glucose (mg/dl)	220	200
	LDH (U/l)	400	350
	AST (U/l)	250	250
During the 48 h of admission	Hematocrit (%)	Fall >10	Fall >10
	BUN (mg/dl)	Increases >2	Increases >5
	Calcium (mg/dl)	<8	<8
	Base deficit (mEq/l)	>	>4
	PaO_2 mmHg	–	<60
	Estimated fluid sequestration (l)	>5	>6

0–2 points; mortality <1%
3–4 points; mortality 15%
5–6 points; mortality 40%
>6 points; mortality 100%

Evidence of systemic inflammatory response syndrome (SIRS)
Age >60 years old
Imaging study reveals pleural effusion
1–2: mild acute pancreatitis
≥3: severe acute pancreatitis

- *Ranson's criteria:* Table 7.1
- *The Apache II score* evaluates the chronic health score and 12 physiologic measurements, but is not specific for AP, and is not designed for day-to-day evaluation in any patient.
- *CT-severity index:* Table 7.2
- *Revised Atlanta criteria:*

  Mild: no local or systemic complication
  Moderate: sterile local complication or transient organ failure <48 h.
  Severe: infected local complication or persistent organ failure >48 h [1–3].

Table 7.2 CT-severity index [1–3]

Degree of acute pancreatitis		Degree of pancreatic necrosis	
Finding	Points	Finding	Points
Normal pancreas	0	No necrosis	0
Enlargement of the pancreas	1	Non-enhancement of ≤30% of the gland	2
Peripancreatic inflammation	2	Non-enhancement of 30–50% of the gland	4
Single fluid collection	3	Non-enhancement of ≥50%	6
Multiple fluid collections or presence of gas in or adjacent to pancreatic tissue	4		

0–3: mild acute pancreatitis
4–6: moderate acute pancreatitis
7–10: severe acute pancreatitis

- **Management:**
  - **Admission** (ICU or ward)
  - **Fluid resuscitation:**

    Early fluid resuscitation is indicated to optimize tissue perfusion targets, without waiting for hemodynamic worsening. Fluid administration should be guided by frequent reassessment of the hemodynamic status, since fluid overload is known to have detrimental effects. Isotonic crystalloids are the preferred fluid [1–3].
  - **Continuous vital signs monitoring** in high dependency care unit is needed if organ dysfunction occurs. Persistent organ dysfunction or organ failure occurrence despite adequate fluid resuscitation is an indication for ICU admission [1–3].
  - **Pain management**

- **Maintain the O_2 delivery:** intubation and mechanical ventilation if indicated
- **Nutrition:**

  Mild: immediate enteral feeding should be initiated as long as the patient is tolerating oral intake.

  Severe: Enteral nutrition is recommended to prevent gut failure and infectious complications. Total parenteral nutrition (TPN) should be avoided but partial parenteral nutrition integration should be considered to reach caloric and protein requirements if the enteral route is not completely tolerated. Both gastric and jejunal feeding can be delivered safely [1–3]
- **Follow-up imaging:**

  Mild: Patients with mild AP do not need a CT in the majority of cases. These patients will require further CT only if there is a change in the patient's clinical status that suggests a new complication

  Severe: In severe acute pancreatitis (computed tomography severity index ≥3), a follow-up CECT scan is indicated 7–10 days from the initial CT scan [1–3].
- **Antibiotic treatment:**

  Routine prophylactic antibiotics are not recommended for all patients with acute pancreatitis.

  Antibiotics are always recommended to treat infected severe acute pancreatitis.

  A CT-guided fine-needle aspiration (FNA) for Gram stain and culture can confirm an infected severe acute pancreatitis and drive antibiotic therapy but is no longer in routine use.

  In patients with infected necrosis, antibiotics known to penetrate pancreatic necrosis should be used, e.g., aminoglycoside, third-generation cephalosporine, and Bactrim.

  In patients with infected necrosis, the spectrum of empirical antibiotic regimen should include both aerobic and anaerobic Gram-negative and Gram-positive microorganisms [1–3].
- **ERCP:**

  Routine ERCP with acute gallstone pancreatitis is not indicated.

  ERCP in patients with acute gallstone pancreatitis and cholangitis or common bile duct stone is indicated [1–3].
- **Cholecystectomy:**

  Mild and moderate acute pancreatitis: laparoscopic cholecystectomy + IOC during the index of hospitalization (if there is a stone in the CBD it can be managed by watchful waiting if the patient is asymptomatic, CBD exploration, or postoperative ERCP)

  Severe: after 6 weeks

  In acute gallstone pancreatitis with peripancreatic fluid collections, cholecystectomy should be deferred until fluid collections resolve or stabilize and acute inflammation ceases [1–3].

• **Management of post-pancreatitis complications:**

1. **Pancreatic pseudocyst:**
   - Acute peripancreatic fluid collection: fluid collection before 4 weeks from the onset of pancreatitis
   - Pancreatic pseudocyst: fluid collection after 4 weeks from the onset of pancreatitis
   - The majority of pseudocysts are asymptomatic.
   - Complications of pseudocyst:

     Obstruction: Intestinal, vascular, or biliary

     Infection

     Rupture; pancreatic ascites

     Hemorrhage; mainly from the splenic artery

     Fistula

- Diagnosis: by the CT scan, MRCP and ERCP to define the ductal anatomy
- Management options:
  - Endoscopic: cysto-gastrostomy or cysto-jejunostomy (less favorable if there is disconnected duct syndrome)
  - Surgical: Roux-en-Y cysto-gastrostomy, Roux-en-Y cysto-jejunostomy, or distal pancreatectomy [4]

2. **Pancreatic necrosis:**
   - Severity of organ failure does not correlate to the degree of pancreatic necrosis.
   - In patients with renal failure, fat-suppressed T1 weighted MRI can be used instead of a CT scan.
   - In presence of necrosis, the best time for intervention is after 4 weeks from the onset of symptoms.
   - In patients with infected necrosis and clinical deterioration, immediate source control is needed and sometimes it can be achieved by percutaneous drainage.
   - Asymptomatic walled-off necrosis does not mandate surgical intervention.
   - In case of other complications such as intestinal ischemia, compartment syndrome, perforated viscus, and acute bleeding that mandate surgical intervention, debridement of sterile necrosis is to be avoided [5].
   - Indication of intervention in sterile necrosis (best time is after 8 weeks):
     - Intractable gastric outlet obstruction
     - Intestinal or biliary obstruction from mass effect
     - Persistent abdominal pain or unwellness
     - Disconnected duct syndrome with persistent symptoms of collection

Table 7.3 Retroperitoneal debridement

Laparoscopic transperitoneal	Video-assisted retroperitoneal debridement
▪ Allow visualization of all compartment of the abdominal cavity ▪ Has the risk of contamination of sterile peritoneal cavity	▪ Currently the preferred method of minimally invasive access ▪ Image-guided drainage through retroperitoneal space, then upsize the tract, rigid nephroscopy or endoscopy is used for visualization

   - In therapeutic intervention is indicated, use the step-up approach:
     A. Initial intervention of choice is image-guided percutaneous drainage (retroperitoneal is the preferred route).
     B. If failed, endoscopic transluminal drainage with the use of EUS (safe alternative to percutaneous drainage)
        - Collection must be located within 2 cm of the stomach or duodenum.
        - Collection is accessed with electrocautery through the posterior wall of the stomach or the medial wall of the duodenum.
        - Transluminal direct endoscopic necrosectomy is another option for minimal invasive necrosectomy.
     C. Laparoscopic transperitoneal and video-assisted retroperitoneal debridement [5]: Table 7.3
     D. Open surgical necrosectomy:
        - Access: standard midline laparotomy or retroperitoneal flank incision
        - Necrotic tissue is debrided manually with blunt and careful dissection.
        - Three ways to manage the patient post necrosectomy [5]:

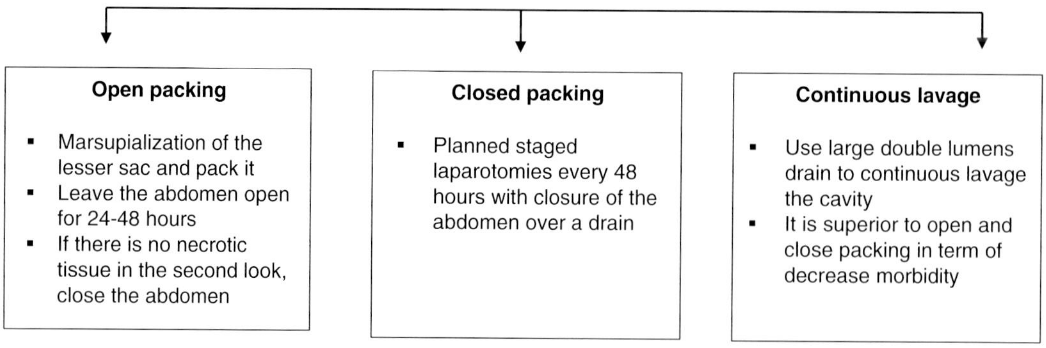

Open packing	Closed packing	Continuous lavage
▪ Marsupialization of the lesser sac and pack it ▪ Leave the abdomen open for 24-48 hours ▪ If there is no necrotic tissue in the second look, close the abdomen	▪ Planned staged laparotomies every 48 hours with closure of the abdomen over a drain	▪ Use large double lumens drain to continuous lavage the cavity ▪ It is superior to open and close packing in term of decrease morbidity

Pancreatic ductal disruption:

- Loss of ductal integrity anywhere in the pancreatic ductal system demonstrated by CT, ERCP, or MRCP
- Pancreatic fistula: internal or external
- **Pancreatic pleural effusion** originates from pancreatic duct disruption "fistulizing" into the retroperitoneum. The location of the ductal disruption determines whether the right or left pleural cavity is the site of collection (i.e., ductal disruption dorsally may accumulate in the right chest whereas a disruption from body and tail may accumulate in the left chest cavity)
- **Disconnected duct syndrome:** proximal and distal sides of the pancreas are separated permanently by pancreatic duct disruption. The common site of disruption is the pancreatic neck.
- **Diagnostic approach:** if the patient with acute pancreatitis is not improving by 1 week of conservative treatment after the onset of symptoms, assessment of the pancreatic duct must be done.
  - CT: identify the presence, location, and size of the pancreatic fluid collection or pancreatic necrosis.
  - ERCP/MRCP with or without secretin administration
  - If the disruption is ventral in the pancreas, the pancreatic juice will collect in the lesser sac.
  - If the disruption in the dorsal of the pancreas, the pancreatic fluid can accumulate in the retroperitoneum [6].
- **Management:**

  CT guided percutaneous drainage using 12 F pigtail drainage catheter. CT scan is obtained after 3 days to observe the status of the collection. The drainage catheter can be removed when the cavity is determined to be collapsed by the CT and the output is minimal.
  - **Indications of percutaneous drainage:** Presence of peripancreatic fluid collection by CT plus:

    Symptoms: refractory abdominal pain despite the use of narcotics, and inability to begin the oral intake

    Clinical signs:
    - Persistent or enlarging fluid collection by CT
    - Persistent abdominal distention/ileus
    - Systemic inflammatory response syndrome ± organ failure
    - Persistent or increase inflammatory data (CRP ± WBCs)
    - Persistent increase in serum amylase or lipase activity
  - **Endoscopic management:** There is no role of endoscopic transluminal drainage for acute peripancreatic fluid collection.
  - **Surgical:** In symptomatic patients with disconnected duct syndrome, especially for those in whom pancreatic juice is leaking from the distal pancreas is not sufficiently drained, distal pancreatectomy is indicated

    Note: the patient with pancreatic duct disruption should be managed by a multidisciplinary team involving intervention radiologists, nurses, dietitians, intensive care specialist, gastroenterologist, and pancreaticobiliary surgeon [6].

7.1.2 Approach to Patient with Chronic Pancreatitis

- **Clinical manifestations:**
  - Abdominal pain
  - Pancreatic exocrine insufficiency, e.g., steatorrhea (fatty malodourous stool)
  - Diabetes mellites type 3: secondary DM occurring in a patient with chronic pancreatitis arises from complete loss of the islet mass [7].
- **Risk factors:**
  - Strong genetic predisposition
  - Toxic metabolites (alcohol, tobacco)
  - Idiopathic (early onset, late onset, and tropical)
  - Autoimmune (isolated or syndromic, e.g., Sjogren's syndrome)
  - Recurrent severe acute pancreatitis
  - Obstruction (pancreatic divisim, IPMNs, ductal adenocarcinoma) [7]
- **Diagnosis:**
  - Clinical presentation
  - Imaging: most common findings are pancreatic duct dilatation, atrophy, calcification, pancreatic duct irregularity, or pancreatic pseudocysts.
  - CT is the primary imaging modality.
  - ERCP: the most sensitive and specific test for diagnosis of chronic pancreatitis.
  - EUS: valuable option especially early in the disease process before the development of ductal abnormality [7]
- **Management:**
  - Medical:

    The aims are to alleviate the pain, replace the pancreatic enzymes, and achieve glucose homeostasis.

    Opioid: the mainstay for pain management

    Pancreatic enzyme replacement to all patient with steatorrhea or excessive weight loss [7]
  - Endoscopic:

    The first line intervention in the setting of obstructive chronic pancreatitis

    ERCP: dilatation of strictured duct, sphincterotomy, placement of stent, or stone extraction
  - Surgical:

    Indicated in case of disabling chronic pain after failure of medical and endoscopic therapies

    Those patients should be evaluated for:
    - Assessment of pancreatic duct dilatation
    - The presence and location of strictures
    - Existence of any malignant mass
    - Presence of correctable anatomic abnormalities, e.g., biliary obstruction, duodenal obstruction, large symptomatic pseudocyst [7]

  The aims of surgery are:
    - Decompression of obstructed duct
    - Pain relief
    - Preservation of pancreatic tissue when possible [7]

  Options:
    - Decompressive procedures like lateral pancreaticojejunostomy
    - Resective procedures like Whipple, distal pancreatectomy, or total pancreatectomy
    - Combination of resection and decompression like duodenum preservation pancreatic head resection with or without lateral pancreaticojejunostomy [7]

  I. **Lateral pancreaticojejunostomy (Puestow procedure):**
    - Indicated in patients with chron.e incised 1 cm from the duodenal wall for at least 7 cm.
    - The duct should be examined for any stones.
    - The jejunum should be divided 15 cm from the ligament of Treitz.
    - The pancreaticojejunostomy should be made by securing the distal end of

the jejunal limb to the tail of the pancreas.
  - The jejujejunostomy should be made 50 cm from the pancreaticojejunostomy and the mesenteric defect should be closed [7].

II. **Duodenal preserving pancreatic head resection (Beger procedure)**
  - Indicated when there is inflammatory mass at the head of the pancreas or severe common bile duct stenosis

III. **Local resection of the head with lateral pancreaticojejunostomy (Frey procedure):**
  - Used in patients with dilated MPD associated with inflammatory mass at the pancreatic head
  - Pancreatic head is not transected.

IV. **Resection only procedure:**
  - Pancreaticoduodenectomy: if malignancy is suspected
  - Distal pancreatectomy is rarely indicated because it is associated with short-term pain relief.
  - Pancreatectomy with islet cell autotransplantation [7]

7.1.3 Approach to Patient with Pancreatic Cystic Lesion

- History and physical examination as described earlier
- Do not forget to ask about:
  - Previous attack of pancreatitis
  - History of abdominal trauma
  - Symptoms of neuroendocrine tumors of the pancreas
  - Symptoms of exocrine insufficiency (DM and steatorrhea)
- Differential diagnosis of pancreatic cysts:
  - Pseudocyst
  - Cyst adenoma
  - Cyst adenocarcinoma
  - Mucinous cyst
  - IPMN
  - Solid pseudopapillary neoplasm
  - Lymphoepithelial cyst
  - Cystic degeneration of solid tumor
  - Hydatid cyst
- Blood investigations:
  - CBC
  - Liver function test
  - Renal function test
  - Electrolyte
  - Blood glucose
  - Amylase/lipase
  - CEA, CA19-9
  - Elisa for echinococcus antibodies
  - CRP and ESR
- Imaging:
  - Pancreatic protocol CT abdomen
  - MRCP/MRI
  - EUS
  - ERCP
- FNA and fluid analysis for amylase, mucin, and CEA (Table 7.4)

Table 7.4 Interpretation of the result of the fluid analysis [8]

Diagnosis	Amylase	CEA	Mucin
Pseudocyst	High	<200	No
IPMN	High	>200	High
Mucinous cyst	Low	>200	High
Cyst adenoma	Low	<200	Low

Cyst adenoma:
- In CT: starburst, cluster of grapes, or honeycomb appearance
- Management:
  - Observation
  - Surgical management if clearly symptomatic or in case of a very large cyst. If it is at the body and tail, managed by splenic preserving distal pancreatectomy, otherwise Whipple procedure [8].

Mucinous cystic neoplasm:
- Has ovarian-type stroma within the cyst capsule
- Diagnosed by CT/MRI, and EUS and FNA
- Risk of malignancy is 5–15%.
- Treatment:
  - All the mucinous cystic neoplasm (MCN) should be surgically resected in the suitable candidate.

- It is usually located in the body and tail and will be managed by distal pancreatectomy with splenectomy. It is important to maintain the integrity of the capsule and complete removal of the cyst.
- If the margins are free, the recurrence of noninvasive MCNs is rare.
- If it is malignant, consider adjuvant therapy and close surveillance similar to adenocarcinoma [8].

Intraductal pancreatic mucinous neoplasm (IPMN):

- Characterized by mucin production, diffuse or segmental involvement of main pancreatic duct or major side branches
- When obstructive jaundice is present, the concern of malignancy is high.
- Not all IPMN need to be resected.
- Risk stratification (Sendai Criteria) [9]:

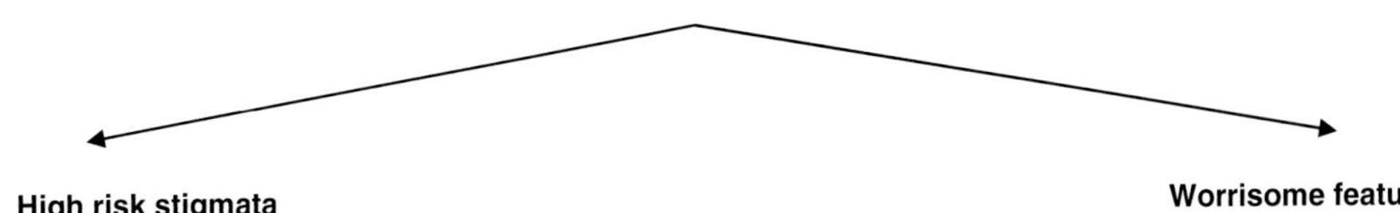

High risk stigmata

- Enhancing solid component
- Main pancreatic duct (MPD) ≥10 mm
- Obstructive jaundice

↓

If present and the patient is fit, for surgery

Worrisome feature

- Size > 3cm
- Thick enhancing cyst wall
- MPD is 5-9 mm
- Symptoms other than jaundice
- Non-enhancing mural nodule

- If it has high-risk stigmata, consider surgery if the patient is fit.
- If it has no high-risk features, check if it has worrisome features, and if any is present, evaluate it with EUS.
- If any of the following is present, consider surgery if the patient is fit:
  - Definite mural nodule
  - MPD with suspicious features (thick wall, mucin, or nodule)
  - Cytology is suspicious or positive for malignancy.
- If the cyst has no worrisome features and no suspicious feature in EUS, management is according to the size of the largest cyst:
  - >3 cm: Close surveillance (alternate MRI/EUS every 3–6 months). Strongly consider surgery in young and fit patient.
  - 2–3 cm: EUS every 3–6 months. Increase the interval and alternate with the MRI as appropriate. Consider surgery in young fit patients who need prolong surveillance [9].
  - 1–2 cm: CT/MRI annually for 2 years, then increase the interval if no change
  - <1 cm: CT/MRI in 2–3 years
- If the patient has worrisome features and a family history, strongly consider the surgery.
- High-risk patient for surgery:
  - MRI/MRCP at 3 months interval and annual EUS for 2 years or until the risk of malignancy weigh more than the risk of surgery.
- Truly unfit patient for surgery, no need for follow-up.
- Surgical options:
  - Pancreaticoduodenectomy
  - Distal pancreatectomy with splenectomy
  - Total pancreatectomy
  - Enucleation is limited for branch duct-IPMN.

- Intraoperative frozen section of the pancreatic neck should be done and if it is positive, re-resection even if required total pancreatectomy [9].
- Complications:
  - Delayed gastric emptying
  - Pancreatic fistula
  - Anastomotic leak
  - Overwhelming post-splenectomy sepsis
  - Bleeding
  - Collection [9]
- Postoperative surveillance:
  - Depends on the final pathology and margins
    - Low and intermediated grade dysplasia: how is the margin? If positive, MRCP every 6 months. If the margin is negative, CT at years 2 and 5 after resection
    - High-grade dysplasia: MRCP or CT every 3–6 months
    - Invasive carcinoma and negative margins: CT every 3 months for 2 years then every 6 months and adjuvant chemotherapy and radiation therapy similar to adenocarcinoma
    - Shorten the interval of surveillance if there is family history, new symptoms developed or worsen of DM, or in the case of positive margins [9]

Autoimmune pancreatitis:

- It appears as a mass effect in the pancreas.
- It mimics pancreatic adenocarcinoma radiographically and clinically [8, 10].
- It has two forms:
  - Type I or lymphoplasmacytic sclerosing pancreatitis [autoimmune pancreatitis without granulocyte epithelia lesions (GELs)]:
  - An IgG4-related systemic disease characterized by elevated serum IgG4 level and extra-pancreatic lesions such as primary sclerosing cholangitis, inflammatory bowel disease, retroperitoneal fibrosis, sarcoid, and others
  - Type II or idiopathic duct centric pancreatitis: characterized by the presence of GELs and relative paucity of IgG4-positive plasma cells
- Clinical picture: jaundice, pancreatitis, progressive pain, endocrine or exocrine pancreatic insufficiency
- On imaging: often appear as if the whole pancreas is full of hypoenhancing mass effect that resembles a sausage with a characteristic enhancing rim, but it can be focal hypoenhancing CT appearance [8, 10].
- ERCP/MRCP: will show structuring of the intrapancreatic CBD as well as focal, segmental, or diffuse strictures of the pancreatic duct
- Serology: elevated IgG4 (in 70% of cases), other markers such as anti-carbonic anhydrase or anti-lactoferrin antibodies
- Histology: EUS-guided FNA is usually inaccurate. Laparoscopic core needle biopsy or open biopsy is sometimes needed [8, 10].
- Mayo clinic extended criteria for autoimmune pancreatitis:
  - Imaging: pancreatic mass or enlargement, pancreatic duct stricture, pancreatic atrophy, pancreatic calcification, or pancreatitis
  - Serology: elevated serum IgG4 level
  - Histology: at least one of the following:
    - Periductal lymphoplasmacytic infiltrate with obliterative phlebitis and storiform fibrosis
    - Lymphoplasmacytic infiltrate with storiform fibrosis and abundant IgG4 positive cells
  - Other organ involvement: hilar or hepatic biliary strictures, persistent distal biliary stricture, parotid or lacrimal gland involvement, mediastinal lymphadenopathy, retroperitoneal fibrosis
  - Response to steroid therapy: resolution or marked improvement of pancreatic or extra-pancreatic manifestation with steroid therapy [8, 10]
- The treatment of both types consists of high-dose systemic corticosteroid (0.6–1 mg/kg) with a reassessment of imaging and CA19-9 after 2 weeks. If successful, repeat imaging at 4–6 weeks.

- In the case of jaundice, biliary strictures are treated first with a temporary endobiliary stent.
- If no change is observed in images or CA19-9 levels, malignancy should be considered [8, 10].

Primary Pancreatic lymphoma:
- It is non-Hodgkin's lymphoma.
- The clinical picture is vague, featuring weight loss, nausea or vomiting, pain.
- Elevated LDH may provide a clue.
- Imaging: nonspecific finding and the appearance of a bulky lesion with considerable local lymphadenopathy
- Definitive diagnosis is made by tissue evaluation either by EUS and FNA or CT guided or operative core biopsy.
- The management and the prognosis depend on the stage and grade of the tumor. The first-line therapy is systemic chemotherapy and surgical resection.
- The prevalent regimen is CHOP (cyclophosphamide, hydroxydoxorubicin, oncovin, and prednisone).
- Complete remission occurs in 75% of patient with early-stage disease [8, 10].

Metastatic pancreatic lesions:
- Less than 1% of all pancreatic tumors
- The most common primary is from renal cell carcinoma (RCC).
- The pancreas appears to be the selective site for metastasis from RCC.
- Other sites like melanoma, lung, colon, gynecological cancers
- Most metastatic tumors in the pancreas appear as hypervascular lesions.
- Diagnosis is made by EUS and FNA.
- As a general rule for all metastatic lesions to the pancreas, surgical interventions are appropriate for instances where the disease is confined to the pancreas and there is no systemic burden otherwise in a good candidate [8, 10].

7.1.4 Approach to Patient with Suspected Periampullary Cancer

The patient may present with either:
- Progressive jaundice
- Pain (advanced disease)
- Gastric outlet obstruction
- Constitutional symptoms (weight loss, anorexia, night sweating, or fever)
- History and physical examination as described earlier
- Do not forget the following points:
- In history:
  - Smoking
  - Alcohol consumption
  - Diet (low fiber high fat diet increases the risk of pancreatic ca)
  - Diabetes mellites type II (new-onset DM can be an early manifestation of otherwise occult pancreatic cancer or sudden increase in the insulin requirement in a patient with preexisting DM)
  - Family history of pancreatic cancer [11]

In examination:
  - Palpable gallbladder (Courvoisier's sign)
  - Virchow lymph node
  - Sister Mary Joseph nodule
  - Ascites
  - Hepatomegaly

Investigations:
  - Blood tests:
    CBC
    Electrolytes
    Coagulation profile
    Blood grouping
    LFT
    Amylase/lipase
    RFT
    Tumor marker, i.e., CA19-9
    Blood glucose
  - Imaging:
    CT Pancreatic protocol
    The finding suggestive of pancreatic ca is a hypodense lesion in the portal phase

surrounding by normal enhancing pancreatic tissue
MRCP if distal cholangiocarcinoma is suspected
EUS
ERCP/brush cytology
– If the images suggest cancer:
Staging CT CAP
Assess resectability
Multidisciplinary team discussion [11]

1. **Distal cholangiocarcinoma:**
   - The second most common cancer of the periampullary region
   - Arises in the CBD between the junction of the cystic duct and the ampulla
   - Accounts for 20–40% of cholangiocarcinoma
   - Affects the patient in the seventh decade of life and has a slight male preponderance
   - Risk factors: primary sclerosing cholangitis, autoimmune disorder, parasitic flatworms, chronic pancreatitis, Hepatitis B and C, and choledochal cysts [11].
2. **Ampullary Adenocarcinoma:**
   - Rare cancer (0.2–0.5% of all GI malignancies)
   - Third common cancer of the periampullary region
   - Most commonly in the sixth to seventh decade of life
   - They present with obstructive jaundice early in disease progression.
   - Higher resectability rate with lower biological aggressiveness
   - Two primary subtypes: intestinal and pancreaticobiliary (prognosis similar to pancreatic adenocarcinoma) [11]
3. **Duodenal Adenocarcinoma:**
   - The least common of periampullary tumors
   - It is the most common site of small bowel adenocarcinoma.
   - More common in the sixth to seventh decades of life and affect both sexes equally
   - It is believed to arise from duodena polyp through the adenoma carcinoma progression pathway
   - The best prognosis among all periampullary tumors
   - 5-year survival between 45% and 71% [11]
4. **Pancreatic adenocarcinoma:**
   - The fourth most common cause of cancer-related death in the USA
   - **Risk factors:**
     – Smoking
     – Heavy alcohol consumption
     – Obesity
     – Chronic pancreatitis
     – Hepatitis B infection
     – Diabetes mellitus (every 0.56 mmol/l increase in the fasting blood sugar is associated with a 14% increase in pancreatic cancer incidence, new-onset DM can be an early manifestation of otherwise occult pancreatic cancer, or sudden increase in the insulin requirement in a patient with preexisting DM)
     – Genetic: familial malignant melanoma syndrome, Lynch syndrome, patient with BRCA1/2 mutation, Peutz–Jegher syndrome, familial pancreatitis [10–13]
   - **Premalignant tumors of the pancreas:** mucinous cystic neoplasms (MCNs) and intraductal papillary mucinous neoplasm (IPMNs) especially that occur in the main duct
   - **Diagnosis:** all patients with suspected pancreatic carcinoma (they may present with symptoms like weight loss, jaundice, floating stool, pain, dyspepsia, nausea, vomiting, and occasionally pancreatitis. As previously noted, sudden onset of DM in patient 50 years or older may be linked to pancreatic cancer; patient with long-standing DM may also develop pancreatic cancer) should undergo initial evaluation by pancreatic protocol CT scan [10–13].
   - **Imaging evaluation:**
     – Pancreatic protocol CT and MRI (submillimetric, axial section using a dual-phase pancreatic protocol with images obtained in the pancreatic and portal venous phase of the contrast enhancement)

- The radiology report should include:
  Morphology: tumor appearance, size, location, as well as the presence of abrupt cutoff pancreatic duct or biliary tree
  Arterial evaluation: assessment of the celiac axis, the SMA, and the common hepatic artery to document if there is any vessel contact, solid soft tissue contact, hazy attenuation, or focal vessel narrowing or contour irregularity.
  Venous evaluation: assessment of the main portal vein and SMV and documentation of any thrombosis within the vein and venous collaterals
  Extra-pancreatic evaluation: for any liver lesions, peritoneal or omental nodule, ascites, suspicious lymph nodes, and other extra-pancreatic disease sites [10–13].
- EUS: the role of EUS in pancreatic cancer is complementary to CT
- ERCP and PTC: can be used in patients who require biliary decompression or for therapeutic stent placement to palliate biliary obstruction when surgery is not elected or must be delayed.
- PET/CT scan may be considered after formal pancreatic CT protocol in high-risk patients to detect extra-pancreatic metastases [10–13].

• **Staging laparoscopy:** can be considered for patients staged with resectable cancer who are considered to be at increased risk of disseminated disease and patients with borderline resectable disease prior to administration of neoadjuvant therapy. Positive cytology from washings obtained at laparoscopy is considered M1 disease [10–13].

• **Biopsy:**
  - Although pathological diagnosis is not required before surgery, it is necessary before the administration of neoadjuvant therapy for a patient staged with locally advanced pancreatic cancer or for metastatic disease.
  - EUS-FNA is preferred over CT-guided FNA (better diagnostic yield, safety, and potentially lower risk of peritoneal seeding).
  - If the biopsy does not confirm a malignancy, at least one repeat biopsy should be performed.
  - Core needle biopsy is recommended, if possible, for patients with borderline resectable disease to obtain adequate tissue for possible ancillary studies.

• **Biomarkers:**
  - CA19-9:
    Although it is not specific to pancreatic cancer, the degree of increase in CA19-9 levels may be useful in differentiating pancreatic adenocarcinoma from an inflammatory condition of the pancreas.
    It has potential uses in diagnosis, screening, staging, determining resectability, as prognostic marker after resection, and as a predictive marker for response to chemotherapy
    National Comprehensive Cancer Network® (NCCN®) recommends measurement of serum CA19-9 level at diagnosis after adequate biliary drainage, after neoadjuvant treatment, prior to surgery, following surgery immediately prior to administration of adjuvant treatment and for surveillance [14]

• **Management:**
  - Criteria defining resectability status at the diagnosis (refer to algorithm)
  - The decision about resectability should be made in consensus at a multidisciplinary meeting.
  - Staging
  - Stage I and II (T1, T2, T3-N0-M0):
    Upfront surgery followed by adjuvant treatment
    Oncological resection of the primary tumor and regional lymph nodes
    For cancers of the pancreas head and uncinate, a pancreaticoduodenectomy is done. For cancers of the pancreas body and tail, distal pancreatectomy with en-bloc splenectomy is done.
    Analysis of the pancreatic neck and bile duct at the time of surgery by frozen section may be considered (it

should be taken approximately 5 mm from the transection margin with clean cut-side facing down, to avoid cautery artifact that may confound analysis and result in a false-negative. If the tumor is located within 5 mm of the margins, further excision of the pancreas should be considered to ensure at least 5 mm of clearance).

The preferred regimens for adjuvant treatment: modified FOLFIRINOX or Gemcitabine + capecitabine [10–13]

- Stage III:

  Borderline resectable: neoadjuvant followed by surgery

  The preferred regimens: FOLFIRINOX ± subsequent chemoradiation or Gemcitabine + albumin-bound paclitaxel ± subsequent chemoradiation

  Locally advanced unresectable: palliative treatment

- Stage IV: no survival benefit from surgery. Systemic treatment and supportive care [10–13].

- Important tips in the management:
  - Correct any coagulopathy preoperatively
  - If the tumor is resectable and the patient is jaundiced, no need for preoperative stenting.
  - If the patient in cholangitis: ERCP and stent (use plastic stent unless it is for palliative treatment use metallic stent) [10–13]
  - If the tumor is borderline resectable and the patient is jaundiced:

    Drain the biliary tree (ERCP and plastic stent)

    EUS and biopsy

    Neoadjuvant chemotherapy

    Reassess the response after 2 months of chemotherapy. If stable disease or improving, continue the neoadjuvant treatment. If still there is no response, resect the tumor. If there is a progression on neoadjuvant to unresectable, stop and start the palliative treatment.

    Restaging after neoadjuvant by CT pancreatic protocol, CA19-9 and performance status [10–13]
  - If the tumor is unresectable by imaging:

    Biliary obstruction: Metallic stent of the CBD or PTD

    Tumor-associated abdominal pain: ultrasound-guided celiac plexus neurolysis

    If there are signs of GI obstruction, insert duodenal stent [10–13]
  - If the tumor is unresectable on operation:

    Biliary obstruction: Hepaticojejunostomy

    GI obstruction: Gastrojejunostomy

    Tumor-associated pain: Celiac plexus neurolysis [10–13]

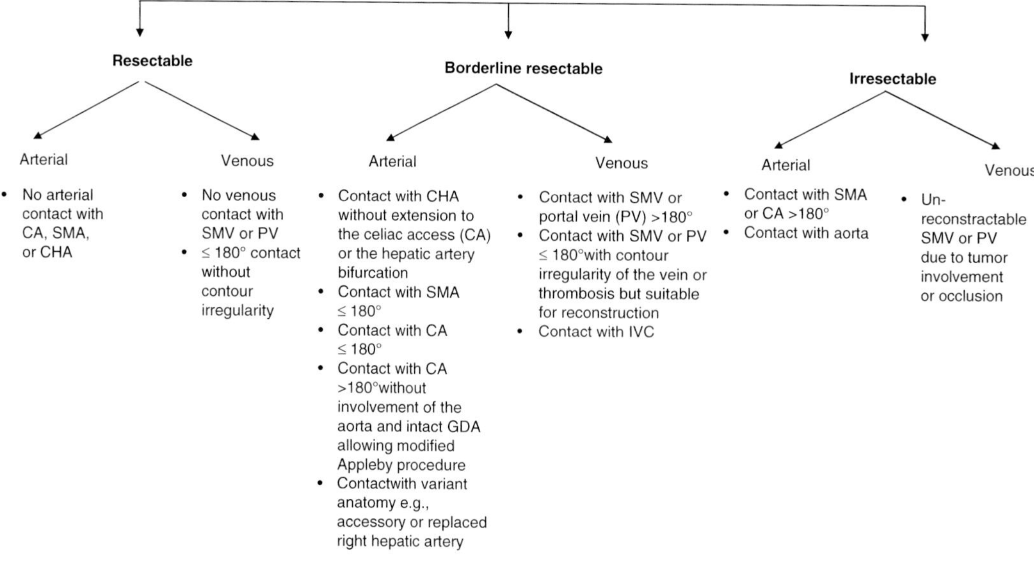

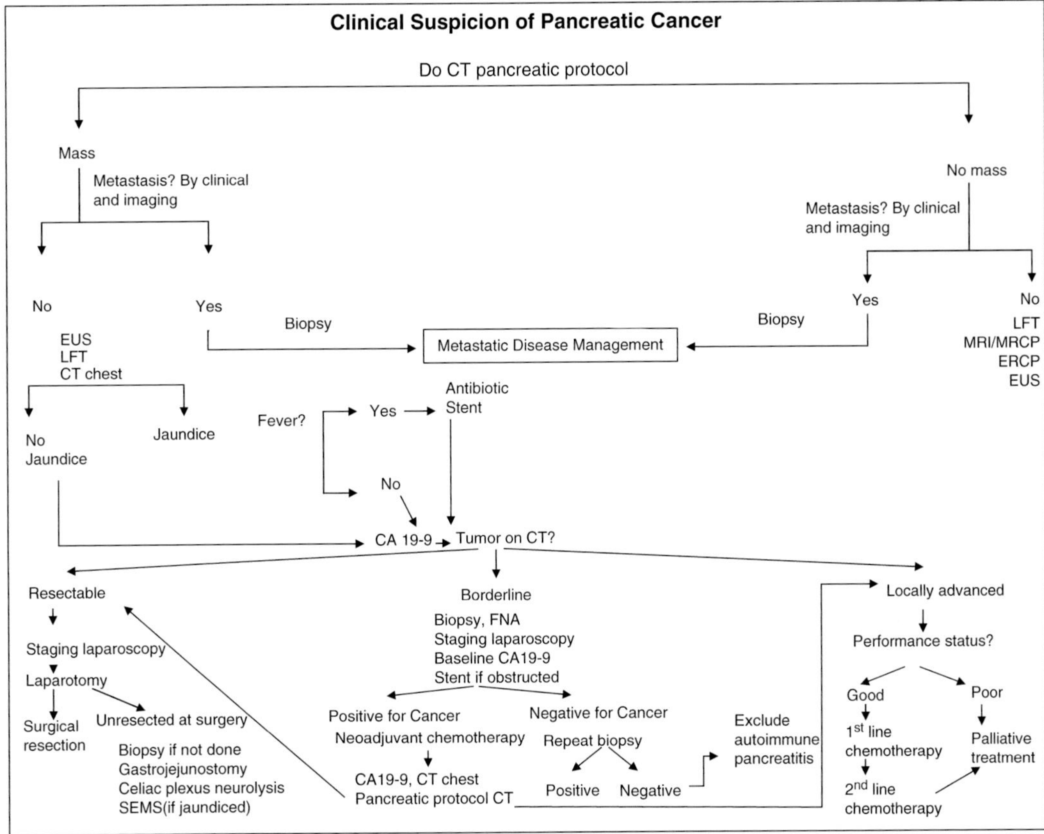

7.1.5 Management of Pancreatic Islet Cell Tumor Excluding Pancreatic Gastrinoma

- Pancreatic neuroendocrine tumors (PNETs) are rare (2–3% of all pancreatic tumors).
- It can be classified as functional and nonfunctional tumors.
- PNETs are usually sporadic but are also associated with autosomal dominant conditions such as MEN1 or with other syndromes like von Hippel–Lindau syndrome and neurofibromatosis.
- Clinical presentation depends on functionality [15].

Functional Tumors: Table 7.5

Nonfunctional tumors:

- 40% of PNETs do not have clinical symptoms.
- Appear as asymptomatic mass or with symptoms of compression due to large size (abdominal pain, anorexia, jaundice, weight loss)
- Diagnosis can be made by the presence of a pancreatic mass without hormonal symptoms, with increase chromogranin A (CGA) or pancreatic polypeptide (PP) or positive somatostatin receptor scan.
- Management:
- Patients with limited disease can undergo curative resection.
- Patients with advanced disease and large tumor burden may undergo cytoreductive surgery for palliative purposes [15].

Table 7.5 Functional tumor of the pancreas [15]

Tumor	Presentation	Diagnosis	Localization	Treatment
Insulinoma	• Age 40–45 years • Symptoms: headache, confusion, visual disturbances, palpitation, sweating, tremor • Whipple's triad: symptoms of hypoglycemia, a plasma glucose <40 mg/dl, and relief of symptoms with administration of glucose	• Elevated insulin to glucose ratio during fasting • Elevated C-peptide • The gold standard test: 72-h fast during which plasma C-peptide, proinsulin, insulin, and glucose levels are drawn every 6 h until symptoms emerge. Failure of insulin suppression in the setting of hypoglycemia supports the diagnosis of insulinoma	• Occur within the pancreas • 80% of tumors smaller than 2 cm • CT/MRI positive in only 20–40% • Somatostatin scan localizes only 25% of cases • EUS: modality of choice if others failed (positive in 70–95% of cases) • Selective angiography and hepatic venous sampling after calcium stimulation has reported high rates of localization • Intraoperative ultrasound + palpation detect the tumor in 92% of cases	• Because of low malignant potential (only 10%), it can be cured enucleation • Enucleation is safe if the tumor is >2–3 mm from the pancreatic duct, otherwise partial resection is indicated • Medical treatment of metastatic insulinoma: small frequent meal, control of hypoglycemia with medication such as diazoxide, somatostatin analogs, and glucocorticoid
Glucagonoma	• Almost exclusively in the pancreas • Malignant in 50–80% of the time • Symptoms and signs: necrolytic migratory erythema (**d**ermatitis), **d**iabetes, **d**iarrhea and **D**VT (4D syndrome)	• Elevated plasma level of glucagon • Biopsy of skin lesions: vacuolated keratinocytes in the epidermis	• CT/MRI is useful in identifying and localizing the tumor	• Surgical resection should be performed whenever possible • Margin: 2 cm • Normalization of glucagon level either by surgery or somatostatin analog usually result in rapid disappearance of the necrolytic migratory erythema • Palliative treatment: somatostatin analog or interferon-alpha

Vasoactive Intestinal polypeptide secreting tumor (VIPoma)	• Located selectively in the body and tail of the pancreas • >70% are malignant • Verner–Morrison syndrome (WDHA): watery diarrhea, hypokalemia, and achlorhydria • Hypercalcemia • Hyperglycemia • Flushing	• Serum level >200 pg/ml	• CT/MRI • Somatostatin scan (90% of VIPoma express somatostatin receptors)	• Correct electrolytes imbalance and volume repletion first • Surgical resection (possible in 80% of cases) to achieve 2 cm negative margins • Somatostatin analogs can control symptoms with or without surgery
Somatostatinoma	• Majority are solitary and large in size at the time of detection • Malignant in 60–70% of cases • Tumor >2 cm is associated with a high risk of metastasis • Higher in the pancreas > proximal small bowel • Diabetes • Diarrhea or steatorrhea • Weight loss	• Fasting plasma somatostatin level greater than three times the normal range + symptoms are diagnostic	• CT/MRI • Somatostatin scan	• Complete surgical resection when possible to achieve 2 cm negative margins • If advanced stage; tumor debulking, chemoembolization of the primary and secondary tumors and chemotherapy

7.1.6 Surgical Aspect of Spleen Disorder

Splenic cysts:

- It is rare.
- Classification:
  - True (with epithelial lining) or false (lacks epithelial lining)
  - Parasitic (hydatid) or nonparasitic
- Primary true splenic cysts account for only 10% of all nonparasitic:
  - They are lined by squamous epithelium.
  - Usually asymptomatic and discovered accidentally
  - Tend to have elevated CEA and CA19-9
  - They are benign in nature.
  - Their clinical importance is attributed to the mass effect and their potential to rupture and bleed profusely.
- Parasitic cysts are caused mainly by *Echinococcus granulosus*:
  - Splenectomy or unroofing of the cyst with marsupialization is described.
  - As with the hydatid cyst in the liver, extreme cautions should be taken while manipulating the cysts to prevent rupture or spillage of the cyst content into the abdominal cavity [16, 17].

Splenic Abscess:

- It is rare but has the potential to evolve into a life-threatening disease with mortality range from 15% to 20%.
- A pyogenic splenic abscess can be seen as an isolated splenic abscess or as a part of systemic multiple abscesses in an immunocompromised patient.
- Most of the splenic abscess originates from the hematogenic spread and some originate from a spread of infection from nearby infected organ, e.g., pancreas, colon, or kidney.
- Gram-positive cocci, e.g., *Staphylococcus* spp or *Enterococcus* and Gram-negative enteric organisms, e.g., *Salmonella* spp typically are involved.
- A unilocular abscess can be drained and treated with antibiotics whereas, a multilocular abscess usually is treated with splenectomy [16, 17].

Splenic Tumors:

- Primary and secondary tumors
- Primary tumors can be benign or malignant and can be categorized further into vascular neoplasm (originating from the red pulp) and lymphoid neoplasm (originating from the white pulp).
- Benign neoplasm of the spleen:
  - Hemangioma: the most common benign tumor of the spleen. They usually are asymptomatic and discovered incidentally. Large hemangioma may rupture and cause significant bleeding.
  - Lymphangioma: benign, slow-growing tumor. This lesion tends to be multiloculated and can be seen as an isolated splenic nodule or as a part of systemic lymphangiomatosis.
  - Hamartoma: rare benign tumor [16, 17]
- Malignant splenic neoplasm:
  - Lymphoma: the most common splenic malignant tumor. Secondary involvement of the spleen is more common than primary involvement.
  - Angiosarcoma: accounts for 1–2% of all soft tissue sarcoma. It is a highly aggressive tumor with a poor prognosis [16, 17].
- Secondary neoplasm of the spleen includes metastases from nearby or distant tumors. Metastatic melanoma, lung, ovarian carcinomas are reported to metastasize to the spleen [16, 17].
- CT scan or MRI is the gold standard for the diagnosis.
- Surgical management:
  - Preoperative planning and preparation are essential.
  - Laparoscopic splenectomy is the standard surgical procedure.
  - Open splenectomy is still indicated in abdominal trauma or in cases where spleen size does not permit safe laparoscopic resection [16, 17].

Splenectomy for Hematologic Disorders:

A. **Autoimmune and Idiopathic Disorders:**

- **Immune thrombocytopenia (ITP):**
  - Characterized by platelet destruction secondary to platelet autoantibodies
  - ITP is the diagnosis of exclusion and other condition that cause secondary ITP such as HIV, SLE, anti-phospholipid syndrome must be considered.
  - Most patients with ITP have asymptomatic thrombocytopenia. Symptoms of bleeding usually do not occur unless platelet count is less than 30,000/mm^3.
  - Platelet type bleeding includes bruising, purpura, petechiae, bleeding from the oral mucosa, epistaxis, menorrhagia.
  - The most severe complication is intracerebral hemorrhage.
  - Patient with persistent thrombocytopenia or platelet count less than 30,000/mm^3 should begin on corticosteroid therapy (1–2 mg/kg/day of prednisone for 2–4 weeks followed by steroid taper).
  - If the platelet counts remain low after 6–8 weeks of steroid therapy, or if the thrombocytopenia recurs after steroid taper, splenectomy should be considered [18].
  - IVIG (1 mg/kg/day for 1–2 days) can be considered for a patient who would benefit from rapid increases in platelet count.
  - Splenectomy is indicated for refractory ITP requiring multiple rounds of therapy or in patient suffer from an unwanted side effect.
  - Splenectomy results in a 75–85% permanent response with no need for further treatment.
  - If perioperative platelet transfusion is indicated, transfusion should be held until the splenic artery has been ligated [18].
- **Thrombotic Thrombocytopenic Purpura (TTP):**
  - Is a disorder in which a deficiency of ADAMS13 protein leads to increased platelet aggregation and subsequent microvascular thrombosis
  - TTP may occur spontaneously but often is precipitated by factors such as chemotherapy agents, cyclosporine, clopidogrel, or pregnancy.
  - Patients often have petechiae, fever, myalgia, and fatigue. Neurological symptoms include headache, mental status changes, seizures, and even coma. Patients can develop congestive heart failure or cardiac arrhythmias.
  - TTP is usually suspected in a patient with microangiopathic hemolytic anemia (MAHA) and thrombocytopenia in the setting of high LDH, elevated bilirubin, a negative Coombs test, and a peripheral blood smear demonstrating schistocytes, nucleated red blood cells, and basophilic stippling.
  - Initial therapy consists of daily plasma exchange. Seventy percent of patients will respond to this therapy.
  - Rituximab and glucocorticoids are second-line therapies.
  - Splenectomy reserved for refractory thrombocytopenia or frequent relapses (response rate for splenectomy is 40%) [18].
- **Autoimmune hemolytic anemia:**
  - Classified as warm autoimmune hemolytic anemia (WAIHA) or cold autoimmune hemolytic anemia (CAIHA) based on direct agglutinin test.
  - should be suspected in any patient with anemia, reticulocytosis, elevated LDH, low haptoglobin, and indirect hyperbilirubinemia
  - in WAIHA, polyclonal IgG autoantibodies directed toward RH antigens,

form a light coat over RBCs that then are removed by the spleen
- In children, the disease is self-limited, occurring after a viral infection and resolving in 2–3 months.
- Initial treatment with steroids usually results in improved hemoglobin levels within several days.
- Splenectomy is indicated for patients who fail to achieve remission by 3 weeks or those in whom hemoglobin levels cannot be maintained with low-dose steroid.
- In CAIHA, monoclonal IgM autoantibodies target RBCS at low temperature and cause hemolysis. RBC destruction is complement-mediated, and RBCs are removed by the liver, rather than the spleen.
- Treatment consists of avoiding cold temperatures. Steroids are usually not an effective treatment. Splenectomy is not indicated for the treatment of CAIHA because the liver is the site of RBCs destruction [18].

B. **Congenital Disease of the Blood:**
- **Hereditary spherocytosis:**
  - It is the most common congenital anemia.
  - Characterized by the presence of spherocytes in the peripheral blood smear, hemolytic anemia, and increased RBCs clearance by the spleen
  - Treatment by splenectomy is curative for almost all patient with dominant forms of spherocytosis and is indicated in the presence of growth retardation, skeletal changes, symptomatic hemolytic disease, anemia-induced organ dysfunction, leg ulcers, or development of extramedullary hematopoietic tumors.
  - Cholecystectomy should be performed at the time of splenectomy for patients with gallstones.
  - Splenectomy usually is delayed until after age 5 to decrease the risk of overwhelming post-splenectomy sepsis (OPSI) [18].
- **Hereditary Elliptocytosis:**
  - A rare disorder resulting from mutation of the RBC membrane skeleton proteins
  - Most patients are asymptomatic with a mild compensated anemia or even no anemia.
  - Splenectomy is indicated in patients with symptomatic anemia and is curative [18].
- **Hereditary Pyropoikilocytosis (HPP):**
  - Autosomal recessive severe hemolytic anemia
  - The disease is usually seen as anemia and jaundice in newborns and infants.
  - Splenectomy is curative for patients with severe anemia [18].
- **Thalassemia:**
  - Autosomal dominant hematologic disorder caused by a defect in the synthesis of one or more of the hemoglobin chains
  - Treatment consists of periodic, lifelong blood transfusion and iron chelation therapy.
  - Splenectomy is reserved for a patient with increased blood transfusion requirements arising in the setting of hypersplenism.
  - Transfusion requirements of more than 180–200 ml/kg/year of PRBCs usually represent excessive RBC requirements and warrants splenectomy.
  - Splenectomy usually is delayed until the age of 4 or 5 to decrease the risk of infectious complication (OPSI) [18].
- **Sickle Cell Anemia (SCA):**
  - Autosomal recessive hemoglobinopathy characterized by an amino acid substitution on the beta chain of the hemoglobin molecule
  - Splenectomy is rarely indicated for sickle cell disease because of autoinfarction of the spleen but can be indicated in case of splenic abscesses and splenic sequestration.
  - Acute splenic sequestration has a high mortality (up to 15%), characterized by

massive splenomegaly, acute exacerbation of anemia, and hypovolemia. This is treated initially with the restoration of blood volume and RBC mass. Splenectomy should be considered to prevent further episodes of sequestration [18].

- **Pyruvate Kinase Deficiency:**
  - Autosomal recessive disease
  - RBC are less deformable and often destroyed in the spleen, leading to splenomegaly.
  - Hemolysis can be exacerbated by acute infection and pregnancy.
  - Splenectomy is indicated for patients with a severe hemolytic variant of pyruvate kinase deficiency or patient requiring a number of transfusions [18].
- **G6PD Deficiency:**
  - Glucose 6 phosphate dehydrogenase deficiency is the most common enzyme deficiency in the world.
  - It is an X-linked disorder.
  - Treatment is directed at the inciting agent.
  - Severe anemia is treated with transfusion.
  - Splenectomy is rarely if ever, indicated for the anemia associated with G6PD deficiency [18].

C. **Neoplasms and Myeloproliferative Disorders:**

- **Hodgkin's Lymphoma:**
  - Primary treatment may consist of chemotherapy and/or radiation.
  - Splenectomy is rarely indicated but may be beneficial for patients who develop thrombocytopenia or symptoms related to splenomegaly [18].
- **Non-Hodgkin's Lymphoma:**
  - Most common type of lymphoma
  - Most common primary splenic neoplasm with splenic involvement occurring in 65–80% of cases
  - Splenectomy is indicated for symptoms related to massive splenomegaly and cytopenias resulting from hypersplenism [18].
- **Hairy Cell Leukemia:**
  - It is a rare type of leukemia.
  - Symptoms include splenomegaly, pancytopenia, neoplastic peripheral mononuclear cell, and bone marrow infiltration.
  - Pancytopenia is caused by hypersplenism and replacement of bone marrow by leukemic cells.
  - Splenectomy is rarely indicated for the treatment of this disease and reserved for cases of incomplete response to first-line therapy, persistent splenomegaly in the absence of bone marrow involvements and severe bleeding from thrombocytopenia [18].
- **Chronic Lymphoid Leukemia:**
  - Represents a B cell leukemia in which there is a progressive accumulation of functionally incompetent lymphocytes
  - Splenic infiltration is common in advanced stages and can lead to severe splenomegaly and substantial cytopenias because of hypersplenism.
  - Splenectomy is indicated to relieve symptoms associated with massive splenomegaly [18].

7.1.7 Pancreatic and Splenic Operation

Preoperative preparation:

- Admission
- Review the images, laboratory results, tumor board decision (for patient required splenectomy, the spleen size can be assessed by ultrasound/CT)
- ECG and Chest-X ray
- ICU consultation
- Anesthesia consultation
- NPO
- IV fluid
- Prophylactic medication (antibiotic, anticoagulant, and stress ulcer)
- Preoperative vaccination for encapsulated bacteria if a splenectomy is to be done.
- Correct coagulopathy

- If the patient has been treated with chronic corticosteroids, a stress dose should be administered with a rapid taper postoperatively.
- Consent

Consent of pancreaticoduodenectomy (Whipple Procedure):

- **The procedure:** under general anesthesia, through an abdominal incision, exploration of the abdomen, and proceed for resection if it is feasible. If the tumor found unresectable at the operation, gastrointestinal and biliary bypass if indicated.
- **Describe if there are any alternatives**
- **Describe the complication:**
  General complication: DVT, PE, MI, Pneumonia, UTI, infection
  Specific: Bleeding, collection, pancreatic leak and fistula, biliary leak, collection, delayed gastric emptying, injury to the nearby structure, and pancreatic insufficiency

Pancreaticoduodenectomy:
Anatomy of the pancreas: Fig. 7.1
Procedure:

- Under general anesthesia and endotracheal intubation
- Epidural analgesia, A-line, central venous line insertion
- Time out, confirm correct patient, correct procedure, surgeon and special instrument (Thompson retractor, GIA, intraoperative ultrasound, or any other required instrument)
- Position: Supine
- Prepping and draping in a usual sterile fashion
- Incision: upper midline incision in a thin patient, or bilateral subcostal incision if the patient is obese.
- Divide the skin and subcutaneous layers, enter the abdominal cavity
- The procedure is divided into three phases:

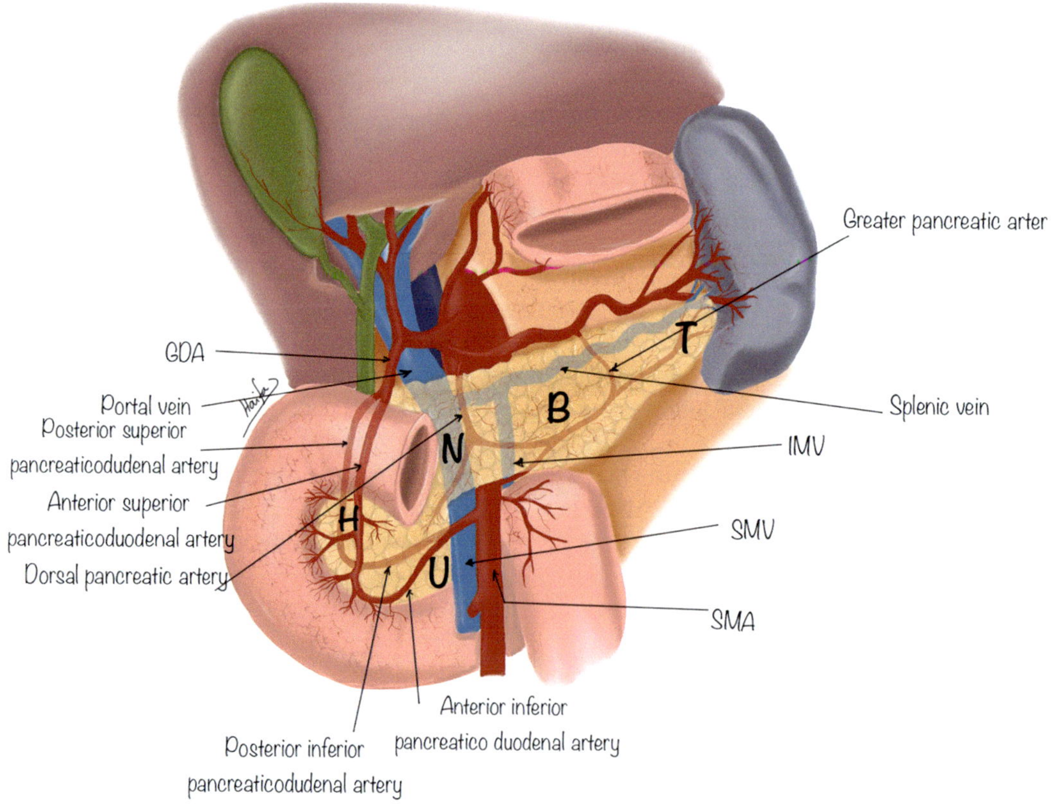

Fig. 7.1 Anatomy of the pancreas

- **Exploration and assessment:**
  The liver and peritoneal surfaces (visceral and partial) are thoroughly assessed, use intraoperative ultrasound if available.
  Open the gastrohepatic ligament and assess the celiac lymph node.
  The base of the transverse colon to the right of the middle colic vessels is examined for tumor involvement.
  Mobilize the right colon and the hepatic flexure off the duodenum and head of the pancreas and reflect it medially.
  Perform extended Kocher maneuver by dissecting behind the head of the pancreas and duodenum.
  Identify the SMV and dissect it toward the lower border of the pancreas.
  Ligate the gastroepiploic vein and artery to prevent any traction injury.
  Assess for any aberrant right hepatic artery by palpating the backside of the hepatoduodenal ligament for any prominent pulsation.
  Examine the ports hepatis, enlarged or firm lymph node can be swept down toward head of the pancreas (it does not preclude resection).
  If the assessment phase reveals no contraindication to Whipple, commence the resection phase [19–21].
- **Resection phase:**
  The proximal hepatic artery is identified by removing the lymph node that lies anterior to the artery, dissect the artery and trace it toward porta hepatis.
  GDA is identified, test clamping is performed to ensure that a strong pulse remains in the proper hepatic before the division of the GDA.
  Once GDA is divided, the hepatic artery retracted medially and the CBD laterally to expose the anterior surface of the portal vein.
  The tunnel under the neck of the pancreas can be completed under direct vision from the inferior and superior.
  Perform cholecystectomy (Fig. 7.2)
  Divide the antrum (Fig. 7.3)

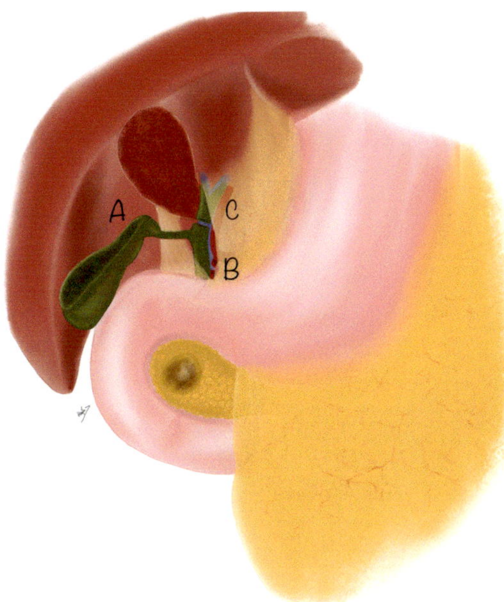

Fig. 7.2 Division of the GDA is followed by cholecystectomy and division of the CHD

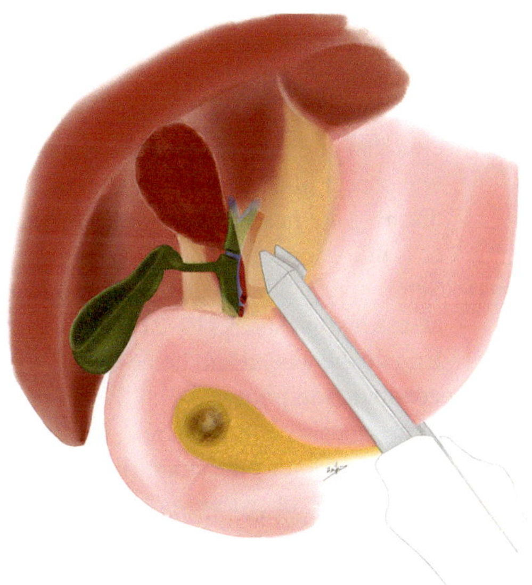

Fig. 7.3 Divide the antrum in standard pancreaticoduodenectomy and the first part of the duodenum in pyloric preserving Whipple's procedure

  Divide the jejunum 10–15 cm distal to the ligament of Treitz.
  Ligate the mesentery until jejunum can be delivered posterior to the superior mesenteric vessels from left to right.

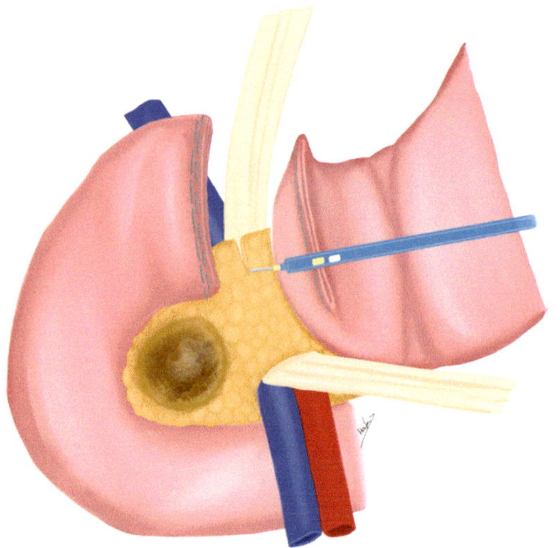

Fig. 7.4 Division the pancreatic neck anterior to the portal vein

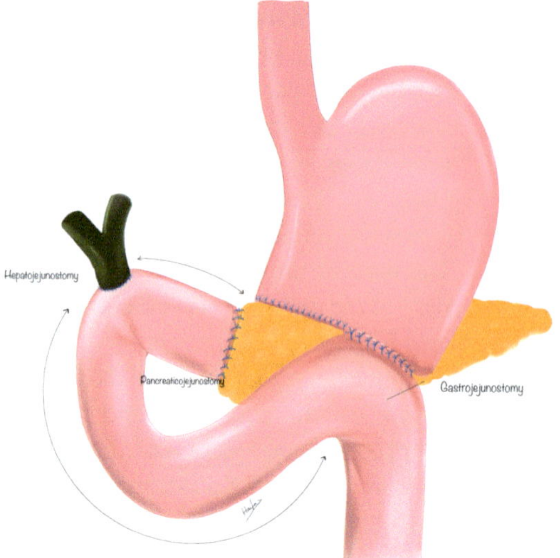

Fig. 7.5 Anastomosis of the pancreas first then biliary and finally the stomach or duodenum in case of pyloric preserving pancreaticoduodenectomy

Divide CHD just above the entrance of the cystic duct and dissect the duct down to the superior margin of the duodenum.

Divide the pancreatic neck anterior to the portal vein (Fig. 7.4).

Pancreatic head and the uncinate process then are dissected off the right lateral aspect of SMV, ligate the branches draining the head and the uncinate process into the portal vein.

Send specimen to histopathology to assess margin status [19–21].

Irrigate the wound and hemostasis.

- **Reconstruction phase:**

  Anastomosis of the pancreas first, then biliary and finally the stomach or duodenum in case of pyloric preserving pancreaticoduodenectomy (Fig. 7.5)

- *Pancreatojejunostomy*:

  Retro-colic, end to side pancreas to the anti-mesenteric border of jejunum in two layers with interrupted 4-0 nonabsorbable monofilament sutures (Fig. 7.6). The other technique is invagination (Fig. 7.7).

  10 cm distal to the pancreaticojejunostomy perform the hepaticojejunostomy as an end to side single anastomosis using interrupted stitches by 4-0 monofilament absorbable suture and close the mesenteric defect (Fig. 7.8).

  Side-to-side gastrojejunostomy performed 30 cm distal to the hepaticojejunostomy (the antecolic is preferred than retrocolic).

  Apply two 10 mm close suction drains near the pancreatic and biliary anastomosis.

  Feeding jejunostomy as indicated

  Close the abdomen in layers [19–21].

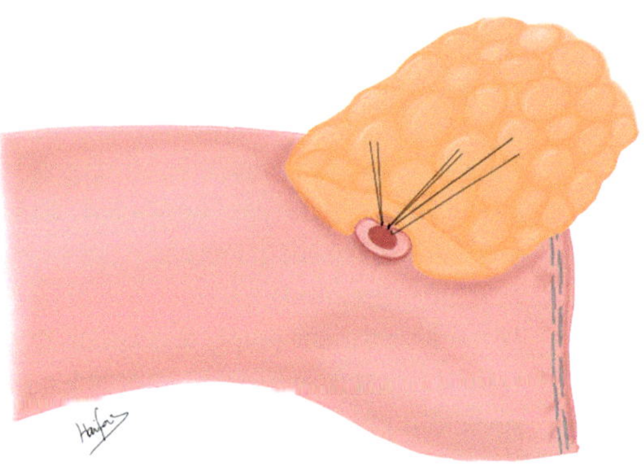

Fig. 7.6 Pancreaticojejunostomy (end to side)

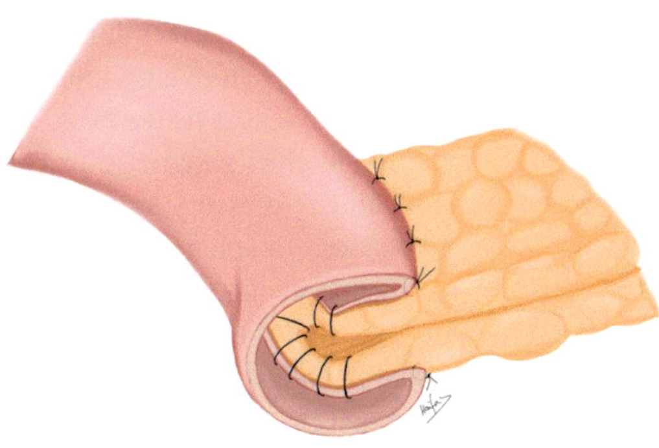

Fig. 7.7 Pancreaticojejunostomy (invagination technique)

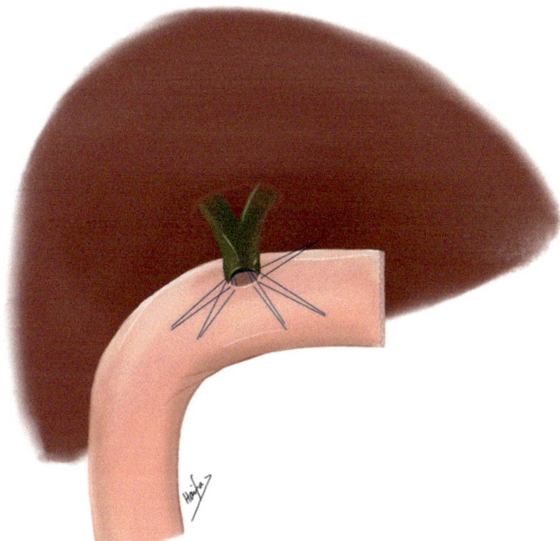

Fig. 7.8 End to side hepaticojejunostomy

Distal pancreatectomy and splenectomy:

- Under general anesthesia, endotracheal intubation, epidural catheter, arterial line, and central line
- Time out and confirm correct patient, correct procedure, and the required instruments
- Prophylaxis (DVT, antibiotics, stress ulcer)
- Position: supine
- Prepping and draping in a usual sterile fashion
- Incisions: bilateral subcostal or upper midline
- Exploration
- Enter the lesser sac by elevating the omentum off the transverse colon
- Expose the body and tail of the pancreas.
- Mobilize the splenic flexure inferiorly, retract the stomach up and the colon caudally
- The peritoneum along the inferior border of the pancreas is incised sharply.
- Mobilize the spleen from lateral to medial along its attachments to the colon, kidney, diaphragm.
- Continue mobilizing the spleen and the pancreas anteromedially from the retroperitoneum
- The splenic artery is identified, and suture ligated as it passes along the posterior superior surface of the pancreas
- The splenic vein is identified inferior and posterior to the splenic artery, ligate it and divide it.
- Stay suture is placed through the superior and inferior border of the pancreas on both sides of the transection plane.
- Divide the pancreas sharply, send the specimen for pathological assessment of the proximal margin
- Alternatively, the pancreas can be divided using a linear stapler provided the pancreas is not too thick (>1 cm).
- Close the pancreatic duct with a fine monofilament nonabsorbable suture in the form of a figure of eight or U-stitch.
- Close the pancreatic remanent by interrupted 3-0 Prolene mattress.
- When the pancreas transected by a stapler, no need for suture closure of the pancreatic duct.
- Irrigation and hemostasis
- Insert close suction drain proximal to the pancreatic end but not in direct apposition [19–21]

Laparoscopic Splenectomy:

- Under general anesthesia, endotracheal intubation
- Position lateral decubitus position or supine position with a bump under the left side, split leg position can be helpful when the patient is supine position and allows the operating surgeon to stand between the legs
- Time out and confirm correct patient, correct procedure, and the required instruments
- Prepping and draping in a usual sterile fashion

- Port placement generally includes a 12-mm periumbilical camera port, a 5-mm right upper quadrant port, a 5-mm left upper quadrant port, and a 12-mm left-sided port placed more inferiorly and laterally to allow passage of the endoscopic stapling device
- Access to the abdomen can be gained using a Veress needle, an optical trocar, or an open approach depending on the preference of the surgeon.
- The patient is generally repositioned in reverse Trendelenburg position with the left side up, after port placement and camera insertion, to facilitate exposure of the spleen.
- For patients with large liver or spleen, the use of a liver retractor can facilitate visualization.
- The abdomen is explored, paying careful attention to identifying accessory spleens that may be present. The liver should be inspected for signs of cirrhosis.
- The splenocolic ligament is mobilized and divided with an energy device. This allows further mobilization and retraction of the splenic flexure of the colon.
- The gastrosplenic ligament and the short gastric vessels then divided using an ultrasonic variational energy device, endoscopic metallic clips, or bipolar energy device.
- This dissection should be carried up the level of the left crus, and the stomach can be retracted to the right.
- The splenorenal ligament then is dissected to identify the splenic artery and splenic vein within the splenic hilum.
- These structures can be divided using a vascular load on an endoscopic linear stapling device taking care not to injure the tail of the pancreas.
- The splenophrenic ligament is divided last because this structure maintains cephalad/lateral retraction of the spleen during the division of the hilar vessels.
- The spleen is then placed into an endoscopic bag. The edges of the bag then are brought through the lateral trocar site. The spleen is morcellated using ring forceps and extracted in a piecemeal fashion.
- After extraction, the splenic bed, hilum, and the greater curvature of the stomach should be inspected thoroughly to insure hemostasis.
- At this point, the abdomen should be examined for splenunculi or accessory spleen. The most common locations of splenunculi are the gastrosplenic ligament and the greater omentum.
- Closure of the abdomen [19–21]

Postoperative complications:

- General complication like DVT, PE, MI, atelectasis, UTI, wound infection, or intraabdominal fluid collection
- Specific complication for pancreatectomy like delayed gastric emptying, pancreatic leak, bile leak, gastrointestinal leak, post-pancreatectomy hemorrhage, endocrine or exocrine insufficiency, overwhelming post-splenectomy sepsis (in case of splenectomy), and injury to the nearby structures [19–21].
- Delayed gastric emptying:
  - Happens in about 14–45% of patients
  - Diagnosed once the mechanical obstruction has been ruled out
  - Management:
    - Supportive
    - NPO
    - NGT decompression
    - Prokinetics
  - If prolonged, consider nutritional support and do CT abdomen to rule out secondary causes like an abscess.
- Postoperative pancreatic fistula:
  - Risk factors:
    - Small pancreatic duct
    - Soft gland
    - Non-pancreatic periampullary tumors
  - Definition:
    - Drain amylase >3 times normal serum level
    - At the third postoperative day or more
    - Regardless of the output volume
  - Treatment:
    - Conservative

NPO or naso-intestinal feeding
Empirical antibiotics
Maintain all the drains
Long-acting somatostatin analog
It usually closes within 4 weeks.

If the patient is unstable, has organ dysfunction, or septic, reexplore and revise the pancreaticojejunostomy [19–21]

- Post pancreatectomy hemorrhage:
  - Time is very important

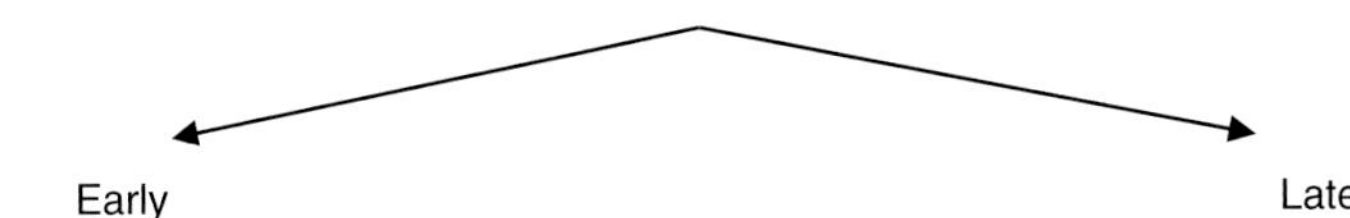

Early

- Within 24 hours
- Failure to achieve good hemostasis
- Best managed by return to OR

Late

- Any time thereafter
- Result from inflammation (pancreatic leak) that cause vascular erosion and formation of arterial pseudoaneurysm prone to bleeding
- Most common sites: GDA stump, Hepatic artery, SMA, or splenic artery
- Best managed by endovascular and embolization (83% success rate)
- Other option: attenuating covered stent to exclude the pseudoaneurysm specially the GDA stump

  - If there is
    Drop in Hb $\geq$ 3 g/dl
    Tachycardia, hypotension or shock
    Transfusion >3 units of PRBCs
    It is considered severe hemorrhage and needs urgent intervention [19–21].

Postoperative care:

Early postoperative period:

- Keep NGT until bowel function resumes
- IV fluid
- Medication:
  - Analgesia
  - Antibiotic as indicated
  - Anticoagulant
  - Stress ulcer prophylaxis
- Monitor CBC, electrolytes, blood glucose, bilirubin, amylase as required.
- If you suspect pancreatic fistula measure the amylase in the drain output.
- Encourage early mobilization
- Incentive spirometry
- Monitor the vital signs
- Pancreatic enzymes supplement may be required.
- Give prokinetic if the patient has delayed gastric emptying

First outpatient visit:

- Check if the patient has any complaint.
- Examine the wound.
- Remove the sutures or clips if there are any.
- Check the final pathology result.
- Arrange for multidisciplinary team discussion.
- Refer to medical oncology or radiation therapy as indicated.

Long-term follow-up (for patients with pancreatic cancer):

- Every 3–6 months history and physical examination for 2 years then every 6–12 months as clinically indicated.
- CA 19-9 and CT CAP every 3–6 months for 2 years after surgical resection
  - MRI of the abdomen and pelvis with contrast is also an option [14].

7.2 Part II: Practice

Do it again. Play it again. Sing it again. Read it again. Write it again. Sketch it again. Rehearse it again. Run it again. Try it again.
Because *again* is practice, and practice is improvement, and improvement only leads to perfection.
—Richelle E.

7.2.1 Case Scenarios for Practice

Tips:

- Practice with a friend and try to mimic the real exam!
  Do not forget to set the timer!
- The clinical data is provided in the answer key section.
- Some twist points are suggested after some cases and can be used to change the scenario to a more difficult one.

Case No. 1

A 43-year-old male patient presented to the ER complaining of upper abdominal area for 3 days.

Questions for discussion:

1. How will you approach the patient?
2. What is your differential diagnosis/provisional diagnosis?
3. What should you do next?
4. What is your final diagnosis?
5. How will you grade its severity?
6. How will you manage the patient?
7. Despite following your management plan, the patient is not improving clinically. What should you do?
8. How will you manage this?
9. After few days in the ICU, the patient develops high-grade fever 39°C and tachycardic 127 bpm. What should you do?
10. The patient's clinical condition is improving and shifted to the floor in a good condition. When will be the appropriate time for cholecystectomy?

Suggested twist points:

- The patient has persistent serous fluid output from the percutaneous drainage. What could be the cause, how will you confirm and manage this condition?
- The patient fails to respond to the percutaneous drainage, what will you do?
- When the patient is in the ICU, he required mechanical ventilation to maintain his oxygenation, became hypotensive with oliguria. What could be the explanation of this and how will you manage it?

Case No. 2

A 70-year-old male patient brought by his family to your clinic as he has jaundice and weight loss for 2 months.

Questions for discussions:

1. How will you approach such a patient?
2. What is your differential diagnosis/provisional diagnosis?
3. What will you do next to confirm your most likely diagnosis?
4. What is your diagnosis?
5. How will you manage this patient?
6. When and how will you assess the response?
7. The patient responds to the chemotherapy, what will you do?
8. What are the possible complications?
9. The patient underwent an uneventful operation and was admitted to the ICU for 48 h and then shifted to the floor. A few days later he complains of abdominal pain and high output from the drain that were placed near the pancreaticojejunostomy. What could be the explanation and how to confirm it?
10. How will you manage this complication?

Suggested twist points:

- The patient started on neoadjuvant chemotherapy and when you assess the response, it

seems the tumor is not responding to chemotherapy. What should you do?
- The patient has metastatic in the liver, what will you do?
- The patient has enlarged para-aortic lymph nodes, what will you do?

Case No. 3

A 49-year-old male patient presented to the clinic complaining of abdominal pain for 2 months.

Questions for discussion:

1. How will you approach the patient?
2. What is your differential diagnosis?
3. What will you do next?
4. How will you confirm the most likely diagnosis?
5. What is your diagnosis?
6. How will you manage this patient?
7. How will you follow the patient postoperative?

Checklist

History	Items	Done	Not done	Not applicable
General	Introduce himself/herself to the patient			
	Patient personal data (name, age, gender nationality)			
	Chief complaint			
	Duration			
Pain	Onset			
	Site			
	Character			
	Radiation/shifting			
	Aggravating/relieving			
	Severity			
	Progression			
	Frequency			
Mass	Onset			
	Site			
	How did the patient notice it?			
	Any change since it was first noticed?			
	Other masses			
Jaundice	Onset			
	Itching			
	Change in stool or urine color			
	Progression			
Associated symptoms	Pain			
	Fever			
	Nausea			
	Vomiting			
	Diarrhea			
	Constipation			
	Change urine or stool color			
	Itching			
	Abdominal distention			
	Dermatitis			
	Sweating			
	Palpitation			
	Fainting			
	Dizziness			

(continued)

History	Items	Done	Not done	Not applicable
Constitutional symptoms	Weight loss			
	Decrease appetite			
	Night sweating			
Symptoms of metastases	Back pain			
	Cough			
	Shortness of breath			
	Abdominal distention			
Risk factors	Gall stone			
	Alcohol			
	Medication: thiazide, steroid, propofol, hormonal replacement therapy			
	Previous hepatobiliary surgery			
	Smoking			
	Previous attack of pancreatitis			
	Recent ERCP			
	Recent increase in insulin requirements			
	New-onset diabetes			
	Diet (low-fiber, high-fat diet)			
	Family history of similar complain or malignancy, MEN syndrome, melanoma			
	Personal history of malignancy			
Differential diagnosis	Chest pain (MI)			
	Cough, SOB (pneumonia)			
	Recent history of trauma			
	Heartburn, gastric reflux			
PMH	Previous similar attack			
	Previous investigation			
	Previous admission			
	Chronic illnesses			
PSH	Previous surgery			
Family history	Of cancers or pancreatic problem			
Social history	Occupation			
	Habits (smoking, alcohol, drugs)			
Other	Medication			
	Allergy			
	Transfusion			
Systemic review				
Physical examination				
General principle	Patient position			
	Exposure			
	Privacy			
	Wash hands			
General examination	Appearance			
	Body built			
	Color			
	Distress/decubitus			
	Environment			
Vital signs	BP, HR, Temperature, RR, SPO_2			
Hand signs	Muscle wasting, palmar erythema, clubbing, flapping tremor, leukonychia, koilonychia			

History	Items	Done	Not done	Not applicable
Eyes	Jaundice, pallor			
Mouth	Jaundice			
Neck	Lymphadenopathy			
	Thyroid or parathyroid swelling			
Chest	Respiratory and CVS examination			
Abdomen: Inspection	Distention			
	Asymmetry			
	Dilated veins			
	Striae			
	Visible peristalsis			
	Scars			
	Signs of retroperitoneal hemorrhage			
Palpation	Superficial then deep palpation			
	Tenderness			
	Palpable masses			
	Organomegaly			
	Cough impulse at hernial orifices			
Percussion	Shifting dullness			
	Fluid thrill			
Auscultation	Bowel sounds			
	Bruit, venous hum			
Groin and hernias				
DRE & proctoscopy				
Back tenderness				
Differential diagnosis	According to the given scenario.			
Investigations				
General laboratory test	CBC with differential			
	Electrolytes			
	Liver function test (ALT, AST, GGT, Albumin, total bilirubin, direct bilirubin)			
	Amylase and lipase			
	LDH			
	Blood glucose			
	Lipid profile			
	Coagulation profile (PT, INR, aPTT)			
	Blood grouping			
	RFT			
	CPR/ESR			
	ABG			
Specific tests	Tumor marker (AFP, CEA, Ca19-9)			
	FNA and fluid analysis (pancreatic cyst)			
Imaging	Ultrasound abdomen			
	Triphasic CT abdomen			
	MRI/MRCP			
	ERCP/choledochoscope			
	EUS and FNA			
Biopsy	If indicated			
Provisional diagnosis	According to the given scenario			

(continued)

History	Items	Done	Not done	Not applicable
Management (depend on the diagnosis)				
Acute pancreatitis	Initial assessment of severity			
	Admission (ICU, ward)			
	Oxygenation			
	NPO/tube feeding/TPN			
	IV fluid			
	Analgesia			
	Prophylaxis (DVT & stress ulcer)			
	Monitor input and output			
	CT pancreatic protocol if indicated			
	Antibiotic if there is a concomitant infection			
	ERCP if there is biliary obstruction			
	Cholecystectomy before discharge if mild biliary pancreatitis			
Infected necrosis	Antibiotics			
	Percutaneous drainage			
	Endoscopic drainage			
	Laparoscopic transperitoneal drainage			
	VARD			
	Open necrosectomy			
Pancreatic pseudocyst	Endoscopic drainage			
	Surgical drainage			
Pancreatic fistula	Recognition (drain amylase)			
	NPO			
	IV fluid			
	Wound care			
	TPN/postpyloric feeding			
	Antibiotic if indicated			
	Octreotide			
	ERCP and sphincterotomy if indicated			
Mucinous cyst	Admission			
	Preoperative preparation			
	Consent			
	Vaccination 2 weeks preoperative			
	Resection (distal pancreatectomy with splenectomy)			
	Check the margins			
	If malignant, consider adjuvant chemotherapy and surveillance			
IPMN	Admission			
	Preoperative preparation			
	Consent			
	Vaccination 2 weeks preoperative if a splenectomy is required			
	Resection if high risk or worrisome features			
	Follow up for small, low-risk lesions			

History	Items	Done	Not done	Not applicable
Pancreatic adenocarcinoma (Resectable)	Staging			
	Tumor board discussion			
	Assess resectability			
	Admission			
	Consent			
	NPO			
	IV fluid			
	Prophylactic medication (DVT and stress ulcer and preoperative antibiotics)			
	Exploration			
	Resection			
	Frozen section of the margins			
	Reconstruction			
Insulinoma	Fasting insulin/glucose ratio			
	C-peptide			
	72 h fasting tests			
	Localization if the diagnosis is confirmed CT/MRI, somatostatin scan, EUS, selective angiography, and hepatic venous sampling			
	Enucleation			
	If metastatic, medical treatment, e.g., diazoxide, somatostatin analog, and glucocorticoid			
Postoperative care				
Early postoperative	Admission to HDU or ICU			
	Early mobilization and DVT prophylaxis			
	Enteral nutrition when possible			
	Analgesia			
	Stress ulcer prophylaxis			
	CBC and LFT daily			
	Coagulation profile especially PT			
	Electrolyte assessment			
	Monitor drain output and the nature of the fluid (blood, bile, serous)			
First outpatient visit	Clinical assessment			
	Remove sutures			
	Review the final pathology report			
	Arrange for multidisciplinary discussion if the case is cancer			
	Refer to oncology if adjuvant treatment is required			
Long term follow-up Pancreatic cancer	Every 3–6 months history and physical examination for 2 years then every 6–12 months as clinically indicated			
	Ca 19-9 and CT CAP every 3–6 months for 2 years after surgical resection			

7.2.2 Answer Key

Case No. 1

A 43-year-old male patient presented to the ER complaining of the upper abdominal area for 3 days.

Questions for discussion:

1. **How will you approach the patient?**
   By obtaining a relevant history and performing a physical examination
   The patient is a 43-year-old male patient who is presenting to the emergency department complaining of epigastric pain that is radiated to the back. The pain is relieved when the patient is leaning forward. It is moderate in severity and progressing since onset. It is associated with nausea and multiple times vomiting. No history of fever, no jaundice, no change in urine or stool color. He is a heavy smoker but not an alcoholic. He has no chest pain or palpitation, no heartburn, no dysphagia. He has no previous similar complaint and has no previous related investigations.
   He is diabetic on insulin. He has no history of previous surgery.
   On examination:
   The patient looks ill but not pale or jaundiced
   His vital signs: BP: 134/85 mmHg, PR: 109 bpm, temperature: 37.3 °C
   He has significant tenderness at the epigastric area but no guarding or rigidity
   Otherwise, unremarkable
2. **What is your differential diagnosis/provisional diagnosis?**
   - **Acute pancreatitis (provisional)**
   - Acute gastritis
   - Complicated PUD
   - Acute cholecystitis
   - Inferior MI
   - Hepatitis
   - Aortic dissection
   - Aortic aneurysm
3. **What should you do next?**
   Give analgesia, IV fluid, and send laboratory investigation for CBC, LFT, RFT, amylase, lipase, inflammatory markers, blood glucose, and LDH. Chest X-ray, ECG, and abdominal ultrasound
   Blood test: Table 7.6
   CXR, ECG: normal
   Ultrasound showed gallstone, otherwise normal finding

Table 7.6 Blood test for Case 1

Test	Result	Normal value
WBC (k/ul)	18	4.8–10.8
HB (g/dl)	13	12.6–16.5
PLT (K/ul)	450	130–400
ALT (U/l)	130	10–130
AST (U/l)	270	10–34
Total bilirubin (mg/dl)	0.8	0–0.8
Direct bilirubin (mg/dl)	0.3	0–0.3
Albumin (g/dl)	3.6	2.4–4
Creatinine (mg/dl)	1	0.7–1.2
PT (seconds)	12	10–13
INR	1	1
Blood glucose (mg/dl)	350	
Amylase (U/ml)	1902	60–180
Lipase (U/ml)	850	0–160
LDH (IU/l)	200	135–214
ESR (mm/h)	17	<15
CRP (mg/l)	75	<3

4. **What is your final diagnosis?**
   Acute biliary pancreatitis
5. **How will you grade its severity?**
   Using one of the pancreatic severity scoring systems, e.g., Ranson's criteria
   He has Ranson's 3
6. **How will you manage the patient?**
   Admission to ICU or HDU
   IV fluid
   Oxygen supplementation
   Enteral feeding if tolerated
   Analgesia
   Antiemetic
7. **Despite following your management plan, the patient is not improving clinically. What should you do?**
   Baseline CT abdomen
   CT: The pancreas is swollen and around 30% of the pancreas is non-enhancing
8. **How will you manage this?**
   Continue supportive care and ICU management

9. **After a few days in the ICU, the patient develops high-grade fever 39 °C and tachycardic 127 bpm. What should you do?**
   - Repeat the CT
     CT result: showed an area of collection around the body of the pancreas with few air bubbles seen inside the collection
   - Drain the collection
   - Start antibiotic
10. **The patient's clinical condition is improving and shifted to the floor in a good condition. When will be the appropriate time for cholecystectomy?**
    After 6 weeks

Suggested twist points:

- **The patient has persistent serous fluid output from the percutaneous drainage. What could be the cause, how to confirm it and manage this condition?**
- It could be a pancreatic fistula. To confirm the diagnosis, send amylase from the drain output. If it is three times higher than the serum level, the diagnosis is confirmed.
- Management is conservative with IV fluid, octreotide, and postpyloric feeding if required
- **The patient fails to respond to the percutaneous drainage, what will you do?**
- Follow the step-up approach with endoscopic drainage, VARD, or open necrosectomy
- **When the patient is in the ICU, he required mechanical ventilation to maintain his oxygenation, became hypotensive with oliguria. What could be the explanation of this and how will you manage it?**
- Compartment syndrome should be ruled out by measuring the intra-bladder pressure. If the diagnosis is compartment syndrome, the patient needs urgent decompressive laparotomy.

Case No. 2

A 70-year-old male patient brought by his family to your clinic as he has jaundice and weight loss for 2 months.

Questions for discussions:

1. **How will you approach such a patient?**
   By obtaining a history and performing a physical examination

The patient is a 70-year-old male patient who is complaining of gradual onset of jaundice that was noticed initially by his wife. It is associated with dark urine, pale stool, itching, poor appetite, and significant weight loss (20 kg over the last 2 months).

He has no abdominal pain, vomiting, or change in bowel habits. He is diabetic and his blood sugar recently become difficult to control with his usual dose of insulin.

He has no significant family history of GI or endocrine malignancy

He is a smoker but not an alcoholic.

He underwent laparoscopic cholecystectomy when he was 45 years old.

On examination

He looks jaundiced, cachectic

Vital signs: BP: 128/65 mmHg, PR: 92 bpm, temperature: 37.1 °C

The abdomen soft, non-tender with palpable round shape mass at the right upper quadrant just below the costal margin at the level of mid clavicular line, smooth surface and it is about 5 × 3 cm in size.

DRE is normal

2. **What is your differential diagnosis/provisional diagnosis?**
   - Pancreatic cancer (provisional)
   - Cholangiocarcinoma
   - Gallbladder cancer
   - Duodenal cancer
   - Liver mass
3. **What will you do next to confirm your most likely diagnosis?**
   Blood investigations: Table 7.7

   CT abdomen pancreatic protocol showed heterogenous mass at the head of the pancreas measuring 4 × 4 cm, it encases the SMV in more than 190° of its circumferences without intravenous thrombosis. Other vessels are not involved by the tumor. There are multiple enlarged peripancreatic lymph nodes. Both intra- and extrahepatic ducts and the gallbladder are dilated.
4. **What is your diagnosis?**
   Pancreatic adenocarcinoma
5. **How will you manage this patient?**
   Staging CT CAP (negative)

Table 7.7 Blood test for Case 2

Test	Result	Normal value
WBC (k/ul)	10	4.8–10.8
HB (g/dl)	9	12.6–16.5
PLT (K/ul)	250	130–400
ALT (U/l)	120	10–130
AST (U/l)	27	10–34
Total bilirubin (mg/dl)	11	0–0.8
Direct bilirubin (mg/dl)	8	0–0.3
Albumin (g/dl)	3	2.4–4
Creatinine (mg/dl)	1.2	0.7–1.2
PT (seconds)	13	10–13
INR	1.2	1
Blood glucose (mg/dl)	435	
CEA (ng/ml)	5	<5
CA 19-9 (u/ml)	878	0–27
AFP	3	<7

Multidisciplinary team approach

Biliary stent (endoscopic plastic stent were inserted)

Staging laparoscopy (negative)

Neoadjuvant chemotherapy

6. **When and how will you assess the response?**
   Repeat the CT abdomen
7. **Patient responds to the chemotherapy, what will you do?**
   Prepare for pancreaticoduodenectomy (Whipple procedure)
8. **What are the possible complications?**
   - Delayed gastric emptying
   - Hemorrhage
   - Pancreatic leak
   - Bile leak
   - Enteric leak
   - Marginal ulcer
   - Stenosis of the anastomoses
   - Pancreatic insufficiency
9. **The patient underwent an uneventful operation and was admitted to the ICU for 48 h and then shifted to the floor. A few days later he complains of abdominal pain and high output from the drain that were placed near the pancreaticojejunostomy. What could be the explanation and how to confirm it?**
   Pancreatic fistula
   Send for fluid amylase if it is three times the serum level the diagnosis is confirmed
10. **How will you manage this complication?**
    - Conservative
    - NPO or naso-intestinal feeding
    - Empirical antibiotics
    - Maintain all the drains
    - Long-acting somatostatin analog
    - It usually closes within 4 weeks
    - If the patient is unstable, has organ dysfunction, or septic, reexplore and revise the pancreaticojejunostomy

Suggested twist points:

- **The patient started on neoadjuvant chemotherapy and when you assess the response, it seems the tumor is not responding to chemotherapy. What should you do?**
- Proceed for resection and venous reconstruction
- **The patient has metastatic in the liver, what will you do?**
- Palliative treatment
- **The patient has enlarged para-aortic lymph nodes, what will you do?**
- Contraindication for resection. Palliative treatment

Case No. 3

A 49-year-old male patient presented to the clinic complaining of abdominal pain for 2 months.

Questions for discussion:

1. **How will you approach the patient?**
   Start by history and physical examination

   The patient is a 49-year-old male patient who is complaining of upper abdominal pain for the last 2 months. It was started gradually and progressing over time. It has no special aggravating or reliving factors. The pain is vague and not radiated or shifted anywhere else.

   He has no previous similar complaint. It is associated with early satiety but no anorexia, weight loss, fever, or jaundice. He has no relevant family history.

   He is not an alcoholic.

   PMH and PSH are unremarkable

   Physical examination:

   There is palpable round shape epigastric mass, 6 × 6 cm, smooth surface, not tender or pulsatile

2. **What is your differential diagnosis?**
   Pancreatic mass
   Pancreatic pseudocyst
   Gastric mass
   AAA
3. **What will you do next?**
   CT abdomen pancreatic protocol:
   Basic labs: within normal limit
   There is a cystic lesion in the body of the pancreas. The distal main pancreatic duct is dilated >1 cm but the proximal duct looks normal
   No abnormal lymph nodes
4. **How will you confirm the most likely diagnosis?**
   EUS and FNA and fluid analysis
   The EUS: showed dilated main pancreatic duct with a well-defined cystic lesion seen at the body of the pancreas. No mural nodule or calcification.
   FNA and fluid analysis and the fluid were positive for mucin, amylase and CEA levels are elevated
5. **What is your diagnosis?**
   IPMN
6. **How will you manage this patient?**
   - Prepare the patient for surgery (distal pancreatectomy with splenectomy)
   - Vaccine against encapsulated bacteria 2 weeks prior to surgery
   - Admission
   - NPO
   - IV fluid
   - Prophylaxis (DVT, antibiotics, and stress ulcer)
   - Anesthesia consultation
   - ECG, CXR
   - Consent
7. **How will you follow the patient postoperative?**
   First outpatient visit:
   - Clinical assessment of the patient's general condition and the wound.
   - Remove sutures/clips
   - Check the final pathology report
     The final pathology confirmed the diagnosis of IPMN with low grade dysplasia and the margin was positive

   Long-term follow-up:
   MRCP every 6 months

References

1. Angela LaFace DD, Velanovich V. The management of acute pancreatitis. In: Cameron J, Cameron A, editors. Current surgical therapy. 12th ed. Canada: Elsevier; 2016.
2. Peter Dixon MP, Kowdley GC, Cunningham SC. The management of gallstone pancreatitis, Part B. In: Cameron J, Cameron A, editors. Current surgical therapy. 12th ed. Canada: Elsevier; 2016.
3. Behrns KE, Hughes SJ. The management of gallstone pancreatitis, Part A. In: Cameron J, Cameron A, editors. Current surgical therapy. 12th ed. Canada: Elsevier; 2016.
4. Nealon WH. The management of pancreatic pseudocyst. In: Cameron J, Cameron A, editors. Current surgical therapy. 12th ed. Canada: Elsevier; 2016.
5. Krezalek MA, Alverdy JC. The management of pancreatic necrosis. In: Cameron J, Cameron A, editors. Current surgical therapy. 12th ed. Canada: Elsevier; 2016.
6. Motokazu Sugimoto DS, Kozarek RA, Traverso LW. Pancreatic ductal disruptions leading to pancreatic fistula, pancreatic ascites, or pancreatic pleural effusion. In: Cameron J, Cameron A, editors. Current surgical therapy. 12th ed. Canada: Elsevier; 2016.
7. Paniccia A, Edil BH. The management of chronic pancreatitis. In: Cameron J, Cameron A, editors. Current surgical therapy. 12th ed. Canada: Elsevier; 2016.
8. Datta J, Vollmer CM. Unusual pancreatic tumors. In: Cameron J, Cameron A, editors. Current surgical therapy. 12th ed. Canada: Elsevier; 2016.
9. Dimou FM, Person JA, Riall TS. Intraductal papillary mucinous neoplasms of the pancreas. In: Cameron J, Cameron A, editors. Current surgical therapy. 12th ed. Canada: Elsevier; 2016.
10. Fisher WE, Anderson DK, Windsor JA, Dudeja V, Brunicardi FC. Pancreas. In: Brunicardi F, editor. Schwartz's principles of surgery. 11th ed. United States: McGraw-Hill Education; 2019.
11. Griffin JF, Poruk KE, Wolfgang CL. The management of periampullary cancer. In: Cameron J, Cameron A,

editors. Current surgical therapy. 12th ed. Canada: Elsevier; 2016.
12. Kadera B, Hines OJ. Palliative therapy for pancreatic cancer. In: Cameron J, Cameron A, editors. Current surgical therapy. 12th ed. Canada: Elsevier; 2016.
13. Tsai S, Evans DB. Neoadjuvant and adjuvant therapy for localized pancreatic cancer. In: Cameron J, Cameron A, editors. Current surgical therapy. 12th ed. Canada: Elsevier; 2016.
14. ["Referenced with permission from the NCCN Clinical Practice Guidelines in Oncology (NCCN Guidelines®) for pancreatic adenocarcinoma V.1.2021. © National Comprehensive Cancer Network, Inc. All rights reserved. Accessed [February 18]. To view the most recent and complete version of the guideline, go online to NCCN.org. NCCN makes no warranties of any kind whatsoever regarding their content, use or application and disclaims any responsibility for their application or use in any way."].
15. Irene Lou HC. The management of pancreatic islet cell tumors excluding gastrinomas. In: Cameron J, Cameron A, editors. Current surgical therapy. 12th ed. Canada: Elsevier; 2016.
16. Park AE, Targarona EM, Weltz AS, CR-OL. Spleen. In: Brunicardi F, editor. Schwartz's principles of surgery. 11th ed. United States: McGraw-Hill Education; 2019.
17. Wiesel O, Fisichella PM. The management of cysts, tumors, and abscesses of the spleen. In: Cameron J, Cameron A, editors. Current surgical therapy. 12th ed. Canada: Elsevier; 2016.
18. John-Paul Bellistri PM. Splenectomy for hematologic disorders. In: Cameron J, Cameron A, editors. Current surgical therapy. 12th ed. Canada: Elsevier; 2016.
19. Zollinger R, Ellison E. Pancreatic cancer: surgical therapy. Zollinger's atlas of surgical operation. 9th ed. United States: McGraw-Hill Education; 2011.
20. Clavien P-A. Liver. In: Clavien P-A, MGS, Fong Y, editors. Atlas of upper gastrointestinal and hepato-pancreatic-biliary surgery. 9th ed. Germany: Springer; 2007.
21. Jean Nicolas Vauthey JS. Liver. In: Fischer JE, editor. Master techniques in general surgery. Hepatobiliary and pancreatic surgery. 9th ed. United States: Lippincott Williams and Wilkins; 2013.

8 Surgical Aspects of Esophageal Diseases for Clinical Board Exams

8.1 Part I: Knowledge

> Any knowledge that doesn't lead to new questions quickly dies out: it fails to maintain the temperature required for sustaining life.
> —Wislawa Szymborska

The Commonest Esophageal Complaints:

- Dysphagia
- Chest pain
- Bleeding

History:

- Introduce yourself to the patient.
- Name, age, occupation, sex, and nationality.
- Chief complaint and duration.
- History of presenting illness:
  - **Analysis of the Chief Complaint**

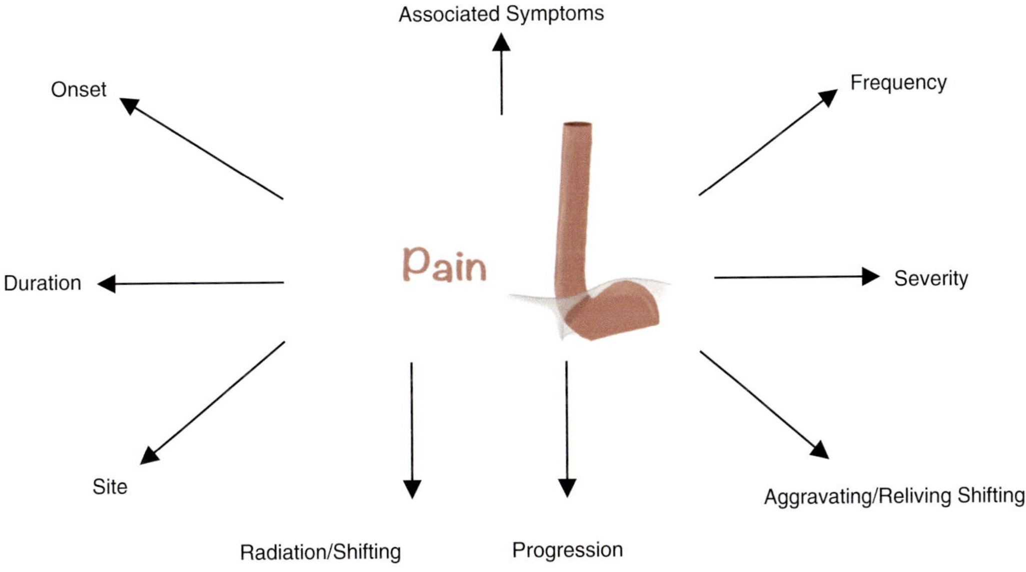

H. Alotaibi, *Study Surgery*, https://doi.org/10.1007/978-981-16-2305-9_8

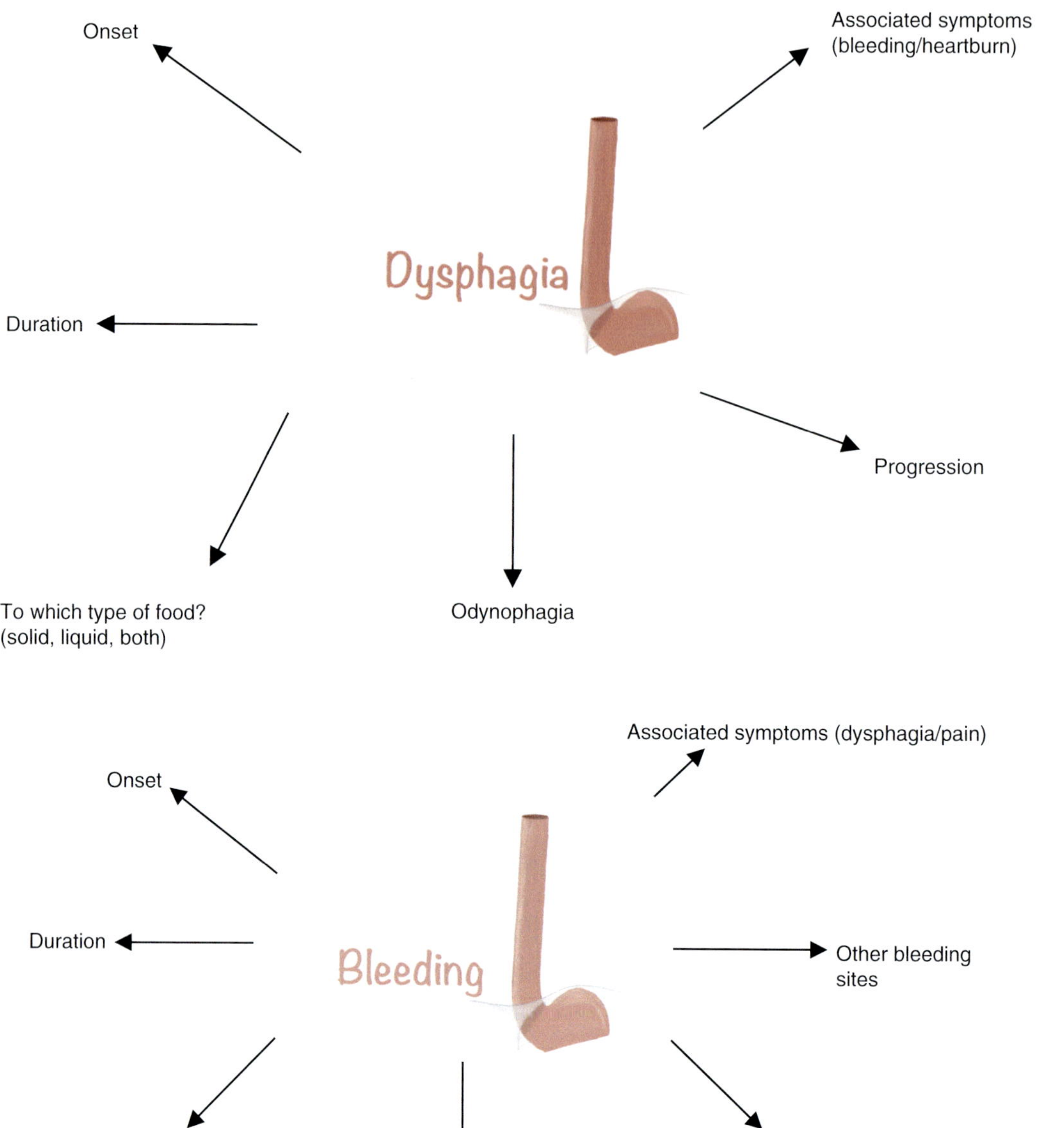

- **Associated Symptoms**
  Pain, fever, nausea, vomiting, diarrhea, change in bowel habits, hematemesis, abdominal distention, dysphagia, regurgitation, stridor, hoarseness, and hiccups
- **Constitutional Symptoms:**
  Weight loss, decrease appetite, night sweating, and fever
- **Symptoms of Metastasis**
  Back pain, abdominal distention, cough, and shortness of breath
- **Risk Factors:**
  Family history of similar complaint or malignancy
  Personal history of cancer
  Smoking

    Alcohol
    Long-standing gastroesophageal reflux disease (GERD)
    History of repeated vomiting/retching
    History of foreign body ingestion/caustic ingestion
  - Previous similar attack, previous admission, previous investigation, or endoscopy (if yes, when was it done and what was the finding?)
  - Systemic review of related system [gastrointestinal tract (GIT)]
    Jaundice, constipation, hematemesis, melena, and history of bleeding
- Past medical history (PMH).
- Past surgical history (PSH).
- Family history.
- Social history.
- Medication, transfusion, and allergy.
- Systemic Review:
  - Central nervous system (CNS): Headache, eye and hearing symptoms, epilepsy, numbness, and paralysis
  - Cardiovascular system (CVS): Chest pain, orthopnea, **paroxysmal nocturnal dyspnea**, lower limb edema, and palpitation
  - Respiratory: Cough, fever, chest pain, and hemoptysis
  - Renal: Dysuria, flank pain, and hematuria
  - Musculoskeletal: weakness, arthritis, and skin erythema

Physical Examination:

- Introduce yourself to the patient.
- Ask permission for examination.
- Assure privacy.
- Position.
- Exposure.
- Handwashing.

General Examination:

- **A**ppearance: ill, well, and dehydrated
- **B**ody built: Cachectic obese
- **C**olor: Pale, Jaundice
- **D**istress
- **E**nvironment and connection to monitors, fluids, drain, and chest tube

Vital signs: Blood pressure (BP), heart rate (HR), temperature, respiratory rate (RR), oxygen saturation (SpO_2)

Hands:

- Pallor
- Palmer erythema
- Koilonychia (iron deficiency anemia)
- Leukonychia (hypoalbuminemia)
- Pulse rate and its characteristics (rhythm, volume, etc.)

Eye:

- Jaundice
- Pallor

Neck:

- Lymphadenopathy

Chest:

- Air entry
- Surgical emphysema
- Signs of pleural effusion

Abdomen:

- Inspection:
  - Distention
  - Asymmetry
  - Visible veins
  - Scars/striae
  - Dilated veins (caput medusa)
  - Hernial orifices
  - Stretch marks
  - Visible peristalsis
- Palpations:
  - Superficial then deep palpation
  - Look for any tenderness
  - Palpable masses
  - Ascites
  - Organomegaly

- Percussion:
  - Shifting dullness
  - Fluid thrill
- Auscultation:
  - Bowel sounds
  - Bruit, venous hum

Groin and hernias
Digital rectal exam (DRE)

8.1.1 Approach to a Patient with Suspected Esophageal Perforation

- History and physical examination
- Investigations
  - Complete blood count (CBC)
  - Chemistry
  - Electrolytes
  - Liver function test (LFT)
  - Renal function test (RFT)
  - Coagulation profile
  - Blood grouping
  - Arterial blood gases (ABG), lactate
  - Erythrocyte sedimentation rate (ESR), C-reactive protein (CRP)
  - Blood culture
- Imaging:
  - Chest X-ray (CXR)
  - Abdominal X-ray (AXR)
  - Gastrografin/computed tomography (CT) with oral and intravenous (IV) contrast
  - Barium
- Endoscopy:
  - If images did not show the perforation, then the patient is highly suspicious for perforation.
- Management:
- Depend on hemodynamic stability and whether the perforation is free or contained

  A. **Nonoperative Management**
  - Criteria:

    Contained perforation
    Normotensive patient
    Pulse rate <100 bpm
    White blood cells (WBC): 12–14 × 10^9/L
    No evidence of ongoing sepsis
  - Admit to intensive care unit (ICU).
  - Nothing per oral (NPO).
  - Broad-spectrum IV antibiotics, antifungal (especially if there is gastric reflux).
  - Proton pump inhibitors (PPI).
  - Total parenteral nutrition (TPN).
  - Chest tube if needed.
  - Repeat imaging 72–96 h.
  - If no leak, start fluid diet with nutritional support.
  - If any deterioration with fever, leukocytosis, change mental status: Operative management is indicated.

  B. **Operative Management:**
  - Depend on location, size, and degree of contamination

    I. **Cervical Perforation:**
    - Left-sided neck incision along the anterior border of sternocleidomastoid muscle.
    - Ligate middle thyroid vein.
    - Retract thyroid and trachea medially.
    - Take care of the recurrent laryngeal nerve.
    - Blunt dissection to drain all the fluid collection.
    - If perforation identified, repair the defect primarily with absorbable suture.
    - The strap muscle can be used to buttress the repair.
    - Patch with strap muscle if you cannot repair primarily.
    - If the patient undergoes repair or patch, do gastrografin on day 5.
    - If the perforation is not identified, insert closed suction drain.

    II. **Abdominal Perforation:**
    - Through upper midline or left thoracotomy if perforation in a large hiatal hernia
    - Debride, repair primarily buttress with omentum, rotational flap, or partial fundoplication

    III. **Thoracic Perforation:**
    - Incision:

- Mid esophagus: right thoracotomy via fifth intercostal space
- Lower esophagus: left thoracotomy via seventh intercostal space
- Mid esophagus:
  - After entering the pleural cavity, open pleura in the area of perforation, debride the edge of perforation, determine the full extent of the injury, and avoid injury to the vagus nerve.
  - For fresh perforation, mucosa may be closed with running absorbable and muscularis with interrupted silk.
  - Irrigate copiously.
  - Buttress the repair by vascularized muscle flap harvested from fifth intercostal muscle (alternatives like pleura, pericardium can be used).
  - Drainage with 32 F chest tube adjacent to injury.
- Lower esophagus:
  - Similar to mid esophagus
  - Buttress with either intercostal or diaphragm
- Repeat the gastrografin in day 5.
- If the patient is unstable, has severe ongoing sepsis, or malignant perforation:
  - Esophageal exclusion: cervical esophagostomy (loop is preferred), gastrostomy, or jejunostomy.
  - Occlude the distal esophagus with 45 mm thoraco-abdominal stapler.
  - Avoid gastrostomy if stomach may be used as conduit later.

– **Esophageal Stent:**

  Patient with limited sepsis from contained leak

  To allow early resumption of enteral feeding

  May need video-assisted thoracoscopy (VATS) in 1–2 days for debridement of the pleural cavity

– **Tips and Tricks:**

  If the perforation happened in patient with achalasia: perform contralateral myotomy.

  If the perforation happened after Nissen fundoplication:

  - The esophagus can be accessed through abdominal approach.
  - Dismantle the fundoplication.
  - Primary repair.
  - Repeat the Nissen repair or use another type of antireflux procedure.

  Intubation in thoracotomy: use double lumen intubation.

  To identify the esophagus, use nasogastric tube (NGT) or Bougie cautiously [1, 2].

8.1.2 Approach to Patient with Variceal Bleeding

- Related to portal hypertension [account for 20% of all upper gastrointestinal (GI) bleeding].
- Causes:
  - Gastroesophageal varices
  - Hypertensive portal gastropathy
  - Isolated gastric varices
- Start resuscitation following the ABC approach:
  - A: Confirm the patency of the air way and assess the level of consciousness, intubate if needed.
  - B: Assess the oxygenation and ventilation.
  - C: Assess the hemodynamic status and start fluid and blood resuscitation.

    Insert two large cannula.

    Draw blood for investigation: CBC, electrolytes, coagulation profile, blood grouping and cross matching, ABG, and lactic acid.

Start fluid resuscitation (ringer lactate).
Start PPI (80 mg bolus followed by infusion 8 mg/h for 72 h).
- History and physical examination after achieving hemodynamic stability.

- Admission to ICU.
- IV fluid.
- IV PPI (infusion).
- Octreotide.
- Vasopressin ± nitroglycerol.
- NGT and Foley's catheter.
- Monitor the fluid input and output.
- Endoscopy (banding or sclerotherapy of the bleeding varices).
- If the bleeding is controlled with endoscopy, repeat the endoscopy to assess if the bleeding recurred or stopped.
- If the bleeding recurs, assess the degree of liver cirrhosis. For child A and B, perform surgical shunt. For child C, perform transjugular intrahepatic portosystemic shunt (TIPS) then liver transplantation later on.
- If the bleeding could not be controlled from the beginning, apply Sengstaken-Blackmore tube followed by TIPS then liver transplantation.
- Refer to the hepatobiliary chapter for more details about TIPS and surgical shunts.

8.1.3 Management of Motility Disorder

A. **Motility Disorder of the Body:**

1. **Diffuse Esophageal Spasm:**
   - Uncoordinated contractions of the esophagus
   - Typical symptoms: chest pain, dysphagia, or both
   - Diagnosis:
     - Radiological (esophagogram): Crock screw appearance (pesudodiverticulosis); indicate advanced disease
     - Manometry:
       Simultaneous multi-peaked contractions of high amplitude >120 mmHg for long duration >2.5 s, normal integrated relaxation pressure
   - Treatment:
     - Medical treatment includes nitrates and sildenafil and typical antidepressants.
     - Endoscopic.
     - Surgical:
       Indicated in patient with intractable chest pain or dysphagia who failed medical and endoscopic treatment or patient with bulging diverticulum of thoracic esophagus.
       Long myotomy through left thoracotomy. The proximal extent is the entire length of abnormal manometry. The distal extent should be the lower esophageal sphincter (LES).
2. **Nutcracker Esophagus:**
   - Characterized by excessive contractility.
   - It is the most painful of all esophageal motility disorder.
   - Diagnosis:
     - Manometry: High pressure (>180 mmHg) or long duration of swallow response (>7 s). Lower esophageal sphincter (LES) pressure is normal.
   - Treatment:
     - Medical: Nitrates, sildenafil, PPIs, and tricyclic antidepressant. Instruct the patient to avoid caffeine, cold, and hot food.
     - Endoscopic: Esophageal dilatation.
     - Role of surgery is questionable.

B. **Motility Disorder of the LES:**
Hypertensive Lower Esophageal Sphincter:

- Esophageal junction outflow obstruction.
- Defined as median integrated pressure >15 mmHg (hypertensive poorly relaxed LES). It differs from achalasia by effective peristalsis.
- Diagnosis:
  - Manometry: LES pressure >26 mmHg with incomplete relaxation
  - Treatment:
  - Endoscopic: Botox injection.

– Surgical: If failed to respond to endoscopic treatment. The operation of choice is modified Heller esophageomyotomy. If normal esophageal motility, add partial fundoplication, that is, Dor or Toupet.

C. **Disorder of both Body and LES:**
   1. **Achalasia:**
      - Primary: Destruction of nerves to LES leads to failure of LES to relax.
      - Secondary: Degenerative of the neuromuscular function of the body, pressurization of esophagus, dilatation, and loss of peristalsis.
      - Types:
        – Type I: Incomplete LES relaxation, aperistalsis, and absence of esophageal pressurization
        – Type II: Incomplete LES relaxation, aperistalsis, and pan-esophageal pressurization
        – Type III: Incomplete LES relaxation and premature contraction in at least 20% of swallow
      - Achalasia is known to be premalignant. The risk of cancer is 8% in 20 years.
      - The classic presentation: Dysphagia, regurgitation, and weight loss.
      - Diagnosis:
        – Esophagogram: Dilated esophagus, bird beak, or sigmoid esophagus
        – Motility study: Aperistalsis, failure to relax LES
        – Endoscopy: To rule out cancer
      - Treatment:
        – Medical: Nitroglycerin, nitrate, and calcium channel blocker
        – Endoscopy: Pneumatic dilatation, Botox injection
        – Surgical: Esophageomyotomy (modified Heller myotomy) ± partial fundoplication, per oral esophageomyotomy (POEM), or esophagectomy (megaesophagus, failure of more than one myotomy, stricture that is not amenable for dilatation)
   2. **Ineffective Esophageal Motility:**
      - Contraction abnormality of distal esophagus.
      - Usually associated with GERD.
      - Diagnosis:
        – Manometry: >50% of swallow are ineffective.
      - Treatment:
        – Best treatment is prevention.
        – Management is similar to GERD.
      - It differs from achalasia by resting LES which is typically low [1, 3, 4].

8.1.4 Management of Gastroesophageal Reflux Disease (GERD)

- Typical symptoms: Heartburn, acid regurgitation, and dysphagia.
- Atypical symptoms: Cough, hoarseness, chest pain, asthma, and aspiration.
- Normal LES characterized by:
  – Resting LES pressure is 13 mmHg.
  – Overall length is 3–6 cm.
  – Intra-abdominal length is 2 cm.
- Defective sphincter defined by one of the following:
  – Resting LES <6 mmHg.
  – Overall sphincter length is <2 cm.
  – Intra-abdominal length is <1 cm.
- The most common cause of defective sphincter is inadequate abdominal length.
- Once the sphincter is defective, it is irreversible.
- Complication of GERD:
  – Esophagitis
  – Stricture
  – Barrett's esophagus (BE)
  – Repetitive aspiration leads to pulmonary fibrosis
- Barrett's esophagus:
- Intestinal metaplasia is defined histologically by presence of goblet cells.
- Treatment:
  – Medical Management:

Instruct the patient to elevate the head of the bed when lying down.

To avoid tight fitting clothes.

To eat small frequent meal.

To avoid eating at nighttime or at least not prior to bedtime.

To avoid alcohol, avoid coffee, avoid chocolate, and peppermint.

Medication: PPIs (high does 40 mg/day), medication to promote gastric emptying.

Most patient will require life-long PPI.

– Surgical Management:

Selection of patient for surgery:

Objectively proven GERD (presence of ulceration esophagitis, abnormal 24-h PH study).

Persistent symptoms of reflux (heart burn, regurgitation) despite adequate medical treatment.

Young patient, unwilling to take life-long medication.

Patient with defective LES should be considered for antireflux surgery regardless of the presence or absence of endoscopic esophagitis.

– *Principles of Surgery:*

The goal is to create antireflux valve at the gastro-esophageal junction (GEJ) while preserving the patient's ability to swallow normally and to belch to relieve gaseous distention.

Operation should place adequate length of distal esophageal sphincter in the positive pressure of the abdomen.

Operation should allow the reconstructed cardia to relax on deglutition to ensure relaxation of the sphincter. Three important factors:

- Only the fundus of the stomach should be used to buttress the sphincter.
- Gastric rap should be placed properly around the sphincter and not to incorporate portion of the stomach.
- Damage to the vagus nerve during dissection of the thoracic esophagus should be avoided.

Fundoplication should not increase the resistance of relaxed sphincter to level that exceeds the peristalsis power of the body of the esophagus.

– *Procedure Selection:*

Nissen is the procedure of choice in all patient with GERD if they have normal or near normal esophageal motility.

Reserve partial fundoplication for use in individual with poor esophageal body motility [1, 5].

8.1.5 Management of Barrett's Esophagus

A. **Barrett's Esophagus (BE) Without Dysplasia:**
   - The patient should be managed like any other patient with GERD.
   - Control GERD (with PPI or antireflux surgery).
   - Berrett's esophagus is not per se an indication for antireflux surgery.
   - The role of mucosal ablation is unproven in patient with nondysplastic BE.
   - In case of long BE (>8 cm), ablation may reduce the complexity of four quadrant surveillance biopsies every 1–2 cm.

B. **Barrett's Esophagus with Low-Grade Dysplasia (LGD):**
   - If the endoscopy showing LGD did not include four-quadrant biopsies, the endoscopy should be repeated to rule out more advanced disease.
   - Start PPI if the patient is not yet on or increase the dose or frequency if he/she is already taking it.
   - Repeat the endoscopic biopsies in 6 months to evaluate for response.
   - Alternatively, the patient can be offered antireflux surgery.

- Persistent BE is an indication for mucosal ablation.

C. **Barrett's Esophagus with High-Grade Dysplasia (HGD):**

- HGD is an indication for intervention given the proven high risk for progression into adenocarcinoma.
- Carefully repeat endoscopy with search for any nodules or lesions in the columnar mucosa. Topical acetic acid spray may help to identify the area of concern.
- Small lesion should be endoscopically resected and sent for pathology evaluation.
- Lesions larger than 1–2 cm should prompt an endoscopic ultrasound (EUS) to evaluate depth of invasion and the presence of enlarged lymph nodes.
- If the endoscopic resection specimen shows adenocarcinoma, it is crucial to determine whether it is T1a (confined to the mucosa) or T1b (has invade the submucosa). Other important features are the presence of lymphovascular invasion and high grade.
- T1a without lymphovascular invasion after endoscopic resection, the options are endoscopic therapy (endoscopic resection of any visible lesions and mucosal ablation for the residual flat columnar mucosa) or an esophagectomy.
- T1b lesions are best treated with an esophagectomy and lymph node dissection.
- Consider esophagectomy for:
  - Long segment of BE.
  - Multifocal adenocarcinoma.
  - Poor esophageal body function with large hiatal hernia or dysphagia.
  - Reflux disease poorly controlled on twice-daily PPI therapy.
- Surveillance endoscopy for BE:
  - Nondysplastic BE: Annual
  - LGD BE every 6 months
  - HGD BE more frequent. Seattle Protocol (four quadrant biopsies at 1 cm interval every 3 months)
  - No BE, no follow-up
  - Esophagitis, start PPIs, and rescope in 3 months [6, 7]

8.1.6 Management of Esophageal Cancer

- Squamous carcinoma of the esophagus accounts for the majority of esophageal carcinoma.
- Smoking, alcohol, and long-standing achalasia are strongly linked to esophageal SCC.
- Adenocarcinoma of the esophagus in the setting of BE.
- Clinical manifestation is mainly dysphagia. Other GI symptoms are non-specific
- Extension of the tumor to the tracheobronchial tree can occur primarily with squamous cell carcinoma and cause stridor, tracheoesophageal fistula resulting in coughing and chocking and aspiration.
- **Diagnosis:**
  - Barium swallow.
  - Esophagogastroduodenoscopy (EGD) "the gold standard": Identify the location of the tumor, its extent, topographic characteristics, and relation to the GE junction and allow for histological evaluation to confirm the diagnosis.
  - CT chest, abdomen, and pelvis (CT-CAP): To assess the locoregional extent and detect any metastasis.
  - Positron emission tomography (PET) scan.
  - EUS: Useful for assessment of the depth of tumor invasion and the presence of paraesophageal lymph nodes.
  - Staging laparoscopy for the tumor near the GE junction.
- **Stage-Based Treatment:**
  - Management depends on the stage at the time of the diagnosis.
  - **High-Grade Dysplasia (Tis, N0, M0), (T1a, N0, M0):**

    HGD carries no risk for lymph node involvement.

    T1a N0 M0 carries low risk for lymph node metastasis (around 2%).

    For those patient, esophageal sparing local therapy can adequately eradicate the neoplastic tissue and that include radiofrequency ablation, photodynamic therapy, cryotherapy, and endoscopic mucosal resection.

Surveillance endoscopy is performed every 3 months for 1 year with adequate four quadrant biopsies at every 1 cm of treated mucosa.

Contraindications to esophageal preserving therapy:

- Presence of multifocal disease
- Presence of submucosal invasion
- Squamous histology resulting from high propensity for lymph node involvement
- Lymphovascular invasion
- Poorly differentiated tumors
- Nodule greater than 3 cm in diameter

– **T1b, N0, M0:**

Esophagectomy with regional lymphadenectomy

– **Locally Advanced Resectable Cancer (T2-4a, Any N, M0):**

Neoadjuvant chemoradiation.

Surgical resection with lymphadenectomy (1 cm margin to achieve R0).

The surgical approach should be individualized depending on the tumor stage, type, location, extent of nodal dissection, patient comorbidities, body habitus, and the surgeon's experience.

Adjuvant treatment is indicated in patient at high risk of local or systemic recurrence. These include patient with T3 or T4 tumors, R1 or R2 resection, or with multiple positive lymph nodes.

– **(T4b, any N any M) or (any T, any N, M1):**

T4b cancers invade structures that cannot be resected, such as the aorta, left atrium, and spine.

Those patients who are not candidates for curative surgical resection should be offered the option of palliative care.

The goal of the palliative care includes the treatment of specific symptoms, delaying the death from metastatic disease, and improving the quality of remaining life.

This can be achieved with systemic chemotherapy, radiation therapy, and/or endoscopic treatment (self-expanding stent, endoscopic dilatation) [1, 8].

Preoperative Preparation:

- Admission.
- Consent.
- NPO.
- IV fluid.
- Deep vein thrombosis (DVT) and stress ulcer prophylaxis.
- Prophylactic antibiotic.
- Confirm the availability of blood intraoperative if needed.
- Anesthesia consultation.
- ICU consultation if required.
- Instruct the patient to take shower the night before surgery.
- Hair removal.

Informed Consent:

A. **Consent for Heller Myotomy:**
   - Explain the procedure to the patient: Under general anesthesia, the surgeon will do division of the inner circular muscular layer of the esophagus through laparoscopic or open approach with or without fundoplication.
   - Mention if there is any other alternative like medication, endoscopic dilatation, or Botox injection.
   - Explain all the possible complications like bleeding, perforation, infection, GERD, Barrett's esophagus, atelectasis, pneumonia, aspiration, or anesthesia complication.

B. **Consent for Fundoplication:**
   - Explain the procedure to the patient: Under general anesthesia, the surgeon will perform 360°/270° (anterior or posterior) fundal wrap around the lower esophageal sphincter with or without lengthening procedure of the abdominal esophagus, and with hiatal hernia repair (if present) via laparoscopic or open technique.
   - Mention if there is any other alternative like medical treatment or application of esophageal device LINX.

- Explain all the possible complications, such as dysphagia, esophagitis, abdominal bloating, heartburn, esophageal perforation, injury to the vagus nerves, need for reoperation, bleeding, infection atelectasis, pneumonia, and anesthesia complications.

C. **Consent for Esophagectomy:**

- Explain the procedure to the patient: Under general anesthesia and through right/left thoracotomy or left cervical incision and mid-line laparotomy, the surgeon will resect part of the esophagus due to presence of malignant tumor. This may require removal of all the draining lymph nodes. The reconstruction will be performed by anastomosing the stomach, jejunum, or part of the colon to the remaining proximal esophagus. This procedure can be done using open or minimal invasive approach.
- Mention if there is any other alternative.
- Explain all the possible complications like bleeding, infection, injury to the recurrent laryngeal nerves, anastomotic leak, chyle leak, acid or bile reflux, respiratory complications like aspiration, stridor, pneumonia, adhesions, hernia, and anesthesia complications.

Antireflux Surgery:

- **Esophageal Surgical Anatomy** (Fig. 8.1)
- **Principles of the Surgical Technique:**
  - Reduction of any hiatal hernia
  - Tension-free restoration of the intra-abdominal esophagus
  - Approximation of the diaphragmatic hiatal crura
  - Performance of a fundoplication (except the Hill repair, which does not include one)
- **Types of Fundoplication:**
  - Nissen fundoplication: 360° fundal wrap (Fig. 8.2)
  - Toupet fundoplication: 270° posterior fundal wrap (Fig. 8.3)
  - Dor fundoplication: 180° anterior fundal wrap (Fig. 8.4)
  - Belsy fundoplication: 270° anterior thoracic fundal wrap

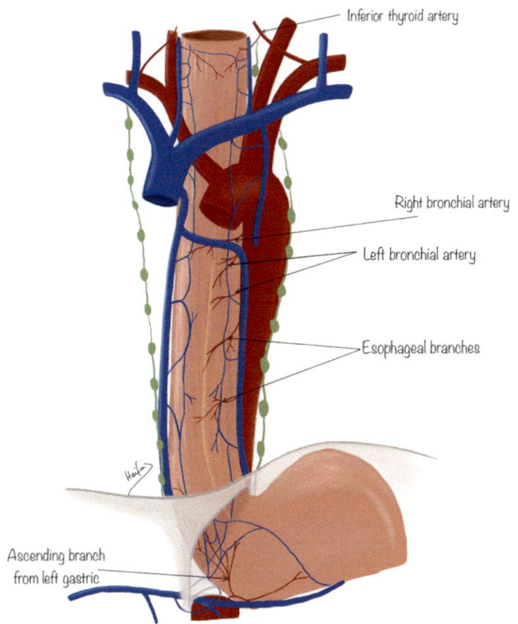

Fig. 8.1 Anatomy of the esophagus

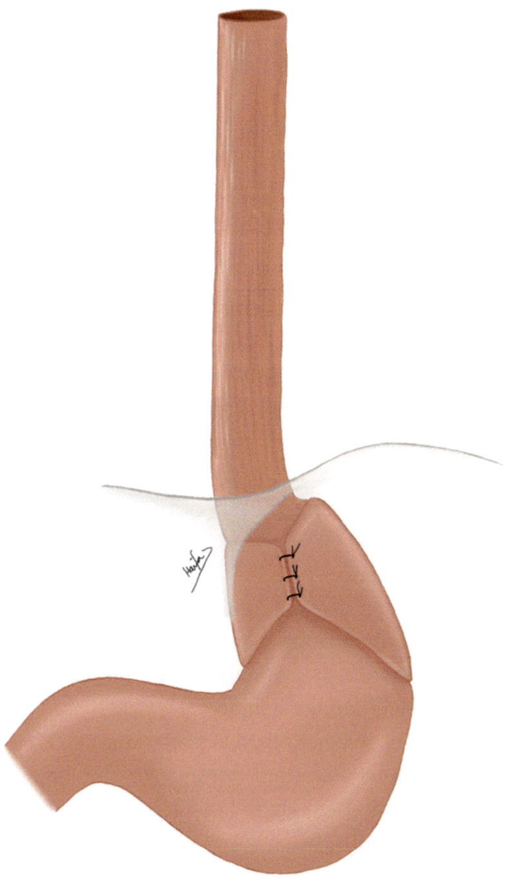

Fig. 8.2 Nissen fundoplication: 360º fundal wrap

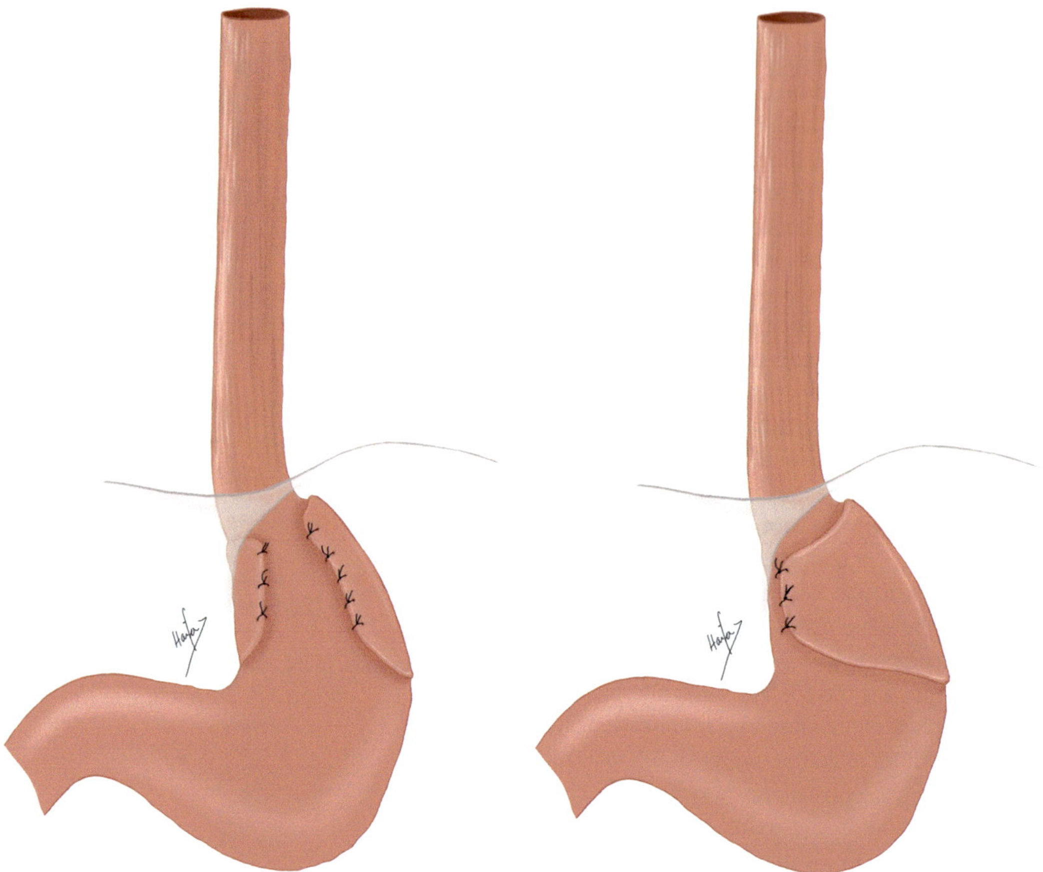

Fig. 8.3 Toupet fundoplication: 270° posterior fundal wrap

Fig. 8.4 Dor fundoplication: 180° anterior fundal wrap

- **Esophageal Lengthening (Collis Gastroplasty):**
  - Collis gastroplasty was first described through a left thoracotomy.
  - A linear stapler is introduced to create a 4- to 5-cm tube of the proximal stomach after passing a bougie (48F–50F) into the stomach and holding it against the lesser curvature.
  - A laparoscopic modification has been described using a circular stapler (35-mm) to create a "buttonhole" in the stomach adjacent to the bougie.
  - A linear stapler then is passed into this buttonhole and fired parallel to the bougie toward the angle of His, creating a neoesophagus.
- **Surgical Approach:**
  - Thoracic approach (left thoracotomy): Preferred in obese patients, hostile abdomen, and for easier creation of Collis gastroplasty
  - Abdominal approach
- **Surgical Technique (Laparoscopic Nissen Fundoplication):**
- Under general anesthesia and endotracheal intubation.
- Position: Supine with arms out and legs separated "semi lithotomy."
- The abdomen is prepped from nipple to the symphysis pubis.
- Patient is draped in sterile fashion.
- Time out: Confirm that correct patient, correct procedure, correct site, and all the required instruments are available.

- Incision: 5 and 10 mm ports incision.
- The patient is placed in a reverse Trendelenburg position (about 30° of elevation to the head of the bed).
  - **Mobilization of the esophagogastric junction (EGJ) and reduction of hiatal hernia:**

    The pars flaccida of the gastrohepatic ligament is divided. Care is taken to preserve any accessory (or rarely completely replaced) left hepatic artery.

    The right crura is identified and the phrenoesophageal ligament is then opened, mobilizing the anterior right crus away from the esophagus with careful blunt dissection.

    This dissection is carried anteriorly and circumferentially toward the left crus, ensuring that the anterior vagus nerve is identified and preserved. The hernia sac and EGJ fat pad are resected.

    The greater omentum then is divided just below the spleen before dividing the short gastric vessels. The surgeon must stay about 1 cm off the greater curvature of the stomach to avoid thermal injury and delayed gastric necrosis.

    The hiatus and both crus along with the posterior vagus nerve are identified posterior to the esophagus. Para-esophageal circumferential dissection is performed into the mediastinum until there is delivery of 3–4 cm into the abdomen without tension.

    Approximation of the crura is then done using three to four nonabsorbable sutures to recreate a hiatus that is nonobstructive (about 2 cm in diameter wider than the EGJ).

    Decision is made at this point regarding the use of onlay mesh.
  - **Creation of the fundoplication**

    A "shoeshine" maneuver then is performed by grasping both sides of the fundus, which then are pulled back and forth as if the back of the esophagus was the vamp of a shoe being shined. This helps to ensure proper orientation and tension. A total fundoplication (Nissen) is made using three nonabsorbable sutures and fashioned as follows:
    - Floppy enough to allow passage of an instrument between the fundus and the esophagus.
    - Short, only 2–3 cm in length.
    - Perfectly straddling the LES and not the stomach.
    - Each stitch must incorporate the esophageal muscularis and the fundal seromuscular layer to prevent slipping of the wrap migration.
  - Hemostasis, closure [5]

Laparoscopic Heller Myotomy:

- Similar to laparoscopic Nissen fundoplication in terms of the trocar placement and exposure and dissection of the hiatus.
- The pars flaccida of the gastrohepatic ligament is divided. Care is taken to preserve any accessory left hepatic artery.
- The right crura is identified and the phrenoesophageal ligament then is opened, mobilizing the anterior right crus away from the esophagus with careful blunt dissection.
- This dissection is carried anteriorly and circumferentially toward the left crus, ensuring that the anterior vagus nerve is identified and preserved. The hernia sac and EGJ fat pad are resected.
- The greater omentum then is divided just below the spleen before dividing the short gastric vessels. The surgeon must stay about 1 cm off the greater curvature of the stomach to avoid thermal injury and delayed gastric necrosis.
- The anterior vagus nerve is swept right laterally along with the fat pad. Once completed, the GEJ and distal 4–5 cm of esophagus should be cleared of any overlying tissue, and generally follows dissection of the GEJ.
- A distal esophageal myotomy is performed. It is generally easiest to begin the myotomy 1–2 cm above the GEJ.

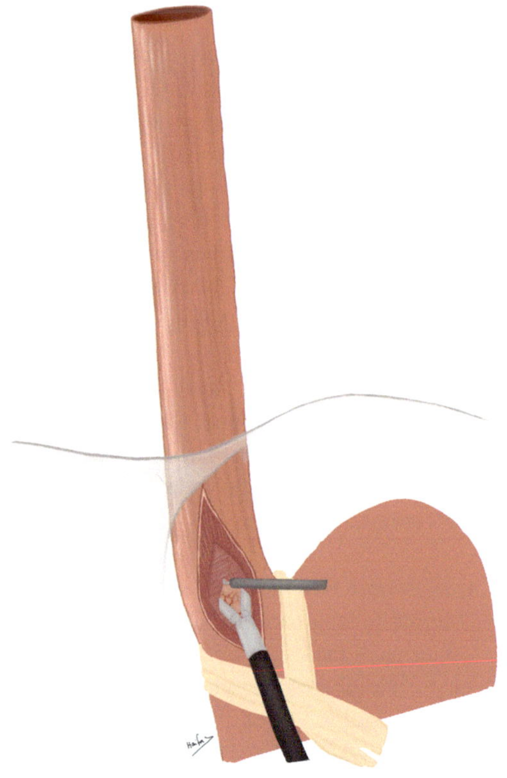

Fig. 8.5 Heller's myotomy is carried across the GEJ and onto the proximal stomach for approximately 2–3 cm, dividing both longitudinal and circular muscle layers

- Either scissors or a hook-type electrocautery can be used to initiate the incision in the longitudinal and circular muscle. Distally, the myotomy is carried across the GEJ and onto the proximal stomach for approximately 2–3 cm (Fig. 8.5).
- After completion, the muscle edges are separated bluntly from the esophageal mucosa for approximately 50% of the esophageal circumference.
- An antireflux procedure follows completion of the myotomy. Either an anterior hemifundoplication augmenting the angle of His (Dor) or posterior partial fundoplication (Toupet) can be performed.
- Hemostasis and closure [1, 3].

Esophageal Resection:
Surgical Options:

- **The Ivor Lewis esophagectomy** (combines a laparotomy with a right thoracotomy): Ideal for adenocarcinoma of the lower and middle third of the esophagus
- **McKeown or Three-Hole Esophagectomy** (combines right posterolateral thoracotomy, laparotomy, and left neck incision): Ideal for adenocarcinoma of the middle or upper third of the esophagus, and for squamous cell carcinoma of the esophagus
- **Transhiatal Esophagectomy**: Ideal in patients who will not tolerate the pulmonary sequela of the thoracic component of an Ivor Lewis or McKeown esophagectomy
- **Left Thoraco-abdominal Esophagectomy**: Ideal for bulky tumors in the region of the hiatus

The Ivor Lewis Esophagectomy:

- Under general anesthesia and endotracheal intubation.
- Position: Supine then left lateral position.
- The abdomen is prepped from nipple to the symphysis pubis.
- Patient is draped in sterile fashion.
- Time out: Confirm that correct patient, correct procedure, correct site, and all the required instruments are available.
- Incision: upper midline laparotomy, right thoracotomy.

The Abdominal Part of the Procedure:

- The abdomen is explored first to rule out undetected metastatic disease and to ascertain resectability.
- Use of a self-retaining upper abdominal retractor is critical for adequate exposure.
- Dividing the triangular ligament and retracting the lateral segment of the liver medially exposes the region of the hiatus.

- The gastrohepatic omentum then is taken down and dissection continued to the right crus taking down the phrenoesophageal ligament.
- The anterior surface of the esophagus then is dissected.
- The greater omentum then is dissected to gain access to the lesser sac.
- Begin the dissection in the clear area of the pars flaccida and proceed cranially dividing the short gastric between the stomach and the spleen.
- Additional dissection of the attachments of the spleen to the diaphragm allows it to fall away from the operative field, exposing the right crus.
- The esophagus now is dissected circumferentially at the hiatus and a Penrose drain placed to provide traction for dissection into the mediastinum.
- The gastrocolic omentum now is divided caudally, taking care to stay wide of the right gastroepiploic vessels so as not to compromise the vascular supply of the conduit.
- The stomach now is reflected upward and medially and dissected free off its posterior attachments to the pancreas and retroperitoneum.
- The lymphatic tissue at the origin of the left gastric vessels is swept into the specimen, and the vessels are divided using a vascular stapler. Care is taken to preserve the right gastric artery.
- Additional mobilization can be achieved by performing a Kocher maneuver
- Augmentation of gastric drainage can be achieved by a variety of methods. One method is to inject 100 units of botulinum toxin onto the pylorus. Alternatively, a pyloromyotomy or pyloroplasty can be performed.
- The gastric conduit then is prepared by several firings of the GIA stapler, ensuring that an adequate distal margin has been obtained and that the conduit will reach the site of anastomosis without tension.
- The hiatus is enlarged to allow the conduit to pass into the posterior mediastinum without compression and possible compromise of the vascular supply.
- A heavy nonabsorbable silk or polyester suture is used to attach the conduit to the esophagogastric specimen.
- A feeding jejunostomy tube is placed, following which the abdomen is closed.

The Thoracic Part of the Procedure:

- The patient then is placed in the left lateral decubitus position to perform a right posterolateral thoracotomy through the fifth or sixth interspace.
- A dual lumen endotracheal tube is used to isolate the right lung.
- The esophagus along with all peri-esophageal tissue and associated lymphatic tissue is resected from the apex down to the hiatus, taking care not to injure the thoracic duct or its major branches.
- Division of the azygous vein greatly facilitates the dissection.
- The esophagogastric specimen and gastric conduit then are drawn into the chest. The proximal esophagus is divided well above the azygous vein.
- Either a stapled or hand-sewn anastomosis is performed after removing all redundancy in the conduit and passing a nasogastric tube past the anastomosis.
- The conduit is then tacked to the diaphragmatic hiatus to prevent visceral herniation.
- A drain is placed alongside the anastomosis, and apicoposterior and basilar chest tubes placed before closure of the chest.

• If the stomach cannot be used as a conduit because of either disease or previous surgery, the colon or jejunum can be used as a conduit.
• For use of the colon as a conduit, complete bowel prep is essential before surgery. The left colon is preferred because of its better size match and more reliable blood supply from the left colic artery [8].

Postoperative Follow-Up:
Early Postoperative:

- NPO and resume the diet gradually once possible or through the feeding jejunostomy.
- Monitor the vital signs.
- Encourage mobilization.
- Consider early removal of Foley's catheter.
- Encourage use of incentive spirometry.
- Analgesia, antibiotic as indicated, stress ulcer, and DVT prophylaxis.

Before Discharge:

- Check that the patient has no significant complaint.
- Tolerates diet
- Check the wound status.

First Outpatient Visit:

- Clinical assessment.
- Examine the wound and remove the sutures.
- Review the final pathology result.
- Discuss in multidisciplinary team when the pathology is cancer.

Long-Term Follow-Up (cancer patients) [9]:

- For esophageal cancer [both squamous cell carcinoma (SCC) and adenocarcinoma]:
  - History and physical examination every 3–6 months for 1–2 years, then every 6–12 months for 3–5 years then annually
  - CBC and chemistry as indicated
  - Imaging study as indicated
  - Upper GI endoscopy as indicated
  - Nutritional assessment and counseling [9]

8.2 Part II: Practice

> Practice like you've never won. Play like you've never lost.
> —Michael Jordan

8.2.1 Case Scenarios for Practice

Tips:

- Practice with a friend and try to mimic the real exam!
- Do not forget to set the timer!
- Clinical data are provided in the answer key section

Case No. 1:
A 35-year-old male patient presented to the clinic complaining of dysphagia and chest pain for 1 year.

Questions for Discussion:

1. How will you approach the patient?
2. What is your differential diagnosis?
3. How will you investigate the most likely diagnosis?
4. How will you manage that?
5. The patient did not response to the initial medical measure. What will you do?
6. Few months later the patient presented with same complaint after a period of improvement. What will you do?

Case No. 2:
A 49-year-old female patient referred from otolaryngology clinic to investigate her heartburn symptoms that may be contributing to her hoarseness of voice.

Questions for Discussion:

1. How will you approach the patient?
2. What will you do further to confirm the diagnosis?
3. How will you manage that?
4. The patient still complaining of the same symptoms despite maximum medical management. What will you do?
5. What are the possible complications of this procedure?

Case No. 3:
A 52-year-old female patient presented to the esophageal reflux (ER) complaining of severe chest pain for 6 h.

Questions for Discussion:

1. How will you approach the patient?
2. What is your differential diagnosis?
3. How will you investigate his condition?
4. What is your final diagnosis?
5. How will you manage that?
6. Intraoperative the patient became unstable. What will you do?

Questions for Discussion:

1. How will you approach the patient?
2. What is your differential diagnosis?
3. How will you investigate his condition?
4. What will you do next?
5. How will you manage his condition?
6. What will be your surgical approach?
7. What are the possible complications?

Case No. 4:

A 62-year-old male patient presented to the clinic complains of dysphagia for 3 months.

Checklist

History	Items	Done	Not done	NA
General	Introduce himself/herself to the patient			
	Patient personal data (name, age, gender, and nationality)			
	Chief complaint			
	Duration			
Pain	Onset			
	Site			
	Character			
	Radiation/shifting			
	Aggravating/relieving			
	Severity			
	Progression			
	Frequency			
Dysphagia	Onset			
	To which type of food?			
	Progression			
	Odynophagia			
Bleeding	Onset			
	Amount			
	Relation to food			
	Fresh blood, coffee ground			
	Proceeding event (cough, vomiting, retching)			
	Another bleeding site			
Associated symptoms	Pain (chest/abdomen)			
	Hematemesis			
	Fever			
	Melena			
	Change in bowel habit			
	Regurgitation			
	Nausea			
	Vomiting			
	Stridor			
	Hoarseness			
	Hiccups			
	Jaundice			

(continued)

History	Items	Done	Not done	NA
Constitutional symptoms	Weight loss			
	Decrease appetite			
	Night sweating			
Symptoms of metastases	Back pain			
	Cough			
	Shortness of breath			
	Abdominal distention			
Risk factors	Smoking			
	Alcohol			
	Family history of similar complaint or malignancy			
	Long-standing GERD			
	History of repeated vomiting, cough, and retching			
	History of foreign body ingestion			
	History of caustic ingestion			
	History of recent endoscopy or instrumentation			
	Personal history of other cancer			
PMH	Previous similar attack			
	Previous investigation or endoscopy			
	Previous admission			
	Chronic illnesses			
PSH	Previous surgery			
Family history	Of similar complain			
Social history	Occupation			
	Habits (smoking, alcohol, drugs)			
Other	Medication			
	Allergy			
	Transfusion			
Systemic review				
Physical Examination				
General principle	Patient position			
	Exposure			
	Privacy			
	Wash hands			
General examination	Appearance			
	Body built			
	Color			
	Distress/decubitus			
	Environment			
Vital signs	BP, HR, Temperature, RR, and SPO_2			
Hand signs	Leukonychia, koilonychia, and pallor			
Eyes	Jaundice and pallor			
Neck	Lymphadenopathy			
Chest	Air entry			
	Surgical emphysema			
	Signs of pleural effusion			

History	Items	Done	Not done	NA
Abdomen: Inspection	Distention			
	Asymmetry			
	Dilated veins			
	Striae			
	Visible peristalsis			
	Scars			
	Cough impulse			
Palpation	Superficial then deep palpation			
	Tenderness			
	Palpable masses			
	Organomegaly			
	Cough impulse at hernial orifices			
Percussion	Shifting dullness			
	Fluid thrill			
Auscultation	Bowel sounds			
	Bruit, venous hum			
Groin and hernias				
DRE				
Back tenderness				
Differential diagnosis	According to the given scenario			
Investigations				
General laboratory test	CBC with differential			
	Electrolytes			
	Liver function test			
	Blood grouping			
	ABG			
	Lactic acid			
	Coagulation profile [prothrombin time (PT), international normalized ratio (INR), activated partial thromboplastin time (aPTT)]			
	RFT			
	CRP/ESR			
Specific tests	Manometry			
	24-h pH study			
Imaging	Chest X-ray			
	Esophagogram			
	EUS			
	CT chest/abdomen/pelvis			
	PET scan			
Endoscopy	EGD			
Biopsy	Biopsy/endoscopic submucosal resection, etc.			
Provisional diagnosis	According to the given scenario			
Management (depend on the diagnosis):				
Esophageal perforation	Admission			
Initial management	NPO			
	IV antibiotics			
	Antifungal			
	PPI			

(continued)

History	Items	Done	Not done	NA
Contained perforation	If the perforation contained start with conservative management			
	Chest tube			
	TPN			
	Repeat imaging in 72–96 h			
	If no leak, start fluid diet			
Non-contained or patient deteriorated	Operative management			
Cervical perforation	Through left neck incision			
	Repair primarily or patch ± buttress the repair			
	Gastrografin on day 5			
	If the perforation not found insert suction drain			
Abdominal perforation	Through upper midline or left thoracotomy (if perforation in large hiatal hernia)			
	Debride the edges			
	Repair primarily + buttress			
Thoracic perforation	Through right thoracotomy if in the middle esophagus or left if in the lower			
	Repair and buttress			
	Drainage with chest tube			
Unstable patient or perforated cancer	Esophageal exclusion			
	Cervical esophagostomy (loop)			
	Close the distal esophagus with stapler			
	Feeding gastrostomy or jejunostomy			
Variceal Bleeding	Admission to ICU			
	Follow ABC approach			
	PPI			
	Octreotide			
	Vasopressin ± nitroglyerol			
	NGT			
	Foley's catheter			
	Endoscopy			
	Sengstaken tube			
	TIPS			
	Surgical shunt			
	Devascularization			
Achalasia	Nitroglycerin			
	Nitrate			
	Calcium channel blocker			
	Pneumatic dilatation			
	Botox injection			
	Heller myotomy/POEM/esophagectomy			
GERD	Medical treatment (PPI)			
	Give the patient instruction for bed elevation			
	To eat small frequent meals			
	Avoid eating at nighttime			
	Avoid tobacco, alcohol, and coffee			
	Surveillance if Barrett's esophagus with dysplasia is there			
	Surgical management if medical treatment failed			

History	Items	Done	Not done	NA
Esophageal cancer	Staging			
	Discussion in multidisciplinary team meeting			
	Break the bad news			
High-grade dysplasia	Endoscopic therapy			
	Surveillance			
Early cancer	Preoperative preparation			
	Esophagectomy with lymphadenectomy			
Resectable locally advanced	Neoadjuvant chemoradiation			
	Revaluation			
	Restaging			
	Preoperative preparation			
	Surgical resection (according to the location)			
	Adjuvant therapy			
Advanced or metastatic	Palliative care			
Postoperative care				
Early postoperative	Admission to high dependency care (HDU) or ICU when needed			
	Early mobilization and DVT prophylaxis			
	NPO or resume feeding orally or through feeding tubes if present			
	Monitor the vital signs			
	Analgesia			
	Stress ulcer prophylaxis			
	CBC and LFT daily			
	Electrolyte assessment			
	Monitor drain output and the nature of the fluid			
First outpatient visit	Clinical assessment			
	Remove sutures			
	Review the final pathology report			
	Arrange for multidisciplinary discussion if the case is cancer			
	Refer to oncology if adjuvant treatment is required			
Long-term follow-up (for adenocarcinoma)	History and physical examination every 3 months for 1–2 years then every 6 months for the 3–5 years then annually			
	Imaging, endoscopy as indicated			

8.2.2 Answer Key

Case No. 1:

A 35-year-old male patient presented to the clinic complaining of dysphagia and chest pain for 1 year.

Questions for Discussion:

1. **How will you approach the patient?**

   A 35-year-old male patient is complaining of dysphagia that was for both solid and food for the last year. It increased in frequency over the last couple of months. It is associated with central chest pain and regurgitation of undigested food. She noticed drop in her weight over the last year (about 15 kg). She has no history of heartburn. No palpitation, no cough, no stridor, no hoarseness, no hematemesis or melena.

   She has no history of traveling or contact with sick patient and no significant family history. She is a smoker but not alcoholic. Her past medical and surgical histories are unremarkable.

   O/E:

   Conscious, alert, and average weight female.

   Vital signs within normal.

Chest and abdominal examinations are normal.

2. **What is your differential diagnosis?**
   Achalasia
   Other motility disorder like diffuse esophageal spasm
   Esophageal carcinoma
   Zenker's diverticulum
   Esophageal ring
   Myocardial infarction (MI)
3. **How will you investigate the most likely diagnosis?**
   Esophagogram: proximal dilatation of the esophagus with distal tapering (bird's peak) with air fluid level in the esophagus
   Esophageal manometry: failure of LES to relax during swallowing with aperistalsis at the esophageal body
   Basic blood investigation: within normal range
   Endoscopy to rule out pseudoachalasia: show lumen narrowing at the distal esophagus but no mass or esophagitis
4. **How will you manage that?**
   Medical treatment: nitroglycerin, nitrate, and calcium channel blocker.
5. **The patient did not respond to the initial medical measure. What will you do?**
   Endoscopy: pneumatic dilatation, Botox injection.
6. **Few months later the patient presented with same complaint after a period of improvement. What will you do?**
   Heller myotomy/POEM.

Case No. 2:
A 49-year-old female patient referred from otolaryngology clinic to investigate her heartburn symptoms that may be contributing to her hoarseness of voice.

Questions for Discussion:

1. **How will you approach the patient?**
   The patient is a 49-year-old female patient who is referred for consultation regarding her new symptom of hoarseness of voice.
   She noticed change in her voice from 1 month, associated with heartburn and regurgitation of gastric acidity into her throat. She noticed that her symptoms got worse when she ate chocolate or drunk coffee or when she lied down immediately after eating.
   No abdominal or chest pain. It is associated with nausea and vomiting sometimes.
   No history of weight loss, hematemesis, stridor, melena. No significant family history or personal history of malignancy.
   Otherwise, she is fit and healthy.
   Physical examination was unremarkable.
   Vocal cord assessment by the otolaryngologist shows bilateral mobile cord with signs of inflammation.
2. **What will you do further to confirm the diagnosis?**
   Upper GI endoscopy shows grade B esophagitis
   Ambulatory 24-h esophageal pH: shows frequent reading of pH less than 4
3. **How will you manage that?**
   - Instruct the patient to elevate the head of the bed when lying down.
   - To avoid tight fitting clothes.
   - To eat small frequent meal.
   - To avoid eating at nighttime or at least not prior to bedtime.
   - To avoid alcohol, avoid coffee, avoid chocolate, and peppermint.
   - Medication: PPIs (high does 40 mg/day).
4. **The patient still complaining of the same symptoms despite maximum medical management. What will you do?**
   She will need antireflux surgery (Nissen fundoplication).
5. **What are the possible complications of this procedure?**
   Dysphagia, esophagitis, abdominal bloating, heartburn, esophageal perforation, injury to the vagus nerves, slipping of the wrap needs reoperation, bleeding, infection atelectasis, pneumonia, and anesthesia complications

Case No. 3:
A 52-year-old female patient presented to the ER complaining of severe chest pain for 6 h.

Questions for Discussion:

1. **How will you approach the patient?**
A 52-year-old female patient presented to ER complaining of severe chest pain that started suddenly after multiple times of vomiting.
It is central chest pain, not radiated or shifted, dull aching, severe enough to prevent her from doing her daily activity. It was not relived by regular analgesic. She has not experienced this pain before. She has history of multiple times vomiting after she ate from outside. No history of palpitation, hematemesis or melena.
No history of fever, no weight loss. She is not smoker or alcoholic.
PMH: Bronchial asthma.
PSH: Open appendectomy.
Not on regular medication and not known allergic.
O/E:
She is conscious, looking ill.
Vital signs:
BP: 117/78 PR: 113 bpm temperature: 37.6°C RR: 20.
Chest: there is surgical emphysema with decrease air entry on the left side.
2. **What is your differential diagnosis?**
Boerhaave syndrome
MI
Pancreatitis
Peptic ulcer disease
Rupture aortic aneurysm
Aortic dissection
3. **How will you investigate his condition?**
Basic blood test
Erect CXR: Left pleural effusion, surgical emphysema
Esophagogram (with water-soluble contrast): Contrast extravasation on the lower esophagus that is leaking freely into the left pleural cavity
4. **What is your final diagnosis?**
Spontaneous esophageal perforation (Boerhaave syndrome).
5. **How will you manage that?**
Admission to ICU
NPO
NGT
Insertion of left chest tube
IV fluid
IV antibiotics
Antifungal
Anesthesia consultation
Consent
Urgent left thoracotomy, primary repair of the perforation, and buttress the repair
6. **Intraoperative the patient became unstable. What will you do?**
Esophageal exclusion
Cervical loop esophagostomy, closure of the distal esophagus by stapler
Feeding gastrostomy or jejunostomy

Case No. 4:
A 62-year-old male patient presented to the clinic complains of dysphagia for 3 months.
Questions for Discussion:

1. **How will you approach the patient?**
A 62-year-old male patient is complaining of dysphagia for the last 3 months. It was initially for solid foods and progress over time to liquid food too. It is associated with significant weight loss (around 20 kg over 3 months), regurgitation, and anorexia. It was not associated with chest or abdominal pain, no hematemesis or melena.
He is a heavy smoker (2 packs/day for 35 years). No significant personal or family history of malignancy. No hoarseness of voice, no stridor.
PMH: diabetes mellitus (DM) and hypertension.
PSH: negative.
On insulin and captopril.
On examination:
Conscious, alert, and cachectic patient.
Vital signs: BP: 132/90, PR: 67 bpm, Temperature: 36.5.
Chest examination: normal.
Abdominal examination: normal.
2. **What is your differential diagnosis?**
Esophageal cancer
Achalasia
Motility disorder
Zenker's diverticulum

3. **How will you investigate his condition?**
   Basic blood test.
   Upper GI endoscopy: Large fungating mass at the lower third of the esophagus, causing lumen narrowing and the scope could not be passed beyond the mass. Biopsy was taken and showed esophageal squamous cell carcinoma.
4. **What will you do next?**
   Staging CT-CAP: No distant metastasis. Lower esophageal intraluminal soft tissue mass with multiple abnormal para-esophageal lymph nodes.
   EUS: Tumor invades the muscularis layer of the esophagus.
   Discuss in multidisciplinary team.
5. **How will you manage his condition?**
   Neoadjuvant chemoradiation followed by surgical resection.
6. **What will be your surgical approach?**
   Left thoracotomy and upper midline laparotomy.
7. **What are the possible complications?**
   Bleeding, infection, injury to the recurrent laryngeal nerves, anastomotic leak, chyle leak, acid or bile reflux, respiratory complications like aspiration, stridor, pneumonia, adhesions, hernia, and anesthesia.

References

1. Jobe BA, Hunter JG, Watson DI. Esophagus and diaphragmatic hernia. In: Brunicardi F, editor. Schwartz's principles of surgery. 11th ed. United States: McGraw-Hill Education; 2019.
2. Robert Maxwell KR. The management of esophageal perforation. In: Cameron J, Cameron A, editors. Current surgical therapy. 12th ed. Canada: Elsevier; 2016.
3. Swanstrom LL, Beard KW. The management of disorders of esophageal motility. In: Cameron J, Cameron A, editors. Current surgical therapy. 12th ed. Canada: Elsevier; 2016.
4. Landreneau RJ, Jobe A, Habib F. The management of achalasia of the esophagus. In: Cameron J, Cameron A, editors. Current surgical therapy. 12th ed. Canada: Elsevier; 2016.
5. Abbas AE-S. The management of gastroesophageal reflux disease. In: Cameron J, Cameron A, editors. Current surgical therapy. 12th ed. Canada: Elsevier; 2016.
6. DeMeester SR. The management of Barrett's esophagus. In: Cameron J, Cameron A, editors. Current surgical therapy. 12th ed. Canada: Elsevier; 2016.
7. Schaheen L, Luketich JD. The endoscopic treatment of Barrett's esophagus. In: Cameron J, Cameron A, editors. Current surgical therapy. 12th ed. Canada: Elsevier; 2016.
8. Jobe BA, Landreneau RJ, Habib F. The management of esophageal cancer. In: Cameron J, Cameron A, editors. Current surgical therapy. 12th ed. Canada: Elsevier; 2016.
9. ["Referenced with permission from the NCCN Clinical Practice Guidelines in Oncology (NCCN Guidelines®) for esophageal cancer V.1.2021. © National Comprehensive Cancer Network, Inc. All rights reserved. Accessed [February,18,]. To view the most recent and complete version of the guideline, go online to NCCN.org. NCCN makes no warranties of any kind whatsoever regarding their content, use or application and disclaims any responsibility for their application or use in any way."].

9 Surgical Aspects of Gastric and Duodenal Diseases for Clinical Board Exams

9.1 Part I: Knowledge

Any knowledge that doesn't lead to new questions quickly dies out: it fails to maintain the temperature required for sustaining life.
—Wislawa Szymborska

The chief complaint could be one of the following:

- Epigastric pain
- Mass
- Bleeding
- Refer to Table 9.1

Table 9.1 Differential diagnosis

Epigastric pain	Upper GI bleeding	Epigastric mass
Gastritis PUD Pancreatitis Gastroenteritis Gastric cancer Pancreatic cancer Inferior MI Abdominal aortic aneurysm (AAA)	Bleeding peptic ulcer Gastritis/duodenitis Mallory Weiss syndrome Esophageal varices Esophagitis Gastric varices Angiodysplasia Arteriovenous malformation	Gastric cancer Pancreatic pseudocyst Pancreatic cancer AAA Lipoma

History:

- Introduce yourself to the patient.
- Name, Age, Occupation, Sex, Nationality.
- Chief complaint and duration.
- History of presenting illness:
  - **Analysis of the chief complaint**

H. Alotaibi, *Study Surgery*, https://doi.org/10.1007/978-981-16-2305-9_9

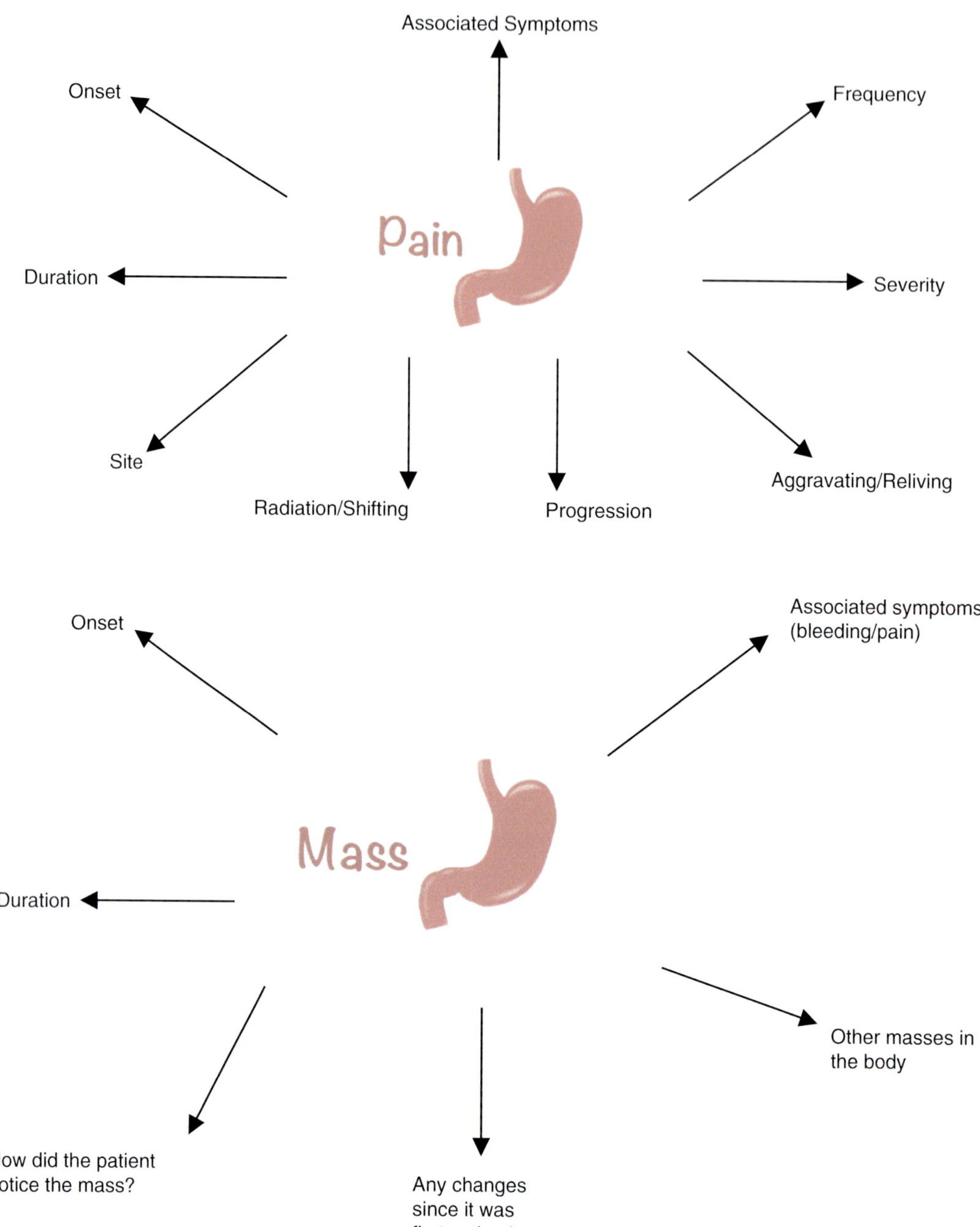
Associated Symptoms
Onset
Frequency
Pain
Duration
Severity
Site
Radiation/Shifting
Progression
Aggravating/Reliving
Onset
Associated symptoms (bleeding/pain)
Mass
Duration
Other masses in the body
How did the patient notice the mass?
Any changes since it was first noticed

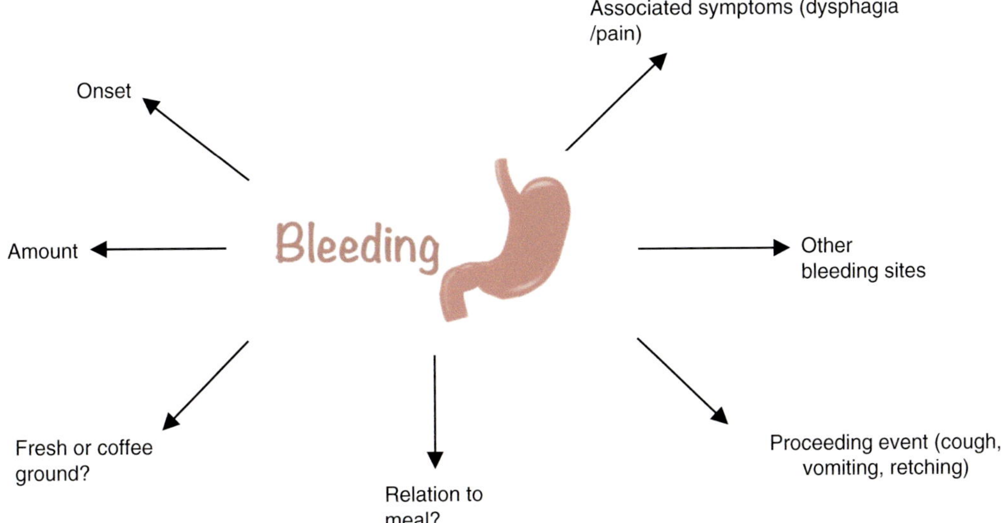

- **Associated Symptoms**
  Pain, fever, nausea, vomiting, diarrhea, change in bowel habits, hematemesis, melena, abdominal distention, dysphagia, symptoms of anemia
- **Constitutional Symptoms:**
  Weight loss, decrease appetite, night sweating, fever
- **Symptoms of Metastasis**
  Back pain, abdominal distention, cough, shortness of breath
- **Risk Factors:**
  Diet (high nitrate, high fat, and high salt)
  Personal history of PUD
  Smoking
  Previous gastric surgery (gastrectomy or gastrojejunostomy)
  Family history of gastric, colon (FAP or HNPCC), or breast cancer (lobular)
  Family history of endocrine syndrome
  Stress or recent surgery (stress gastritis)
  NSAID intake (PUD)
- **Differential Diagnosis:**
  History of eating from outside (gastroenteritis)
  Contact with sick patient (gastroenteritis)
  History of gall stone, alcohol (pancreatitis)
  Cough, SOB (lower lobe pneumonia)
  Chest pain, palpitation (inferior MI)
- **Previous Similar attack**, previous admission, previous investigation or endoscopy (if yes, when was it done and what was the finding?)
- **Systemic Review of related system (GIT)**
  Jaundice, constipation, diarrhea, dysphagia, history of bleeding

• **PMH.**
• **PSH.**
• **Family history.**
• **Social history.**
• **Medication, blood transfusion, allergy history.**
• **Systemic Review:**
  - **CNS:** headache, eye and hearing symptoms, epilepsy, numbness, paralysis
  - **CVS:** chest pain, orthopnea, paroxysmal nocturnal dyspnea, lower limb edema, palpitation

- **Respiratory:** cough, fever, chest pain, hemoptysis
- **Renal:** dysuria, flank pain, hematuria
- **MSK:** weakness, arthritis, skin erythema

Physical Examination:

- Introduce yourself to the patient.
- Ask permission for examination.
- Assure privacy.
- Position: supine.
- Exposure: nipple to mid-thigh.
- Handwashing.

General Examination:

- Appearance: ill, well, dehydrated
- Body Built: Cachectic, obese
- Color: Pale, Jaundice
- Distress
- Environment and connection to monitors, fluids, etc.

Vital signs: BP, HR, Temperature, RR, SPO_2

Hands:

- Pallor
- Palmar erythema
- Koilonychia (iron deficiency anemia)
- Leukonychia (hypoalbuminemia)
- Pulse rate and its characteristics (rhythm, volume)

Eye:

- Jaundice
- Pallor

Neck:

- Lymphadenopathy (left supraclavicular lymph node, Virchow lymph node)
- Acanthosis nigricans
- Thyroid or parathyroid swelling in case MEN syndromes is suspected

Chest:

- Respiratory system
- Cardiovascular
- Axilla: Irish lymph node in patient with gastric cancer

Abdomen:

- Inspection:
  - Distention
  - Asymmetry
  - Visible veins
  - Scars/Striae
  - Dilated veins (caput medusa)
  - Umbilical nodule (Sister Mary Josef)
  - Hernial orifices
  - Stretch marks
  - Visible peristalsis
- Palpations:
  - Superficial then deep palpation
  - Look for any tenderness
  - Palpable masses
  - Ascites
  - Cough impulse at hernial orifices
  - Organomegaly
- Percussion:
  - Shifting dullness
  - Fluid thrill
  - Organomegaly
- Auscultation:
  - Bowel sounds
  - Bruit, venous hum

Groin

DRE

- Bloody stool
- Look for any palpable hard nodule anteriorly

Lower Limb:

- Edema, peripheral neuropathy

Back:

- Tenderness

9.1.1 Peptic Ulcer Disease (PUD)

- *Helicobacter pylori* (*H. pylori*) predispose to peptic ulcer by increased acid hypersecretion and compromised the mucosal defect.

Risk Factors:

- *H. pylori* infection (duodenal ulcer more than gastric ulcer).
- Chronic use of NSAIDs increases the incidence of PUD by fivefolds and upper GI bleeding by twofolds.
- Complications of PUD are much more common in patients taking NSAIDs.
- Factors that increase the risk of NSAIDs induced GI complications:
  - Age >60 years
  - Prior GI event
  - Concurrent steroids intake
  - Concurrent anticoagulation
- Smoking increases the risk of PUD by twofolds due to increased gastric acid secretions, increases duodenogastric reflux, and decreases the prostaglandin and bicarbonate production.
- Head trauma leads to Cushing ulcer.
- Burn leads to Curling ulcer.
- Cocaine use increases the risk of juxta pyloric peptic ulcer [1–3].

Clinical Manifestations:

- Duodenal ulcer: pain 2–3 h after meal and at night. Two-thirds of patients have pain that awake them from sleep.
- Gastric ulcer: pain occur with eating. It less likely to awake patient at night [1–3].

Diagnosis:

- **Young patient with dyspepsia without alarm symptoms:**
  - Initiate PPI without endoscopy or supper GI series.
  - *H. pylori* should be ruled out.
  - NSAIDs should be stopped.
  - Patient with persistent symptoms or cannot stop NSAIDs or Aspirin, do upper endoscopy.
- **Any patient has these symptoms:**
  - Age >55 years with new onset dyspepsia
  - Weight loss
  - Persistent or recurrent vomiting
  - Progressive dyspepsia
  - Odynophagia
  - Iron deficiency anemia
  - Palpable mass or lymph node
  - Family history of upper GI malignancy

    All those patients regardless the age should have endoscopy
- All gastric ulcer should be biopsied, and any site of gastritis should be biopsied to rule *H. pylori*.
- Test for *H. pylori*.
- If the peptic ulcer is in unusual site (distal duodenum or jejunum), baseline serum gastrin level to rule out gastrinoma [1–3].
- Complications of PUD: Table 9.2.
- Types of peptic ulcer: Table 9.3.

Medical Management of PUD:

- PPI, H_2 blocker, sucralfate
- *H. pylori* regimen:
  - Bismuth quadrant therapy for 10–14 days:

    PPI
    Bismuth subsalicylate 300 mg QID
    Tetracycline 500 QID
    Metronidazole 250 mg QID
  - Clarithromycin triple therapy for 14 days:

    PPI
    Clarithromycin 500 mg twice/day
    Amoxicillin 1 g twice/day or metronidazole 500 mg TID
    Restricted to areas with known low clarithromycin resistance (<15%)
  - Metronidazole triple therapy for 14 days:

    PPI
    Metronidazole 500 mg TID
    Amoxicillin 1 g BID

Table 9.2 Complications of PUD [1–3]

Bleeding	Perforation	Obstruction
• Most common cause of upper GI bleeding (PUD) • NGT aspiration for confirmation • Early endoscopy is important • Three fourth of bleeding respond to PPI and NPO • Risk stratification: – Forrest classification – Latch ford – Rockall score (use endoscopic criteria) • Persistent bleeding or rebleeding, repeat endoscopy • Surgery is indicated after failure of endoscopy • Deep bleeding ulcer on duodenal bulb or lesser curvature • Consider early operation for high-risk patient	• Presented as acute abdomen • Chest X-ray will show 80% positive for air under diaphragm • If the diagnosis confirmed: – Analgesia – Antibiotics – Fluid – Take the patient to OR • Sealed perforation confirmed by contrast CT and no peritonitis, conservative management	• >5% in patient due to duodenal or pre-pyloric disease • May be acute or chronic • Non-bilious vomiting, hypokalemia, hypochloremia, metabolic alkalosis • Succession splash may be evident in physical examination • Diagnosis confirmed by endoscopy • Cancer must be rule out • Treatment: – NGT – Hydration – Electrolytes correction – PPI – Balloon dilatation or surgery

Table 9.3 Types of peptic ulcer (Johnson classification) [1–3]

Johnson classification:		
Type I	Near the angularis incisura on the lesser curvature, close to the border between antral and corpus mucosa	Fig. 9.1
Type II	Associated with active or quiescent duodenal ulcer. Normal or increase gastric acid	Fig. 9.2
Type III	Pre-pyloric ulcer with normal or increase gastric acid	Fig. 9.3
Type IV	Near the GE junction with normal or low acid secretion	Fig. 9.4
Type V	Medication induced and may occur anywhere in the stomach	Fig. 9.5

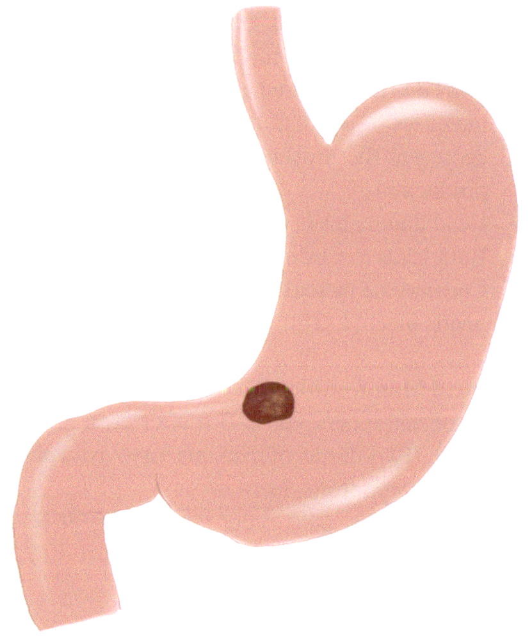

Fig. 9.1 Type I peptic ulcer

- Levofloxacin triple therapy for 14 days:
  PPI
  Amoxicillin 1 g BID
  Levofloxacin 500 m OD [1–5]

Surgical Treatment:

- Indicated for medically refractory disease or intractability.
- Highly selective vagotomy (HSV):
  - Inhibits the vagal nerve supply to proximal two-thirds of the stomach and preserves innervation to antrum and pylorus (preserving the nerve of Latarjet)
  - Decreases the total gastric acid secretion by 75%
- Truncal vagotomy and pyloroplasty/gastrojejunostomy (vagotomy and drainage):
  - Can be performed safely and quickly.
  - Main disadvantage (10% dumping and diarrhea).

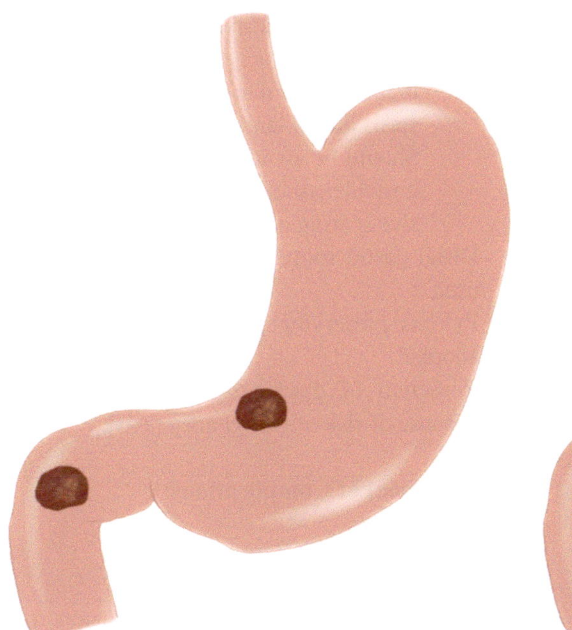

Fig. 9.2 Type II peptic ulcer

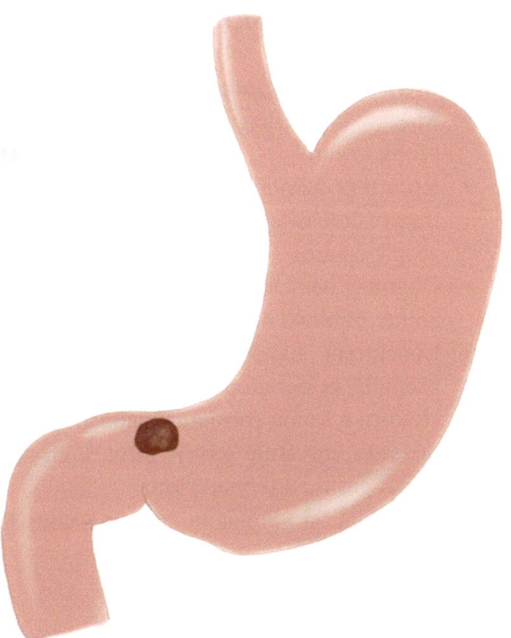

Fig. 9.3 Type III peptic ulcer

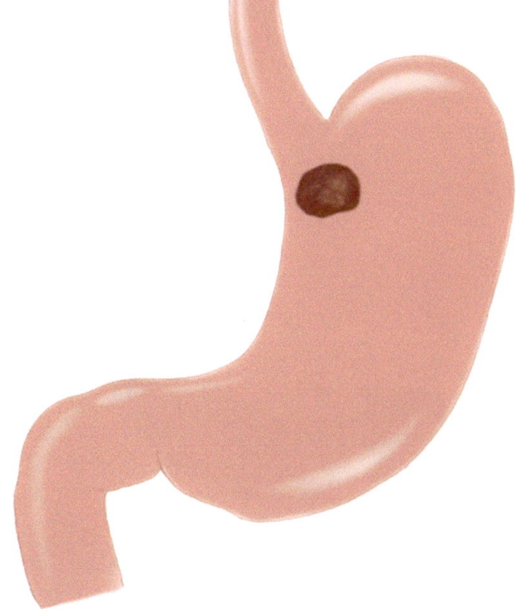

Fig. 9.4 Type IV peptic ulcer

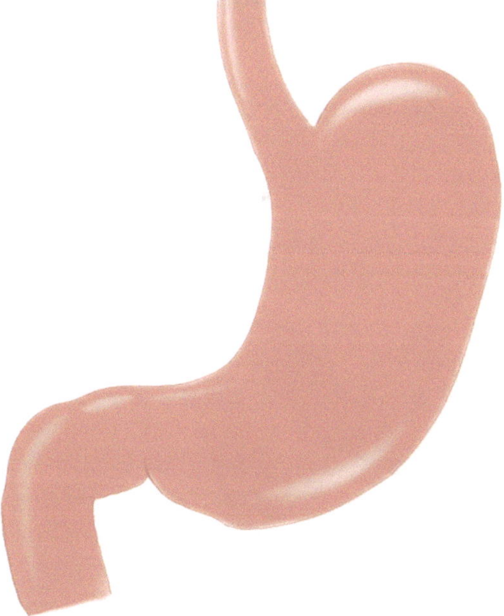

Fig. 9.5 Type V peptic ulcer

  - Intraoperative frozen section to contain at least two vagal trunks is important.
- Vagotomy and antrectomy:
  - Associated with very low recurrence
  - Higher operative mortality
  - Irreversible
  - Reconstruction: Billroth I and II (Figs. 9.6 and 9.7)

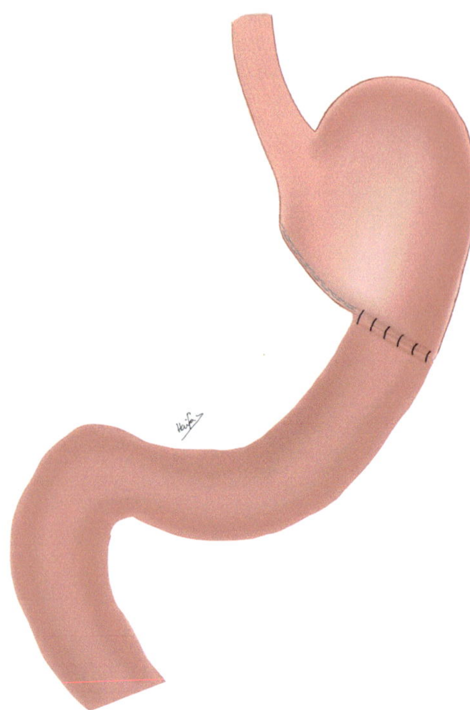

Fig. 9.6 Billroth I (gastroduodenostomy)

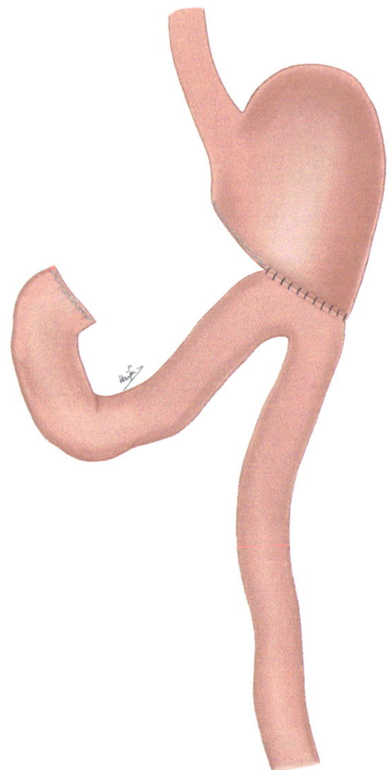

Fig. 9.7 Billroth II (gastrojejunostomy)

Routine reconstruction with Roux-en-Y gastrojejunostomy should be avoided; predispose to marginal ulcer and gastric stasis due to large gastric remnant.

Should be avoided in hemodynamically unstable patient and patient with extensive scaring of proximal duodenum.

- Distal gastrectomy without vagotomy: rarely used.
- Pylorus preserving gastrectomy: not widely adopted.
- Resection of gastric ulcer is the standard because of risk of malignancy [1–3].

Management of Complications:

A. **Bleeding:**
- Endoscopic and PPI
- Surgery if uncontrolled
- Options: suture ligation of bleeder and definitive non-resective operation (HSV or vagotomy and drainage)
- Gastric resection
- If ulcer is not resected, biopsy

Indications of Operation:

- Massive hemorrhage unresponsive to endoscopic control
- Recurrent hemorrhage requiring multiple transfusion after two attempts at endoscopic control
- Ongoing hemorrhage with limited availability of blood or lack of endoscopist
- Concurrent indication for surgery, for example, perforation
- High-risk lesion (posterior duodenal ulcer or lesser curvature gastric ulcer, high risk of left gastric artery erosion)
- Requiring >4 units is in 24 h or 8 units in 48 h
- Ulcer >2 cm in diameter

Operations for Bleeding Duodenal Ulcer:

- Oversewing the ulcer ± vagotomy and drainage
- Vagotomy and antrectomy (avoid if patient in shock or unstable)

Operations for Gastric Ulcer:

- Distal gastric resection to include the bleeding ulcer is the procedure of choice.
- Second best is vagotomy and drainage with over-sewing the bleeding and biopsy.
- Biopsy and over-sewing followed by acid suppression is acceptable approach in high risk and unstable patient [1–3].

B. **Perforated Peptic Ulcer:**

- Almost always surgery is indicated.
- Non-surgical management for stable patient, with no peritonitis, and has a radiological that confirmed sealed perforation.
- Patient with acute perforation and GI blood loss should be suspected to have second ulcer or gastric cancer.

Operations for Perforated Duodenal Ulcer:

- **Simple patch closure:** most common procedure of choice in unstable patient or perforation happens more than 24 h (Fig. 9.8).
- **Patch closure + HSV:** if the patient is stable, free perforation <12 h, the patient has chronic symptoms of PUD or after failure medical treatment.
- **Patch closure + vagotomy and drainage:** acceptable approach but the side effect is disabling.

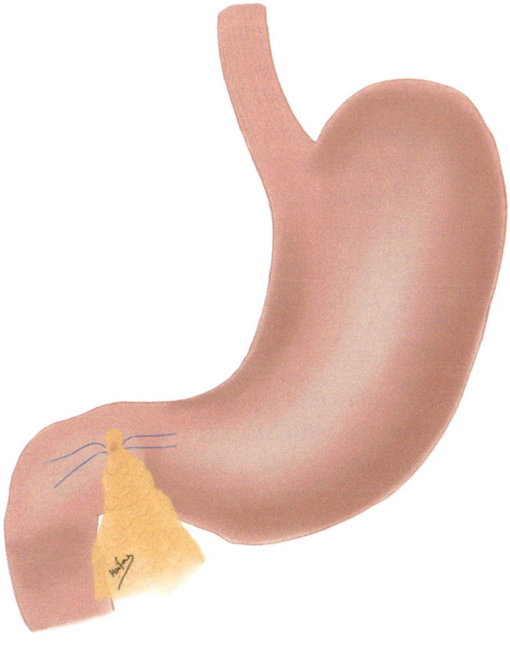

Fig. 9.8 Graham's patch closure for perforated duodenal ulcer

Operation for Perforated Gastric Ulcer:

- Biopsy and patch: in unstable and high-risk patient
- Wedge excision and vagotomy with drainage: in unstable or high-risk patient
- Distal gastrectomy: in stable patient without operative risk factors, add vagotomy if type II or III ulcer

C. **Obstructed Peptic Ulcer:**

- Acute ulcer with obstruction due to edema or motor dysfunction. Managed by antisecretory therapy and NGT

Chronic Ulcer Needs Interventions

- **Endoscopic balloon dilatation:** a temporary measure
- **Vagotomy and antrectomy:** the standard approach
- **Vagotomy and gastrojejunostomy:** when difficult duodenal stump is suspected

D. **Intractable Nonhealing Ulcer:**

- Should raise red flag for surgeon (cancer, noncompliant patient, use of NSADs, *H. pylori* infection or Zollinger-Ellison syndrome)
- Management:
  - Gastric resection (definitive)
  - HSV and gastrojejunostomy: if duodenal ulcer
  - HSV and wedge resection: indicated in thin patient
  - Vagotomy is not indicated in type I or IV ulcers [1–3]

9.1.2 Approach to Patient with Suspected Gastrinoma

- History and physical examination as described earlier
- **Investigations:**

- CBC, electrolyte, coagulation profile.
- Blood grouping.
- Liver function test (LFT).
- Renal function test (RFT).
- Amylase, lipase.
- CXR, ECG.
- Endoscopy: (findings may be esophagitis, gastric and duodenal ulcer, or atypical presentation like multiple ulcers, jejunal ulcer) should raise the suspicious of gastrinoma.
- If patient on PPI or histamine receptor, antagonist must be discontinued.
- Fasting serum gastrin (>1000 pg/ml) and basal acid output (>15 mmol/h) are diagnostic for gastrinoma.
- If serum gastrin (150–1000 pg/ml):
  - Confirm diagnosis by secretin stimulation test:
  - Give IV bolus of secretin 2 U/kg, and check gastrin level before and after. If there is increase in serum gastrin of 200 or more, the diagnosis is gastrinoma.
- If patient is diagnosed with gastrinoma:
  - Screen for MEN 1
  - Serum calcium and PTH
- If MEN-1 is confirmed, perform parathyroidectomy before addressing the gastrinoma [6].

- **Localization of Gastrinoma:**
  - 80% of primary tumor found in the gastrinoma triangle (Fig. 9.9).
  - CT abdomen can localize gastrinoma in 50% of patient specially if the lesion is >2 cm.
  - EUS (can localize gastrinoma in 43–85% of patient).
  - Octreotide scan (can detect it in 71% of patient).
  - DOTATOC PET/CT (localize 90% of gastrinoma).
  - All patients with sporadic gastrinoma should be considered for surgical exploration:
    - Explore gastrinoma triangle, other sites like liver, small bowel, mesentery, and pelvis.
    - Mobilize duodenum and pancreas.
    - Use intraoperative ultrasound IOUS.

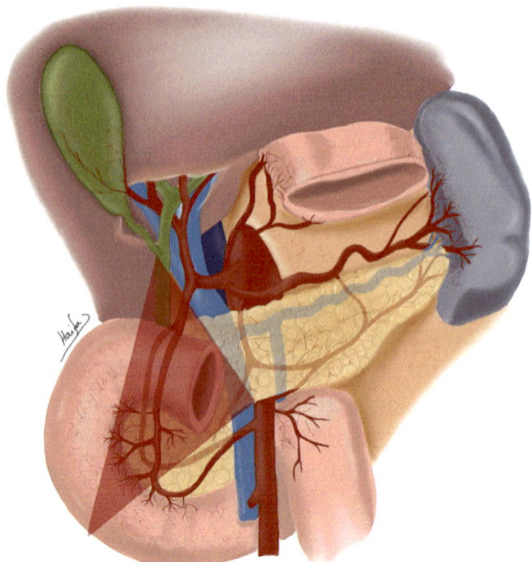

Fig. 9.9 Gastrinoma triangle (between the junction of common hepatic and cystic ducts, between junction of neck and body of the pancreas, to the junction between second parts of the duodenum)

    - Intraoperative EGD.
    - If sill cannot be found, longitudinal duodenotomy is indicated with inspection and palpation of duodenal wall.
  - If found the management is:
    - Duodenal gastrinoma: resection with adequate margin + lymphadenectomy (periportal, portal, pancreatic, celiac lymph nodes)
    - If there are hepatic metastases, managed by ablation
    - Body and tail of pancreas: distal pancreatectomy + lymphadenectomy
    - Head of pancreas:
      - Enucleation if not involving major duct or vessels
      - Pylorus preserving Whipple procedure if bulky tumor [6]

- **Gastrinoma with MEN1:**
  - Multiple, small, and high risk of metastasis.
  - Surgery is seldom curative in (0–10%).
  - Surgery is recommended only if there is tumor >2 cm
    - If in the body and tail of pancreas: resect
    - If in the head of pancreas: enucleation

If in the duodenum: longitudinal duodenotomy and excision of duodenal tumor
– Otherwise, medical treatment: High dose of PPI or HSV [6].

9.1.3 Management of Non-variceal Bleeding

- Start resuscitation following the ABC approach:
  – A: confirm the patency of the air way and assess the level of consciousness, intubate if needed.
  – B: assess the oxygenation and ventilation.
  – C: assess the hemodynamic status and start fluid and blood resuscitation.
    Insert two large IV cannulas.
    Draw blood for investigation: CBC, electrolytes, coagulation profile, blood grouping and cross matching, ABG, and lactic acid.
    Start fluid resuscitation (Ringer's lactate).
    Start PPI (80 mg bolus followed by infusion 8 mg/h for 72 h).
  – History and physical examination after achieving hemodynamic stability.
- Admission to ICU.
- IV fluid.
- IV PPI (infusion).
- NGT, Foley's catheter.
- Erect chest X-ray to rule out concomitant perforation.
- Monitor the fluid input and output.
- Endoscopy within 24 h to identify the source of bleeding and assess the risk of rebleeding using Forrest classification (Table 9.4).

Table 9.4 Forrest classification [7]

Forrest	Finding
Ia	Spurting hemorrhage
Ib	Oozing hemorrhage
IIa	Nonbleeding visible vessel
IIb	Adherent clot
IIc	Hematin covered lesion
III	Flat spot, clean base

- **For Forrest I a, I b, II a, II b:**
  – Endoscopic therapy (cautery, clipping, epinephrine injection).
  – If the bleeding continues, take the patient to surgery.
  – If the bleeding stops, monitor the patient and repeat the endoscopy if bleeding recurs.
  – Rebleeding after second endoscopic attempt is an indication for surgery.
- **For Forrest II c or III:**
  – Assess for *H. pylori* and start treatment with PPI and follow with endoscopy if gastric ulcer.
- **Surgical Management of Bleeding Ulcer: Indications:**
  – Massive hemorrhage unresponsive to endoscopic control
  – Recurrent hemorrhage after two attempts of endoscopic treatment
  – Ongoing bleeding with limited availability of blood or lack of endoscopist
  – Concurrent indication of surgery
  – High-risk lesions (posterior duodenal ulcer or lesser curvature gastric ulcer)
  – Require >4 units in 24 h or >8 units in 48 h
  – Ulcer >2 cm in diameter
- **Surgical options**: as described earlier in the PUD section [1–3, 7]

9.1.4 Management of SMA Syndrome

- Compression of the third, or transverse, portion of the duodenum between the aorta and the superior mesenteric artery. This results in chronic, intermittent, or acute complete or partial duodenal obstruction.
- The superior mesenteric artery usually forms an angle of approximately 45° (range, 38–56°) with the abdominal aorta
- Any factor that sharply narrows the aortomesenteric angle to approximately 6–25° can cause entrapment and compression of the third part of the duodenum as it passes between the superior mesenteric artery and aorta, resulting in SMA syndrome.

- The aortomesenteric distance in superior mesenteric artery syndrome is decreased to 2–8 mm (normal is 10–20 mm).
- **Clinical Presentation:**
  - Abdominal pain, nausea, eructation, voluminous vomiting (bilious or partially digested food), postprandial discomfort, early satiety, and sometimes, subacute small bowel obstruction.
  - The symptoms are typically relieved when the patient is in the left lateral decubitus, prone, or knee-to-chest position, and they are often aggravated when the patient is in the supine position.
- **Causes:**
  - Constitutional factors:
    - Thin body build
    - Exaggerated lumbar lordosis
    - Visceroptosis and abdominal wall laxity
    - Depletion of the mesenteric fat caused by rapid severe weight loss due to catabolic states such as cancer, surgery, burns, trauma, or psychiatric problems
  - Severe injuries, such as head trauma, leading to prolonged bedrest
  - Dietary disorders
    - Anorexia nervosa
    - Malabsorption
- **Diagnosis:**
  - CT scan: aortomesenteric angle of less than 22° and an aortomesenteric distance of less than 8–10 mm.
  - Upper GI endoscopy may be necessary to exclude mechanical causes of duodenal obstruction.
- **Management:**
  - Conservative treatment: adequate nutrition, nasogastric decompression, and proper positioning of the patient after eating (i.e., left lateral decubitus, prone, knee-to-chest position, or Goldthwaite maneuver).
  - Enteral and parenteral nutritional support may be needed.
  - The patient's weight should be monitored daily.
  - Surgical intervention is indicated when conservative measures are ineffective, A trial of conservative treatment should be instituted for at least 4–6 weeks prior to surgical intervention.
  - Options for surgery:
    - Duodenojejunostomy
    - Gastrojejunostomy to bypass the obstruction
    - Duodenal derotation procedure (the Strong procedure) to alter the aortomesenteric angle and place the third and fourth portions of the duodenum to the right of the superior mesenteric artery [8]

9.1.5 Management of Gastric Gastrointestinal Stromal Tumor (GIST)

- Most common sarcoma of the GIT.
- Due to mutation in protooncogene KIT.
- Cell of origin is intestinal cell of Cajal.
- Disease of adult with slight male predominance.
- Stomach is the most common site for GIST (around 40–60%).
- It grows from the muscular layer.
- Erosion of the mucosa can cause bleeding in 25% of patient.
- Metastasis typically involve the liver or peritoneal cavity.
- Lymph node metastasis is rare in GIST <5% [9].
- Workup:
  - CT abdomen and pelvis with oral and IV contrast: enhancing mass arising in the wall of the stomach. Large mass may exhibit heterogenous enhancement resulting from necrosis.
  - Endoscopy: submucosal mass.
  - FNA: spindle cells that are CD117 positive. It helps to differentiate GIST from leiomyoma, lymphoma, or adenocarcinoma [9].
- Risk stratification:
  - Tumor size >5 cm.
  - Mitotic rate 5/50 HPF.
  - Tumor site: nongastric site has poor prognosis [9].
- Surgery for the primary disease:
  - 70% of patients with 3 cm tumors are cured by surgery.

- NCCN guideline recommends surgery for GIST larger than 2 cm and observe smaller lesions (with no high-risk EUS features) with serial endoscopy or imaging.
- High-risk EUS features include irregular border, cystic spaces, ulceration, echogenic foci, and heterogeneity.
- General technical aspects:
  Explore the liver and the peritoneal cavity.
  Once the tumor identified, manipulation should be done with care because the tumors are friable (especially after neo-adjuvant treatment).
  In laparoscopy use non-touch technique and remove the specimen by bag to prevent tumor seeding.
  Peritoneal rupture whether spontaneous or iatrogenic is associated with almost inevitable peritoneal recurrence [9].

• Site-specific consideration:
  - Complete R0 is the goal.
  - Margin is 1 cm.
  - For GE junction:
    Neoadjuvant imatinib.
    CT after 4 weeks from initiation of imatinib to assess the response and then repeat the imaging in every 8–12 weeks.
    Neoadjuvant imatinib and other tyrosine kinase inhibitors (TKI) can be continued up until the time of surgery without compromising the wound healing.
    Open surgery is preferred particularly for posterior aspect of GE junction. Use bougie (50 F) during reconstruction.
  - Large tumor adherent to spleen, colon, pancreas:
    Neoadjuvant imatinib if recognized preoperative
    Enbloc resection
  - Duodenal GIST:
    Neoadjuvant imatinib unless the tumor is small and away from the pancreas.
    Extensive Kocher maneuver is required.
    Tumor near the ampulla requires pancreaticoduodenectomy.
    Small lateral tumor: wedge resection.
    Tumors in third and fourth parts of the duodenum: resection with either direct anastomosis to jejunum or Roux-en-Y [9].

• Adjuvant imatinib:
  - Improve in the recurrence free survival (RFS).
  - Indicated in patient with high risk for recurrence.
  - Duration is at least for 3 years.

• Resection of liver GIST should be approached as colorectal liver metastases.

• Surveillance after resection:
  - CT abdomen and pelvis every 3–6 months for 3–5 years then annually [9].

9.1.6 Management of Gastric Neuroendocrine Tumors (NETs)

• Around 1% of all NETs and <2% of gastric neoplasm.

• Arise from gastric enterochromaffin-like cells (ECL).

• Carcinoid tumor is a well-differentiated neuroendocrine tumor.

• Types: Table 9.5

• Diagnosis:
  - Endoscopy and biopsy.
  - Determine the type depend on the presence or absence of atrophic gastritis, gastric PH, and gastrin level.
  - Chromogranin A.
  - CT abdomen.
  - Octreotide scan for staging.

• Management:
  - **Type I and II:** follow up with serial endoscopy.
    Small lesions <1 cm can be treated with endoscopic mucosal resection if there is <5 lesions.
    Large lesion 1–2 cm should be managed by local excision.
  - **For type III and large lesion >2 cm**: D1 or D2 gastrectomy.
  - Somatostatin analogue may delay the progression of metastatic disease [3].

Table 9.5 Types of gastric NETs [3]

Type I	Type II	Type III
• Most common type >75% • Occur in patient with chronic hypergastrinemia secondary to pernicious anemia or atrophic gastritis • More common in female • Usually small and multiple lesions • Has <5% malignant potential	• Associated with MEN1 and ZES • Small and multiple lesions • Higher malignant potential (around 10%) • Uncommon with sporadic ZES • The presence of high gastric acidity, hypergastrinemia, and gastric NET suggest gastrinoma until proven otherwise	• Solitary • >2 cm • Common in males • Not associated with hypergastrinemia • Usually, the patient has lymph nodes or distant metastasis at the time of the diagnosis • Patient can present with carcinoid syndrome: flushing, diarrhea, heart failure

9.1.7 Management of Gastric Lymphoma

- 4% of all gastric malignancy.
- Stomach is the most common site of primary GI lymphoma.
- More than 95% are non-Hodgkin's lymphoma.
- Types:
  1. Low-grade lymphoma MALT (mucosa-associated lymphoid tissue):
     - Associated with chronic gastritis.
     - Can undergo malignant degeneration.
     - When *H. pylori* eradicated and gastritis improved, MALT disappears.
     - It is not a surgical lesion.
     - Careful follow up is necessary particularly in those lesions with t (11:18) translocation.
     - If persistent after *H. pylori* eradication, radiation therapy should be considered for disease confined to the stomach. Chemotherapy without radiotherapy for more advanced lesions.
  2. High-grade lymphoma:
     - Requires aggressive oncologic treatment for cure.
     - The patients present with symptoms similar to gastric cancer.
     - Diagnosed by endoscopy and biopsy.
     - Much of the tumors are submucosal.
     - Primary lymphoma is nodular with enlarged gastric folds.
     - Diffuse infiltrative like linitis plastica is a more aggressive form of secondary gastric involvement by lymphoma and search for extra gastric lesions.
     - Treatment is chemoradiotherapy.
     - For patient presented with bleeding or perforation, D2 gastrectomy if limited to stomach and adjacent lymph nodes [3].

9.1.8 Approach to Patient with Suspicion of Gastric Cancer

- History and physical examination as described earlier
- **Investigations:**
  - CBC.
  - Electrolyte.
  - Coagulation profile.
  - Blood grouping.
  - Liver function test.
  - Renal function test.
  - Nutritional assessment.
  - LDH.
  - CXR.
  - ECG.
  - Endoscopy.
  - Biopsy if there is any mucosal lesion. If the diagnosis is cancer, the type (intestinal/diffuse), the differentiation degree, and the biomarker should be reported.
  - If positive for cancer:

    Staging CT CAP with IV contrast

    EUS to stage the tumor locally (especially for early gastric cancer), FNA if there is suspicions lymph node

Staging laparoscopy and peritoneal lavage

Discuss in multidisciplinary team meeting

PET scan if high risk or locally advance before any major resection

- **Management:**
  - Admission.
  - Noting per oral (NPO).
  - IV fluid.
  - IV medication (antibiotics prophylaxis, PPI, DVT prophylaxis).
  - Consent.
  - ICU consultation.
  - Anesthesia consultation.
  - Review blood tests, make sure of blood grouping, cross match, and stand by blood.

Surgical Anatomy of the Stomach (Fig. 9.10)
Depend on the Staging:

- **Clinical (c) Tis—c T1a:**
  - Nonsurgical candidate: endoscopic resection.
  - Surgical candidate: endoscopic resection or surgery.
  - If endoscopic resection is performed, follow with endoscopic surveillance.
- **Loco-regional Disease (c M0):**
  - Medically fit patient, potentially resectable:

    c T1b: surgery

    c T2 or higher, N positive: either surgery, neoadjuvant chemotherapy (preferred), or neoadjuvant chemoradiation therapy
  - Surgically unresectable:

    Chemoradiation

    Systemic therapy

    Or palliative management
  - Nonsurgical candidate:

    Chemoradiation (definitive)

    Palliative management
- **Metastatic disease:** palliative management
- **Surgical Options:**
  - Distal gastrectomy
  - Subtotal gastrectomy
  - Total gastrectomy
- **Lymphadenectomy**
  - D1 lymphadenectomy is indicated for:

    cT1a tumors that do not meet the criteria for EMR/ESD (refer to Table 9.6).

    cT1b N0 tumors that are histologically of differentiated type and 1.5 cm or smaller in diameter.
  - D1+ lymphadenectomy is indicated for cT1N0 tumors other than the above.
  - D2 lymphadenectomy is indicated for potentially curable cT2–T4 tumors as well as cT1N+ tumors.
  - **Total Gastrectomy**

    D0: Lymphadenectomy less than D1

    D1: No. 1–7

    D1+: D1 + No. 8a, 9, 11p

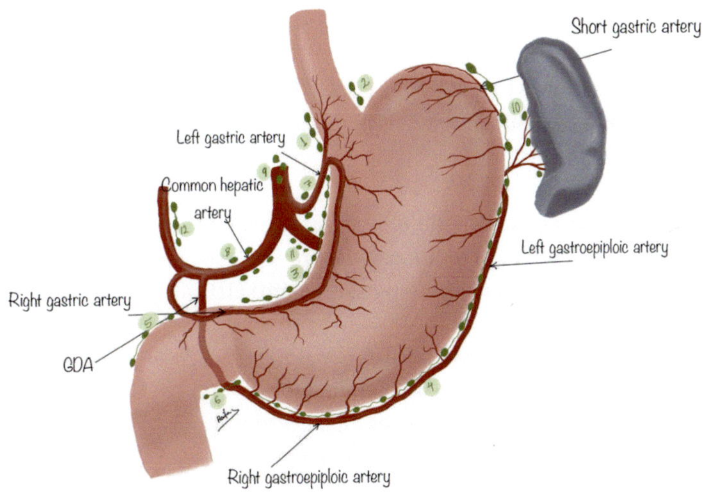

Fig. 9.10 Surgical anatomy of the stomach (arterial and lymphatic)

D2: D1 + No. 8a, 9, 11p, 11d, 12a
- **Distal Gastrectomy**
  D0: Lymphadenectomy less than D1
  D1: No. 1, 3, 4sb, 4d, 5, 6, 7
  D1+: D1 + No. 8a, 9
  D2: D1 + No. 8a, 9, 11p, 12a
- **Gross Margin:**
- For T1 tumors: 2 cm
- For ≥T2:
  Bormann types 1 and 2: at least 3 cm
  Bormann types 3 and 4: 5 cm
- Send frozen section to confirm negative margin.
- Number of harvested lymph node is 15 lymph nodes.
- **Criteria of Unresectability for Cure:**
  - Loco-regional advanced tumor:
    Infiltration of the root of the mesentery or para-aortic lymph nodes
    Invasion or encasement of major vascular structure excluding splenic
  - Distant metastasis or peritoneal seeding
- **Palliative Resection:**
  - For palliation of symptoms (obstruction, or uncontrolled bleeding) in patient with incurable disease.
  - If resection is done for palliation, lymph node dissection is not required.
- If patient was assigned to receive neoadjuvant chemoradiation or perioperative chemotherapy, do restaging CT CAP:
  - If improve or persistent: surgical resection
  - If progress to unrespectable or metastatic: palliative treatment
- **Endoscopic Mucosal Resection (EMR) or Endoscopic Submucosal Dissection (ESD)** (Table 9.6)

If anyone of the criteria is not met, resection consider incomplete (additional therapy by gastrectomy and lymphadenectomy is required) [10].

- **Surveillance Post Successful EMR:**
  - History and physical examination every 3–6 months for 1–2 years then every 6–12 months for 3–5 years then annually
  - EGD every 6 months for 1year then annually for 3 years
  - Routine laboratory investigations and imaging as clinically indicated

- **Neoadjuvant Chemotherapy:**
- Three cycles preoperative and three cycles postoperative
- Regimen: fluoropyrimidine and oxaliplatin
- **Preoperative Chemoradiation:**
- All should be given preoperative.
- Regimen: fluorouracil, oxaliplatin.
- **Adjuvant Chemoradiation:**
  - The patients undergone less than a D2 dissection with ≥pT3, any N, or any pT, N+ tumors.
  - The patients received less than a D2 dissection with pT2, N0 and high-risk futures (poorly differentiated, lymphovascular invasion, neural invasion, age <50 years)
  - All patients following R1 and R2 resection
- **Post Resection Follow-up:**
  - History and physical examination every 3–6 months for 1–2 years then every 6–12 months for 3–5 years then annually
  - EGD as clinically indicated
  - Laboratory investigations and CT as clinically indicated if stage I and every 6–12

Table 9.6 Criteria for EMR, ESD [10]

Absolute indications of EMR or ESD
1. A differentiated-type adenocarcinoma. 2. No ulcerative findings (UL0). 3. Depth of invasion clinically diagnosed as T1a (mucosal stage). 4. The diameter is ≤2 cm.
Absolute indications of ESD
1. A differentiated-type adenocarcinoma. 2. Without ulcerative findings (UL0). 3. The depth of invasion is clinically diagnosed as T1a. 4. The diameter is >2 cm. Or 1. A differentiated-type adenocarcinoma. 2. With ulcerative findings (UL1). 3. The depth of invasion is clinically diagnosed as T1a. 4. The diameter is ≤3 cm.
Expanded indications
1. An undifferentiated-type adenocarcinoma. 2. Without ulcerative findings (UL0). 3. The depth of invasion is clinically diagnosed as T1a. 4. The diameter is >2 cm.

months for 2 years then annually if stage II or III
- Monitor nutritional deficiency and treat it as indicated [3, 10, 11]

9.1.9 Approach to the Surgical Management of Obesity

- The international classification of adult overweight and obesity according to body mass index (BMI):
  - Normal range: 18.50–24.99 kg/m^2
  - Pre-obese: 25.00–29.99 kg/m^2
  - Class I obesity: 30.00–34.99 kg/m^2
  - Class II obesity: 35.00–39.99 kg/m^2
  - Class III obesity: ≥40 kg/m^2
- **Indications for Bariatric Surgery:**
  - BMI ≥ 40 kg/m^2 with no comorbid conditions.
  - BMI ≥ 35 kg/m^2 with obesity-associated comorbidity.
  - Patients with T2DM and BMI of 30–34.9 kg/m^2 (class I obesity) if blood sugar is inadequately controlled despite optimal medication treatment [12].
- **Contraindications of Bariatric Surgery:**
  - Prohibitive surgical risk, ASA IV, reversible endocrine, or other disorders that can cause obesity
  - Current drug or alcohol misuse
  - Uncontrolled severe psychiatric illness
  - Uncontrolled severe bulimia
  - Lack of comprehension of risks, benefits, expected outcomes, alternatives, and lifestyle changes [12]
- **Preoperative Issues:**
  - **Patient Selection:**

    Patient selection for surgery should be based on a multidisciplinary team approach.
  - **Assessment of the Nutritional Status:**

    The preoperative assessment of the patient for bariatric surgery must include input from the nutritionist as an important independent evaluation.

    Careful assessment of the patient's eating habits, knowledge, self-awareness, and insight.

    Estimation of the patient's motivation to change eating habits is important.

    The operation to be performed requires specific nutritional counseling and education [12].
  - **Psychological Assessment**
  - **Obstructive Sleep Apnea (OSA) Assessment:**

    The Epworth Sleepiness Scale, a standard set of questions evaluating daytime sleepiness, is often used as a screening tool for OSA.

    Standard preoperative management of obese patients with OSA using continuous positive airway pressure (CPAP) is recommended [12].
  - **Hypoventilation Syndrome:**

    Hypoventilation syndrome of obesity is defined as resting arterial partial pressure of oxygen less than 55 mmHg and partial pressure of carbon dioxide greater than 47 mmHg, with accompanying pulmonary hypertension and polycythemia.

    Pulmonary consultation is indicated for patients with hypoventilation syndrome.

    Postoperative intensive care unit hospitalization is indicated.
  - **Preoperative Weight Loss:**

    Preoperative weight loss can reduce liver volume/size and may help improve the technical aspects of surgery in those people with extreme central obesity and an enlarged liver.

    Ten percent total body weight loss (TBWL) with energy-restricted diets has been associated with a reduction in hepatic volume.
  - **Glycemic Control:**

    Preoperative glycemic control should be optimized using diet, physical activity, and medications, as needed.

Target hemoglobin A1c value of 6.5–7.0% or less, a fasting blood glucose level of ≤110 mg/dl, and a 2-h postprandial blood glucose concentration of ≤140 mg/dl.

- **Assessment of GERD:**
  For patients with active GERD on medication, a preoperative screening upper endoscopy to rule out Barrett's esophagus and to rule out intrinsic lesions of the stomach or duodenum is recommended. This is especially true for patients planning LRYGB, where the distal stomach and duodenum will be precluded from easy inspection postoperatively.
  The presence of Barrett's esophagus is a contraindication to SG, which is a reflux-inducing operation. The presence of a hiatal hernia detected on preoperative EGD will alert the surgeon for the need to perform intraoperative repair [12].
- **Assessment of DVT Risk:**
  Patients with a history of DVT or cor-pulmonale should undergo a diagnostic evaluation for DVT.
  The overall risk of venous thromboembolism (VTE) after surgery is 0.42%, and over 70% of these events occur after hospital discharge, most within 30 days after surgery.
  The risk of VTE is greater in patients undergoing Roux-en-Y gastric bypass (RYGB) than in those undergoing laparoscopic adjustable gastric banding (LAGB) and is more frequent following open surgery.
- **Pregnancy:**
  Candidates for bariatric surgery should avoid pregnancy preoperatively and for 12–18 months postoperatively and women who become pregnant after bariatric surgery should be counseled and monitored for appropriate weight gain, nutritional supplementation, and for fetal health.
- **Consent:**
  The risks and benefits, procedural options, and the need for long-term follow-up and vitamin supplementation (including costs required to maintain appropriate follow-up) [12].

- **Bariatric Surgery Procedures:**
  - **Laparoscopic Roux-en-Y Gastric Bypass (LRYGB)**
    It is an appropriate operation for consideration for most patients eligible for bariatric surgery.
    Relative contraindications specifically for LRYGB include previous gastric surgery, previous antireflux surgery, severe iron deficiency anemia, distal gastric or duodenal lesions that require ongoing future surveillance, and Barrett's esophagus with severe dysplasia [12].

Procedures:

- Proximal gastric pouch of small size (<20 ml) that is totally separated from the distal residual stomach.
- A Roux limb of proximal jejunum is brought up and anastomosed to the pouch.
- The pathway of that limb can be anterior to the colon and stomach, posterior to both, or posterior to the colon and anterior to the stomach.
- The length of the biliopancreatic limb from the ligament of Treitz to the distal enteroenterostomy is 20–50 cm, and the length of the Roux limb is 75–150 cm [12] (Fig. 9.11).

Procedure Specific Complications:

- **Anastomotic leak:** is the single serious complication after RYGB, either open or laparoscopic. Tachycardia, tachypnea, fever, and oliguria are the most common symptoms that should arouse suspicion for this problem. The treatment is surgical, except in

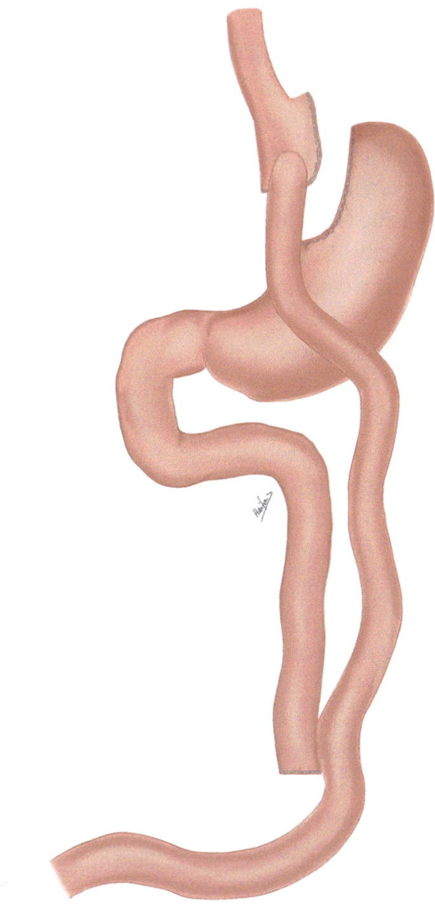

Fig. 9.11 Roux-en-Y gastric bypass

rare circumstances where a drain is already in place, no hemodynamic or clinical deterioration is present, and the leak is contained. Usual surgical treatment involves repair as feasible, drainage, and creation of a reliable feeding access through a distal Stamm gastrostomy [12].

- **VTE**
- Wound infection
- Marginal ulcer: The patient presents with pain in the epigastric region that is not altered by eating. Diagnosis is by endoscopy. Treatment is medical with proton pump inhibitors, which are effective in 90% of cases. Only those with a gastrogastric fistula to the distal stomach, severe stenosis of the lumen of the gastrojejunostomy, or acute perforation require surgical therapy. Treatment of a perforated marginal ulcer is a laparoscopic Graham patch.
- **Bowel obstruction:** This is because the etiology of the bowel obstruction after LRYGB is often an internal hernia from inadequate or non-closure of the mesenteric defects by the surgeon at the time of operation. Cutoff of passage of contrast on CT scan at the enteroenterostomy is particularly suggestive of this diagnosis. It should be managed by emergent operation. If the bowel is viable, suturing the mesenteric defect is all that is needed for treatment.
- Anastomotic stenosis: Stenosis of the gastrojejunostomy has been reduced by the use of the linear stapling technique. Stenosis symptoms usually appear from 6 to 12 weeks postoperatively, but less commonly can occur later. Diagnosis is by upper endoscopy. Treatment is circumferential balloon dilatation.
- Early and late dumbing.
- Nutritional complications: Iron deficiency anemia, vitamin B12, vitamin D deficiencies [12].

– **Laparoscopic Sleeve Gastrectomy (LGS):** Patients who have longstanding severe GERD may not be good candidates for SG as GERD is worsened by the anatomical configuration of the SG. Barrett's esophagus is also a contraindication for performing SG.

Procedure:

- Devascularizing the greater curvature of the stomach, beginning 3–5 cm proximal to the pylorus.
- A complete mobilization of the fundus in and division of posterior fibrous attachments to the antrum and body of the stomach.

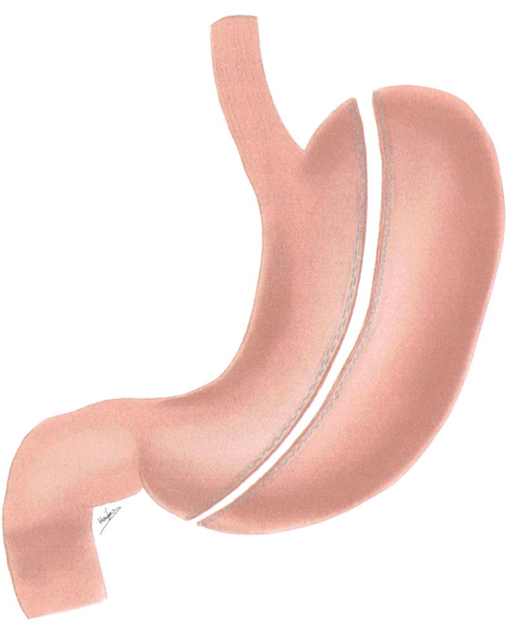

Fig. 9.12 Sleeve gastrectomy

- Stapled division of the stomach starting from 2 cm lateral to the incisura up to the angle of His.
- A 32- to 40-French bougie and position it along the lesser curvature of the stomach. This bougie then serves as a guide for further gastric division [12] (Fig. 9.12).

Procedure-Related Complications:

- **Stapler Line Leak:**
  - Distal staple line leaks: earlier presentation, related to mechanical failure of the staple line to securely approximate the thicker distal gastric tissue are more amenable to successful repair with a reoperation.
  - Proximal leaks: late presentation, due to high intraluminal pressure and better managed by drainage of the collection endoscopy dilatation of the stenosis or stenting.
- **Stap**ler line bleeding
- GERD
- VTE **[12]**

– **Laparoscopic Adjustable Gastric Banding (LAGB)**

Patients who have had previous upper gastric surgery, such as a Nissen fundoplication, and those with severe GERD are relatively poor candidates for LAGB due to altered proximal gastric anatomy interfering with proper band placement or worsening of GERD symptoms.

Procedure:

- LAGB involves placement of an inflatable silicone ring around the proximal stomach.
- The band is attached to a reservoir system that allows adjustment of the tightness of the band.
- This reservoir system is accessed through a subcutaneously placed port [12].

Procedure-Specific Complications

- **Gastric Prolapse:**
  - Acute gastric prolapse:
  - It is the most common emergent complication that requires reoperation after LAGB. Acute, severe pain with immediate dysphagia, vomiting, and inability to take oral food or liquid is the typical presentation. Vomiting may predispose or exacerbate this problem. Either anterior or posterior prolapse may occur. Initial treatment for an acute or chronic prolapse is to remove all the fluid from the system. This often allows reduction of the prolapse and resolution of symptoms. If prolapse persists, then reoperation laparoscopically to reduce the prolapse and re-suture the band in place is indicated.
  - Chronic gastric prolapse is more subtle. The band retains its normal oblique angle, but there is sym-

metric dilation of the gastric pouch above the band. These are initially managed with fluid removal and monitoring of symptoms.

- Band slippage
- Band erosion
- Port and tubing complications [12]
  - **Biliopancreatic Diversion and Duodenal Switch:**

Currently, BPD and DS represent together less than 1–2% of bariatric operations performed in the United States. Patients who undergo either BPD or DS must be prepared for the consequences of a malabsorptive operation [12].

Preoperative Preparation:

- Admission.
- Consent.
- NPO.
- IV fluid.
- DVT and stress ulcer prophylaxis.
- Prophylactic antibiotic.
- Confirm the availability of blood intraoperative if needed.
- Anesthesia consultation.
- ICU consultation if required.
- Instruct the patient to take shower the night before surgery.
- Hair removal.

Informed consent:

Gastrectomy and Lymphadenectomy:

- *Describe the Procedure to the patient:* under general anesthesia the surgeon will resect part or the whole stomach along with the draining lymph nodes due to the presence of gastric cancer. The continuity of the GIT will be performed by reconnecting the proximal stomach or the esophagus to the jejunum.
- *Mention if there is any alternative.*
- *Mention all the possible complications:* bleeding, infection, subphrenic fluid collection, anastomotic leak, injury to pancreas, spleen or colon, dumbing syndrome, post vagotomy diarrhea, marginal ulcer, vitamins deficiency, alkaline reflux, anemia, adhesions, hernia, atelectasis, pneumonia, MI, DVT, PE.

Open Subtotal Gastrectomy

- 75% of the stomach is resected.
- Reconstruction between remaining stomach and proximal jejunum either as an omega loop or as Roux en Y reconstruction.

Procedure:

- Under general anesthesia and endotracheal intubation.
- Position: supine.
- Time out: confirming correct patient, correct procedure, surgeon, and any special instrument, for example (self-retaining retractors, GIA, feeding tube).
- Confirm DVT and antibiotics are given as indicated.
- Prepping and draping in usual sterile fashion.
- Through midline incision, skin and subcutaneous tissue divided till the fascia is reached. Divide the fascia and enter the peritoneal cavity.
- Exploration of the abdominal cavity, liver, peritoneum in case of gastric cancer.
- Identify the gastric lesion.
- Apply the retractors.
- Dissect the greater omentum of the stomach from the transverse colon exposing the posterior wall of the stomach and opening the lesser sac.
- Pylorus is freed from adjacent connective tissue.
- The omentum is opened along the lesser curvature taking care not to injure the left hepatic artery.
- Left gastric artery and coronary vein are identified, ligated, and transected, these lymphatic tissue along lesser and greater curvature included in the specimen.
- Right gastric artery and vein are ligated and transected as well as the right gastroepiploic artery and vein at the greater curvature, preserving the arcade vessels of the proximal part of the stomach.

- Resection margins are set at the pyloric region about 1 cm distal to the pylorus and proximal third of the stomach.
- Duodenum is divided with stapler device, invert the suture line with seromuscular stitches.
- Transect the stomach using stapler device, send margins for frozen if the case is cancer [13].

Reconstruction: BillrothII(OmegaLoopGastrojejunostomy):

- Choose loop of proximal jejunum that can easily be mobilized to distal part of the posterior wall of the remnant stomach.
- Can be done in antecolic or retrocolic fashion.
- Prepare a small passage in mesentery of the transverse colon and pull the omega loop through the mesentery mind that no lesion on the mesentery when loop is in place.
- Open the closure of the distal gastric remnant and the antimesenteric side of the omega loop.
- To avoid anastomotic stricture, the gastrojejunostomy should be performed over 5–6 cm.
- The inner layer of the anastomosis is performed using a running suture, beginning in the back wall and coming around the corner in front, the anastomosis completed with an anterior row of interrupted sutures.
- Close the mesenteric defect.
- Close the fascia with non-absorbable suture and skin by stapler [13].

Open Subtotal Gastrectomy with Lymphadenectomy:

- Under general anesthesia and endotracheal intubation.
- Position: supine.
- Time out: confirming correct patient, correct procedure, surgeon and any special instrument, for example, (self-retaining retractors, GIA, sutures).
- Confirm DVT and antibiotics are given as indicated.
- Prepping and draping in usual sterile fashion.
- Through midline incision or bilateral subcostal incision, skin and subcutaneous tissue divided till fascia is reached. Divide the fascia and enter the peritoneal cavity.
- Exploration of the abdominal cavity looking for any sign of metastasis (liver, peritoneum, lymph node, penetration to pancreas, spleen, and colon).
- Apply the retractors.
- The entire gastrocolic ligament (omentum) is separated from the transverse colon through avascular plane.
- Elevate the omentum from the transverse colon to expose the anterior surface of the pancreas.
- Perform Kocher maneuver and separate duodenum from anterior surface of pancreas carefully.
- Retract the liver, divide the lesser omentum. If present, a replaced left hepatic artery will be identified at this time and should be preserved.
- Retract the stomach inferiorly to expose the abdominal esophagus and incise the peritoneal and phrenoesophageal membrane.
- Identify both crura and clear them.
- Dissect around the esophagus and encircle it with Penrose drain.
- Divide the vagal nerves.
- Greater omentum is released from splenic flexure, dissect and divide the short gastric vessels.
- Divide the right gastroepiploic and right gastric arteries and the posterior wall of the duodenum is freed.
- Transect the duodenum 2 cm distal to the pylorus.
- Oversaw the stapler line.
- Retract the stomach upward and to the left, which allow for optimal exposure.
- Start D2 lymphadenectomy by removing all lymph nodes along the common hepatic artery, nodes around and along the celiac trunk, trunk of the splenic artery and cranial margin and surface of pancreas.
- All arteries are freed from areolar and lymphatic tissue and secured with vessel loops.

- Identify left gastric artery, isolate it, ligate it, and divide it.
- Divide the coronary vein (just caudal to the artery).
- After mobilization of entire stomach, the esophagus is then divided just above the cardia.
- Right-angled clamp is placed distal to the lower esophagus and the esophagus is divided by electrocautery.
- Send the specimen to the pathology to confirm adequacy of the margins before reconstruction [14].

Reconstruction:
Roux-en-Y Esophagojejunostomy:

- Retrocolic Roux-en-Y end to side esophagojejunostomy.
- Divide the jejunum 20 cm distal to ligament of Treitz. Adequate length can be achieved with division of one or two of the arcades.
- Small incision is made in avascular plane of the transverse mesocolon to the left of the middle colic artery.
- The Roux limb is brought through this opening and positioned next to the esophagus, with staple end facing to the left. Adequate length is verified, avoid twisting or kinking of the jejunal mesentery.
- Align the jejunum limb with the esophageal opening.
- An antimesenteric incision is made in the end of the jejunum, its length corresponding to the diameter of the esophagus.
- To avoid blind end syndrome, this incision is made close (1–2 cm) to the jejunal stapler line.
- Apply two corner sutures.
- Perform the posterior layer of the anastomosis by using 3-0 silk suture placed in interrupted fashion, from one corner stitch to the other (knots are tied intraluminal).
- After completion of posterior wall, pass the NGT.
- The anterior layer is then closed with interrupted 3-0 silk tied extra luminal.
- Perform the jejunojejunostomy 60 cm distal to esophagojejunostomy, side to side using GIA.
- Close the mesenteric defect.
- Assure hemostasis and insert drain if needed.
- Close the abdomen in layers [14].

Gastrostomy Tube:

- Percutaneous (endoscopic): PEG tube
- Surgical: using either Stamm's or Janeway's techniques
- Indications:
  - Feeding (neurological disease, trauma, extensive burns, aerodigestive tract malignancy)
  - Decompression (unresectable malignant obstruction with life expectancy >4 weeks)
- Strategy:
  - Stamm: fast, relatively safe. When the tube is no longer needed, removal of the tube result in prompt closure of the tract.
  - Janeway: Long-term gastric tube feeding. Its construction does not need indwelling tube.
- Technique (Stamm Gastrostomy):
  - Incision: small upper midline or if it is part of other procedure through the same incision
  - Location: mid portion of the stomach, closer to the greater curvature more than the lesser curvature
  - Steps:

    Make two purse string sutures with diameter 1.5 cm using 2.0 silk.

    Raise the left side of the Lina alba using Kocher forceps.

    Make stab wound through the middle third of the left rectus muscle at the level of the purse string sutures.

    Pass a Kelly hemostat through the stab from the peritoneum outward and grasp the tip of 18 F Foley, Malecot, or mushroom catheters and draw the catheter into the abdominal cavity.

    Insert the catheter into the stomach, tighten the purse string and tie it to invert the gastric serosa using the second purse string.

    If Foley's catheter is used, inflate the balloon.

    Insert lambert sutures using silk sutures in the four quadrants around the catheter

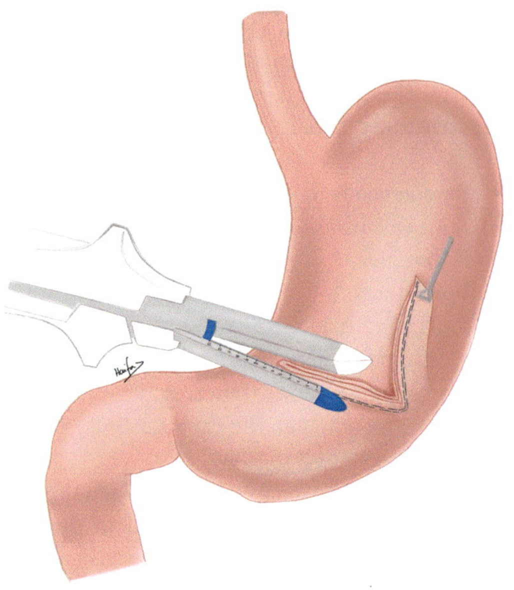

Fig. 9.13 Janeway's technique for gastrostomy tube

to sew the stomach to the anterior abdominal wall around the stab wound.
Closure of the abdominal wall incision in layers.

– Technique (Janeway):
Incision: 10–12 cm midline incision in the mid epigastrium.
Apply two Babcock clamps to the anterior stomach wall near the lesser curvature.
Apply cutting linear stapling device, fire the device and incise for a distance of 4 cm (it will provide a tunnel of mucosa about 4 cm in length) (Fig. 9.13).
Reinforce the line of staples with a layer of continuous or interrupted 3-0 atraumatic seromuscular lambert suture to invert the staples.
Make vertical incision about 1.5 cm in the skin over the middle third of the left rectus muscle.
Deepen the incision through the rectus muscle with the aid of electrocautery then dilate it by insertion of the index finger.
Grasp the gastric nipple and draw it to the outside by passing a Babcock clamp. This brings the gastric wall into contact with the anterior abdominal wall, to which it should be fixed with two lambert sutures with 2-0 suture.
Transect the tip of the gastric nipple, leaving enough gastric tissue to reach the skin level.
Insert 18 F catheter into the stomach to assess the channel.
Mature the gastrostomy using 3-0 interrupted suture.
Close the skin incision in layers [15].

Postoperative Care:

- Nothing per oral (NPO).
- If patient has feeding tube, feeding can be started.
- IV fluid.
- IV medication
  - Analgesia
  - Antibiotics if needed
  - DVT prophylaxis
  - PPI
- Investigations as indicated
- Monitor vital sign
- Mobilization
- Incentive spirometry
- Contrast study on postoperative day 5–6

Complications:

- Short term:
  - Intra-abdominal bleeding
  - Subphrenic abscess
  - Anastomotic leak
  - Pancreatic fistula
  - Duodenal stump leak
  - Injury to colon or spleen
- Long term:
  - Weight loss
  - Anemia
  - Diarrhea
  - Vitamin deficiency
  - Dumping

– Alkaline reflux
- General complications:
  – DVT
  – PE
  – MI
  – Pneumonia

9.2 Part II: Practice

Practice doesn't make perfect. Practice reduces the imperfection.
—Toba Beta, Master of Stupidity

9.2.1 Case Scenarios for Practice

Tips:
- Practice with a friend and try to mimic the real exam!
- Do not forget to set the timer!
- The clinical data is provided in the answer key section.

Case No. 1:
A 32-year-old male patient presented to the emergency department complaining of severe upper abdominal pain for 12 h.

Questions for Discussion:

1. How will you approach the patient?
2. What is your differential diagnosis?
3. What will you do next to confirm the most likely diagnosis?
4. How will you manage the patient?
5. The exploration shows small duodenal perforation at the first part of the duodenum. What will you do?
6. How will you follow the patient in the immediate postoperative period?
7. On the fourth postoperative day, the patient is complaining of abdominal pain, fever and on examination he is febrile and has tenderness and guarding at the epigastric area. His recent laboratory investigation shows raising in his WBC and CRP. What will you do?
8. CT shows contrast leak and intra-abdominal collection. What will you do?
9. The patient's condition deteriorates despite percutaneous drainage of the fluid. What will you do?
10. On exploration the duodenal repair was dehiscent, and the perforation size increased, the tissue was friable, and you could not repair or patch the hole. The hemodynamic status of the patient is not stable. What will you do?

Case No. 2:
A 45-year-old male patient presented to the clinic complaining of epigastric discomfort for 2 months.

Questions for Discussion:

1. How will you approach the patient?
2. What is your differential diagnosis?
3. How will you investigate his condition?
4. What is your diagnosis?
5. How will you manage his condition?

Case No. 3:
A 50-year-old male patient presented to the emergency department complaining of three times coffee ground vomiting followed by one time vomiting of bright red blood.

Questions for Discussion:

1. How will you approach the patient?
2. What will you do next?
3. What is your differential diagnosis?
4. How will you manage the patient?
5. The endoscopic findings as described. What is the Forrest classification?
6. The patient has another attack of hematemesis. What will you do?
7. The endoscopist could not control the bleeding in the second endoscopic attempt. How will you manage that?

Case No. 4:
A 55-year-old male patient presented to the clinic complaining of epigastric pain for 3 months.

Questions for Discussion:

1. How will you approach the patient?
2. How will you investigate his condition?
3. What will you do next?
4. How will you manage him?
5. The patient responds well to the given treatment. What will you do?
6. How will you follow the patient?

Case No. 5:
A 49-year-old female patient presented to the clinic complaining of epigastric pain and weight loss for 4 months.

Questions for Discussions:

1. How will you approach the patient?
2. What is your differential diagnosis?
3. How will you investigate the most likely diagnosis?
4. The result of the requested investigation as given. How will you manage that?
5. Few weeks later, the patient presented to the emergency department with upper GI bleeding. After initial resuscitation, how will you manage her condition?

Checklist

History	Items	Done	Not done	Not applicable
General	Introduce himself/herself to the patient			
	Patient personal data (name, age, sex, nationality, occupation)			
	Chief complaint			
	Duration			
Pain	Onset			
	Site			
	Character			
	Radiation/shifting			
	Aggravating/relieving			
	Severity			
	Progression			
	Frequency			
Mass	Onset			
	How did the patient notice the mass?			
	Any changes since it was first noticed?			
	Any other lumps in the body?			
Bleeding	Onset			
	Amount			
	Relation to food			
	Fresh blood, coffee ground			
	Proceeding event (cough, vomiting, retching)			
	Another bleeding site			
Associated symptoms	Pain			
	Hematemesis			
	Fever			
	Melena			
	Change in bowel habit			
	Regurgitation			
	Nausea			
	Vomiting			
	Heartburn			
	Jaundice			
	Symptoms of anemia			

History	Items	Done	Not done	Not applicable
Constitutional symptoms	Weight loss			
	Decrease appetite			
	Night sweating			
Symptoms of metastases	Back pain			
	Cough			
	Shortness of breath			
	Abdominal distention			
Risk factors	Smoking			
	Diet (high fat, high nitrate, or high salt)			
	Personal history of PUD			
	Previous gastric surgery			
	Family history of gastric, colon (FAP or HNPCC) or breast cancer (lobular)			
	Family history of endocrine syndrome			
	Stress or recent surgery (stress gastritis)			
	NSAID intake			
	Personal history of other cancer			
Differential diagnosis	History of eating from outside (gastroenteritis)			
	Contact with sick patient (gastroenteritis)			
	History of gall stone, alcohol (pancreatitis)			
	Cough, SOB (lower lobe pneumonia)			
	Chest pain, palpitation (inferior MI)			
PMH	Previous similar attack			
	Previous investigation or endoscopy			
	Previous admission			
	Chronic illnesses			
PSH	Previous surgery			
Family history	Of similar complain			
Social history	Occupation			
	Habits (smoking, alcohol, drugs)			
Other	Medication			
	Allergy			
	Transfusion			
Systemic review				
Physical examination				
General principle	Patient position			
	Exposure			
	Privacy			
	Wash hands			
General examination	Appearance			
	Body built			
	Color			
	Distress/decubitus			
	Environment			
Vital signs	BP, HR, temperature, RR, SPO_2			
Hand signs	Leukonychia, koilonychia, pallor			
Eyes	Jaundice, pallor			
Neck	Lymphadenopathy (left supraclavicular lymph nodes)			
	Acanthosis nigricans			
	Thyroid or parathyroid swelling (in case of MEN syndromes is suspected)			

(continued)

History	Items	Done	Not done	Not applicable
Chest	Respiratory system			
	Cardiovascular			
	Axilla: Irish lymph node in patient with gastric cancer			
Abdomen: Inspection	Distention			
	Asymmetry			
	Dilated veins			
	Umbilical nodule (Sister Mary Josef)			
	Striae			
	Visible peristalsis			
	Scars			
	Cough impulse			
Palpation	Superficial then deep palpation			
	Tenderness			
	Palpable masses			
	Organomegaly			
	Cough impulse at hernial orifices			
Percussion	Shifting dullness			
	Fluid thrill			
	Organomegaly			
Auscultation	Bowel sounds			
	Bruit, venous hum			
Groin				
DRE (bloody stool, look for any palpable hard nodule anteriorly)				
Back tenderness				
Differential diagnosis	According to the given scenario.			
Investigations				
General laboratory test	CBC with differential			
	Electrolytes			
	Liver function test			
	Amylase and lipase			
	Blood grouping			
	ABG			
	Lactic acid			
	Coagulation profile (PT, INR, aPTT)			
	RFT			
Specific tests (as indicated)	Serum gastrin level			
	Chromogranin A			
	LDH			
	ECG			
	Octreotide scan			
	DOTA scan			
Imaging	Chest X ray			
	Esophagogram			
	EUS			
	CT chest/abdomen/pelvis with IV contrast			
	PET scan			
Endoscopy	EGD			
Biopsy	FNA			
	Biopsy/endoscopic submucosal resection			
H. pylori	*H. pylori* test			

History	Items	Done	Not done	Not applicable
Provisional diagnosis	According to the given scenario			
Management (depend on the diagnosis):				
PUD Non-complicated	PPI			
	H. pylori regimen if positive			
	Endoscopic follow up if gastric ulcer			
	Confirm the eradication of H. Pylori			
	Surgical treatment if indicated			
Perforated PUD	Admission			
	IV fluid			
	IV PPI			
	IV antibiotic			
	IV antifungal			
	Conservative management if sealed perforation in stable patient			
	Surgical options for perforated duodenal ulcer (simple patch closure, patch closure+ HSV, or patch closure+ vagotomy and drainage)			
	Surgical options for perforated gastric ulcer (biopsy and patch, wedge excision and vagotomy with drainage, or distal gastrectomy)			
Bleeding ulcer	Admission			
	IV fluid and blood products			
	IV PPI			
	IV antibiotic			
	Endoscopy			
	Surgery if the bleeding is not controlled by endoscopy			
Obstructing ulcer	Admission			
	IV fluid			
	IV PPI			
	IV antibiotic			
	NGT decompression			
	Endoscopic balloon dilatation			
	Operative management			
Gastrinoma	Admission			
	Localization: endoscopy			
	CT abdomen			
	EUS			
	Octreotide scan			
	DOTA scan			
	Surgical resection if sporadic gastrinoma			
	Medical management if metastatic or familial			
Upper GI bleeding	Start resuscitation with ABC approach			
	Insert two large cannulas			
	Draw blood for investigation			
	Start fluid and blood resuscitation			
	PPI bolus then IV infusion			
	Admission to ICU			
	NGT, Foley's catheter			
	Endoscopy			
	Surgical management if bleeding could not be controlled by endoscopy			

(continued)

History	Items	Done	Not done	Not applicable
GIST	Admission			
	Multidisciplinary team			
	Neoadjuvant imatinib if indicated			
	Follow up CT scan			
	Prepare the patient surgery			
	Resection with 1 cm margin			
Gastric NETs	Admission			
	Multidisciplinary team			
	Endoscopic resection if small lesion, type I or II			
	Prepare the patient surgery			
	Resection			
Gastric lymphoma	Admission			
	Multidisciplinary team			
	If low-grade lymphoma (MALT), eradication of H. Pylori			
	If high-grade lymphoma: chemoradiation therapy			
	Surgical treatment for complication			
Gastric cancer	Staging CT CAP			
	Staging laparoscopy and peritoneal lavage			
	Multidisciplinary team			
	PET scan if high risk or locally advanced before any major resection			
	Neoadjuvant treatment (if indicated)			
	Prepare for operation			
	Operative management: total or subtotal gastrectomy ± D1 or D2 lymphadenectomy			
Postoperative care				
Early postoperative (gastric cancer)	Admission to HDU or ICU when needed			
	Early mobilization and DVT prophylaxis			
	NPO or resume feeding orally or through feeding tubes if present			
	Monitor the vital signs			
	Analgesia			
	Stress ulcer prophylaxis			
	CBC and LFT daily			
	Electrolyte assessment			
	Monitor drain output and the nature of the fluid			
First outpatient visit	Clinical assessment			
	Remove sutures			
	Review the final pathology report			
	Arrange for multidisciplinary discussion if the case is cancer			
	Refer to oncology if adjuvant treatment is required			
Long-term follow-up (for adenocarcinoma)	History and physical examination every 3–6 months for 1–2 years then every 6–12 months for the 3–5 years then annually			
	EGD as clinically indicated			
	Laboratory investigations and CT as clinically indicated if stage I and every 6–12 months for 2 years then annually if stage II or III			
	Monitor nutritional deficiency and treat it			

9.2.2 Answer Key

Case No. 1:

A 32-year-old male patient presented to the emergency department complaining of severe upper abdominal pain for 12 h.

Questions for Discussion:

1. **How will you approach the patient?**

   The patient is a 32-year-old male patient who is complaining of sudden onset severe epigastric pain that was started 12 h ago. It does not radiate elsewhere and is not shifted. It has a severity of 9/10 scores and the pain increase when he moves. It is sharp pain and progressive since its onset. It is associated with multiple times vomiting of clear gastric content. He has no history of fever, jaundice, chest pain, or GI bleeding. He is a heavy smoker (2 packs per day for the last 12 years). Last week he fell while he was playing football and sprain his ankle for which he is taking ibuprofen.

   He is otherwise a healthy man with no previous surgical history.

   On examination:

   He is conscious, looks ill.

   Not pale or jaundiced.

   Vital signs: Bp: 119/76 mmHg PR: 100 bpm, temperature 38 °C, RR: 19.

   Abdomen: rigid on palpation with diffuse severe tenderness.

2. **What is your differential diagnosis?**
   - Perforated viscus (PUD)
   - Pancreatitis
   - Gastritis
   - MI
   - Rupture AAA
   - Aortic dissection
3. **What will you do next to confirm the most likely diagnosis?**

   Blood test: Table 9.7

   Chest X-ray (erect): pneumoperitoneum

Table 9.7 Blood test for case 1

Test	Result	Normal value
WBC (k/ul)	18	4.8–10.8
HB (g/dl)	12	12.6–16.5
PLT (K/ul)	405	130–400
ALT (U/l)	120	10–130
AST (U/l)	31	10–34
Total bilirubin (mg/dl)	0.7	0–0.8
Direct bilirubin (mg/dl)	0.2	0–0.3
Albumin (g/dl)	3.6	2.4–4
Creatinine (mg/dl)	1	0.7–1.2
Na (mEq/l)	135	135–145
K (mEq/l)	3.4	3.5–5.1
PT (seconds)	12	10–13
INR	1	1

4. **How will you manage the patient?**
   - Admission
   - IV fluid
   - IV antibiotics
   - IV antifungal
   - Analgesia
   - Antiemetic
   - Blood culture
   - Consent
   - Urgent laparotomy exploration
5. **The exploration shows small duodenal perforation at the first part of the duodenum. What will you do?**
   - Generous peritoneal wash
   - Graham patch repair
6. **How will you follow the patient in the immediate post-operative period?**
   - NPO.
   - Continue IV medication (fluid, antibiotic, analgesic, PPI, DVT prophylaxis).
   - Encourage early mobilization.
   - Incentive spirometry.
   - Resume oral diet gradually after 24 h if the patient is stable and no abdominal complain.
   - Remove the drain if the patient tolerated orally and no obvious leak from the drain.
7. **On the fourth postoperative day, the patient is complaining of abdominal pain, fever and on examination he is febrile and has tenderness and guarding at the epigastric area. His recent laboratory investigation shows raising in his WBC and CRP. What will you do?**

   CT abdomen with IV and oral contrast.

8. **CT shows contrast leak and intra-abdominal collection. What will you do?**
   CT guided percutaneous drainage
   NPO
   IV fluid and continue antibiotics
9. **The patient's condition deteriorates despite percutaneous drainage of the fluid. What will you do?**
   Re-exploration and redo the repair.
10. **On exploration the duodenal repair was dehiscent, and the perforation size increased, the tissue was friable, and you could not repair or patch the hole. The hemodynamic status of the patient is not stable. What will you do?**
   Pyloric exclusion and triple drainage (gastrostomy, retrograde duodenostomy and feeding jejunostomy).

Case No. 2:
A 45-year-old male patient presented to the clinic complaining of epigastric discomfort for 2 months.

Questions for Discussion:

1. **How will you approach the patient?**
   A 45-year-old male patient who is complaining of epigastric discomfort for 2 months. It started gradually at the epigastric area. It is dull aching, not radiated or shifted, no specific aggravating or relieving factor. It became more frequent over the past few weeks. It is associated of vomiting three times over the last week. He has no history of nausea, anorexia or significant weight loss. He has no personal or family history of malignancy and no history of GI bleeding, heartburn, regurgitation, flushing, diarrhea or fever.
   He is not alcoholic or smoker.
   PMH, PSH are unremarkable.
   Not on regular medication.
   On examination:
   Conscious, looks comfortable in the bed.
   Not pale or jaundice.
   Vital signs: normal.
   Abdominal examination: soft abdomen with mild tenderness with deep palpation over the epigastrium. There is hard non-pulsatile palpable mass at the epigastric area, round shape, 4 × 5 cm, smooth surface. No cervical or axillary palpable abnormal lymph nodes.
   DRE: unremarkable.
2. **What is your differential diagnosis?**
   - GIST
   - NETs
   - Gastric cancer
   - Pancreatic mass
   - AAA
   - Lipoma
   - Hernia
3. **How will you investigate his condition?**
   Blood test: see Table 9.8.
   CT abdomen: shows 5 × 5 cm exophytic gastric lesion
   with heterogenous density and no abnormal lymph nodes.
   Endoscopy: shows submucosal lesion at the body of the stomach.
   FNA was taken and shows spindle cells that is positive for CD117.
4. **What is your diagnosis?**
   GIST.
5. **How will you manage his condition?**
   - Discuss the plan in multidisciplinary team.
   - Inform the patient.
   - Admission.
   - NPO.
   - IV fluid.
   - Prophylaxis (antibiotic, DVT, stress ulcer).
   - Anesthesia consultation.

Table 9.8 Blood test for case 2

Test	Result	Normal value
WBC (k/ul)	12	4.8–10.8
HB (g/dl)	10	12.6–16.5
PLT (K/ul)	260	130–400
ALT (U/l)	120	10–130
AST (U/l)	31	10–34
Total bilirubin (mg/dl)	0.6	0–0.8
Direct bilirubin (mg/dl)	0.1	0–0.3
Albumin (g/dl)	3	2.4–4
Creatinine (mg/dl)	1	0.7–1.2
Na (mEq/l)	139	135–145
K (mEq/l)	4	3.5–5.1
PT (seconds)	12	10–13
INR	1	1

- CXR.
- Consent.
- Operative management: wide local excision with 1 cm margin.
- Adjuvant imatinib.

Case No. 3:
A 50-year-old male patient presented to the emergency department complaining of three times coffee ground vomiting followed by one time vomiting of bright red blood

Questions for Discussion:

1. **How will you approach the patient?**
Start with resuscitation following the ABC approach.
A: ensure the patency of the air way and assess the level of consciousness.
B: assess the breathing and oxygenation.
C: insert two large IV cannulas.
Draw labs for investigation (ABG, CBC, blood grouping, cross match, electrolyte, RFT, LFT, coagulation profile).
Fluid and blood products administration, PPI IV bolus 80 mg.
2. **What will you do next?**
After stabilization of the patient hemodynamics. Obtain a history and perform a physical examination.
He is a 50-year-old male patient who complains of coffee ground vomiting since morning and another attack of vomiting fresh blood. It was moderate in amount and not related to meal, not proceeded by non-bloody vomiting or coughing. No current history of abdominal or chest pain.
Over the last few months, he had recurrent attack of epigastric abdominal pain that was relieved by eating.
He has no history of weight loss, decrease appetite, dysphagia, or fever.
He is smoker for 2 years and is not alcoholic.
PMH: diabetic on insulin.
PSH: laparoscopic cholecystectomy 15 years ago.
On examination:
Conscious, pale, lethargic
Vital signs after the initial resuscitation: BP: 98/66 mmHg, PR: 114 bpm
Abdomen: no stigmata of chronic liver disease, soft with mild tenderness with deep palpation
DRE: showed melena on the examining finger
3. **What is your differential diagnosis?**
    - Bleeding peptic ulcer
    - Bleeding varices
    - Angiodysplasia
    - Mallory Weiss syndrome
    - Arteriovenous malformation
    - Gastric cancer
4. **How will you manage the patient?**
    - Admission to ICU or HDU
    - NGT
    - NPO
    - IV fluid and blood resuscitation
    - PPI infusion
    - Mechanical DVT prophylaxis
    - IV antibiotics
    - Urgent upper GI endoscopy: showed gastric ulcer (at the greater curvature of the body of the stomach) with diffuse bleeding that was managed endoscopically, and the bleeding stopped
5. **The endoscopic finding as described. What is the Forrest classification?**
Class I b.
6. **The patient has another attack of hematemesis. What will you do?**
Resuscitate and repeat EGD.
7. **The endoscopist could not control the bleeding in the second endoscopic attempt. How will you manage that?**
Operative management with options either to oversew the bleeding vessel or wedge resection.

Case No. 4:

A 55-year-old male patient present to the clinic complaining of epigastric pain for 3 months.

Questions for Discussion:

1. **How will you approach the patient?**

   A 55-year-old male patient is complaining of epigastric pain for 3 months.

   It started gradually, dull aching pain, mild in severity but increased in frequency over the last month. He did not notice a specific aggravating or relieving factors. It is associated with anorexia and weight loss (more than half of his weight in 3 months). No history of hematemesis but he noticed that his stool is black. He is a smoker and his diet composed mostly of smoked meat.

   His mother died due to breast cancer when she was 55 years old.

   He has no history of dysphagia, odynophagia, or change in bowel habit.

   PMH and PSH: unremarkable.

   Not on regular medication.

   On examination:

   He looks underweight, with obvious muscle wasting, and appears pale.

   Vital signs: normal.

   Abdomen: soft with a palpable mass at the epigastric area about 4 × 4 cm.

   No succession splash. No abnormal supraclavicular, axillary lymph nodes.

   DRE: empty rectum with no palpable masses.

2. **How will you investigate his condition?**

   Blood test: see Table 9.9.

   Endoscopy, EUS: large ulcerated mass at the body of the stomach. By EUS the mass invading up to the muscularis layer of the stomach.

   Biopsy taken and showed: moderated differentiated adenocarcinoma (intestinal type with HER-2 positive).

3. **What will you do next?**
   - CT CAP staging: shows intragastric mass with peri-gastric enlarged lymph nodes, no distant metastasis or invasion to the nearby structure.
   - Laparoscopic staging and peritoneal lavage: negative for metastasis.
   - Multidisciplinary team approach.
   - Break the bad news to the patient.
   - Describe the management plan.

4. **How will you manage him?**

   Neoadjuvant chemotherapy followed by surgery and adjuvant therapy.

5. **The patient responds well to the given treatment. What will you do?**

   Total gastrectomy with D2 lymphadenectomy

   Send margins for frozen section

6. **How will you follow the patient?**
   - History and physical examination every 3–6 months for 1–2 years then every 6–12 months for 3–5 years then annually.
   - EGD as clinically indicated.
   - Laboratory investigations and CT as clinically indicated if stage I and every 6–12 months for 2 years then annually if stage II or III.
   - Monitor nutritional deficiency and treat it as indicated.

Table 9.9 Blood test for case 4

Test	Result	Normal value
WBC (k/ul)	9	4.8–10.8
HB (g/dl)	8	12.6–16.5
PLT (K/ul)	260	130–400
ALT (U/l)	120	10–130
AST (U/l)	31	10–34
Total bilirubin (mg/dl)	0.6	0–0.8
Direct bilirubin (mg/dl)	0.1	0–0.3
Albumin (g/dl)	2	2.4–4
Creatinine (mg/dl)	1	0.7–1.2
Na (mEq/l)	135	135–145
K (mEq/l)	3.7	3.5–5.1
PT (seconds)	12	10–13
INR	1	1

Case No. 5:

A 49-year-old female patient presented to the clinic complaining of epigastric pain and weight loss for 4 months.

Questions for Discussions:

1. **How will you approach the patient?**
   A 49-year-old female patient who is presenting to the clinic with complaint of epigastric pain that was started gradually over the past 4 months. It was a squeezing pain at the epigastric area increased by eating and is associated with heartburn, nausea and occasional vomiting. She has no history of GI bleeding, weight loss, or fever.
   She noticed that she has excessive sweating while she is sleeping.
   She has no personal or family history of malignancy.
   Her past medical and surgical history were unremarkable.
   Physical examination detects no abnormal findings.
2. **What is your differential diagnosis?**
   - Peptic ulcer disease (gastric)
   - Gastritis
   - Esophagitis
   - GERD
   - Gastric lymphoma
   - Gastric cancer
3. **How will you investigate the most likely diagnosis?**
   Blood test: Table 9.10
   EGD:

Table 9.10 Blood test for case 5

Test	Result	Normal value
WBC (k/ul)	8	4.8–10.8
HB (g/dl)	11	12.6–16.5
PLT (K/ul)	240	130–400
ALT (U/l)	110	10–130
AST (U/l)	34	10–34
Total bilirubin (mg/dl)	0.8	0–0.8
Direct bilirubin (mg/dl)	0.1	0–0.3
Albumin (g/dl)	3	2.4–4
Creatinine (mg/dl)	1.1	0.7–1.2
Na (mEq/l)	135	135–145
K (mEq/l)	3.7	3.5–5.1
PT (seconds)	12	10–13
LDH (IU/l)	290	135–214
INR	1	1

   Multiple focal area of gastric erosions and ulceration involving the entire stomach. Multiple biopsies were taken and was positive for H. pylori and area of atrophic gastritis and mucosa-associated lymphoid tissue (MALT) lymphoma.
4. **The result of the requested investigation as given. How will you manage that?**
   PPI
   Eradication of *H. pylori*
   Follow up with EGD
5. **Few weeks later, the patient presented to the emergency department with upper GI bleeding. After initial resuscitation, how will you manage her condition?**
   Operative management: gastric resection.

References

1. Lightner AL, F. Charles. The management of benign gastric ulcers. In: Cameron J, Cameron A, editors. Current surgical therapy. 12th ed. Canada: Elsevier; 2016.
2. Dempsey DT. The management of duodenal ulcers. In: Cameron J, Cameron A, editors. Current surgical therapy. 12th ed. Canada: Elsevier; 2016.
3. Roses RE, Dempsey TD. Stomach. In: Brunicardi F, editor. Schwartz's principles of surgery. 11th ed. United States: McGraw-Hill Education; 2019.
4. Fallone CA, Moss SF, Malfertheiner P. Reconciliation of recent Helicobacter pylori treatment guidelines in a time of increasing resistance to antibiotics. Gastroenterology. 2019;157(1):44–53.
5. Fallone CA, Chiba N, van Zanten SV, Fischbach L, Gisbert JP, Hunt RH, et al. The Toronto Consensus for the treatment of Helicobacter pylori infection in adults. Gastroenterology. 2016;151(1):51–69.e14.
6. Norton JA, Krampitz GW, Jensen RT. The management of the Zollinger-Ellison syndrome. In: Cameron J, Cameron A, editors. Current surgical therapy. 12th ed. Canada: Elsevier; 2016.
7. Tavakkoli A, Ashley SW. Acute gastrointestinal hemorrhage. In: Mattox CTRDBBMEK, editor. Sabiston textbook of surgery. 20th ed. Elsevier; 2016.
8. Karrer FM. Superior Mesenteric Artery (SMA) syndrome treatment and management: medscape. 2018. https://emedicine.medscape.com/article/932220-treatment#d7.
9. Cavnar MJ, DeMatte RP. The management of gastrointestinal stromal tumors. In: Cameron J, Cameron A, editors. Current surgical therapy. 12th ed. Canada: Elsevier; 2016.

10. Japanese Gastric Cancer A. Japanese gastric cancer treatment guidelines 2018 (5th edition). Gastric Cancer. 2021;24(1):1–21.
11. McFadden DW, Brenner MB. The management of gastric adenocarcinoma. In: Cameron J, Cameron A, editors. Current surgical therapy. 12th ed. Canada: Elsevier; 2016.
12. Couroculas AP, Schauer PR. The surgical management of obesity. In: Brunicardi F, editor. Schwartz's principles of surgery. 11th ed. United States: McGraw-Hill Education; 2019.
13. Wayne JD, Bell RH, Jr. Gastrectomy: Subtotal or Partial. In: Bell RH, DBK, editors. Northwestern handbook of surgical procedures. 11th ed. United States: LANDES BIOSCIENCE; 2005.
14. Sener SF, Bilimoria MM. Gastrectomy: total. In: Bell RH, DBK, editors. Northwestern handbook of surgical procedures. 11th ed. United States: LANDES BIOSCIENCE; 2005.
15. Zollinger R, Ellison E. gastric cancer: surgical therapy. Zollinger's Atlas of surgical operation. 9th ed. United States: McGraw-Hill Education; 2011.

10 Surgical Aspects of Small Bowel Diseases for Clinical Board Exams

10.1 Part I: Knowledge

> Knowing is not enough; we must apply. Willing is not enough; we must do.
> —Johann Wolfgang von Goethe

The presenting complaint could be one of the following:

- Central abdominal pain
- Abdominal mass

History:

- Introduce yourself to the patient.
- Name, age, occupation, gender, and nationality.
- Chief complaint and duration.
- History of presenting illness:
  - **Analysis of the chief complaint**

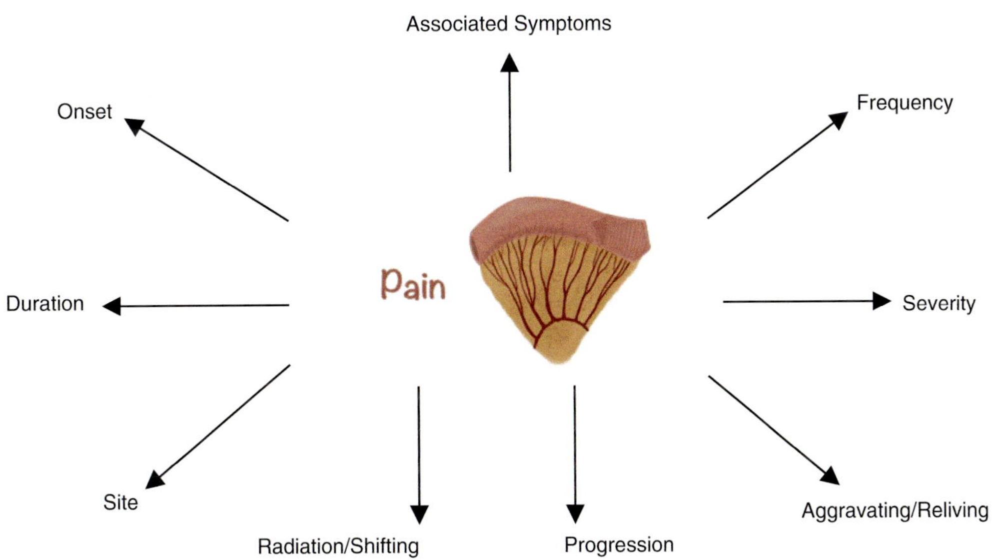

H. Alotaibi, *Study Surgery*, https://doi.org/10.1007/978-981-16-2305-9_10

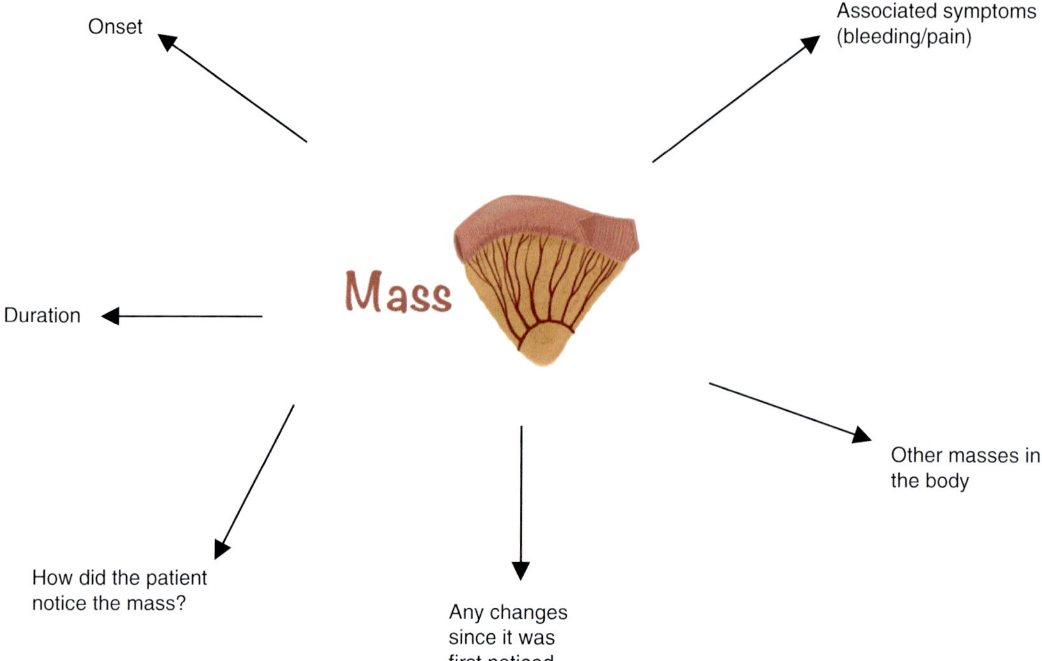

- **Associated symptoms:**
  Hematemesis, heartburn, dysphagia, odynophagia, nausea, vomiting, change in the bowel habit, constipation, diarrhea, bleeding per rectum, abdominal distention, fever, or jaundice. If the pain in the lower abdomen, ask about urinary symptoms like frequency, urgency, and dysuria. If the patient is female, ask about gynecological symptoms like vaginal discharge and last menstrual period.
- **Constitutional symptoms:**
  Weight loss, decrease appetite, night sweating, and fever.
- **Symptoms of metastasis:**
  Back pain, cough, and shortness of breath.
- **Risk factors:**
  Smoking.
  Contact with TB patient.
  Family history of malignancy, IBD, and TB.
  Cardiac disease (atrial fibrillation, valvular disease, and mural thrombus).
  Low flow state (heart failure, shock, and hemodynamic instability).
- **Symptoms/factors related to differential diagnosis:**
  History of eating from outside (gastroenteritis).
  Contact with sick patient (gastroenteritis).
  History of gall stone and alcohol (pancreatitis).
  Cough and SOB (lower lobe pneumonia).
  Chest pain and palpitation (inferior MI).
- **Previous similar attack**, previous admission, previous investigation, or endoscopy (if yes, when was it done and what was the finding?).

- **PMH**
- **PSH**
- **Family history**
- **Social history**
- **Medication, transfusion, and allergy**
- **Systemic review:**
  - **CNS:** headache, eye and hearing symptoms, epilepsy, numbness, and paralysis
  - **CVS:** chest pain, orthopnea, PND, lower limb edema, and palpitation
  - **Respiratory:** cough, fever, chest pain, and hemoptysis

- **Renal:** dysuria, flank pain, and hematuria
- **MSK:** weakness, arthritis, and skin erythema

Physical examination:
- Introduce yourself to the patient
- Ask permission for examination
- Ensure patient's privacy and ask for Chaperon
- Position: supine
- Exposure: from nipple to mid-thigh
- Hand washing

General examination:

- **A**ppearance: ill/well, dehydrated
- **B**ody built: cachectic and obese
- **C**olor: pale and Jaundice
- **D**istress and decubitus (lying down not moving or moving from one side to another—writhing pain)
- **E**nvironment and connection to monitors, IV fluids, or drains

Vital signs: BP, HR, temperature, RR, and SPO_2

Hands:

- Pallor
- Palmer erythema
- Koilonychia (iron deficiency anemia)
- Leukonychia (hypoalbuminemia)
- Pulse rate and its characteristics (rhythm, volume, etc.)

Eye:

- Jaundice
- Pallor

Mouth: aphthous ulcer

Neck:

- Lymphadenopathy

Chest:

- Respiratory system
- Cardiovascular

Abdomen:

- Inspection:
  - Distention
  - Asymmetry
  - Visible veins
  - Scars/striae
  - Dilated veins (caput medusa)
  - Hernial orifices
  - Stretch marks
  - Visible peristalsis
- Palpations:
  - Superficial palpation (start away from the tender area):
    Tenderness
    Masses
  - Deep palpation:
    Palpable masses
    Organomegaly
- Percussion:
  - Ascites: shifting dullness and fluid thrill
  - Tympany
- Auscultation:
  - Bowel sounds
  - Bruit and venous hum
  - **Groin:**
    Examine the hernial orifices: assess the presence of any hernia and its features like reducibility and strangulation.

DRE

- Bloody stool, sphincter tone, any palpable masses (describe it if mass is felt), and assess the prostate in males

Lower limb:

- Edema and peripheral neuropathy

Table 10.1 Differential diagnosis of central, lower abdominal pain and abdominal mass

Central abdominal pain	Lower abdominal pain		Abdominal mass
	Right side	Left side	
Gastroenteritis IBD Mesenteric ischemia Small bowel obstruction Infectious enteritis Intussusception Internal hernia TB peritonitis	Appendicitis Diverticulitis Typhlitis IBD (Crohn's disease) Gynecological diseases Meckel's diverticulitis Urinary problems Bowel or appendicular neoplasm	Diverticulitis Colitis (infectious, inflammatory, and ischemic) Colonic neoplasms Gynecological disease Urinary problems	Mesenteric cyst Duplication cyst Small bowel neoplasm GIST NETs Inflammatory mass

Back:

- Tenderness

Extraintestinal manifestations (in case of inflammatory bowel disease):

- Dermatological: erythema nodosum and pyoderma gangrenosum
- Ocular: conjunctivitis, uveitis, iritis, and episcleritis
- Rheumatological: arthritis and ankylosing spondylitis
- Hepatic: primary sclerosing cholangitis

Differential diagnosis: Table 10.1

10.1.1 Approach to a Patient with Suspected Small Bowel Crohn's Disease (CD)

- History and physical examination as described above. Focus on symptoms and signs related to CD such as whether the patient is known to have CD or not, prior attacks, medications, and previous surgical history.
- Diagnostic investigations:
  - Blood tests:
    CBC with differential
    Electrolytes
    LFT
    RFT
    Coagulation profile
    Blood group
    ESR and CRP
    Serology (ANCA, PANCA, and ASCA)
    Fecal calprotectin
    Stool analysis
  - Imaging:
    Chest and abdominal X-ray
    ECG
    CT scan of the abdomen and pelvis with oral and IV contrast
    MRE
    CT enterography
  - Colonoscopy with intubation of the terminal ileum:
    Preparation: fluid diet and mechanical bowel preparation
    The whole colon and terminal ileum should be examined, looking for any masses and inflammation. If there is any lesion, biopsy it.
    Finding like: aphthous ulcer, cobblestone appearance, skip lesions, and pseudopolyps
  - Biopsy: noncaseating granuloma and transmural inflammation (if the specimen is surgical)
    No single symptoms or sign or diagnostic test establishes the diagnosis. Clinical, radiological, endoscopic, and pathological findings together can help in diagnosing Crohn's disease.

Management of Small Bowel Crohn's Disease
Types:

- Fibrostenotic
- Fistulizing
- Aggressive inflammatory disease

Treatment:

- No curative therapies
- Medical management:
  - **Mild active disease:**
    5-ASA
  - **Induction of remission:**
    Corticosteroids
    Infliximab (should not be used in septic patient)
    Infliximab and azathioprine (drug of choice for patient with fistula)
    Neobiologic
  - **Maintain of remission:**
    Methotrexate
    Azathioprine
    6-mercaptopurine
    Biologic
- Nutritional support
- Surgical management:
  - Principles:
    Measure the length of healthy bowel.
    Resect only the segment(s) causing symptoms.
    Determine whether resection or stricturoplasty is appropriate.
    Bypass can be considered if there was duodenum involvement, since the resection is technically difficult, or there is risk of short bowel syndrome [1].
  - Indications:
    Acute onset of severe disease.
    Failure of medical therapy.
    Development of complication like obstruction (most common), perforation, fistulas, hemorrhage, and risk of malignancy.
  - If elective surgery is indicated:
    Exploration.
    Segmental resection with end ileostomy is the preferred option, other options like primary anastomosis with or without diversion depend on other factors like, hemodynamic stability of the patient, nutritional status, and medication.
    Microscopic evidence of Crohn's disease at the margin does not compromise a safe anastomosis.
    Stricturoplasty (alternative to resection): especially in patient with extensive disease and fibrotic strictures [1].

Stricturoplasty:

- The affected segment opened longitudinally and biopsied.
- Reconstruction depends on the size (Table 10.2).
- Stricturoplasty site should be marked with metallic clips.
- Contraindication to stricturoplasty:

Table 10.2 Types of stricturoplasty [2]

Short length	Intermediate length	Long segment
Heineke-Mikulicz technique: • For stricture ≤7 cm • Longitudinal incision on the antimesenteric side of the small bowel wall extending 2 cm proximal and 2 cm distal to the stricture (Fig. 10.1) • The enterotomy is closed in transverse fashion in one or two layers (Fig. 10.2)	**Finney stricturoplasty:** • For stricture >7 cm and ≤15 cm • The bowel loop is folded over itself as U-shape • Longitudinal enterotomy halfway between the antimesenteric and mesenteric borders (Fig. 10.3) • Opposed edges are sutured together to create side-to-side isoperistaltic enteroenterostomy (Fig. 10.4)	**Michelassi (side-to-side isoperistaltic stricturoplasty):** • For stricture >15 cm • Strictured segment is divided at its midpoint • Side-to-side isoperistaltic enteroenterostomy (Fig. 10.7) • If there is any area of suspicion, send for frozen section
Judd stricturoplasty: • For short stricture with fistula • Enterotomy encompass the fistula opening • Debridement of the opening • Closure like Heineke-Mikulicz	**Jaboulay stricturoplasty:** • For stricture 15–20 cm • The strictured loop is folded as U-shape • Two enterotomies • The enterotomy not extended to the tip of the folded loop like in Fenny (Fig. 10.5) • Side-to-side enteroenterostomy (Fig. 10.6)	

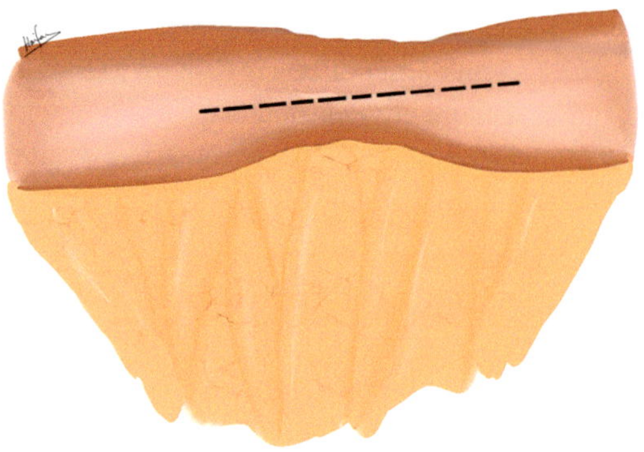

Fig. 10.1 Heineke-Mikulicz stricturoplasty; longitudinal incision on the antimesenteric side of the small bowel wall extending 2 cm proximal and 2 cm distal to the stricture

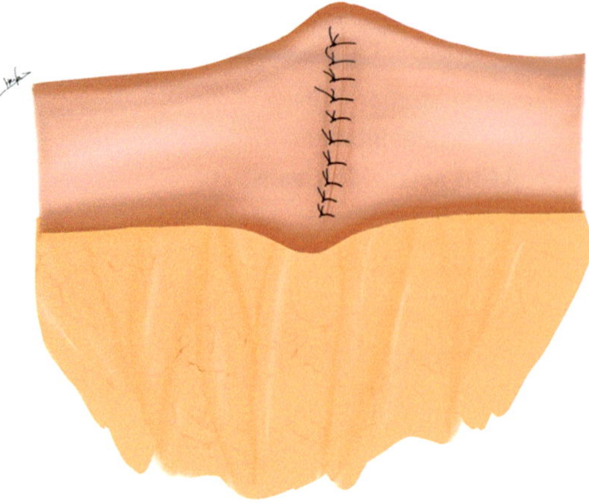

Fig. 10.2 Heineke-Mikulicz stricturoplasty; closure in transverse fashion in one or two layers

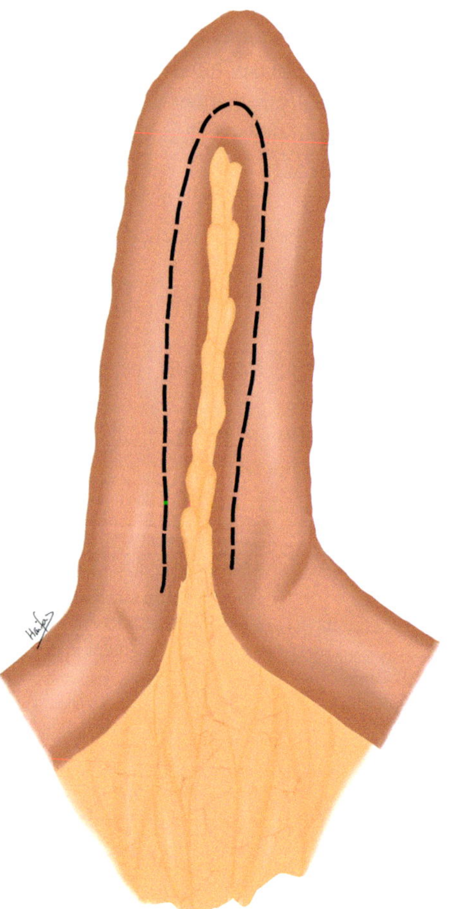

Fig. 10.3 Finney stricturoplasty; longitudinal enterotomy halfway between the antimesenteric and mesenteric borders

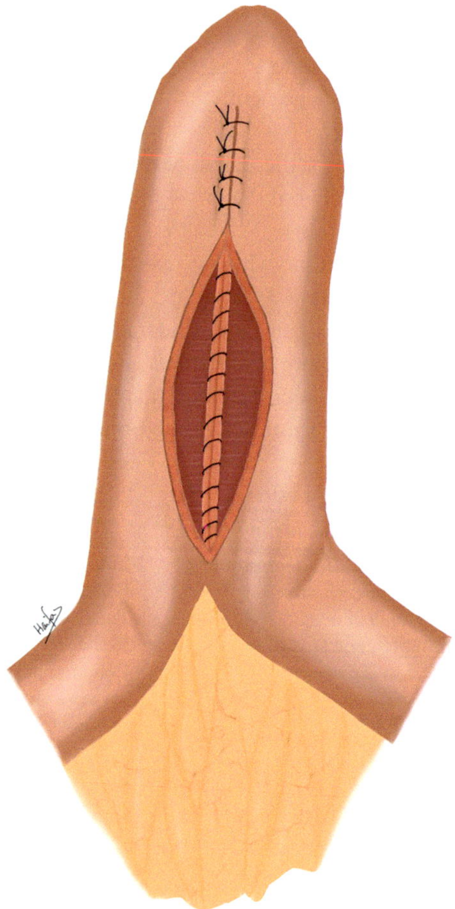

Fig. 10.4 Finney stricturoplasty; opposed edges are sutured together to create side-to-side isoperistaltic enteroenterostomy

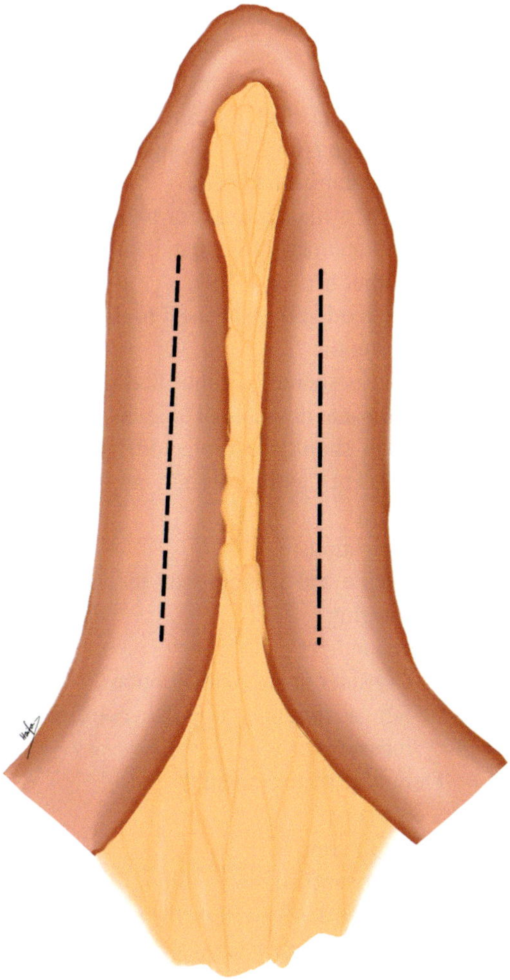

Fig. 10.5 Jaboulay stricturoplasty; two enterotomies and the enterotomy are not extended to the tip of the folded loop like in Fenny

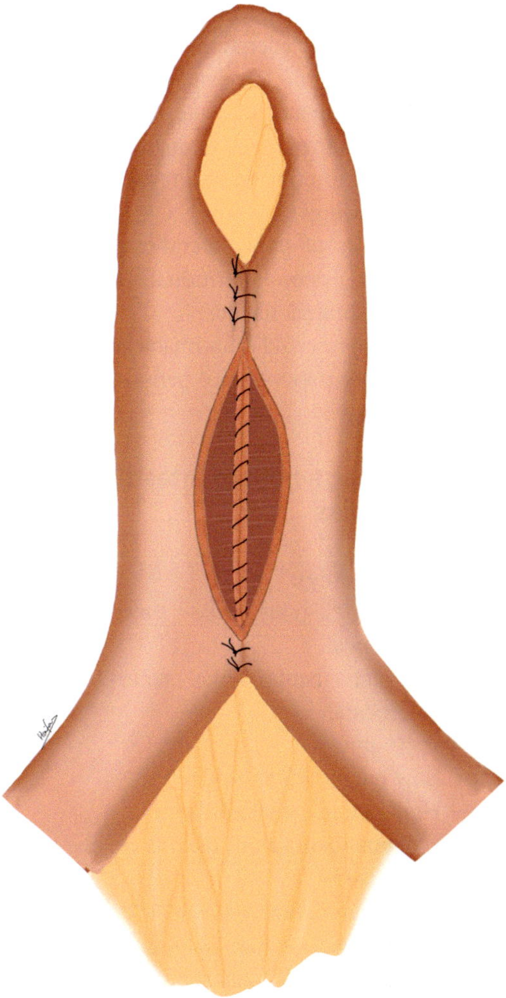

Fig. 10.6 Jaboulay stricturoplasty; side-to-side enteroenterostomy

- Absolute:
    - Dysplasia or cancer at stricture site (if suspected, send intraoperative biopsy and resect if positive)
    - Hemorrhage
    - Locoregional sepsis: phlegmon, abscess, and peritonitis
- Relative:
    - Impaired nutritional status
    - Fistula
    - Stricture close to area of resection

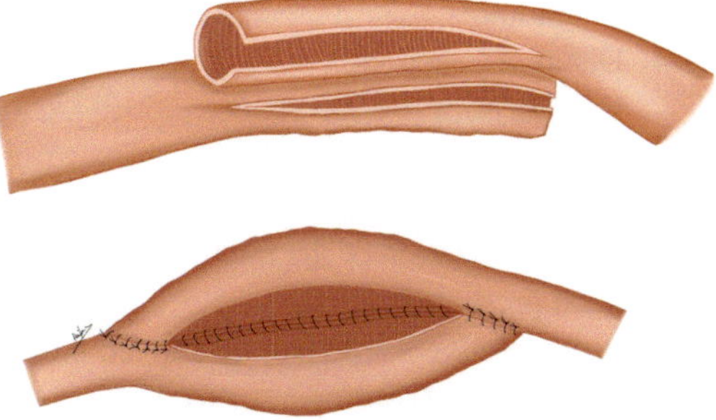

Fig. 10.7 Michelassi (side-to-side isoperistaltic stricturoplasty); sided-to-side isoperistaltic enteroenterostomy

Long stricture with thick intestinal wall
- Preoperative considerations:
  - Assessment of the extent of the disease. Magnetic resonance enterography (MRE) is the preferred study to distinguish inflammatory from fibrotic stricture.
  - Colonoscopy.
  - Predictors of poor outcome: preoperative steroids, poor nutritional status, and intraabdominal fistula.
  - Azathioprine and infliximab can be continued in the perioperative period [2].

10.1.2 Management of Intestinal Fistulas

- Types (anatomy):
  - Internal fistulas like enterocolic or colovesical.
  - External fistulas like rectovaginal or enterocutaneous.
- Types (output):
  - Low output: <200 ml/day.
  - High output: >500 ml/day.
- 80% of enterocutaneous fistulas are due to iatrogenic causes.
- 20% of enterocutaneous fistulas are spontaneous, for example, Crohn's disease.
- Factors that inhibit spontaneous closure:
  - Malnutrition.
  - Sepsis.
  - IBD.
  - Cancer.
  - Radiation.
  - Distal obstruction.
  - Foreign body.
  - High output.
  - Short tract <2 cm.
  - Epithelialization of the tract.
- Clinical presentation:
  - Postoperative fistula will be noticed mostly on day 5 to 10 postoperatively.
  - Fever, prolonged ileus, tenderness, and wound infection are the most frequent symptoms and signs.
- Diagnosis:
  - CT with contrast is the initial test of choice.
  - Enteroclysis.
  - Fistulogram.
- Management:
  - Stabilization:

    Fluid and electrolytes resuscitation.

    Nutrition usually through total parenteral nutrition (TPN).

    TPN is mainly used for high output fistula and oral intake can be used for low output fistula.

    Octreotide may be used to decrease the secretion.

    Sepsis should be controlled with antibiotics and drainage of abscess.

    Skin should be protected from fistula effluent with ostomy appliance or drain.
  - Investigations:

    Define the anatomy of the fistula by imaging.
  - Decision:

    Consider the available options.

    Set a timeline for the conservative measures.
  - Definitive management:

    Surgery.
  - Rehabilitation
- Timing for surgical intervention:
  - 3–6 months of conservative management before considering surgical intervention.
  - 30% of intestinal fistula will close spontaneously.
  - 90% of that 50% will close within 5 weeks.
  - If fistula fails to resolve during this period, resection of the fistula along with segment of intestine from which it originates is nescessary [3].

10.1.3 Management of Small Bowel Tumors

- Primary small bowel tumors are rare.
- Clinical presentation: vague abdominal pain, nausea, vomiting, weight loss, and anemia. Location of the tumor influence its presentation.
- Risk factors:

- Genetic cancer syndromes such as FAP, HNPCC, and Peutz-Jeghers syndrome
- Chronic inflammation like Crohn's and celiac diseases
- Structural abnormalities including Meckel's diverticulum
- Dietary factors like high sugars, smoked meats, and increase in alcohol consumption

- Work up:
  - Endoscopy: push enteroscopy, double-balloon endoscopy, and video capsule endoscopy
  - Imaging: CT scan of the abdomen and pelvis, and fluoroscopic imaging (upper GI series with small bowel follow through, Enteroclysis) [4, 5]

Malignant Small Bowel Tumors

A. **Neuroendocrine tumors:**
  - It arises from enterochromaffin cells.
  - Characterized by the expression of somatostatin receptors.
  - Risk factors: MEN1, neurofibromatosis, somatostatinoma, presence of breast and colorectal cancers, and smoking.
  - Clinical presentation: depend on the site of origin and the production of bioactive substances.
  - Carcinoid syndrome occurs when the tumor is bulky or metastatic (most commonly to the liver).
  - Diagnosis:
    - Biochemical evaluation: chromogranin A, pancreatic polypeptide, and urinary 5-HIAA (a metabolite of serotonin).
    - Structural imaging: CT scan, DOTA scan, and octreotide scan.
  - Management:
    - For resectable tumors: exploratory laparotomy, and segmental resection of the involved bowel with lymphadenectomy. Cholecystectomy is recommended at the time of laparotomy, especially if the need of octreotide therapy is anticipated.
    - Nonresectable tumors: palliation with resection may be done in addition to octreotide treatment for patient with carcinoid syndrome.
    - Surgery should be considered for recurrent locoregional and metastatic disease.
    - For hepatic metastasis, resection with curative intent should be considered if:
      Resectable, well-differentiated tumor burden in the liver with acceptable morbidity and mortality
      Absence of right heart insufficiency
      Absence of extra abdominal or diffuse peritoneal disease [4, 5]

B. **Adenocarcinoma:**
  - Risk factors: genetic, smoking, alcohol use, and presence of peptic ulcer disease.
  - Clinical presentation may be recurrent partial small bowel obstruction, intussusception, or GI bleeding.
  - Work up should include CEA and Ca19-9, CT CAP, and upper and lower endoscopy to rule out synchronous lesions.
  - Staging is based on TNM system
  - Management:
    - Surgical resection with curative intent is recommended.
    - The goal of surgical resection is complete resection with negative margins and lymphadenectomy (at least 8–10 lymph nodes).
    - For distal ileal disease, right hemicolectomy may be required [4, 5].

C. **Lymphoma:**
  - The patients usually present with nonspecific abdominal pain, anorexia, weight loss, diarrhea, or palpable abdominal mass.
  - Most common histologic diagnosis is non-Hodgkin's lymphoma.
  - Work up for suspected or confirmed small bowel lymphoma should include CT neck, chest, abdomen, and pelvis as well as PET scan in addition to endoscopic evaluation of the entire GIT.
  - Biochemical evaluation should include LDH and beta-2 microglobulin.
  - Bone marrow biopsy is required.
  - Management:
    - Multidisciplinary team approach.
    - Localized disease can be managed with surgical resection and adjuvant chemotherapy.

- Advanced disease require chemotherapy alone.
- Presence of complications like obstruction or bleeding requires urgent surgical intervention [4, 5].

D. **Gastrointestinal stromal tumors:**
- Most patients with GIST are symptomatic.
- Symptoms include nausea, vomiting, early satiety, melena, anemia, abdominal pain, distention, or fever.
- Surgical intervention depends on overall health of the patient, presence or absence of metastatic disease, the size of the primary tumor, and the difficulty of resection.
- The goal is resection to achieve negative margin with no rupture of the tumor capsule.
- No lymphadenectomy is necessary.
- Resectable tumors with high-risk features should be excised followed by adjuvant tyrosine kinase inhibitors (TKI).
- High-risk features are tumor size >2 cm, mitotic index >5 mitosis per HPF, intraoperative tumor rupture, and inability to achieve R0 resection.
- TKI can be given as neoadjuvant treatment when the resection of the tumor is technically difficult [4, 5].

10.1.4 Management of Acute Mesenteric Ischemia

- Types:
  - Embolic occlusion of the mesenteric vessels.
  - Acute thrombosis of mesenteric vessels.
  - Nonocclusive mesenteric ischemia (NOMI).
  - Mesenteric venous thrombosis [6].
- Clinical presentation:
  - Sudden-onset mid-abdominal pain that is out of proportion to the physical finding is the hallmark of mesenteric ischemia.
  - Recent history of cardiac events, for example, myocardial infarction, atrial fibrillation, mural thrombus, mitral valve disease, or left ventricular aneurysm is suggestive of embolic occlusion.
  - Presence of chronic mesenteric ischemia (postprandial abdominal and history of food avoidance leading to significant weight loss) in addition to the new onset of sudden abdominal pain is suggestive of thrombotic occlusion as well as other manifestations of diffuse atherosclerotic disease such as coronary or peripheral artery disease.
  - The pain with NOMI is usually not sudden and tends to wax and wane depending on the patient's hemodynamic stability. If the patient is in ICU and cannot appreciate the pain, the diagnosis may be suggested by progressive abdominal distention with worsening acidosis.
  - Patients with mesenteric venous thrombosis have nonspecific symptoms like nausea, vomiting, diarrhea, cramping, and nonlocalized abdominal pain [6].
- Diagnosis:
  - Laboratory test: CBC, ABG, and lactic acid.
  - Imaging:

    Plain abdominal graph and duplex ultrasound are of less help.

    CT angiography: Finding suggestive of mesenteric ischemia like bowel wall thickening, nonenhanced bowel segment, filling defect in the mesenteric vessels, pneumatosis intestinalis, portal vein gas, or perforation and pneumoperitoneum.

    Angiography [6].
- Treatment:
  - Initial treatment:

    Fluid resuscitation.

    Correction of metabolic acidosis.

    Antibiotics.

    Anticoagulant [6].
  - The goals of surgical treatment:

    Restore the normal pulsatile flow to the superior mesenteric artery.

    Resect any nonviable intestine.

    Restore the intestinal continuity once mesenteric revascularization achieved [6].
  - Assessment of bowel viability:

    Visual: color and peristalsis.

    Palpation: of mesenteric pulsation.

Tests: Doppler imaging, fluorescein injection, and Wood's lamp inspection.

If still the viability is questionable, a second look operation after 24–36 h [6].

- Revascularization options:

  Percutaneous embolectomy.

  Exposure of SMA: either lateral or anterior approach.

  Longitudinal arteriotomy and embolectomy balloon catheter is used to ensure removal of the embolus.

  Bypass procedure which may be in either an antegrade or retrograde manner [6].
- Management of NOMI is mainly nonoperative and supportive with fluid resuscitation, improvement of cardiac output, and elimination of vasopressors. Selective catheterization of the SMA with direct intraarterial infusion of vasodilator such as papaverine (30–60 mg/h) may be used as adjunctive therapy.
- In patient with mesenteric venous occlusion, surgery is indicated in patient with signs of bowel infarction. Surgery should be limited to bowel resection [6].

10.1.5 Management of Intestinal Tuberculosis

- **Risk factors:** Cirrhosis, HIV infection, diabetes mellitus, underlying malignancy, treatment with antitumor necrosis factor (TNF) agents, and use of peritoneal dialysis [7].
- **Forms:**
  - Abdominal TB can involve any of the following sites: peritoneum, esophagus, stomach, intestinal tract, hepatobiliary tree, pancreas, perianal area, and lymph nodes.
  - The most common forms of disease include involvement of the peritoneum, intestine, and/or liver [7].
- **Pathogenesis:**
  - Tuberculosis of the abdomen may occur via reactivation of latent TB infection or by ingestion of tuberculous mycobacteria. In the setting of active pulmonary TB or military TB, abdominal involvement may develop via hematogenous spread [7].
- **Clinical manifestations:**
  - Fever, abdominal pain and/or distension, ascites, hepatomegaly, diarrhea, bowel obstruction, and abdominal mass.
  - Intestinal colic, abdominal distension, chronic diarrhea, nausea, vomiting, constipation, and bleeding.
  - Ascites, lymph node enlargement, and tubo-ovarian symptoms.
  - Fatigue, weight loss, and night sweats [7].
- **Diagnosis:**
  - CT imaging: concentric mural thickening in the ileocecal region, with or without proximal intestinal dilatation, and asymmetric thickening of the medial cecal. Lymphadenopathy with hypodense centers (representing caseous liquefaction) may be present in the adjacent mesentery.
  - Patient with ascites should undergo paracentesis. The fluid should be sent for routine tests (cell count and differential, albumin and protein concentration, and Gram stain) as well as adenosine deaminase (ADA) level, AFB smear, mycobacterial culture, and, if available, Nucleic acid amplification test (NAAT) for *M. tuberculosis*.
  - Endoscopic findings of intestinal TB may include ulcers, strictures, nodules, pseudopolyp, fibrous bands, fistulas, and/or deformed ileocecal valve.
  - Histopathology (presence of caseating granulomas, with or without demonstration of acid-fast bacilli [AFB]) is suggestive of tuberculosis but is not pathognomonic [7].
- **Management:**
  - Antituberculosis therapy.
  - Surgery may be warranted for patients with complications such as perforation, abscess, fistula, bleeding, and/or high-grade obstruction.

- The surgical resection should be as conservative as possible; in some cases, multiple strictures of the small bowel may be amenable to stricturoplasty to avoid major resection.
- Bypass surgery for obstructing lesions should be avoided because of complications related to blind loop syndrome [7].

10.1.6 Small Bowel Operation

10.1.6.1 Preoperative Preparation

- Admission.
- Consent.
- NPO.
- IV fluid.
- DVT and stress ulcer prophylaxis.
- Prophylactic antibiotic.
- Confirm the availability of blood intraoperative if needed.
- Anesthesia consultation.
- ICU consultation if required.
- Instruct the patient to take shower the night before surgery.
- Stoma marking.
- Hair removal.

10.1.6.2 Informed Consent:

Consent for small bowel resection:

- *Describe the procedure to the patient:* under general anesthesia, the surgeon will perform resection of part of the small bowel due to (specify the reason). The continuity of the GIT will be restored by primary anastomosis or ileostomy.
- *Mention if there is any alternative.*
- *Mention the possible complications:* bleeding, infection, anastomotic leak, fistula, injury to the nearby structure, adhesion, hernia, or short bowel syndrome. General complications like DVT, PE, atelectasis, pneumonia, and MI.

10.1.6.3 Small Bowel Resection and Anastomosis

- **Principles:**
  - Gentle handling of the tissues is imperative with anastomosis of grossly healthy tissue only.
  - Open anastomosis may be used, and the risk of infection and later anastomotic leaks minimized by the use of appropriate antibiotics and limiting spillage of the intestinal contents at the time of anastomosis.
  - Adequate resection of the involved segment beyond the area of pathology is important in some diseases, including a 5–6 cm margin of tissue, especially for malignant tumors.
  - One must be very cautious when attempting an anastomosis in segments of bowel that are dilated. An increased incidence of leakage may occur depending upon the degree of dilatation.
- **Details of procedure:**
  - Under general anesthesia and endotracheal intubation.
  - Position: supine.
  - The abdomen is prepped from nipple to the symphysis pubis.
  - Patient is draped in a sterile fashion.
  - Time out: confirm that correct patient, correct procedure, correct site, and all the required instruments are available.
  - Incision: midline incision.
  - Systematic exploration of the abdomen should be done.
  - The area of small bowel containing the pathology should be isolated along with the appropriate section of mesentery. Towels can be used to wall off the area from the general abdominal cavity.
  - Noncrushing intestinal clamps can be applied at some distance from the proposed resection lines to minimize spillage of the intestinal contents.
  - A small opening in the mesentery immediately adjacent to the bowel wall should be made at the proposed proximal and distal resection sites, being careful to adequately expose the serosa of the bowel wall at the proposed resection sites.
  - The peritoneum overlying the mesenteric leaf should be scored with scissors to outline the proposed line of resection of the mesentery.
  - This resection line should extend from the small aperture adjacent to the bowel wall in

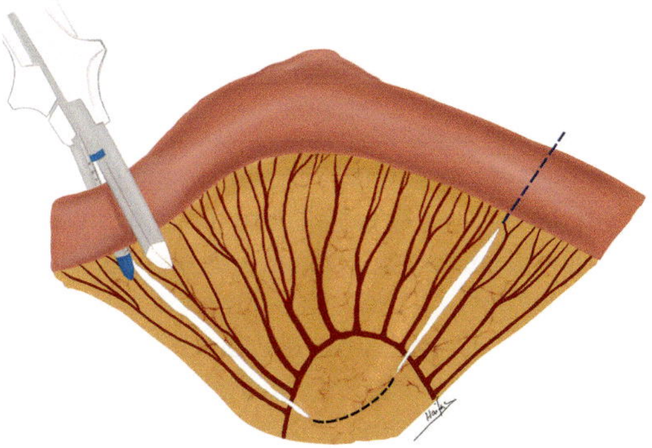

Fig. 10.8 Resection of the small bowel using linear stapler

a U-shaped fashion toward the other proposed resection margin.

- During this step it is important to transilluminate and/or palpate the mesenteric vessels so that only that portion of the vascular supply that is supplying the area of the proposed resected bowel is removed.
- Starting with the space adjacent to the bowel at the proximal resection margin, the mesentery is divided between fine clamps along the U-shaped area to separate the mesentery of the resected bowel from the mesentery to be left behind. Alternatively, LigaSure can be used.
- The extent of the mesenteric resection will depend on the amount of bowel to be removed. If a malignancy is present or suspected, an appropriate en bloc resection of mesenteric nodal tissue is required.
- The segment of the bowel to be removed is transected at each end with a linear stapler (Fig. 10.8).
- The bowel is flattened and emptied, then the device is placed in a scissor-like fashion around the bowel wall and the staples fired.
- The two ends of the bowel are placed adjacent to one another, and two seromuscular sutures are placed to approximate the bowel loops.
- Care must be taken not to twist the mesentery of the bowel.

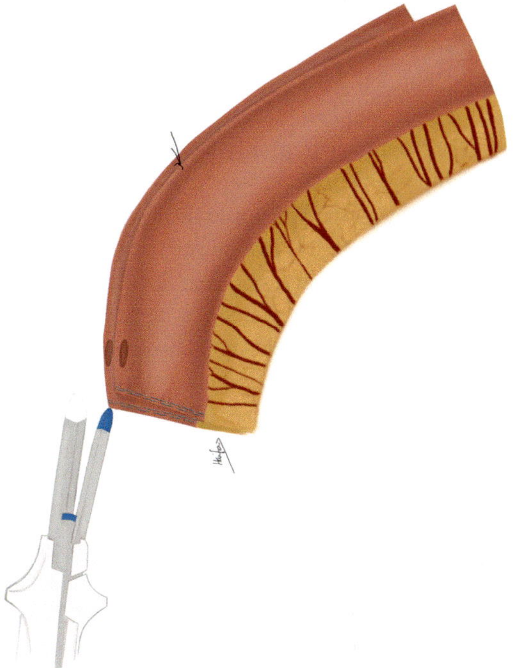

Fig. 10.9 Side-to-side small bowel anastomosis

- The bowel openings should be large enough to introduce one anvil of the linear stapler into each limb of bowel.
- The instrument is closed, and the staples are fired (Fig. 10.9).
- After the instrument is removed, it is very important to inspect the staple line for any bleeding.
- The common bowel opening is closed using a 55-mm double-row stapling instrument.
- One must avoid direct apposition of the anastomotic staple lines.
- The lumen is checked for patency and any leaks. The adequacy of the blood supply to the bowel at the suture lines is checked.
- The mesenteric opening is carefully closed with absorbable 4-0 suture, being careful not to injure the vessels to the bowel at the area of the anastomosis.
- Cover the anastomosis with omentum.
- Hemostasis and closure of the abdomen [8, 9].

10.1.6.4 Loop Ileostomy (Open)

- Under general anesthesia and endotracheal intubation.
- Position: supine.
- The abdomen is prepped from nipple to the symphysis pubis.
- Patient is draped in sterile fashion.
- Time out: confirm that correct patient, correct procedure, correct site, and all the required instruments are available.
- Incision: midline incision (most of the times ileostomy will be part of another procedure).
- If the operation requires a bowel resection or drainage of pelvic sepsis, this is carried out first.
- Just prior to closing the abdominal incision, the segment of ileum to be exteriorized is chosen.
- Typically, this is 10–15 cm proximal to the ileocecal junction. When the loop ileostomy is used in conjunction with proctocolectomy and ileoanal anastomosis, the surgeon should identify the most distal segment of ileum which has sufficient mesenteric laxity to comfortably reach the surface of the abdomen at the previously marked stoma site.
- An oval of skin and the underlying subcutaneous fat are excised at the stoma site. The anterior rectus fascia is incised in a cruciate fashion and the loop of ileum is drawn through the abdominal wall, passing through the rectus abdominis muscle (Fig. 10.10). Care is taken to maintain the proper orientation of the loop and avoid twisting or angulation when exteriorizing the bowel.
- The loop is supported at the skin surface with a plastic rod slipped through a small opening in the mesentery adjacent to the bowel wall.
- The primary abdominal incision is closed completely. Then, the loop ileostomy is matured by incising the distal limb transversely for about three quarters of its circumference and folding it back over the proximal limb (Fig. 10.11). The full thickness of the opened edge of bowel wall is then sewn to the dermis circumferentially with absorbable suture. Make sure to spout the proximal end (Fig. 10.12).
- A stoma appliance is cut to the corresponding size and placed over the newly fashioned stoma [9, 10].

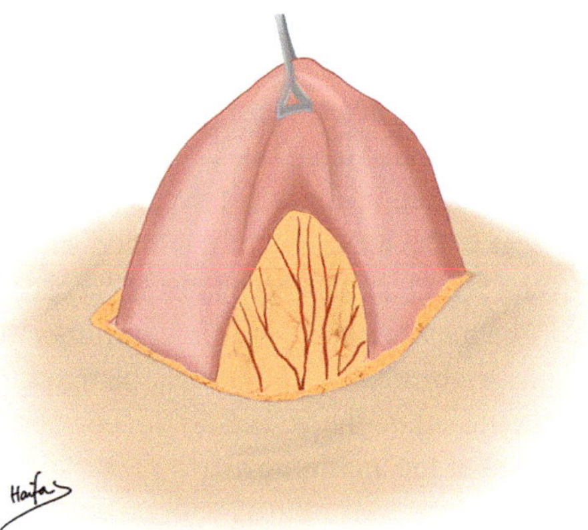

Fig. 10.10 Delivering the ileal loop through the anterior abdominal wall

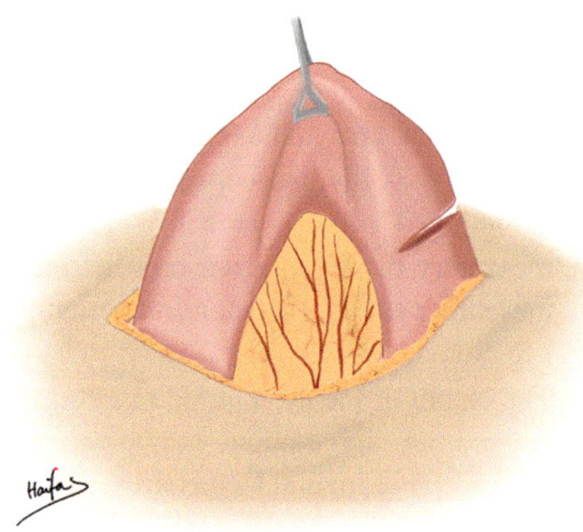

Fig. 10.11 Incising the distal limb transversely for about three quarters of its circumference and folding it back over the proximal limb

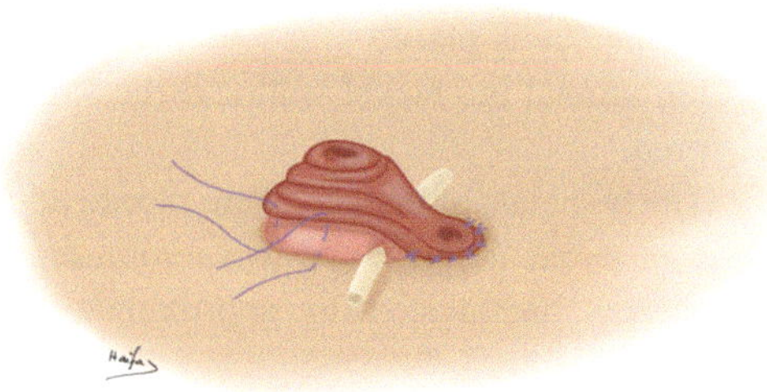

Fig. 10.12 Maturation of the stoma and suturing the bowel to the dermis

10.1.6.5 Postoperative Follow-up

Early postoperative:

- NPO and resume the diet gradually once possible.
- Monitor the vital signs.
- Encourage mobilization.
- Consider early removal of Foley's catheter and NGT.
- Encourage use of incentive spirometry.
- Analgesia, antibiotic as indicated, stress ulcer, and DVT prophylaxis.
- Stoma care when indicated.

Before discharge make sure that:

- The patient has no significant complaint.
- Tolerating oral diet.
- Stoma is functioning.
- Check the wound status.
- If the patient has stoma, he/she should be seen by the enterostomal nurse.

First outpatient visit:

- Clinical assessment.
- Examine the wound and remove the sutures.
- Review the final pathology result.
- Discuss in multidisciplinary team when the pathology is cancer.

Genetic counselling if indicated.

10.2 Part II: Practice

> You need to put what you learn into practice and do it over and over again until it's a habit
> —Brett Hoebel

10.2.1 Case Scenarios for Practice

Tips:

- Practice with a friend and try to mimic the real exam!
- Do not forget to set the timer!
- The clinical data are provided in the answer key section.

Case no. 1:

A 65-year-old male patient presented to the emergency department due to sudden-onset severe abdominal pain for 8 h.

Questions for discussion:

1. How will you approach the patient?
2. What is your differential diagnosis?
3. How will you investigate the patient?
4. What will you do next?
5. The intraoperative findings as given. What will you do?
6. When you will operate again?
7. The patient was taken again to OR and the findings as given. What will you do?

Case no. 2:

A 23-year-old male patient presented to the emergency department due to right lower abdominal pain for 2 days.

Questions for discussion:

1. How will you approach the patient?
2. What is your differential diagnosis?
3. What will you do next?
4. How will you manage the patient?
5. The intraoperative finding as given. How will you manage that?
6. Few days later the patient has offensive large amount of fluid discharge from the surgical site. What will you do?
7. How will you manage this complication?
8. Four months later, the patient condition did not resolve. What will you do?

Case No. 3:

A 44-year-old male patient who presented to the emergency department with acute-onset lower GI bleeding for 1 day.

Questions for discussion:

1. How will you approach the patient?
2. What will you do next?
3. What further investigation will you do?
4. What is your differential diagnosis?
5. How will you manage the patient?
6. How will you follow the patient?

Checklist

History	Items	Done	Not done	NA
General	Introduce himself/herself to the patient			
	Patient personal data (name, age, gender, and nationality)			
	Chief complaint			
	Duration			
Pain	Onset			
	Site			
	Character			
	Radiation/shifting			
	Aggravating/relieving			
	Severity			
	Progression			
	Frequency			
Mass	Onset			
	Site			
	How did the patient notice it?			
	Any change since it was first noticed?			
	Other masses			
Associated symptoms	Pain			
	Fever			
	Nausea			
	Vomiting			
	Diarrhea			
	Constipation			
	Hematemesis			
	Melena			
	Abdominal distention			
	Jaundice			
	Skin or wound discharge			
Constitutional symptoms	Weight loss			
	Decrease appetite			
	Night sweating			
Symptoms of metastases	Back pain			
	Cough			
	Shortness of breath			
	Abdominal distention			
Risk factors	Smoking			
	Contact with patients having TB			
	Family history of malignancy, IBD, or TB			
	Cardiac disease			
	Low flow state (hear failure, sepsis, or shock)			
Symptoms or factors related to differential diagnosis	History of eating from outside (gastroenteritis)			
	Contact with sick patient (gastroenteritis)			
	History of gall stone and alcohol (pancreatitis)			
	Chest pain and palpitation (MI)			
PMH	Previous similar attack			
	Previous investigation or endoscopy			
	Previous admission			
	Chronic illnesses			
PSH	Previous surgery			

History	Items	Done	Not done	NA
Family history	Of similar complain			
Social history	Occupation			
	Habits (smoking, alcohol, and drugs)			
Other	Medication			
	Allergy			
	Transfusion			
Systemic review				
Physical examination				
General principle	Patient position			
	Exposure			
	Privacy			
	Wash hands			
General examination	Appearance			
	Body built			
	Color			
	Distress/decubitus			
	Environment			
Vital signs	BP, HR, temperature, RR, and SPO_2			
Hand signs	Leukonychia, koilonychia, and pallor			
Eyes	Jaundice and pallor			
Mouth	Aphthous ulcer			
Neck	Lymphadenopathy			
Chest	Respiratory and CVS examination			
Abdomen: Inspection	Distention			
	Asymmetry			
	Dilated veins			
	Striae			
	Visible peristalsis			
	Scars			
Palpation	Superficial then deep palpation			
	Tenderness			
	Palpable masses			
	Organomegaly			
Percussion	Shifting dullness			
	Fluid thrill			
Auscultation	Bowel sounds			
	Bruit and venous hum			
Groin and Hernias				
DRE and proctoscopy				
Lower limb	Edema and peripheral neuropathy			
Back tenderness				
Extraintestinal manifestations	Erythema nodosum			
	Arthritis			
	Sacroiliitis			
	Ankylosing spondylitis			
Differential diagnosis	According to the given scenario			
Investigations				

(continued)

History	Items	Done	Not done	NA
General laboratory test	CBC with differential			
	Electrolytes			
	Liver function test			
	Blood grouping			
	Coagulation profile (PT, INR, and aPTT)			
	RFT			
	CPR/ESR			
	Blood culture			
	ABG			
	Lactic acid			
Specific tests (as indicated)	Tumor marker (CEA)			
	LDH			
	Fecal calprotectin			
	Serology (ANCA, PANCA, and ASCA)			
	Stool analysis			
Imaging (as indicated)	X-ray			
	ECG			
	CT abdomen/CT staging			
	CT angiogram/angiography			
	CT/MRI enterography			
	Fistulogram			
	Octreotide/DOTA scan			
Endoscopy	Colonoscopy			
Biopsy	Biopsy			
Provisional diagnosis	According to the given scenario			
Management (depend on the diagnosis):				
Management of small bowel Crohn's disease	Admission			
	NPO			
	IV fluid			
	Antibiotics			
	IV steroid			
	Antipyretic			
	Prophylaxis (DVT and stress ulcer)			
	If the patient presents with complication like bleeding or fibrotic stricture, surgical management is indicated			
	Consent			
	Stoma marking			
	Operative management			
Fistula	Admission			
	Nutrition: TPN/enteral feeding			
	Antibiotics			
	Fluid replacement and electrolytes correction			
	Octreotide if indicated			
	Drainage of collection			
	Skin and wound care			
	Conservative management			
	Surgical treatment if failed to close spontaneously			
	Surgery (resection of the fistula along with the related bowel segment)			

History	Items	Done	Not done	NA
Mesenteric ischemia	Admission			
	NPO			
	IV fluid			
	Analgesia			
	Anticoagulant			
	Antibiotics			
	Stress ulcer prophylaxis			
	Operative management if acute arterial ischemia:			
	o Consent			
	o Stoma marking			
	o Laparotomy exploration			
	o Resect the nonviable bowel and assess the viability of the rest			
	o Revascularization if needed			
	o Reconstruction or second look			
Postoperative care				
Early postoperative	Admission to HDU or ICU			
	Early mobilization and DVT prophylaxis			
	Enteral nutrition as early as possible			
	Analgesia			
	Stress ulcer prophylaxis			
	CBC and LFT daily			
	Electrolyte assessment			
	Monitor drain output and the nature of the fluid			
	Monitor the stoma itself and its output			
First outpatient visit	Clinical assessment			
	Remove sutures			
	Review the final pathology report			
	Arrange for multidisciplinary discussion if the case is cancer			
	Refer to oncology if adjuvant treatment is required			

10.2.2 Answer Key

Case no. 1:

A 65-year-old male patient presented to the emergency department due to sudden-onset severe abdominal pain for 8 h.

Questions for discussion:

1. **How will you approach the patient?**

   By obtaining a focused medical history and performing a physical examination.

   The patient is a 65-year-old male patient who is complaining of sudden onset of severe central abdominal pain, colicky in nature, and no specific aggravating or relieving factors. The pain is not radiated or shifted to another site. The patient describes the severity of pain to be 10/10. It is associated with multiple times vomiting. No fever and no change in bowel habit.

   He is known case of atrial fibrillation but noncompliant on his medication. He is diabetic and hypertensive.

   He has no previous surgical history, and he is a smoker for the last 30 years.

   Physical examination:

   Conscious and in pain.

   Vital signs:

Table 10.3 Blood test for case 1

Test	Result	Normal value
WBC (k/ul)	12	4.8–10.8
HB (g/dl)	13	12.6–16.5
PLT (K/ul)	360	130–400
ALT (U/l)	123	10–130
AST (U/l)	29	10–34
Total bilirubin (mg/dl)	0.7	0–0.8
Direct bilirubin (mg/dl)	0.2	0–0.3
Albumin (g/dl)	3	2.4–4
Creatinine (mg/dl)	1.2	0.7–1.2
Na (mEq/l)	135	135–145
K (mEq/l)	3.5	3.5–5.1
PT (seconds)	12	10–13
INR	1	1
PH	7.30	
HCO_3	11	
Pco_2	40	
Lactic acid	3	

BP: 140/79, PR: 125 bpm (irregular), and temperature: 36.8 °C.

Abdominal examination reveals no abnormality.

2. **What is your differential diagnosis?**
   - Mesenteric ischemia
   - Gastroenteritis
   - Gastritis
   - MI
   - DKA
3. **How will you investigate the patient?**
   Blood test: Table 10.3.
   CT angiography:
   Filling defect of the SMA distal to the origin of first jejunal branches. The distal jejunum and the ileum are edematous, and the wall is not enhanced.
4. **What will you do next?**
   - Admission
   - NPO
   - IV fluid
   - Anticoagulation with heparin
   - IV antibiotics
   - Prepare the patient for emergency laparotomy exploration
   - Consent

   Intraoperatively, the small bowel from the distal jejunum till 20 cm proximal to the ileocecal valve is black with obvious necrosis and thinning of the bowel wall. The right colon up to the proximal transverse colon is questionable. After resection of the small bowel, the hemodynamic status of the patient is deteriorating, and he is in severe metabolic acidosis.
5. **The intraoperative findings as given. What will you do?**
   Keep the resected ends of the bowel closed and close the skin and shift the patient to the ICU for second look after correction of his acidosis and improve his hemodynamics.
6. **When you will operate again?**
   24–48 h.
   After 48 h, the abdomen reexplored. The questionable colon has no signs of ischemia.
7. **The patient was taken again to OR and the findings as given. What will you do?**
   Anastomosis of the small bowel and definitive closure of the abdomen.

Case no. 2:

A 23-year-old male patient presented to the emergency department due to right lower abdominal pain for 2 days.

Questions for discussion:

1. **How will you approach the patient?**
   The patient is a 23-years-old male patient who has this right lower abdominal pain from 2 days. He describes the pain as sharp pain at the right iliac fossa and progress to be diffuse today. It is associated with repeated vomiting, fever, and anorexia. He has three times diarrhea for 1 day. The patient has recurrent right lower abdominal pain for 6 months, but he had never been investigated. No urinary symptoms. No recent history of upper respiratory tract infection.
   The patient is otherwise healthy with negative surgical history.
   On examination:
   He looks ill and toxic.
   Vital signs: BP: 123/76 mmHg, PR: 123 bpm, and temperature: 38.7 °C.
   Abdomen: tender with guarding all over the lower half.

Table 10.4 Blood test for case 2

Test	Result	Normal value
WBC (k/ul)	19	4.8–10.8
HB (g/dl)	13	12.6–16.5
PLT (K/ul)	390	130–400
Creatinine (mg/dl)	1	0.7–1.2
Na (mEq/l)	137	135–145
K (mEq/l)	3.9	3.5–5.1
PT (seconds)	12	10–13
INR	1	1
CRP (mg/l)	89	<3

2. **What is your differential diagnosis?**
   Crohn's disease
   Acute complicated appendicitis
   Perforated PUD
   Gastroenteritis
   Typhlitis
3. **What will you do next?**
   - Blood investigation: Table 10.4.
   - Chest X-ray: no pneumoperitoneum.
   - CT abdomen: diffuse inflammatory process at the ileocecal area with free fluid in the abdomen and pneumoperitoneum.
4. **How will you manage the patient?**
   - Admission.
   - NPO.
   - IV fluid.
   - IV antibiotics.
   - Prophylaxis (stress ulcer and DVT prophylaxis).
   - Consent.
   - Take the patient for emergency appendectomy.

   Intraoperatively, the terminal ileum, cecum, and appendix are inflamed with perforation at the antimesenteric border of the terminal ileum 15 cm from the ileocecal valve.
5. **The intraoperative finding as given. How will you manage that?**
   Ileocecal resection with ileocolonic anastomosis.
6. **Few days later, the patient has offensive large amount of fluid discharge from the surgical site. What will you do?**
   - Open few stitches.
   - Drain if there is any collection.
   - Take swab for culture.
   - CT abdomen to rule out any collection and detect any fistula and determine its anatomy (there is enterocutaneous fistula connecting the anastomotic site to the anterior abdominal wall. No intraabdominal collection).
7. **How you will manage this complication?**
   - Fluid and electrolytes resuscitation.
   - Nutrition usually through total parenteral nutrition (TPN).
   - Octreotide may be used to decrease the secretion.
   - Sepsis should be controlled with antibiotics and drainage of abscess.
   - Skin should be protected from fistula effluent with ostomy appliance or drain.

   The final pathology of the resected small bowel confirms the diagnosis of Crohn's disease and the patient was seen and started on medical management from the gastroenterologist side.
8. **Four months later, the patient condition did not resolve. What will you do?**
   Operative management (take down the fistula and resection of the affected bowel segment with primary anastomosis).

Case no. 3:

A 44-year-old male patient was presented to the emergency department with acute-onset lower GI bleeding for 1 day.

Questions for discussion:

1. **How will you approach the patient?**
   - Airway: assess the patency of airway.
   - Breathing: ensure good ventilation and oxygenation.
   - Circulation:
     – Insert two large cannulas
     – Draw blood for investigation (CBC, electrolytes, coagulation profile, blood group and cross match, ABG, and lactic acid)
     – Start IV fluid, for example, Ringer lactate
2. **What will you do next?**
   After initial stabilization, obtain medical history and perform physical examination.

The patient is 44-year-old male patient who presented to the emergency department due to one-time passage of large amount of blood per rectum. It was fresh blood mixed with clots. Not related to defecation and associated with mild vague lower abdominal pain. No other bleeding site and no previous similar complaint. He has no family or personal history of malignancy.

He is otherwise healthy with no significant PSH and not on any regular medication.

On examination:

He is conscious and pale.

Vital signs: BP: 99/67 mmHg and PR: 115 bpm.

Abdomen soft and mild tenderness over the lower abdomen.

DRE: no obvious anal pathology apart from blood on the gloved finger.

3. **What further investigation you will do?**
   Insert NGT to rule out upper GI cause brought greenish fluid.

   Bowel preparation and colonoscopy: no obvious colonic pathology. Intubation of the terminal ileum shows blood in the small bowel but no obvious pathology.
4. **What will you do?**
   CT angiography: shows exophytic small bowel lesion at the mid-jejunum about 10 × 5 cm with active intraluminal extravasation of the IV contrast.
5. **How will you manage the patient?**
   Prepare for surgical exploration and small bowel resection and anastomosis.
6. **How will you follow the patient?**
   Early postoperative:
   - NPO and resume the diet gradually once possible.
   - Monitor the vital signs.
   - Encourage mobilization.
   - Consider early removal of Foley's catheter and NGT.
   - Encourage use of incentive spirometry.
   - Analgesia, antibiotic as indicated, stress ulcer, and DVT prophylaxis.

   Before discharge that:
   - The patient has no significant complaint.
   - Tolerating oral diet.
   - Check the wound status.

   First outpatient visit:
   - Clinical assessment.
   - Examine the wound and remove the sutures.
   - Review the final pathology result: **GIST tumor with mitotic index 6 mitosis per HPF. The resection margins are free of the tumor.**
   - Discuss in multidisciplinary team and refer to oncology for adjuvant TKI treatment.

References

1. Talamini MA. The management of Crohn's disease of the small bowel. In: Cameron J, Cameron A, editors. Current surgical therapy. 12th ed. Canada: Elsevier; 2016.
2. Heather Yeo FM. Strictureplasty in Crohn's disease. In: Cameron J, Cameron A, editors. Current surgical therapy. 12th ed. Canada: Elsevier; 2016.
3. Fischer JE. The management of enterocutaneous fistulas. In: Cameron J, Cameron A, editors. Current surgical therapy. 12th ed. Canada: Elsevier; 2016.
4. Tavakkoli A, Ashley SW, Zinner MJ. Small intestine. In: Brunicardi F, editor. Schwartz's principles of surgery. 11th ed. United States: McGraw-Hill Education; 2019.
5. Helmink BA, Bailey CE, Tarpley JL. The management of small bowel tumors. In: Cameron J, Cameron A, editors. Current surgical therapy. 12th ed. Canada: Elsevier; 2016.
6. Eslam MH. Acute mesenteric ischemia. In: Cameron J, Cameron A, editors. Current surgical therapy. 12th ed. Canada: Elsevier; 2016.
7. Ahuja V. Abdominal tuberculosis. In: Sanjiv Chopra JB, editor: uptodate 2021.
8. Caprini JA. Small bowel resection and anastomosis (enterectomy): open. In: Bell RH, DBK, editors. Northwestern handbook of surgical procedures. 11th ed. United States: LANDES BIOSCIENCE; 2005.
9. Zollinger R, Ellison E. Zollinger's Atlas of surgical operation. 9th ed. United States: McGraw-Hill Education; 2011.
10. Stryker SJ. Ileostomy: open loop. In: Bell RH, DBK, editors. Northwestern handbook of surgical procedures. 11th ed. United States: LANDES BIOSCIENCE; 2005.

11 Surgical Aspects of Colon and Rectal Diseases for Clinical Board Exams

11.1 Part I: Knowledge

> Real knowledge is intrinsic, and it's built from the ground up.
> —Naval Ravikant

The presenting complaint might be any of the following:

- Abdominal pain
- Lower gastrointestinal bleeding
- Colonic obstruction

History:

- Introduce yourself to the patient.
- Name, age, occupation, gender, nationality
- Chief complaint and duration
- History of presenting illness:
  - **Analysis of the chief complaint**

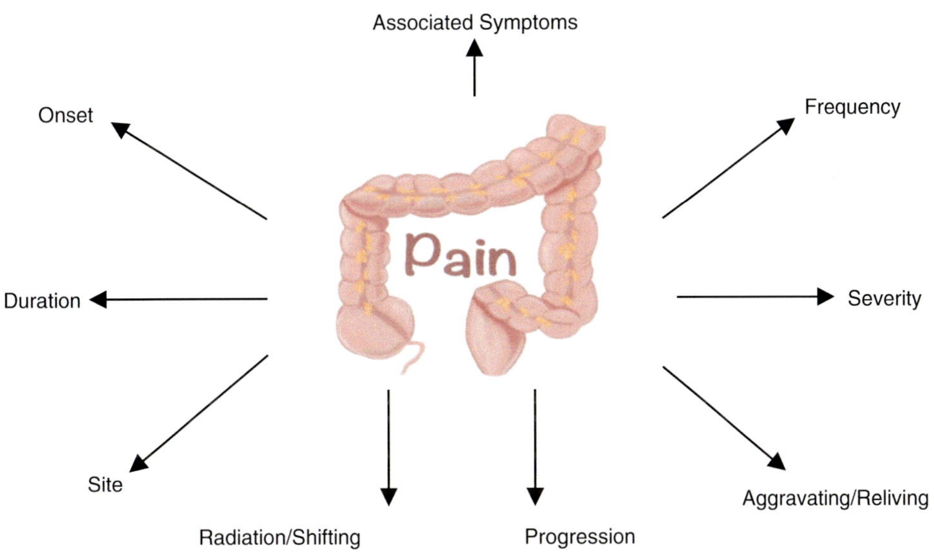

H. Alotaibi, *Study Surgery*, https://doi.org/10.1007/978-981-16-2305-9_11

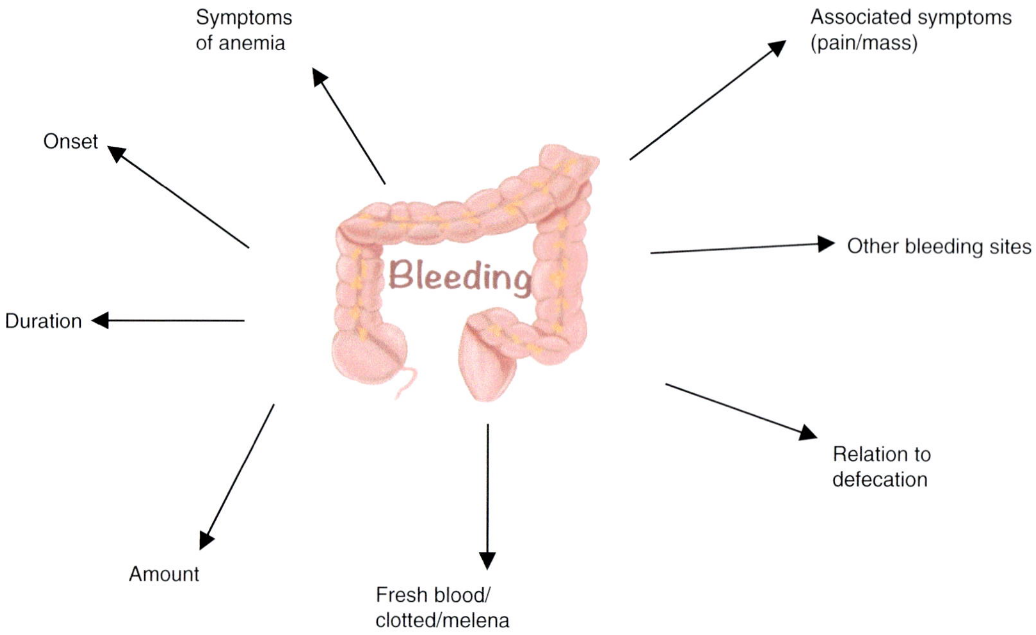

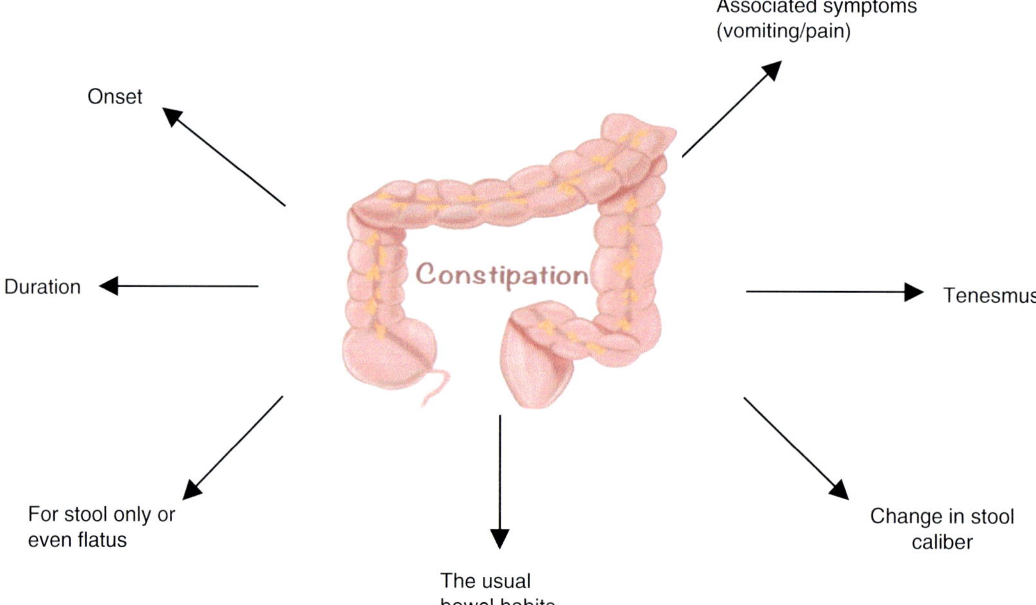

- **Associated Symptoms**
  Pain, fever, nausea, vomiting, dysphagia, hematemesis, diarrhea, change in bowel habits, constipation, abdominal distension, tenesmus, change stool caliber, incontinence, jaundice, fecaluria, pneumaturia, hematuria
- **Constitutional Symptoms:**
  Weight loss, decrease appetite, night sweating, fever
- **Symptoms of Metastasis**
  Back pain, abdominal distention, cough, shortness of breath

- **Risk factors:**
  Diet
  Family history of similar complain or malignancy (colon cancer, breast, endometrial)
  Personal history of cancer
  History of inflammatory bowel disease
  Smoking
- **Symptoms or factors related to differential diagnosis**
  Chest pain (MI)
  Cough, fever, SOB (pneumonia)
  Recent history of trauma
  Heartburn, gastric reflux (GERD, Peptic ulcer disease)
- Previous Similar attack, previous admission, previous investigation or colonoscopy (if yes, when was it done and what was the finding?)

- PMH
- PSH
- Family history
- Social history
- Medication, blood transfusion, allergy
- Systemic Review
  - CNS: Headache, Eye and Hearing symptoms, Epilepsy, numbness, paralysis.
  - CVS: Chest pain, orthopnea, PND, lower limb edema, Palpitation.
  - Respiratory: Cough, Fever, chest pain, hemoptysis.
  - Renal: Dysuria, Flank pain, Hematuria.
  - MSK: weakness, arthritis, skin erythema.

Physical examination:

- Introduce yourself to the patient.
- Ask permission for examination.
- Ensure patient's privacy and ask for a chaperon
- Position: Supine
- Exposure: from nipple to midthigh
- Wash hands

General Examination:

- **A**ppearance: ill/well, dehydrated
- **B**ody Built: Cachectic, obese
- **C**olor: Pale, Jaundice
- **D**istress, **d**ecubitus
- **E**nvironment and connection to monitors, IV fluids, drains

Vital signs: BP, HR, Temperature, RR, SPO_2

Hands:

- Pallor
- Palmer erythema
- Koilonychia (Iron deficiency anemia)
- Leukonychia (Hypoalbuminemia)
- Pulse rate and its characteristics (Rhythm, Volume, etc.)

Eye:

- Jaundice
- Pallor

Mouth:

- Jaundice in the mucus membrane, below the tongue
- Fetor Hepaticus

Neck:

- Lymphadenopathy
- Thyroid swelling

Chest:

- Respiratory and CVS examination

Abdomen:

- Inspection:
  - Distention
  - Asymmetry
  - Visible veins
  - Scars/Striae
  - Dilated veins (Caput medusa)
  - Stretch marks
  - Visible peristalsis
- Palpations:
  - Superficial palpation (away from the tender area)
    Tenderness

Temperature
Superficial masses
- Deep palpation:
  Palpable masses
  Organomegaly
- Percussion:
  - Ascites:
    Shifting dullness
    Fluid thrill
  - Tympany/dullness
- Auscultation:
  - Bowel Sounds
  - Bruit, venous hum

Groin: Examine the hernial orifices and when there is a hernia, assess the type, reducibility, incarceration, and the presence of strangulation

DRE:

- Any obvious pathology (hemorrhoids, fissure, fistula)
- Introduce the finger and assess the tone, any palpable mass (if yes, estimate the distance and assess if it is circumferential or not).
- Assess the prostate in men.

Proctoscopy:

- For the presence of internal hemorrhoids
- Internal opening of the fistula
- If there is any mass, clarify the position, distance, appearance, and the circumference

Lower limbs: edema, swelling, skin rash, weakness

If IBD or polyposis syndromes are suspected, look for the extraintestinal manifestation.

Back: for tenderness

Anatomy of the colon: Fig. 11.1

Differential diagnosis: Table 11.1

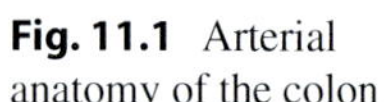

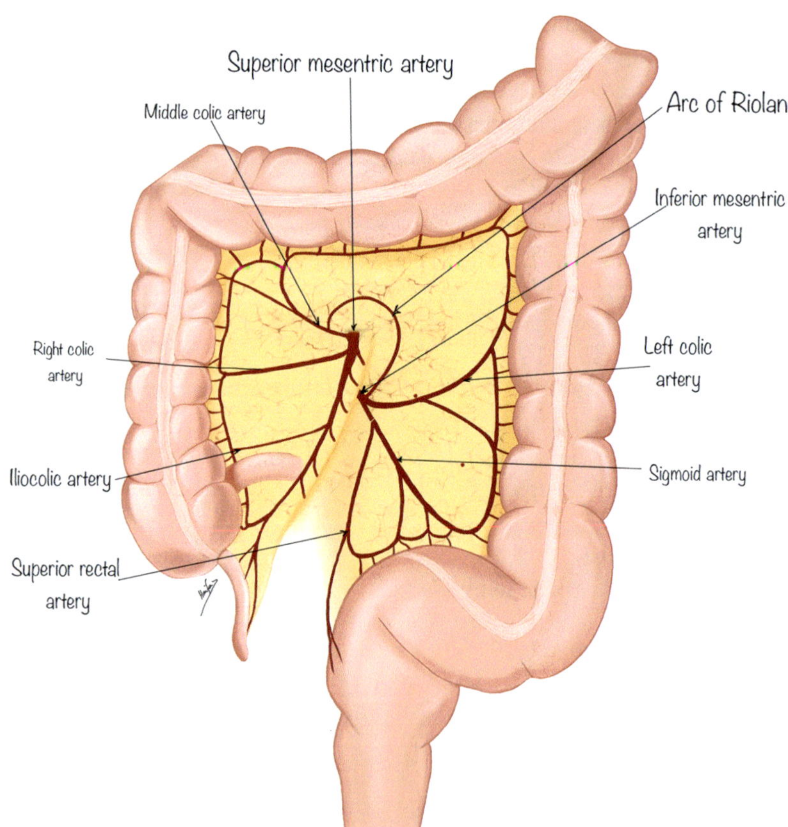

Fig. 11.1 Arterial anatomy of the colon

Table 11.1 Differential diagnosis of central and lower abdominal pain, bleeding per rectum, and large bowel obstruction

PR bleeding	Obstruction	Pain		
		Right lower abdomen	Left lower abdomen	Central
■ Hemorrhoids ■ Fissure ■ Neoplasm ■ Diverticulosis ■ Angiodysplasia ■ Colitis ■ Upper gastrointestinal bleeding ■ IBD	■ Neoplasm ■ Hernia ■ Adhesion ■ Volvulus ■ Pseudo-obstruction ■ Foreign body ■ Stool impaction ■ Intussusception	■ Appendicitis ■ Diverticulitis ■ Typhlitis ■ IBD (Crohn's disease) ■ Gynecological diseases ■ Meckel's diverticulitis ■ Urinary problems ■ Colonic or appendicular neoplasm	■ Diverticulitis ■ Colitis (infectious, inflammatory, ischemic) ■ Colonic neoplasms ■ Gynecological disease ■ Urinary problems	■ Gastroenteritis ■ IBD ■ Mesenteric ischemia ■ Small bowel obstruction ■ Infectious enteritis ■ Intussusception ■ Internal hernia

11.1.1 Approach to Patients with Suspected Inflammatory Bowel Disease (IBD)

- History and examination as described earlier. Focus on whether the patient is diagnosed with inflammatory bowel disease or not. If the patient is known to have it, ask about the previous attacks, his/her medication, and previous surgeries.
- Laboratory investigation:
  - Blood tests:
    CBC
    Electrolytes
    LFT
    Lipase, amylase
    RFT
    Coagulation profile
    Blood group
    ESR, CRP
    Serology: ANCA, PANCA, ASCA (if the patient is not diagnosed yet)
    Fecal calprotectin (if the patient is not diagnosed yet)
    Stool analysis (to rule out other differentials such as infectious colitis)
    Toxin A and B if Clostridium difficile (if suspected)
  - Imaging:
    Chest and abdominal X-ray
    ECG
    CT/MRI abdomen and pelvis
  - Colonoscopy:
    The gold standard in diagnosis and follow-up.
    Preparation: fluid diet, mechanical bowel preparation
    The whole colon should be examined, looking for any masses, polyps, diverticulosis. If there is any lesion, biopsy and tattooing if required
  - Biopsy

11.1.2 Management of Colonic Inflammatory Bowel Disease

A. **Ulcerative Colitis:**
- Peaks in the third decade of life and again in the seventh (bimodal)
- A multifactorial condition that includes environmental, genetic, and immune causal elements
- Cigarette smoking is protective in ulcerative colitis but is a risk factor for Crohn's colitis.
- The ulcerative colitis may affect the rectum (proctitis), rectum and sigmoid (proctosigmoiditis), rectum and left colon (left-sided colitis), or rectum and varying

involvement of the colon proximal to the splenic flexure (pancolitis).

- Terminal ileum may demonstrate inflammatory changes (backwash ileitis).
- Diagnosis is almost always made endoscopically; proctoscopy may be adequate to establish the diagnosis (because the inflammation always starts in the rectum).
- The earliest manifestation is mucosal edema, which results in the loss of vascular pattern.
- In advanced disease, mucosal ulceration, pus, and mucus may be present.
- Mucosal biopsy is diagnostic in the chronic phase but in acute phase will often reveal nonspecific inflammation
- In acute flare-up, diagnosis with colonoscopy and biopsy is contraindicated because there is a risk of perforation.
- Long-standing disease, the colon will appear as lead pipe.
- Stricture is highly uncommon because inflammation is purely mucosal.
- Any stricture diagnosed in ulcerative colitis is malignant until proven otherwise (24% risk).
- Ulcerative colitis patients present to surgeon due to:
  - Severe disease that is not responding to medication, whether it be in the hospital or as an outpatient
  - Have significant side effects of medications used to treat their colitis
  - The presence of colonic neoplasia (dysplasia or colorectal cancer) [1].
- Definitions:
  - Severe colitis: bloody diarrhea, weight loss, volume depletion, fever, and severe anemia
  - Fulminant colitis: severe colitis + progressive symptoms of toxicity
  - Toxic colitis: fulminant colitis + fever, tachycardia, and leukocytosis
  - Toxic megacolon: toxic colitis + the transverse colon >8 cm on X-ray
- Toxic colitis and toxic megacolon are surgical emergencies if the patient failed to improve after 48–96 h of medical management (bowel rest, IV fluid, IV steroids, and IV antibiotics)
- Medical management of Ulcerative colitis: 5-ASA. Corticosteroids, antipyrine or anti-pyrimidine components, and TNF alpha antibodies
- Indications of surgery:
  - Emergency:

    Life-threatening hemorrhage: it is rare (about 4–5%)

    Toxic megacolon

    Fulminant colitis who failed to respond to medical therapy within 24–48 h
  - Elective:

    Intractability despite maximal medical treatment (defined as poorly controlled symptoms, poor quality of life, or growth failure)

    High-risk medical therapy complications, e.g., aseptic necrosis of joints due to steroids

    Risk of developing colorectal carcinoma:

    - Carcinoma arises from an area of flat dysplasia. For this reason, it is recommended that patients with long-standing ulcerative colitis undergo colonoscopic surveillance with multiple (at least 32 biopsies), four quadrants random biopsies at 10-cm intervals to identify dysplasia.
    - Colonoscopic surveillance should be done while in remission.
    - Surveillance should start annually after 8 years in a patient with pancolitis and after 15 years from left-sided colitis.
    - Patient with cancer or high-grade dysplasia should go for proctocolectomy.
    - Patients with low-grade dysplasia should be advised to undergo elective prophylactic proctocolectomy. If the patient refused, close surveillance every 3–6 months.

Extracolonic manifestations:

- Proctocolectomy for ulcerative colitis is beneficial for erythema nodosum (most responsive), arthritis, eye diseases (episcleritis, uveitis, iritis, and conjunctivitis)
- Proctocolectomy does not affect the outcome for primary sclerosing cholangitis and ankylosing spondylitis [2–4].

- Surgical options:
  - Emergency:

    Total abdominal colectomy with end ileostomy with or without mucus fistula is better than proctocolectomy (avoid difficult and time-consuming pelvic dissection in critically ill patients).

    Definitive surgery to be done once the patient is fully recovered

    Complex technique, such as ileal pouch-anal anastomosis generally is contraindicated

    Massive bleeding that includes bleeding from the rectum may require proctectomy [2–4].
  - Elective:

    Total proctocolectomy with end ileostomy: acceptable option in patients who have a risk for pouch failure, impaired anal sphincter, previous anoperineal disease

    Total proctocolectomy and continent ileostomy "Kock's pouch": has significant morbidity

    Total proctocolectomy with ileal pouch-anal anastomosis:
    - Can be done as a single-stage procedure, two-staged procedure, or three-staged procedure.
    - It requires a good sphincter tone.
    - It is contraindicated in patients with metastatic disease.
    - If radiation therapy is required, it should be before pouch creation.
    - J-pouch: limb of the J pouch should be 15–18 cm in length. If the distal aspect of the pouch reaches 6 cm below the pubic symphysis without tension, the pouch can be created.
    - Hand sewing versus stapled ileal pouch-anal anastomosis: if the patient has rectal dysplasia or rectal cancer, mucosectomy with hand sewing anastomosis is appropriate.

    Abdominal colectomy with ileorectal anastomosis may be appropriate in patients with indeterminate colitis or young patient who wants to preserve fertility. It is contraindicated in patients with moderate or severe rectal inflammation, dysplasia or cancer of the rectum, perianal disease, or patient with anal incontinence [2–4].
- Post-operative complications:
  - Obstruction
  - Sexual dysfunction (including infertility)
  - Pelvic sepsis: should be treated aggressively with IV antibiotics and drainage of abscess
  - Stricture: managed with repeated dilatation under anesthesia
  - Hemorrhage: mostly occur within 7 days of surgery and the majority are self-limited. If the bleeding persists, irrigation of the pouch with adrenaline
  - Pouchitis: treated by oral metronidazole or ciprofloxacin, probiotics, budesonide enema. If it is not responding, may need diversion or pouch excision [2–4].

B. **Crohn's Colitis:**

- Bimodal Incidence (15–30 years and ages 60–70 years)
- It is a multifactorial condition that includes environmental, genetic, and immune causal elements.
- Tobacco use is an important risk factor in the etiology and exacerbation of Crohn's disease.
- The endoscopic appearance of Crohn's colitis is characterized by deep ulcers and a "cobblestone" appearance. Skip lesions and rectal sparing are common.

- Extraintestinal manifestations: Primary sclerosing cholangitis (more common with ulcerative colitis), sacroiliitis, arthritis, ankylosing spondylitis, erythema nodosum, pyoderma gangrenosum, or ocular lesions.
- The patients can be classified as either high risk or low risk.
  - High-risk patients:
    Diagnosed at age <30 years
    Using tobacco
    Elevated CRP/fecal calprotectin levels
    Deep ulcers on colonoscopy
    Long segments of bowel involvement
    Perianal disease
    Extraintestinal manifestations
    History of bowel resection
  - Low-risk patients:
    Has no or mild symptoms
    Normal or mild elevation in CRP/fecal calprotectin levels
    Diagnosed at age >30 years
    Limited distribution of bowel inflammation
    Superficial or no ulceration on colonoscopy
    Lack of perianal complications
    No prior intestinal resection
  - **Non-operative management:**
    Nutrition: patients with IBD are often malnourished. Abdominal pain and obstructive symptoms may decrease oral intake. Diarrhea causes significant protein loss. Parenteral nutrition should be strongly considered early in the course of therapy for IBD. The nutritional parameters such as serum albumin, prealbumin, and transferrin should be assessed. In a severely malnourished patient who is also being treated with corticosteroid, the creation of a stoma is often safer than a primary anastomosis.
    Two medical approaches: bottom-up approach (start with a less potent agent and go further according to the patient response), and top-down approach (put the patient on more potent drugs as a first-line therapy)
    Low-risk patients are often managed by step-up approach (bottom-up).
    Top-down approach is appropriate for high-risk patient.
    Medications: see Table 11.2 [3, 5, 6]

Indications of surgery in Crohn's disease:

1. **Massive lower GI bleeding:**
   - Initial resuscitation, localization of the source of bleeding
   - Stable patient can be managed endoscopically or with angiography.
   - Instability requires surgical resection [6].
2. **Sever colitis, fulminant colitis, or toxic megacolon:**
   - Managed by hemodynamic resuscitation, bowel rest, IV antibiotics
   - If deteriorate, total abdominal colectomy with ileostomy is required.
   - Morbidity and mortality increased with colonic perforation.
3. **Stricture and obstruction:**
   - Symptomatic stricture should be resected.
   - If asymptomatic, consider resection because it is difficult to rule out cancer.
4. **Perforation, fistula, and abscess:**
   - If the fistula is between two segments of the bowel and both segments have active disease, resect both segments.
   - If one segment is diseased and the other one is healthy, resect the diseased and repair the secondary involved segment.
5. **Risk or development of malignancy:**
   - 2–3 times more than the general population.
   - Surveillance: every 1–3 years and not later than 8 years after the diagnosis
   - Patient with primary sclerosing cholangitis, pseudopolyp, or stricture needs more frequent evaluation.

Table 11.2 Medical treatment of inflammatory bowel disease [3, 5]

Salicylates	Antibiotics	Corticosteroids	Immunomodulating drugs			Biologic agents
			Inhibition of nucleic acid synthesis	Immunosuppressive Interference with T-lymphocyte function	Folate antagonists	
• E.g., Sulfasalazine, 5-acetyl salicylic acid (5-ASA) • First-line agents in medical treatment of IBD • Decrease inflammation by inhibition of cyclooxygenase and 5-lipogenase in the gut mucosa • They require direct contact with affected mucosa	• E.g., Metronidazole or Fluoroquinolones • Used to decrease the luminal bacterial load in Crohn's disease and management of perianal disease	• Either oral or parenteral • A key component of the treatment of an acute exacerbation of IBD • The use of this agent should be limited to the shortest course possible.	• Azathioprine and 6-mercaptopurine • Useful in the treatment of patients who failed to respond to salicylate therapy or who are dependent or refractory to steroids. • The onset of action takes 6–12 weeks and concomitant use with corticosteroids almost always is required.	• E.g., cyclosporine • Is occasionally used to treat exacerbation of Crohn's disease • Long-term use of cyclosporine is limited by its toxicity (e.g., nephrotoxicity, hirsutism, gum hypertrophy)	• Methotrexate • Although the efficacy of this agent is unproven, there are reports that more than 50% of patents will improve with administration of these drugs	• Inhibition of TNF-alpha • The ultimate goal is mucosal healing. • Infliximab is partially consisting with of mouse antibodies and human antibodies against it can mitigate the efficacy of this drug • Adalimumab and cetrolixumab have no nonhuman component and can be administered subcutaneously

- Dysplasia-associated lesion or mass (DALM) is an indication for resection due to the high risk of malignancy [2, 4].

6. **Extracolonic manifestation:**
   - Pyoderma gangrenosum and erythema nodosum improved with surgery
7. **Intractability**
8. **Complications of medical therapy**
   - Ileal pouch-anal anastomosis is not recommended in those patients because of the risk of inflammation.
   - Anal and perianal Crohn's disease:
     - Most common perianal lesion in Crohn's disease is skin tag.
     - Fissures are typically deep, multiple, broad (anal ulcer), and located laterally.
     - Perianal fistulas are usually complex.
     - Skin tags and hemorrhoids should not be excised unless they are extremely symptomatic because of the risk of chronic nonhealing wounds.
     - Lateral sphincterotomy is a relative contraindication. In absence of active Crohn's proctitis, one can proceed cautiously with partial internal sphincterotomy if EUA reveals a classic posterior or anterior anal fissure.
     - A rectovaginal fistula is a difficult problem and may be managed with rectal or vaginal flap if mucosa appears healthy and scaring of the rectovaginal septum is minimal. Occasionally, proctectomy is the best option for women with highly symptomatic rectovaginal fistula.
     - It is important to drain any and all abscesses before starting immunosuppressive therapy such as corticosteroids or biologic agents [2, 4].

11.1.3 Management of Diverticular Disease

- They are false diverticula.
- The sigmoid colon is the most common site of diverticulosis.
- Asymptomatic diverticulosis can be managed by diet alteration.
- It can be inflamed, cause obstruction, bleeding, or fistula with the nearby organ [3, 7].

Diverticulitis:

- Due to microscopic or macroscopic perforation of the diverticulum
- **Non-complicated:**
  - Left lower quadrant pain and tenderness
  - CT scan will show pericolic soft tissue stranding, colonic wall thickening (>4 mm) with or without phlegmon.
  - Majority of patients can be managed as outpatients with oral antibiotics for 7–10 days and a low residue diet.
  - Ciprofloxacin and Metronidazole are usually effective.
  - Some patients will present with severe pain and tenderness that require hospitalization and IV antibiotics.
  - Failure to improve after 3 days suggests the presence of an abscess.
  - Most patient with noncomplicated diverticulitis will recover without surgery.
  - Indications of elective sigmoid colectomy
- It is no longer depended on the number of attacks, but the decision should be individualized. It is recommended in immunocompromised patients or patients with significant medical comorbidities even after the first attack of noncomplicated diverticulitis.
- Inability to rule out malignancy
  - Colonoscopy is recommended after 4–6 weeks after recovery to rule out carcinoma.
  - If elective sigmoid colectomy is indicated:
- Resection + primary anastomosis
- The proximal extent of resection should include all thickened or inflamed bowel and the distal resection margin is the proximal rectum [3, 7].
- **Complicated Diverticulitis:**
  - Includes diverticulitis with abscess, obstruction, diffuse peritonitis, or fistula between the colon and adjacent structures
  - The modified Hinchey staging system is used to describe the severity of diverticulitis:

Stage 0: mild diverticulitis
Stage I: colonic inflammation associated with pericolic phlegmon (Ia) or abscess (Ib)
Stage II: colonic inflammation associated with distant intraabdominal, retroperitoneal or pelvic abscess
Stage III: inflammation associated with purulent peritonitis
Stage IV: inflammation associated with fecal peritonitis

– Treatment depends on the patient's overall general condition, degree of infection, and presence of peritonitis:
  Small abscess <4 cm can be treated with parenteral antibiotics.
  A larger abscess can be treated with CT-guided percutaneous drainage.
  Urgent or emergent laparotomy may be needed if an abscess is inaccessible to percutaneous drainage or if the patient presents with perforation and peritonitis.
  Sigmoid colectomy with primary anastomosis can be done in Hinchey I or II.
  Hartmann's pouch for patients with larger abscess, peritoneal contamination or peritonitis
  If the patient is extremely unstable, can be managed by proximal diversion and local drainage.
  Revision of Hartmann's can be done after 3–6 months [3, 7].
– Obstruction: Patient with incomplete obstruction can be managed fluid resuscitation, nasogastric suction, and gentle low volume water Gastrografin enemas. Obstruction that does not respond to medical management mandates laparotomy and Hartmann's pouch.
– Fistula between the colon and adjacent organs can develop in 5% of patients with complicated diverticulitis. Colovesical fistulas are the most common followed by Colovaginal and Coloenteric fistulas.
– It is important to define the anatomy of the fistula and exclude other diagnoses before any operative management. Resection of the affected segment of the colon with diverticulitis and simple repair of the secondarily involved organ is the procedure of choice to manage patients with fistula [3, 7].
– Perforation:
  Represent 1% of patients with complicated diverticulitis
  Almost exclusively in the first attack
  Required operative intervention
  The mainstay of treatment is the Hartmann procedure.
  One-third of patients never undergo reversal [3, 7].
– Hemorrhage:
  Bleeding from a diverticulum is caused by erosion of the peri-diverticular arteriole and may result in massive hemorrhage.
  The exact bleeding source is sometimes difficult to identify.
  Most of the bleeding will stop spontaneously.
  Clinical management should be focused on resuscitation and localization of the bleeding site.
  Colonoscopy may identify the bleeding diverticulum that may then be treated with epinephrine injection or cautery.
  RBC scan can detect as low as 0.1 ml/min and it is useful in patients with intermittent bleeding.
  Angiography may be diagnostic and therapeutic at the same time. It detects bleeding at a rate of 0.5 ml/min.
  Requirement of >4–6 units of PRBCs within 24 h, continuous bleeding after 72 h, or rebleeding within 1 week of the first episode are indications for surgical treatment [3, 7].

- **Right-sided diverticula:**
  – True diverticula (congenital), false diverticula (acquired)
  – Occur more often in young patient and more in people of Asian descent
  – Most are asymptomatic
  – If are symptomatic may be mistaken with acute appendicitis

- Sometimes the diagnosis is made intraoperative. If there is a single large diverticulum and minimal inflammation, a diverticulectomy may be performed or ileocecal resection [3, 7].

11.1.4 Management of Ischemic Colitis

- Disease of small blood vessels
- Arch of Riolan (*meandaring mesenteric artery*) is a collateral vessel that is not often present. It connects the proximal SMA with the proximal IMA at the base of the mesentery.
- The marginal artery of Drummond forms a continuous arterial arcade that runs along the distal mesentery near the colonic wall and serves as a connection between SMA and IMA.
- Despite these collaterals specific areas of the colon are more susceptible to ischemia
- These areas are:
  - Right colon: because it is vulnerable to ischemia from low flow states caused by hypotension.
  - Splenic flexure (Griffth's point): because its location at the distal extent of arterial supply to the left colon (IMA) and the middle colic artery (SMA)
  - Rectosigmoid junction (Sudeck's point): because it receives blood supply from the distal branches of sigmoid artery branches and from the superior hemorrhoidal artery (both are terminal branches from the IMA) (Fig. 11.2)
- The signs and symptoms of ischemic colitis are nonspecific such as abdominal pain, urgent desire to defecate, hematochezia that begins after 24 h of pain. Other symptoms like nausea, vomiting, and low-grade fever happen less frequently.
- Medical history is important especially cardiovascular risk factors, history of hypercoagulability, prior surgery especially aortic, and presence of low flow states.
- Ischemic colitis tends to be segmental based on the affected blood supply, the splenic flexure is the most commonly affected segments.

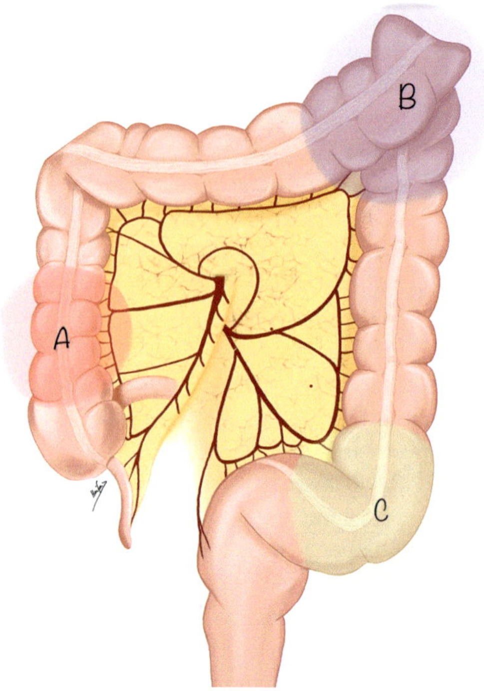

Fig. 11.2 Watershed areas of the colon, A: right colon, B: splenic flexure (Griffith's point), and C: rectosigmoid junction (Sudeck's point)

- Most episodes of ischemic colitis are mild and self-limited. A small proportion of patients will continue to have chronic colitis lasting more than 3 months.
- Diagnosis is made initially by CT abdomen with IV and oral contrast that can show the involved area, severity of colitis, and exclude the presence of other diseases. Presence of pneumatosis, portal vein gas, and megacolon indicate severe disease.
- Colonoscopy is the gold standard for diagnosis. It allows for visualization of colonic mucosa and the presence of edema, erythema, petechial, and ulceration.
- Biopsy should be taken from the involved area and it shows mucosal infarction and the presence of ghost cells.
- The initial treatment of the patient with IC focus on determining the severity of the ischemia and whether surgery is required or not.
- Patients with mild or moderate ischemic colitis respond to medical management with bowel rest, aggressive fluid resuscitation as

needed. An empiric antibiotic is recommended for at least 1 week. Serial abdominal radiographs may be used to follow colonic dilatation. Cardiac output should be optimized. Colonoscopy may be repeated to reevaluate for signs of worsening ischemia.

- Indication of surgical management:
  - Peritonitis
  - Pneumoperitoneum or signs of transmural necrosis on abdominal imaging including pneumatosis or portal vein gas
  - Deterioration despite initial medical treatment (leukocytosis, acidosis, oliguria, or signs of sepsis)
- Surgical intervention should include a thorough exploration of the abdomen. Clear necrotic or perforated bowel should be resected. Questionable viability of any segment of bowel should be assessed intraoperative using visual examination, intravenous injection of fluorescein followed by illumination with ultraviolet light (Woods lamp), or intraoperative infrared angiography. Creation of anastomosis after resection is not advised in acute setting because of the presence of potential tenuous blood flow to the newly created anastomosis [8].

11.1.5 Management of *Clostridium Difficile* Colitis

- *Clostridium difficile* is a Gram-positive, spore-forming anaerobic bacillus that is the leading cause of nosocomial infectious colitis.
- **Primary risk factors:**
  - Age >65 years old
  - Antibiotic treatment within the last 3 months. Almost all antibiotics can cause it but most frequently is Fluroquinolone and Cephalosporin.
  - Hospitalization [9]
- **Secondary risk factors:**
  - Proton pump inhibitors
  - Female
  - Double occupying rooms
  - Post-pyloric feeding
  - Chemotherapy
  - Immunocompromised
  - Inflammatory bowel disease
- Asymptomatic carries 3% [9]
- **Clinical manifestation:**
  - Most common presentation is mild antibiotics associated diarrhea <10 times non-bloody stool/day.
  - Moderate to severe disease consists of profuse diarrhea, fever, nausea, abdominal pain, leukocytosis, distension, and varying degree of abdominal tenderness and peritonitis.
  - Fulminant colitis in 1–8% and characterized by severe systemic inflammatory response [9].
- **Diagnosis:**
  - Stool analysis: enzyme immunoassay for toxin A and B (very specific) PCR to identify DNA coding for the toxins (very sensitive)
  - Imaging:

    X-ray: to assess the presence of megacolon, ileus, colonic wall edema

    CT: can detect localized or diffuse bowel wall thickening, megacolon, pericolic fat stranding, or ascites.
  - Endoscopic: colonoscopy is preferred over sigmoidoscopy because colitis is limited to the right side in one-third of patients. It may be used for decompression and placement of a long colonic tube for vancomycin irrigation [9].
- **Management:**

  A. **Medical:**
  - Depend on the severity
  - Asymptomatic carrier requires no treatment, only contact precaution and hand hygiene with soap and water, i.e., alcohol is not adequate.
  - Symptomatic patient:

    Stop the antibiotic.

    Avoid antidiarrheal agents and narcotic. They lead to megacolon.

    Metronidazole tablet 500 mg TID for 14 days or vancomycin tablet 125 mg QID for 10–14 days.

    IV metronidazole when the enteric route is not available

IV vancomycin does not result in an adequate intraluminal level.

Vancomycin enema or irrigation through the colonic tube may be of benefit in these patients.

Fidaxomicin 200 mg PO BID for 10 days is equivalent to vancomycin with decreased recurrence.

Intravenous tigecycline is useful in the patient who needs a broad-spectrum coverage that also active against *C. difficile* [9].

B. **Surgery:**
   - Around 20% of patient will need surgery.
   - Total colectomy and end ileostomy
   - Anastomosis is not recommended.
   - Immediate surgical intervention:
     Peritonitis
     Perforation
     Fulminant colitis
     Recalcitrant severe colitis
   - Surgery if not improving within 12 h:
     Severe colitis with megacolon
     Severe colitis with inflammatory bowel disease
     Severe colitis and age >65 years
   - Surgery if not improving within 12–24 h:
     Severe colitis [9]

- **Recurrent Infection:**
  - Within the first 2 weeks
  - If first time recurrence, repeat standard doses.
  - If subsequent recurrence, consider additional treatment such as tapering and pulsed antibiotic strategies, combination or adjunct drug regimen [9].

11.1.6 Management of Large Bowel Obstruction

- Large bowel obstructions most often due to neoplastic processes.
- Malignant obstruction most commonly occurs in the descending colon and rectosigmoid.
- **Clinical presentation:** the patient typically presents with abdominal pain, distention, and obstipation. Vomiting is usually late unless there is a concomitant small bowel obstruction. Fever, tachycardia, peritonitis, point tenderness, and pain out of proportion to examination suggest perforation, strangulation, or ischemia and indicate a surgical emergency and the need for an urgent laparotomy.
- Supine and upright abdominal X-ray is a quick and useful tool for diagnosing large bowel obstruction.
- If the patient is stable, additional imaging can be performed. CT abdomen and pelvis with contrast enema is the preferred imaging of choice.
- Large cecal diameter >12 cm or greater is associated with increased risk of ischemia and risk of perforation [10].
- **Initial management:**
  - Emergent laparotomy should be performed in any patient with signs of perforation, close loop obstruction, ischemia, or peritonitis.
  - In patients who are stable, preoperative preparation is essential to improve the outcome.
  - Fluid resuscitation and correction of electrolytes abnormalities
  - Close monitoring of urine output is important for the evaluation of adequate fluid resuscitation.
  - Decompression with a nasogastric tube should be performed early.
  - Appropriate antibiotics (to cover anaerobic and aerobic organisms)
  - Preoperative stoma marking [10]
- **Surgical options:**
  - **Colostomy:**
    Loop colostomy proximal to the obstruction is a good option in urgent operations for patients who are acutely ill, septic, have signs of peritonitis, hemodynamic instability, have gross contamination because of perforation or immunocompromised as a means to decompress the colon [10].

- **Segmental colectomy:**
  Segmental colectomy with primary anastomosis is a good option if the patient is stable and the proximal bowel is not hugely dilated.
  Primary anastomosis with proximal loop ileostomy is a good option in high-risk patients.
  In unstable patient or high-risk patient with left-sided obstruction, Hartmann Procedure is the procedure of choice.
- **Subtotal colectomy:**
  Subtotal colectomy with the removal of the compromised, dilated colon can be performed with either an ileo-sigmoid or ileorectal anastomosis or end ileostomy [10].
  This procedure is usually for patients with medically refractory functional large bowel obstruction. It is rarely used for mechanical large bowel obstruction unless there is a concern of synchronous lesion [10].
- **Endoscopic stenting:**
  Can be used for palliation or as a bridge to surgery
  Complications include stent migration, regrowth into stent, and perforation.
  When it is used as a bridge to surgery, it helps in avoiding emergency operations [10].

11.1.7 Management of Colonic Volvulus

- It causes 10–15% of large bowel obstruction.
- Sigmoid volvulus manifests as large bowel obstruction, while cecal volvulus manifests as small bowel obstruction.
- The patient may present with relapsing chronic recurrent obstruction, i.e., intermittent episodes of pain and distention followed by sudden relief of the pain and the distention.
- Late presentation manifest as tachycardia, decreased urine output, hypotension, sepsis, and change in mental status [11].
- **Diagnosis:**
  - Patient with peritonitis and abdominal film demonstrating large bowel obstruction should be taken to the operating room after resuscitation.
  - In patients with less urgent symptoms, CT abdomen is accurate for diagnosis [11].
- **Treatment options:**
  - Depend on the location
  - All patient should be resuscitated, and comorbid condition maximized in an urgent manner if possible.
  - Analgesia, antibiotics
  - Nasogastric tube decompression
  - Stoma marking
  - Sigmoid volvulus can be managed by endoscopic or surgical detorsion.
  - Endoscopic decompression alone is associated with an extremely high rate of recurrence.
  - Decompression can be done using a rigid or flexible endoscope.
  - After successful endoscopic decompression, the patient can be prepared for surgical management.
  - There are two options for surgery: either resection or fixation. However, resection is the best method to address the acute and chronic sigmoid volvulus.
  - Cecal volvulus is managed by surgery, detorsion, and either resection or colopexy.
  - Depend on the patient factors and the condition of the abdominal cavity (perforation or gross contamination), surgical resection can be followed by primary anastomosis, end stoma, or primary anastomosis and diverting loop ileostomy [11].
- Other colonic volvulus like transverse colon or splenic flexure are rare. However, the surgical management resection of the affected

segment and diversion or anastomosis is chosen based on the patient condition at the time of operation [11].

11.1.8 Management of Acute Appendicitis

- One of the most common causes of acute surgical abdomen worldwide.
- The appendix is a hollow viscus with a blind-ending tip and a base located at the confluence of the three taenia coli of the cecum.
- The appendix may be positioned adjacent to the ileocecal valve, retrocecal or pelvic, and these different locations often result in diverse presenting signs and symptoms.
- Clinical presentation:
  - History: Onset of vague abdominal discomfort, cramping, nausea, progressing to right lower quadrant pain, with associated anorexia, vomiting, and general malaise
  - Physical examination: Right lower quadrant tenderness, voluntary and involuntary guarding, fever, tachycardia, occasionally palpable mass
- Diagnostic tests:
  - Laboratory investigations: Typically, leukocytosis, normal urinalysis, negative pregnancy testing
  - Imaging: Ultrasound (to rule out other differential diagnoses) and CT abdomen and pelvis
- Management:
  - Noncomplicated appendicitis: the standard treatment is appendectomy.
  - Complicated (perforated) appendicitis:

    The presence of a perforated appendix on preoperative imaging does not preclude up-front surgery.

    In patients with generalized peritonitis or septic shock, immediate appendectomy is indicated, and the initial approach should still be laparoscopic.

    Patients with complicated appendicitis with phlegmon or abscess formation can be considered for treatment by antibiotics and radiographically guided percutaneous drainage.

    Empiric intravenous antibiotics (broad Gram-negative coverage), and conversion to oral antibiotics when a regular diet is tolerated.

    Antibiotic choice may be narrowed based on operative cultures.

    If source control is successfully achieved by radiographically guided percutaneous drain placement, antibiotics should be continued for 4 days only.

    If patients fail to improve clinically with antibiotics and drainage, operative intervention may be indicated.
  - Nonoperative management of acute appendicitis (current controversies):

    Several randomized trials have compared appendectomy with a nonoperative approach that involves treatment with antibiotics alone.

    Results show that up to 37% of patients do end up requiring appendectomy within the first year after antibiotic treatment.

    Additionally, they found no advantage to nonoperative management with regard to the length of hospital stay, duration of pain, and time off work.

    An important limitation is that all studies excluded immunocompromised and pregnant patients.
  - Interval appendectomy: Removal of the appendix is considered safe after 6 weeks or so, by which time the acute inflammatory process will have settled down.
  - Appendicitis in pregnancy:

    The position of the appendix is changed during pregnancy (more cephalad).

    Multidisciplinary team approach

    Appendectomy is highly recommended over nonoperative treatment.

    Laparoscopic appendectomy (apply the general laparoscopic principles in pregnancy for the appendectomy, i.e., access, port sites and minimize the pressure) [12].

11.1.9 Polyposis Syndromes

A. **Adenomatous Polyposis syndromes:**
   1. **Familial adenomatous polyposis (FAP):**
      - Autosomal dominant
      - Inherited mutation of APC gene "tumor suppressor gene" on 5q21
      - >100 polyps or <100 polyps with a family history
      - Polyps found predominantly in the rectum and left colon
      - If left untreated, the risk of colorectal cancer is 100% by the age of 35–40 years.
      - The most common presentations are bleeding, diarrhea, abdominal pain, and mucus discharge.
      - For patients with a family history or identified APC gene mutation, screening colonoscopy should be performed at 10–12 years of age and continue annually.
      - Because polyps are predominantly found on the rectum and left colon, annual flexible proctosigmoidoscopy can be done instead of formal colonoscopy and if polyps found, formal colonoscopy can be done [13].
      - **Extracolonic intestinal manifestation:**
        - 80–90% of patient will have gastric fundic gland hyperplastic polyps with very low malignant potential.
        - Gastric adenomas are rare (10%).
        - Duodenal adenoma most commonly found around the ampulla. It develops 15 years after the colonic polyp. Duodenal cancer diagnosed around the age of 50 years and it is the second leading cause of death in patients with FAP
        - Screening EGD is typically performed at age of 20 years and Spigelman severity score is used to determine the surveillance interval.
        - Small tubular adenomas as well as those with low-grade dysplasia, can undergo biopsies and observation.
        - High-risk adenomas (villous), >1 cm, severe polyposis, or high-grade dysplasia, should offer pancreatic preserving duodenectomy.
        - Patient with cancer is managed by pancreaticoduodenectomy.
        - Chemoprevention with NSAID (Sulindac, Celecoxib), can result in polyp regression in patients with less polyp burden although the effect is minimal [13].
      - **Extraintestinal manifestations:**
        - Osteoma
        - Congenital hypertrophy of retinal pigment epithelium (CHRPE)
        - Epidermoid cyst
        - Desmoid tumors:
          In 15–30% of patients
          Locally invasive abdominal wall, intrabdominal, retroperitoneal myofibroblastic tumors
          Typically develop 2–3 years after surgery and occur around 30 years of age
          They can develop spontaneously.
          The third most common leading cause of death in patients with FAP
          Risk factors include female gender, presence of other extraintestinal manifestation, and family history of desmoid tumor
          Extra-abdominal desmoid can be managed with surgical excision with a 1-cm margin.
          Intra-abdominal and retroperitoneal desmoid can invade through the mesentery and surrounding structure resulting in obstruction, hemorrhage, fistulaization, ischemia, and perforation. The primary treatment is medical with NSAID (Sulindac, Celecoxib). Estrogen antagonist (Tamoxifen), chemotherapy (e.g., Methotrexate, Vinblastine, Doxorubicin), and radiation therapy

Surgical removal is difficult and sometimes impossible. Non-resective procedures such as diversion or bypass can be done. Ureteral obstruction can be managed with stenting [13].

2. **Attenuated Familial Adenomatous Polyposis (aFAP):**
   - Occur at later age 30–40 years
   - Less than 100 polyps
   - Found predominantly in the right colon
   - If left untreated, the risk of malignancy is 100% at 59 years old.
   - Extracolonic and extraintestinal manifestations are typically absent.
   - For those patients with a family history or identified APC mutation suggesting aFAP, the screening colonoscopy should begin at age of 20 years and be repeated every 1–2 years.
   - The endoscopic screening should be formal colonoscopy because polyps predominantly in the right side [13].
3. **Mutation Y-Homolog-Associated Polyposis:**
   - Autosomal recessive inherited form of FAP
   - Result from mutation in MYH gene
   - Number of polyps are variable (10–100)
   - Polyps mainly in the left colon and occur at a median age of 48 years old.
   - If left untreated, the risk of malignancy is 80% by age of 70 years.
   - Extraintestinal manifestations are exceedingly rare.
   - Genetic testing for MYH typically is performed when:
     - <100 polyps
     - Family history irrelevant or do not reveal the dominant mode of inheritance.
   - There is no define endoscopic screening criteria.
   - Colonoscopy and esophagogastroduodenoscopy (EGD) starting from around 25–30 years of age and to be repeated every 3–5 years if no polyp identified [13]

- **Chemoprevention:**
  - NSAID (Sulindac, Celecoxib):
    Decrease the size and number of adenomas in the colon and rectum
    There is no appreciable reduction in the risk of cancer.
  - It is not recommended as primary therapy and is not an alternative to surgery.
  - Can be used in:
    Treating ileal pouch-anal anastomosis (IPAA) polyp
    High family risk of desmoid
    When delayed surgery is indicated
    Unwilling or inability to tolerate polypectomy or completion proctectomy [13]
- **Surgery:**
  - The primary goal to prevent colorectal cancer
  - Severe polyposis more than 1000 colonic polyps or more than 20 rectal polyps, APC mutation
  - Those with a high risk of desmoid disease, surgery should be delayed as long as possible.
  - For patients with classic FAP, surgery occur around 16–20 years of age [13].
  - **Surgical options are:**
    1. **Total proctocolectomy with end ileostomy**
       - Low rate of complications
       - Indications: low rectal cancer requiring postoperative radiation, when APR is indicated. Inability to create IPAA (inadequate mesenteric length, and in patients with poor sphincter function)
       - The procedure should follow an oncological approach because of the risk of unrecognized cancer.
       - The ideal projection of the stoma is 2.5 cm [13].
    2. **Total proctocolectomy with ileal pouch-anal anastomosis (restorative proctocolectomy):**
       - Indicated in severe polyposis, rectal polyp >3 cm, dysplastic colonic or rectal polypin a patient with intact sphincter and willing to adhere to close follow-up.

- Restorative pouch can be fashioned in two limbs (J pouch), three limbs (S pouch), four limbs (W pouch), or isoperistaltic (H pouch).
- The J pouch is the most commonly used because it is easy to construct and excellent function outcome.
- If the proposed apex of the pouch can be advanced to 3–4 cm below the inferior edge of the pubis, one can feel confidant of successful reach of the anastomosis [13].
- The strategies to decrease the tension:
  - Complete mobilization of the bowel mesentery to the root of SMA cephalad to head of the pancreas
  - Proximal division of the ileocolic artery
  - Relaxing incision of the mesentery over the tension point along SMA
- Without evidence of adenoma in the anal transition zone or lower rectum, the double stapled IPAA can be fashioned otherwise anal mucosectomy and hand-sewn IPAA [13].

3. **Total abdominal colectomy with ileorectal anastomosis:**
   - Only in attenuated or mild polyposis
   - Rectal polyp <3 cm
   - No colorectal dysplasia or cancer
   - Distensible and compliant rectum
   - Intact sphincter
   - The patient is willing for follow up (every 6–12 months)
   - The risk of rectal carcinoma is 40% by age 30 [13]

- **Postoperative Surveillance:**
  - Annual endoscopic surveillance for adenoma dysplasia or carcinoma will continue the lifetime.
  - Biopsy and histological assessment
  - Frequent surveillance is performed to increase the number or size of polyps.
  - Severe dysplasia and villous adenoma or >1 cm, proctocolectomy in patients with ileorectal anastomosis [13].

B. **Other polyposis syndromes:**

1. Peutz–Jegher Syndrome:
   - Autosomal dominant
   - Hamartomas polyps found throughout the GIT but most commonly in the small intestine
   - Extraintestinal: mucocutaneous hyperpigmentation (perioral, buccal region, eyes, nostril, perioral, finger, toes, hand, and feet)
   - Risk of malignancy increases with age
   - EGD and colonoscopy around 10 years of age.
   - If there are polyps, repeat it every 2–3 years
   - If there are no polyps, repeat the endoscopic and capsule endoscopic at age of 20 years and repeat it 2–3 years.
   - Any polyp >1.5 cm should be removed.
   - Surgery: Reserved for symptomatic patients
   - Clean sweep technique for small bowel to detect any other polyps to minimize future intervention [13]
2. Juvenile polyposis syndrome:
   - Autosomal dominant inherited
   - Polyps can be found through the colon
   - Extraintestinal manifestations present in 15% like cleft lip and palate, polydactyl, and intestinal malrotation
   - Lifetime risk of colorectal carcinoma is 39%.
   - Screening colonoscopy at age of 15 years and repeat it every 2–3 years if there are no polyps
   - EGD at age of 25 years [13]
3. Serrated polyposis syndrome (SPS):
   - Multiple polyps (hyperplastic or serrated)
   - WHO criteria (any of the following)
     - At least five serrated polyps, proximal to the sigmoid colon, and two of which >10 mm
     - Any number of serrated polyps, proximal to the sigmoid colon in individuals with first degree relative with serrated polyposis

- More than 20 serrated polyps of any size distributed throughout the colon
- Risk of colon cancer is 30–50% at age of 50–60 years.
- Strict surveillance with colonoscopy every 1–2 years starting at age 40 years

4. Other syndromes like Cowden's syndrome (high risk of colon, breast, and thyroid cancers), Bannayan–Riley–Ruvalcaba syndrome, and Cronkite–Canada Syndrome [13]

11.1.10 Management of Colonic Polyps

1. *Non-neoplastic polyps:*
   A. **Hyperplastic polyps:**
   - Most common non-neoplastic polyps
   - Result due to normal epithelial cells accumulating on the mucosal surface creating a pale appearance
   - They are typically sessile.
   - Most common frequently reported polyps in sigmoidoscopy and found most often in the rectum
   - <10 mm hyperplastic polyp limited to sigmoid or rectum are considered benign and should not shorten the 10 years interval of screening [14].

   B. **Mucosal polyps:**
   - Caused by prolapse of the mucosa
   - They have no clinical significance [14].

   C. **Inflammatory polyps:**
   - Occur with IBD
   - Typically found in clusters, may be associated with surrounding dysplasia (this area must be biopsied to rule out DALM) [14]

   D. **Hamartomatous polyps:**
   - When sporadic are called juvenile polyps (because they are commonly found in children)
   - Non-sporadic polyps, occur with three syndromes (Juvenile polyposis, Peutz–Jegher, and Cowden's syndromes)
   - They are not malignant polyps, but all the above syndromes increase the risk of colon cancer [14].

2. *Neoplastic Polyps:*
   A. **Adenomas**
   - Differ from hyperplastic polyps, they have cellular atypia and consider as a precursor for invasive colorectal carcinoma
   - Most common neoplastic polyps found on colonoscopy
   - Histologically classified as tubular (65–85%), tubulovillous (10–25%), and villous adenomas (10%)
   - Advanced adenoma defined as adenoma >1 cm, villous, severe dysplasia, or focus of invasion
   - Adenoma carcinoma sequence:
     - 80% of colorectal cancer develop from adenoma
     - The average time of development of adenoma to carcinoma is 7–10 years and shortened for advanced adenoma
     - Risk of cancer increase if >1 cm, high-grade dysplasia, or villous type [14]

   B. **Sessile serrated adenomas (SSA)**
   - 0.5–4% of colorectal polyps
   - Difficult to distinguish from normal mucosa and their margin may be difficult to delineate endoscopically
   - Larger than 5 mm
   - More often in the right colon
   - Increase incidence in female
   - Progression to adenocarcinoma is rapid and more than the adenoma-carcinoma sequence for tubular adenoma [14]

Guideline for Colonoscopy Screening and Surveillance

1. **Average risk individual:**
   Ten-years interval is appropriate after negative finding on baseline colonoscopy which should be done at the age of 45 years.
2. **Individual with first degree relative with colorectal cancer or high-risk adenoma at an age younger than 60 years:**

Screening should start early and continue at 5-years interval and stop screening at the age of 75–85.

3. **Distal small hyperplastic polyps:**
   Interval remains 10 years
4. **One or two tubular adenomas, smaller than 10 mm, low-grade dysplasia:**
   Repeat colonoscopy in 5–10 years
5. **High-risk adenoma (3–10 adenomas, one tubular adenoma ≥1 cm, or villous feature, high-grade dysplasia of any size):**
   Repeat colonoscopy in 3 years
6. **Large sessile polyps, removed in piecemeal fashion:**
   Repeat colonoscopy in less than a year (3–6 months)
7. **>10 adenomas:**
   Repeat endoscopy <3 years and do genetic consultation
8. **Single SSA <1 cm with no dysplasia:**
   Repeat colonoscopy in 5 years
9. **Multiple SSA, >1 cm, or dysplastic:**
   Repeat colonoscopy in 3 years [14]

11.1.11 Approach to Malignant Polyp

- 5% of polyps contain a focus of invasive cancer.
- Malignant polyp defined as adenocarcinoma that invades into but not deeper than the submucosal layer representing T1 (it differs from carcinoma in situ which is high-grade dysplasia)
- Depth of the submucosal invasion found on polypectomy can be used to predict the risk of lymph node metastasis.
- Submucosal invasion in a sessile polyp classified as:
  - Sm1: invasion to upper third of the submucosa
  - Sm2: invasion up to middle third of submucosa
  - Sm3: invasion up to the lower third of submucosa (indication for formal resection)
- Other risk feature for lymph node metastasis:
  - High tumor grade
  - Extensive tumor budding (presence of a cluster of malignant cells in the submucosa remote from the main site of submucosal invasion)
  - Lymphovascular invasion
- Without risk features, the risk of lymph node metastasis is <1%, with single risk feature is around 20%, and with two risk features is 36%
- Haggitt's level (Fig. 11.3), submucosal invasion in:
  1. Polyp head
  2. Polyp neck
  3. Polyp stalk
  4. Polyp base
- Close surveillance after endoscopic polypectomy is enough if:
  1. Complete endoscopic excision
  2. Microscopic free margin is >2 mm
  3. Well to moderate differentiated adenocarcinoma
  4. Haggitt's level 1, 2, 3 or Sm1 or Sm2

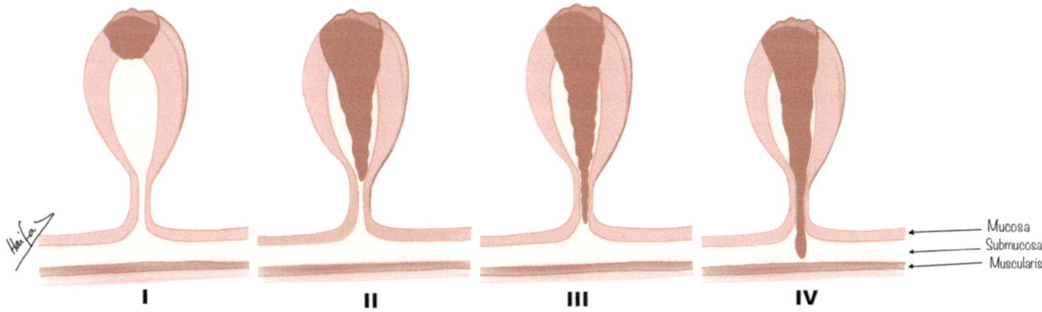

Fig. 11.3 Haggitt's levels

- Otherwise, the patient needs formal resection [14].

Lynch syndrome (hereditary nonpolyposis colon cancer):

- It accounts for approximately 3% of all cases of colorectal cancer and for approximately 15% of these cancers in patients with a family history of colorectal cancer.
- Autosomal dominant
- Tumors are typically microsatellite unstable MSI-H.
- The most common clinical variants are Muir–Torre syndrome and Turcot's syndrome.
- Before the genetic mechanisms underlying the Lynch syndrome were understood, it was defined by the Amsterdam criteria, which required three criteria for the diagnosis:
  - Colorectal cancer in three family members (first-degree relatives)
  - Involvement of at least two generations
  - At least one affected individual being younger than 50 years at the time of diagnosis
- The modified Amsterdam criteria expanded the cancers to be included to not only colorectal but also endometrial, ovarian, gastric, pancreatic, small intestinal, ureteral, and renal pelvic cancers.
- Colorectal cancer, or a Lynch syndrome-related cancer, arising in a person younger than 50 years should raise suspicion for this syndrome.
- Genetic counseling and testing should be offered. If the individual proves to have Lynch syndrome by identification of a mutation in one of the known MMR genes.
- It is usually recommended that a program of surveillance colonoscopy begin at the age of 20 years.
- Colonoscopy is repeated every 2 years until the age of 35 years and then annually thereafter.
- In women, periodic vacuum curettage is begun at age 25 years, as are pelvic ultrasound and determination of CA-125 levels.
- Annual tests for occult blood in the urine should also be carried out because of the risk for ureteral and renal pelvic cancer [15].

11.1.12 Approach to Patient with Suspicion of Colorectal Cancer

- History and physical examination as described earlier.
- Investigations:
  - CBC
  - Electrolytes
  - Coagulation profile
  - Blood grouping and cross match
  - RFT
  - X-rays (erect chest X-ray, abdomen in erect and in supine positions)
  - ECG
  - Colonoscopy after colonic preparation if possible. The whole colon should be examined for any masses, polyps, diverticulosis, the exact site of any detected abnormality should be determined and biopsied and marked if needed.
  - If colonoscopy could not be completed due to partial obstruction: CT colonography is indicated.
  - Consider endoscopic stent if there is a malignant obstruction in the colon as a bridge to surgery.
  - If colonoscopy cannot be performed due to complete obstruction: intraoperative colonic lavage and colonoscopy. If it is not possible, intraoperative palpation of the rest of the colon and full colonoscopy to be done postoperative when feasible.
  - If the biopsy is positive for cancer:
    - Staging CT-CAP
    - Tumor marker (CEA)
    - MRI pelvis or endorectal ultrasound in case of rectal cancer
    - Multidisciplinary team discussion
    - Break the bad news for the patient and explained the management
- If the patient is for upfront surgery

- Refer to the preoperative and operative section
- If the patient for Neoadjuvant chemotherapy
  - Refer him/her to the oncology and radiotherapy teams
  - Reevaluation
  - Restaging
  - Prepare for operation

Management of Colon cancer
General principles:

- The goals of surgery are:
  - Complete removal of the tumor
  - Adequate tumor-free margin
  - Anatomically complete lymphadenectomy of draining lymph nodes
  - En bloc resection of involved organs
  - Avoidance of contamination of the surgical field with tumor cells
  - The extent of colonic resection determined by the vascular pedicle
  - Minimal 12 lymph nodes should be harvested
- All curable intent procedure should include thorough exploration for evidence of metastatic disease (peritoneal surface, omentum, para-aortic lymph nodes)
- Tumors of the ascending colon and cecum are managed with right hemicolectomy
- Tumors of the transverse colon are managed with either extended right or extended left hemicolectomy.
- Tumors of the descending colon are managed with left hemicolectomy.
- Sigmoid colon tumors are managed with either sigmoid colectomy or left hemicolectomy.
- Laparoscopic is similar to open resection in term of oncological efficacy, nodal harvest, survival, and locoregional recurrence.

Management of colon cancer based on clinical stage:

- **Stage 0 (Tis "carcinoma in situ," N0, M0)**
  - Polyps containing carcinoma in situ or high-grade dysplasia
  - Managed by endoscopic polypectomy
  - Polyps should be excised completely.
  - Pathological margin should be free of dysplasia.
  - The patient should be followed with colonoscopy to ensure that polyp has not recured.
  - If polyp was not completely removed, it requires segmental resection [3, 16, 17].
- **Stage I (T1 "malignant polyp," N0, M0)**
  - See the approach to malignant polyp
- **Stage II (T1-3, N0, M0):**
  - Formal oncological resection
  - Adjuvant chemotherapy for selected patient
    Young patients
    High-risk features such as the presence of lymphovascular invasion, poorly differentiated, bowel perforation, inadequate margins, low nodal count [3, 16, 17]
- **Stage III (any T, N1-2, M0):**
  - Formal oncological resection
  - Adjuvant chemotherapy [3, 16, 17]
- **Stage IV (any T, any N, M1):**
  - Almost all cases need systemic chemotherapy.
  - The most common site of metastasis is the liver, hepatic resection of synchronous metastasis from colorectal cancer may be performed in one or two stages.
  - The second common site is lung metastasis, and it is rarely resectable.
  - If stage IV cannot be cured surgically, focus on palliation. For obstructed patients, palliation can be achieved by stenting, diverting stoma, or bypass. If the patient has bleeding, it can be controlled with angioembolization [3, 18].

Management of Rectal cancer
General Principles

- History and physical examination including proctoscopy (assess the orientation of the tumor and the circumferential involvement)
- **Full colonoscopy is important:**
  - 5% of patients have synchronous lesions
  - If the colonoscopy is not possible, do CT colonography [3, 16, 17].
- **Pelvic MRI:**
  - Better modality to distinguish T2 from T3
  - Determine the relationship of the tumor to the mesorectal fascia

- Provide information about the pelvic anatomy and the relationship of the tumor to adjacent pelvic organs [3, 16, 17]
- **Endorectal ultrasound (ERUS):**
  - The main advantages, it can distinguish T0, T1, and T2
- MRI is superior to ERUS in evaluating the mesorectal fascia and pelvic lymph node
- PET scan is not recommended as a routine workup, but if there is suspicion for distant metastasis found in CT or MRI [3, 16, 17].
- **Local excision techniques:**

  A. *Transanal excision (TAE):*
  - The tumor must be accessible from the anal canal.
  - It must be below the peritoneal reflection.
  - The proximal limit of resection is usually 6–8 cm from the anal verge.
  - The goal of the TAE is full-thickness excision of the rectal lesion with negative margins.

  B. *Transanal endoscopic microsurgery and Transanal minimally invasive surgery (TEM and TAMIS):*
  - For tumors located in the mid or upper rectum
  - Tumor as high as 10 cm anteriorly, 15 cm laterally and 18 cm posteriorly can be excised with the TEM approach
  - Limitations of TEM and TAMIS are very distal lesions <5 cm from the anal verge and inadvertent entry to the abdominal cavity.
- All the three local excision techniques (TAE, TEM, TAMIS) have a higher recurrence rate for T1 and T2 adenocarcinoma compared with radical resection [3, 16, 17].
- **Radical resection:**
  - Resection of the tumors and blood supply along with draining lymphatics
  - Sphincter preserving low anterior resection (LAR) is the preferred approach and it is appropriate for tumor located more than 1 cm from the upper portion of the anorectal ring.
  - Contraindication to LAR:

    Invasion to anal sphincter or levator muscles

    Impaired preoperative anorectal function
  - Abdominoperineal resection (APR) is preferred when a margin-negative resection would result in loss of anal sphincter function leading to fecal incontinence [3, 16, 17].
- **Total Mesorectal excision:**
  - Defined as complete excision of the visceral mesorectum with pelvic nerve preservation; the mesorectum refers to the fatty tissue that encompasses the rectum and it contains the lymphatic drainage from the rectum.
  - In the middle and low rectal cancer, the entire mesorectum is mobilized and resected.
  - Cancer of upper rectum, 10 cm from anal verge, can be treated with tumor-specific excision in which the mesorectum is divided at a right angle to bowel 5 cm distal to the mucosal edge of the tumor [3, 16, 17].
- **Autonomic nerve preservation:**
  - *Sympathetic nerves:*

    Originate from the T12 to L3 ventral roots which form superior hypogastric plexus distal to the aortic bifurcation.

    The superior hypogastric plexus gives rise to hypogastric nerves and these may be associated intimately with the visceral fascia of the mesorectum.

    Damage to sympathetic hypogastric nerves result in increased bladder tone, decrease bladder capacity, and retrograde ejaculation [3, 16, 17]
  - *Parasympathetic nerves:*

    Arise from the S2 to S4 ventral roots and join the sympathetic hypogastric nerves on the pelvic sidewall to form the inferior hypogastric plexus.

    Injury to the parasympathetic nerves leads to voiding difficulty from increase the tone in the neck of the bladder, erectile dysfunction in men, and impaired vaginal lubrication in women [3, 16, 17].

- **Circumferential resection margin (CRM):**
  - Is referred to the adequacy of the surgical resection margin relative to the 360-degree radial extension of the primary tumor, which may include extension into the mesorectum and adjacent extrarectal soft tissue
  - CRM <2 cm is associated with local recurrence in 16% of patients.
  - And CRM ≥2 cm is associate with local recurrence in 6% of patients [3, 16, 17].
- **Distal resection margin (DRM):**
  - The required free distal margin is 2 cm.
  - 1 cm margin may not compromise the oncological outcome.
  - Histologically negative DRM <1 cm is acceptable in a carefully selected patient in the absence of adverse histological feature [3, 16, 17].
- **Reconstruction options after LAR:**
  - Straight coloanal anastomosis (end to end or side to end)
  - Creation of colonic reservoir (colonic J pouch or transverse coloplasty pouch) [3, 16, 17]
- **Temporary diversion after LAR:**
  - Decrease anastomotic leak rate and leak related complications
  - Risk factors for the leak after LAR
    - Male gender
    - Low anastomosis ≤6 cm from the anal verge
    - Preoperative radiation therapy
    - Presence of adverse intraoperative events
  - Ileostomy reversal 3 months after the surgery. When chemotherapy is required, postpone the reversal for several weeks after chemotherapy.
  - Before reversal
    - Do DRE.
    - Contrast-enema study with water-soluble contrast is recommended to ensure that the anastomosis is patent and no evidence of leak before closure [3, 16, 17].
- **APR:**
  - Abdominal and perineal approach to resect the rectum, mesorectum, surrounding perineal soft tissue, and pelvic floor musculature
  - Permanent end colostomy
  - APR is indicated when:
    - The tumor is directly invading the sphincter muscle.
    - Adequate margin cannot be obtained during a restorative resection.
    - If the patient already has fecal incontinence preoperatively [3, 16, 17]

Management of Rectal Cancer based on clinical stage:

- **Carcinoma in situ and T1-N0 rectal cancer:**
  - The goal is total excision of the tumor without attempting to remove regional lymph nodes
  - Criteria of local excision of rectal cancer:
    - Location and size: within 15 cm from the anal verge, diameter <3 cm, involve <1/3 of the circumference, mobile non-fixed tumor, and T1N0 in MRI or ERUS
    - Histology: well to moderate differentiated tumor, no lymphovascular invasion, no mucinous or signet cells, and T1 on the final histology examination
  - Local recurrence is 11–29%.
  - If the patient treated initially with local excision and later needed resection or salvage procedure due to local recurrence or final pathology revealed more invasive cancer, it is worse prognosis than comparable stage who underwent surgery initially.
  - Local excision is indicated in:
    - Low-risk patient
    - Significant medical contraindication to major surgery
    - Unwilling to accept the risk of permanent or temporary stoma [3, 16, 17]
- **T2 N0 Rectal cancer:**
  - Standard treatment is radical resection with TME.

- If the lymph node found to be involved in the final pathology, the patient is indicated for adjuvant chemoradiotherapy (CRT).
- Very selected patient with clinically T2N0 is indicated for Neoadjuvant chemoradiotherapy when bulky tumor found in proximity to the upper part of anorectal sphincter preclude sphincter preservation surgery [3, 16, 17].

- **Locally advanced rectal cancer (T3-4/N0/M0 or any T/N1-2/M0):**
  - The standard treatment is neoadjuvant CRT followed by radical resection and adjuvant chemotherapy.
  - Locally advanced tumor is now treated with either short-course radiation therapy (5 Gy/day × days) followed by surgery within 1 week, or long course chemoradiation (1.8–2.0 Gy/day over 5–6 weeks to a total dose of 45–50 Gy along with %-fluorouracil-based intravenous or oral capecitabine chemotherapy) followed by surgery 8–12 weeks later.
  - Both courses reduced the local recurrence, but the benefit of overall survival is less clear [3, 16, 17].
- **Distant metastasis M1 disease:**
  - Three important factors to consider:
    - The primary tumor (related symptoms and resectability)
    - The extent of metastasis (site and resectability)
    - The age of the patient and the comorbidities
  - If both, the primary and the secondary, are limited and resectable:
    - Systemic chemotherapy
    - Restaging
    - Resection of both either in combined or staged procedures
  - Upfront surgery either single or combined procedures can be considered in patients with limited metastatic disease.
  - For patients with advanced disease palliation can be done with chemotherapy or chemotherapy and surgery for symptomatic primary [3, 16, 17].

11.1.13 Management of Lower GI Bleeding

- In more than 95% of patients with lower GI bleeding, the source of hemorrhage is the colon.
- The incidence of lower GI bleeding increases with age, and the cause is often age related.
- The clinical presentation of lower GI bleeding ranges from severe hemorrhage with diverticular disease or vascular lesions to a minor inconvenience secondary to anal fissure or hemorrhoids.
- Lower GI bleeding typically is manifested with hematochezia that can range from bright red blood to old clots. If the bleeding is slower or from a more proximal source, lower GI bleeding often is manifested as melena.
- Differential diagnosis of lower GI bleeding includes diverticular disease, anorectal disease, ischemia, neoplasia, IBD, post polypectomy, radiation, Dieulafoy lesion, ectopic varices, and angiodysplasia.
- **Initial resuscitation**:
  - Airway: assess the patency of airway
  - Breathing: ensure good ventilation and oxygenation
  - Circulation
    - Insert two large cannulas
    - Draw blood for investigation (CBC, electrolytes, coagulation profile, blood group and cross match, ABG, lactic acid)
    - Start IV fluid, e.g., Ringer lactate
- After initial stabilization, obtain a relevant medical history and perform a physical examination.
- **Localization:**
  - Rule out anorectal bleeding by DRE and anoscopy.
  - Rule out upper GIT source. An NG aspirate that contains bile and no blood effectively rules out upper tract bleeding in most patients. However, when emergent surgery for life-threatening hemorrhage is being contemplated, preoperative or intraoperative EGD is usually appropriate.

- Subsequent evaluation depends on the magnitude of the hemorrhage and the hemodynamic stability of the patient.
- An unstable patient who continues to bleed and requires ongoing aggressive resuscitation should be taken to the operating room for expeditious diagnosis and surgical intervention.
- Moderate bleeding and stable patient after resuscitation, colonoscopy is the main diagnostic and therapeutic tool. Gentle preparation can improve visualization. Because the majority of lower GI bleeds are self-limited, the timing of colonoscopy (within 24 h).
- Findings may include an actively bleeding site, clot adherent to a focus of mucosa or a diverticular orifice, or blood localized to a specific colonic segment. Polyps, cancers, and inflammatory causes can frequently be seen. Unfortunately, angiodysplasias are often difficult to visualize, particularly in the unstable patient with mesenteric vascular constriction.
- Tc 99m (99mTc-labeled RBC) is the most sensitive but least accurate method for localization of GI bleeding. The RBC scan can detect bleeding as slow as 0.1 ml/min.
- Selective angiography, using either the superior or inferior mesenteric arteries, can detect hemorrhage in the range of 0.5–1.0 ml/min and is generally employed only in the diagnosis of ongoing hemorrhage. Catheter-directed vasopressin infusion can provide temporary control of bleeding, permitting hemodynamic stabilization. It can also be used for embolization.

• **Management of most common causes:**
  - *Diverticular bleeding:*

    The bleeding stops spontaneously in 75% of patients

    If the bleeding diverticula identified in colonoscopy, injection of epinephrine, electrocautery, or endoscopic clip may stop the bleeding.

    If none of the endoscopic methods stop the bleeding, highly selective angiography and embolization can stop the bleeding in 90% of cases.

    If the bleeding continues, colonic resection is indicated.

    Blind hemicolectomy associated with a recurrence rate of up to 50% and subtotal colectomy does not eliminate the risk.
  - *Angiodysplasia:*

    Most commonly cecum and ascending colon

    Risk factor include old age, medical comorbidity, anti-platelets and anticoagulant

    During colonoscopy, they appear as red stellate lesions with a surrounding rim of pale mucosa and can be treated with sclerotherapy or electrocautery.

    Angiography demonstrates dilated, slowly emptying veins and sometimes early venous filling.

    In acutely bleeding patients, they have been successfully treated with intra-arterial vasopressin, selective gel foam embolization, endoscopic electrocoagulation, or injection with sclerosing agents.

    If these measures fail or bleeding recurs and the lesion has been localized, segmental resection, most commonly right colectomy, is effective.
  - *Neoplasia:*

    The bleeding is usually painless, intermittent, and slow in nature. Frequently, it is associated with iron deficiency anemia.

    The best diagnostic tool is colonoscopy.

    If the bleeding is attributable to a polyp, it can be treated with endoscopic therapy.
  - *Anorectal bleeding:*

    Anorectal hemorrhage is low-volume bleeding that is bright red blood per rectum seen in the toilet bowl and on the toilet paper. Most hemorrhoidal bleeding arises from internal hemorrhoids.

    Internal hemorrhoids should be treated with bulking agents, increased dietary fiber, and adequate hydration. A variety of office-based interventions, including rubber band ligation, injectable sclerosing agents, and infrared coagulation, have also been used. If these measures fail, surgical hemorrhoidectomy may be needed. Most anorectal bleeding is self-limited and responds to dietary and local measures [19].

11.1.14 Colorectal Operations

Preoperative preparation:

- Admission
- Consent
- NPO
- IV fluid
- DVT and stress ulcer prophylaxis
- Prophylactic antibiotic
- Bowel preparation (mechanical and oral antibiotics)
- Confirm the availability of blood intraoperative if needed
- Anesthesia consultation
- ICU consultation if required
- Urology consultation for insertion of ureteric stent if indicated
- Instruct the patient to take shower the night before surgery
- Stoma marking
- Hair removal

Informed Consent:

- **Explain the procedure:**
  - If the surgery is for a neoplastic lesion, explain that it will start with exploration and what would be the action in case a more advanced disease is found.
  - Removal of the (right colon/left colon/sigmoid/rectum/the entire colon/the entire colon and rectum) through (midline incision/laparoscopic) approach. Reconstruct the remaining colon by performing (ileocolic, colocolic, colorectal, coloanal) anastomosis or perform (ileostomy or colostomy).
  - Mention whether the stoma (if performed) is temporary or permanent.
- **Mention if there is any alternative procedure**, e.g., endoscopic excision
- **Mention the possible complications:**
  - General complication: DVT, PE, atelectasis, pneumonia, MI
  - Specific complication: bleeding, anastomotic leak, wound infection, fistula, wound dehiscence, stricture or stenosis of the anastomosis, injury to the ureter, small bowel, autonomic nerve injury (sexual and bladder dysfunction) in case of rectal surgery, and local recurrence and metachronous metastasis.
  - Stoma complications: skin excoriation, electrolyte imbalance, dehydration in case of ileostomy. Prolapse, retraction, necrosis for both colostomy and ileostomy.

A. **Right hemicolectomy:**
  - **General Principles:**
    - It is defined as removal of the distal 10–15 cm of the ileum, cecum, ascending colon, hepatic flexure and the proximal one-third of the transverse colon (Fig. 11.4). If extended right hemico-

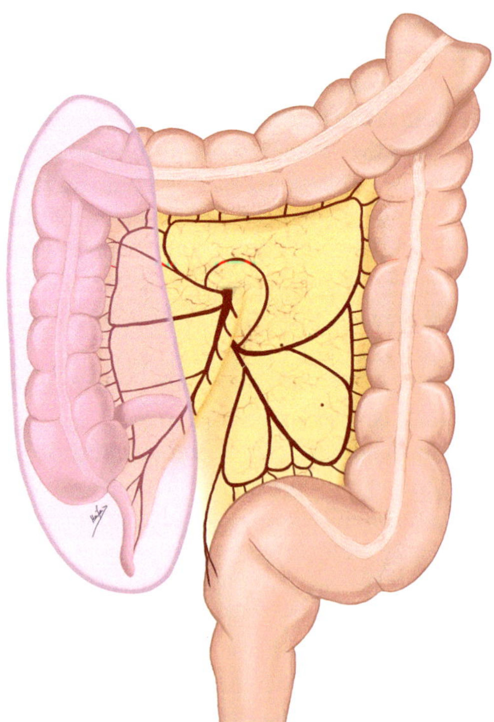

Fig. 11.4 Right hemicolectomy

lectomy to be performed include the transverse colon to the splenic flexure (ligate the left branches of the middle colic artery too).
  - Oncological Resection is to perform high ligation of mesenteric vessels to include the lymph nodes draining this part of the colon.
  - The required number of harvested lymph node is at least 12 lymph nodes.
  - No preoperative bowel preparation is required for right hemicolectomy
  - Preoperative ileostomy marking (in case it is needed intraoperatively)
  - Approaches: medial to lateral, lateral to medial.
- **Details of the procedure (open lateral to medial approach):**
  - Under general anesthesia and endotracheal intubation
  - Position: supine
  - The abdomen is prepped from the nipple to the symphysis pubis.
  - Patient is draped in a sterile fashion.
  - Time out: confirm that correct patient, correct procedure, correct site, and all the required instruments are available
  - Incision: midline incision
  - Explore all the abdomen and palpate the liver and rest of the colon
  - Apply the retractors.
  - The peritoneal attachments to the cecum are incised with electrocautery (Fig. 11.5).
  - The colon is retracted anteriorly and medially so that electrocautery can be used to further release the lateral peritoneal attachments along the right gutter. Blunt dissection with a sponge can be used to divide any remaining thin attachments to the retro-peritoneum.
  - Identify and preserve the right ureter (it courses from the posterior aspect of the duodenum toward the bifurcation of the iliac vessels), duodenum, and the gonadal vessels.

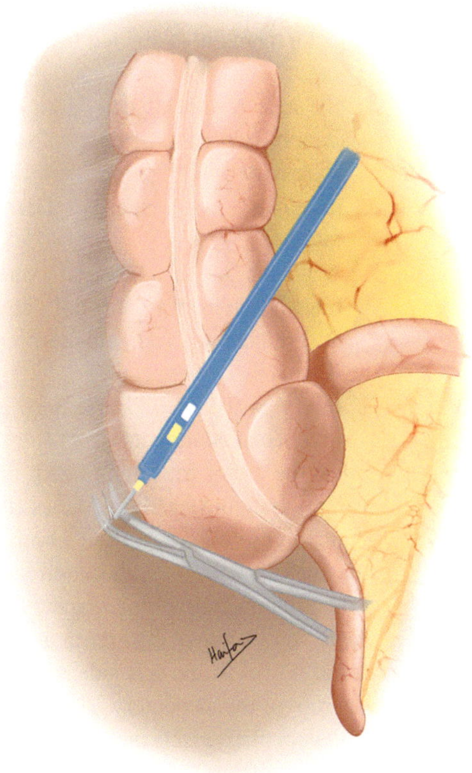

Fig. 11.5 The colon is retracted anteriorly and medially, and electrocautery can be used to further release the lateral peritoneal attachments along the white line of Toldt

  - Continue with hepatic flexure mobilization and avoid excessive traction on the duodenum.
  - Mobilization of the right colon is completed when the hepatic flexure is freed superiorly from the liver and posteriorly from the duodenum. The duodenum and head of the pancreas can be visualized when the hepatic flexure dissection is completed.
  - The reno-colic ligament that anchors the hepatic flexure may be thick and either be ligated with 2-0 silk or divided with ultrasonic shears or electrothermal bipolar device.
  - Dissect distally through the gastrocolic ligament is encountered and dissect through it.

- Once the lesser sac is opened, the gastrocolic ligament is divided from left to right.
- Three areas require caution during cephalad mobilization of the right colon:
  Excessive mobilization deep to the mesentery and entering Gerota's fascia
  Avulsion of a collateral venous branch between the inferior pancreaticoduodenal and middle colic veins
  Injury to the second and third portion of the duodenum
- Once the colon fully mobilized, identify the lymphovascular pedicles (ileocolic, right colic, and right branch of the middle colic vessels require ligation at their origins for adequate oncologic procedures) by retracting the small bowel to the left side to expose the root of the mesentery.
- The ileocolic vessels are located at the caudal portion of the root of the mesentery.
  Identify the superior mesenteric artery to prevent injury or inadvertent ligation.
- Incise the peritoneum over the vascular pedicle and ligate the vessels close to their origins.
- Divide the ileal mesentery between artery hemostats applied serially proximal and distal.
- Protect the wound with abdominal packs and resect the bowel.
- Options for restoring bowel continuity include a side-to-side or an end-to-side anastomosis closure of the mesenteric defect, the abdominal cavity may be irrigated with sterile saline.
- Insert drain if indicated.
- Hemostasis is confirmed and omentum is positioned over the anastomosis, followed by closure [20].

B. **Left hemicolectomy:**

- **General Principles:**
  - It is defined as the removal of the distal one-third of the transverse colon, splenic flexure, descending colon (Fig. 11.6). If extended left hemicolectomy is to be performed include the proximal transverse colon to the splenic flexure (ligate the right branches of the middle colic artery too).
  - Oncological resection is to perform high ligation of mesenteric vessels to include the lymph nodes draining this part of the colon.
  - The required number of harvested lymph node is at least 12 lymph nodes.
  - Preoperative bowel preparation is required for left colon surgery (mechanical and with oral antibiotic).
  - Preoperative ileostomy/colostomy marking (in case it is needed intraoperatively).
  - Two approaches: medial to lateral or lateral to medial.

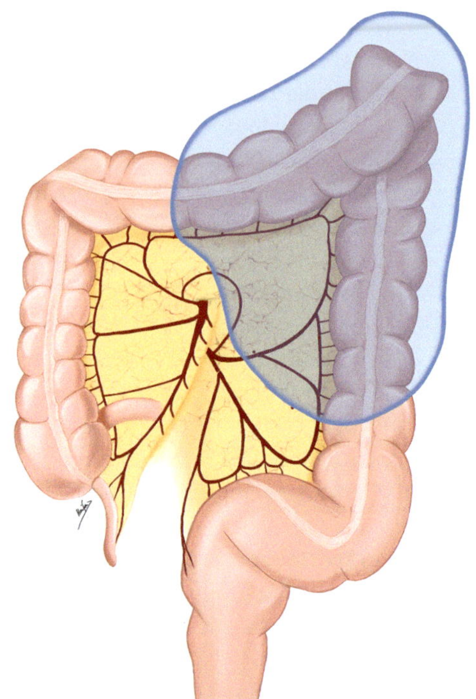

Fig. 11.6 Left hemicolectomy

- **Details of the procedure (open lateral to medial approach):**
  - Under general anesthesia and endotracheal intubation

- Position: The patient is placed in a modified lithotomy position using Allen's stirrups with sequential compression devices in place, bladder catheter in place, and the rectum is irrigated to clear the rectum of any solid stool.
- The abdomen is prepped from the nipple to the symphysis pubis.
- The patient is draped in a sterile fashion.
- Time out: confirm that correct patient, correct procedure, correct site, and all the required instruments are available.
- Incision: midline incision
- Explore all the abdomen and palpate the liver and rest of the colon.
- Bookwalter retractor is placed for exposure and opened widely.
- The small bowel is retracted to the right upper quadrant and upper midline.
- Mobilize the left colon starting at the level of sigmoid until you reach the splenic flexure proximally and the rectosigmoid junction distally. The exposed areolar tissue plane allows dissection anterior to the retroperitoneum. Blunt dissection frees the left colon from the retroperitoneum and exposes the ureter and gonadal vassals.
- The ureter and the gonadal vessels should be identified at this stage crossing the iliac artery. The left kidney and its Gerota's fascia should be visible; then divide the colorenal attachment.
- Free the omentum from the distal 10–12 cm of the transverse colon.
- Now once the lesser sac is exposed, you can use the transverse colon as a guide and divide the Colo pancreatic and colosplenic ligament, now the splenic flexure should be free and fully mobile.
- The left colon is lifted from the abdomen and is pulled to the patient's left, exposing the medial aspect of the left colon mesentery over the aorta.
- The inferior mesenteric artery is encountered at the level of the aorta just above the bifurcation of the common iliac artery. The inferior mesenteric vein (IMV) is identified at the level of the ligament of Treitz at the base of the mesentery of the left colon above a window of clear peritoneum along the anterior surface of the aorta.
- The inferior mesenteric artery and vein are isolated at their origins and divided between ties.
- The left colon is stretched all the way to the pelvis bringing the splenic flexure to near the pelvic brim. This allows the left colon to be evaluated for point of transection removing adequate proximal and distal margins from the lesion.
- Protect the wound and resect the colon.
- Options for restoring bowel continuity include a side-to-side colosigmoid anastomosis, end-to-end colorectal anastomosis or stoma, and close the mesenteric defect.
- The abdominal cavity may be irrigated with sterile saline.
- Insert drain if indicated
- Hemostasis is confirmed and omentum is positioned over the anastomosis, followed by closure [21].

C. **Low anterior resection:**
   - **General principles:**
     - Low anterior resections are performed to treat upper and mid rectal cancer (Fig. 11.7).
     - Assess the quality of the anal sphincter and whether the patient is a candidate for restorative surgery.
     - Adequate preoperative staging of the patient with rectal cancer involves the determination of tumor level from the dentate line, depth of penetration, lymph node involvement, and distant metastases.
     - The timing of surgery after neoadjuvant is 8 weeks.
     - Patients who undergo anterior resection should be informed of specific

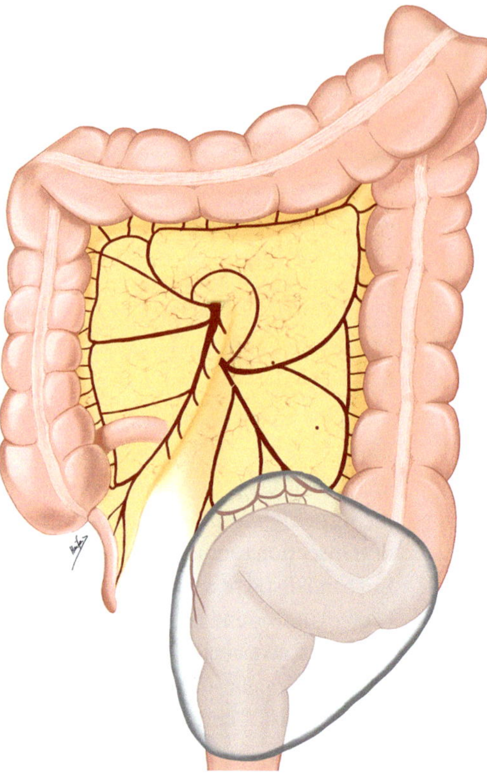

Fig. 11.7 Low anterior resection

risks involved with the surgery, especially potential injuries to the pelvic autonomic nerves resulting in sexual and bladder dysfunction.
  - Patients should have some understanding of function after restorative proctectomy, with an expectation for increased frequency and urgency in the early postoperative period.
  - Patients are seen preoperatively by the enterostomal nurse for stoma education and optimal stoma site marking.
  - The proximal margin is 5 cm while the distal margin can be as little as 2 cm.
  - All patients receive a preoperative full mechanical bowel preparation. Perioperative antibiotics are administered for 24 h.
- **Details of the Procedure:**
  - Under general anesthesia and endotracheal intubation
  - Position: The patient is placed in the modified lithotomy position with careful attention to adequate padding to avoid injury to the peroneal nerve that may result in postoperative foot drop.
  - The abdomen is prepped from nipple to the symphysis pubis.
  - The patient is draped in a sterile fashion.
  - Time out: confirm that correct patient, correct procedure, correct site, and all the required instruments are available.
  - Incision: midline incision
  - Explore all the abdomen and palpate the liver and rest of the colon.
  - Bookwalter retractor is placed for exposure and opened widely.
  - The small bowel is retracted to the right upper quadrant and upper midline.
  - The sigmoid and descending colon are mobilized medially, and the left ureter is identified.
  - The splenic flexure mobilization is facilitated with the operating surgeon standing between the legs of the patient in the modified lithotomy position.
  - The peritoneum on both sides of the rectum is incised at the level of the sacral promontory, with care to avoid injury to the ureters and to the sympathetic nerves.
  - The dissection is carried underneath the superior rectal artery, and the superior rectal artery is dissected to the level of the left colic artery and inferior mesenteric artery.
  - Division at level just inferior to the left colic artery, with preservation to the left colic artery, will result in more predictable blood supply to the anastomosis, but may not give sufficient length especially when most of the sigmoid colon is resected.
  - Proximal division of superior mesenteric artery and vein will typically ensure sufficient length for the anastomosis

- Protect the wound and using GIA 60 stapler transect the colon at the sigmoid colon junction.
- Use the transected sigmoid as a guide by upward and superior traction to guide your dissection toward the rectum and the presacral fascia.
- The proper plane of dissection is initiated by following the posterior aspect of the superior rectal artery until a shiny, filmy membrane is an encounter at the pelvic brim. This plane lies between the fascia propria of the rectum containing the mesorectum and its vessels and lymph nodes and the endopelvic fascia which cover the hypogastric nerves and pelvic plexuses.
- The dissection proceeds posteriorly along this plane, keeping in mind that the fascia propria may be tethered to the presacral fascia at the level of the fourth sacral vertebra.
- At this point, it is important to avoid entering the presacral fascia for fear of injuring the presacral veins, which may result in significant bleeding.
- The dissection is carried posteriorly as far as can be accomplished safely under direct vision. Avoid blunt dissection as this technique may result in a breach of the fascia propria and incomplete mesorectal excision.
- The anterolateral dissection is initiated by incising the peritoneum in the pouch of Douglas and dividing the remaining peritoneum laterally, avoiding injury to the pelvic sidewall and its vessels.
- The anterior dissection is carried out in front of the Denonvillier's fascia, which lies posterior to the prostate and seminal vesicle in males and vault of the vagina in females.
- It is important to recognize that immediately anterior to the Denonvillier's fascia lies the parasympathetic nerve that supplies the corpora and erectile function in males.

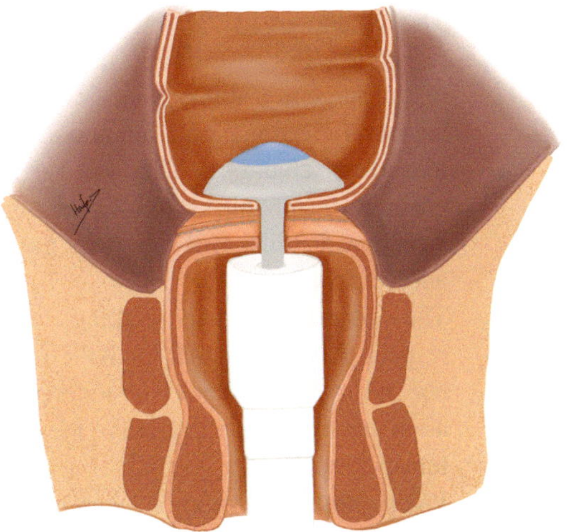

Fig. 11.8 Coloanal anastomosis using a circular stapler

- If there is enough margin (distal resection margin of 1 cm), transect and prepare for the anastomosis.
- Make sure there is no tension, good vascular healthy edges.
- The anastomosis is created with the circular stapler, using the double-stapled technique (Fig. 11.8).
- Test the anastomosis by checking the donut, air-tight test, and by sigmoidoscopy to assess it from inside.
- If indicated, after completion of the anastomosis, a location is selected in the terminal ileum for exteriorization as a diverting loop ileostomy.
- The abdominal cavity may be irrigated with sterile saline
- Insert drain if indicated
- Hemostasis is confirmed followed by closure [22].

D. **Abdominoperineal resection:**

- **General principles**
  - Abdominoperineal resection (APR) is generally performed for patients who have a rectal adenocarcinoma but may also be performed for benign conditions such as inflammatory bowel diseases or incontinence and is sometimes appropriate for other low anorectal and pelvic malignancies or as a salvage procedure for anal canal cancers.

- The choice of APR versus anterior resection (AR) is primarily dependent on the surgeon's ability to achieve distal mural clearance of 2 cm and distal mesorectal clearance of 5 cm and to perform a reliable sphincter-sparing anastomosis that will preserve good anorectal function.
- The ultimate decision-making with respect to selecting AR or APR may not be possible until intraoperative assessment and mobilization of the rectum are complete.
- Preoperative consultation with other specialty colleagues to plan the optimal treatment, achieve the optimal oncologic outcome with the least morbidity, and implement a coordinated and safe operation is essential.
- If there is the involvement of the genitourinary tract or sacrum, preoperative consultation with a urologist, neurosurgeon, or orthopedic surgeon is advised.
- Patients with distal or mid rectal cancer should be seen preoperatively by an enterostomal therapist for counseling and marking of the abdominal wall for any potential stomas. In cases where it is not clear whether the procedure will be an APR versus AR and low anastomosis with a diverting ileostomy, both sides of the abdomen should be marked.
- Perineal wound closure may require plastic surgical consultation to plan a rotational myocutaneous nap.
- Mechanical bowel preparation is required (mechanical and oral antibiotics)

• **Details of the procedure:**
  - Under general anesthesia and endotracheal intubation
  - A bladder catheter is inserted, and a ureteric stent may be used to facilitate the identification of the ureters.
  - Position: the patient is placed in the modified lithotomy position with buttocks brought down to the edge of the table and legs placed into Allen or Yellow Fin stirrups. In general, the hips should be slightly flexed and abducted with feet positioned flat within the stirrups.
  - The abdomen and perineum, including the vagina in females, should be prepped into the field.
  - The patient is draped in a sterile fashion.
  - Time out: confirm that correct patient, correct procedure, correct site, and all the required instruments are available like Bookwalter or Omni-track retractors.
  - Incision: midline incision
  - Explore all the abdomen and palpate the liver and rest of the colon.
  - Bookwalter retractor is placed for exposure and opened widely.
  - The patient is placed in a slightly Trendelenburg position, small bowel is retracted to the right upper quadrant and upper midline.
  - **Step 1: mobilization of the colon**
  - The sigmoid colon is retracted to the right, and the peritoneal attachment to its left is incised along the white line of Toldt distally into the pelvis and proximally as needed to ensure sufficient mobilization so that tension-free end descending colostomy can be created.
  - Left ureter and gonadal vessels are identified and preserved by using sharp and gentle blunt dissection to separate the retroperitoneal tissue from the left colonic mesentery.
  - **Step 2: ligation of inferior mesenteric artery**
  - The mobilized rectosigmoid is retracted anteriorly to the left to expose the inferior mesenteric artery (IMA).
  - Transillumination of the mesentery facilitates the identification of an avascular space adjacent to the IMA at the base of the mesentery.
  - IMA is ligated and divided (there is not enough evidence to recommend high

vs low ligation of IMA in APR over the other).

- The descending-sigmoid junction where the colon is then divided with a linear stapler.
- Step 3: total mesorectal excision and mobilization of the levator
- Use the transected sigmoid as a guide by upward and superior traction to guide your dissection toward the rectum and the presacral fascia.
- The proper plane of dissection is initiated by following the posterior aspect of the superior rectal artery until a shiny, filmy membrane is an encounter at the pelvic brim. This plane lies between the fascia propria of the rectum containing the mesorectum and its vessels and lymph nodes and the endopelvic fascia which cover the hypogastric nerves and pelvic plexuses.
- The dissection proceeds posteriorly along this plane, keeping in mind that the fascia propria may be tethered to the presacral fascia at the level of the fourth sacral vertebra.
- At this point, it is important to avoid entering the presacral fascia for fear of injuring the presacral veins, which may result in significant bleeding.
- The dissection is carried posteriorly as far as can be accomplished safely under direct vision. Avoid blunt dissection as this technique may result in a breach of the fascia propria and incomplete mesorectal excision.
- The anterolateral dissection is initiated by incising the peritoneum in the pouch of Douglas and dividing the remaining peritoneum laterally, avoiding injury to the pelvic sidewall and its vessels.
- The anterior dissection is carried out in front of the Denonvillier's fascia, which lies posterior to the prostate and seminal vesicle in males and vault of vagina in females.
- It is important to recognize that immediately anterior to the Denonvillier's fascia lies the parasympathetic nerve that supplies the corpora and erectile function in males.
- The dissection is stopped at the proximal level of the levator muscles just as the mesorectum begins to taper and thin
- This transition is usually occurring at the level of the fifth sacral vertebra. At this level, the rectum is mobilized in the posterior to lateral direction.
- A conscious effort is made to avoid dissecting centrally into the pelvis along the levator or distally beyond the proximal levator
- As the pelvic surgeon initiates the perineal dissection as described below, the abdominal surgeon may proceed with additional distal dissection and complete the abdominal part of the procedure.
- End colostomy is created.
- Step 4: Perineal dissection
- The anus is closed with a purse-string suture to minimize the risk of spillage into the operative field.
- In the absence of local spread beyond the anorectum, the landmarks used for dissection include the coccyx posteriorly, the perineal body anteriorly, and the ischial tuberosities laterally.
- An elliptical incision is made incorporating these landmarks.
- A Lone Star retractor is placed to separate the skin edges and the incision is deepened to the level of the ischiorectal fat bilaterally.
- Branches of the inferior rectal vessels within the ischiorectal fossa typically can be controlled with electrocautery.
- To assure adequate lateral clearance and avoid the "waist" problem, the surgeon directs the dissection in each ischiorectal fossa through the fat to the levator ani muscles laterally and the coccyx posteriorly.
- The posterior dissection is performed first beginning in the midline, leaving

the more challenging anterior dissection until last.

- The anorectum is retracted anteriorly, and the postanal space is entered by sharply dividing the anococcygeal ligament at the tip of the coccyx. If needed for exposure, a coccygectomy can easily be done usually with electrocautery and heavy scissors or a periosteal elevator.
- Once the true pelvis is entered posteriorly, a finger can be inserted to "hook" the levator ani muscles, which are then divided along the pelvic bone posterolaterally and then laterally.
- While some surgeons divide the muscle with cautery, some prefer to maintain absolute hemostasis by either using the LigaSure device or by clamping, dividing, and suture ligating the coccygeus, iliococcygeus, pubococcygeus, and puborectalis.
- At this point in the operation, the perineal dissection has merged with the previously performed abdominal presacral dissection. The lateral resection margin is extended anterolaterally. When about two-thirds of the planned resection is complete, we generally find it convenient to retrieve the mobilized rectosigmoid with the attached drain and gently deliver it through the large posterior pelvic wound.
- This maneuver provides better exposure for the remaining anterior dissection, which is often the most challenging part of the APR.
- The anterior perineal incision is deepened using the posterior border of the superficial transversa perineal muscle as the guide to the rectoprostatic or rectovaginal plana.
- Allis clamps are used to maintain countertraction between the perineal body anteriorly and the everted specimen posteriorly as the surgeon develops the anterior dissection plane.
- The rectovaginal septum is dissected proximally, often with a guiding digit in the vagina to avoid inadvertent vaginal perforation.
- In a male patient, anterior dissection is facilitated by palpating the Foley catheter to help avoid injury to the urethra and the prostate. The median raphe of the rectourethralis and puborectalis is divided, and the remaining attachments are divided.
- Step 5: perineal wound closure
- The pelvis is irrigated, and the hemostasis is ensured.
- The transabdominal drain is trimmed to fit into the pelvis, and the abdomen is closed.
- Primary perineal wound closure may be undertaken in several layers with 2-0 and 3-0 absorbable sutures, but, because the levator muscles were divided laterally along with the pelvic bones, it is only possible to re-approximate the subcutaneous tissues and the skin. This excision leaves a large "dead space" deep in the pelvis that predisposes to postoperative morbidity.
- To overcome the perineal wound morbidity, we increasingly use myocutaneous flaps [23].

E. **End colostomy creation:**
   - A circular incision (2.5 cm in diameter) is made at the previously marked stoma site, usually in the left lower quadrant of the abdominal wall.
   - A folded lap pad is placed on the underside of the abdominal beneath the stoma site and pushed upwards.
   - The skin aperture, subcutaneous tissue, and fascia are kept in alignment to create a straight tract.
   - The subcutaneous fat is cored out or separated to expose the anterior rectus fascia that is opened in cruciate incision.
   - The rectus muscle is split with a clamp to expose the posterior rectus fascia, which is then opened to create the aperture of ade-

quate size (typically two finger breadths) to accommodate passage of the appropriate mobilized descending colon.

- A Babcock clamp is placed through the aperture to deliver the staple-closed end of the descending colon through the abdominal wall.
- Care should be taken to avoid twisting the colonic mesentery.
- Tension-free elevation of the descending colon 2–3 cm above the skin level is ideal to ensure that an adequate stoma can be created.
- Once the fascia and skin have been closed, the stapled end of the colon is opened, and the edges of the stoma are sutured to the skin using 3-0 (Vicryl) [23].

Postoperative follow-up:
Early postoperative:

- NPO and resume the diet gradually once possible
- Monitor the vital signs
- Encourage mobilization
- Consider early removal of foley's catheter and NGT
- Encourage use of incentive spirometry
- Analgesia, antibiotic as indicated, stress ulcer & DVT prophylaxis
- Stoma care when indicated

Before discharge make sure that:

- The patient has no significant complaint
- Tolerating oral diet
- Stoma is functioning
- Check the wound status
- If the patient has a stoma, he/she should be seen by the enterostomal nurse.

First outpatient visit:

- Clinical assessment
- Examine the wound and remove the sutures
- Review the final pathology result
- Discuss in a multidisciplinary team when the pathology is cancer
- Genetic counseling if indicated

Long-term follow-up (cancer patients)

- History, physical examination, and CEA every 3 months for 2 years and then every 6 months for the next 3 years.
- Annual CT CAP
- Colonoscopy after 1 year (6 months if was not completed preoperative) and then every 3 years if normal

11.2 Part II: Practice

Case No. 1:
A 49-year-old male patient presented to an outpatient clinic due to blackish discoloration of stool and fatigue for 3 months

Questions for discussion:

1. How will you approach the patient?
2. What will you do next?
3. What will be your next step?
4. How will you manage the patient?
5. How will you prepare the patient for operation?
6. The patient underwent an uneventful right hemicolectomy with ileocolic anastomosis and discharge home after few days of hospitalization. How will you follow the patient postoperatively (short term)?
7. The final pathology report shows poorly differentiated adenocarcinoma of the cecum, 5 × 6 cm in its greatest dimensions, that invade through but not beyond the muscularis propria with lymphovascular and perineural invasion. Four out of 13 lymph nodes were positive for metastasis. What further management you should over the patient?
8. How will you follow the patient (long term)?
9. After 2 years of follow-up, you discover a single liver lesion about 2 × 2 cm at segment II. How will you manage that?

Case No. 2:

A 52-year-old female patient presented to the emergency department complaining of left-sided abdominal pain for 2 days

Questions for discussion:

1. How will you approach the patient?
2. What is your differential diagnosis?
3. How will you investigate that?
4. What is your most likely diagnosis?
5. Laboratory investigation and the requested imaging as given. What will be your management?
6. How will you follow the response to your management?
7. The follow-up CT scan shows resolution of the collection with residual mass at the descending colon-sigmoid junction with multiple abnormal pericolic mesenteric lymph nodes. What will you do?
8. The biopsy shows adenocarcinoma of the colon, what will you do?
9. Staging CT scan is negative, and the CEA is 339 ng/ml. What is the clinical stage for this patient?
10. How will you manage the patient?
11. How will you prepare her for OR?
12. She underwent left hemicolectomy with colorectal anastomosis and the final pathology report shows a T4 poorly differentiated adenocarcinoma of the colon measuring 5 × 2 cm in its greater dimensions. Lymphovascular and perineural invasion are seen. Seven out of 13 lymph nodes harvested were positive for malignancy. What further management should you consider for this patient?

Case No. 3:

A 77-year-old male patient presented to the emergency department complaining of abdominal pain and constipation for 4 days

Questions for discussion:

1. How will you approach the patient?
2. What will you do next?
3. How will you manage the patient?
4. The endoscopic detorsion of the colon was successful. What will be your definitive management?
5. The patient underwent uneventful sigmoid resection with primary colorectal anastomosis. Seven days post-operative he has discharge from the wound that is brown in color and has a bad smell. What will you do?
6. How to confirm the most likely diagnosis?
7. How to manage that?

Case No. 4:

A 44-year-old male patient presented to the outpatient clinic complaining of bleeding per rectum for 1 month.

Questions for discussion:

1. How will you approach the patient?
2. How will you confirm the most likely diagnosis?
3. What will you do?
4. How will you manage this patient?
5. The patient completed his neoadjuvant chemoradiation and referred back to surgery. What will you do?
6. Intraoperative you could not achieve distal 1 cm free margin without compromising the anal sphincter. What will you do?
7. What are the possible complications?

Case No. 5:

A 23-year-old female patient presented to the clinic asking for screening as she noticed multiple cases of colorectal cancer in her family.

Questions for discussion:

1. How will you approach the patient?
2. What will you do next?
3. How will you manage this patient?
4. What further screening is required for such a patient?
5. She underwent an uneventful total proctocolectomy with ileal pouch-anal anastomosis. Two years later she presented to the ER with a picture of bowel obstruction. What could be the cause?

6. CT abdomen reveals presence of intrabdominal mass, near the root of the mesentery that causing obstruction to the small bowel. How will you manage that?

Case No. 6:
A 35-year-old male patient presented to the emergency department complaining of constipation, abdominal distention, and vomiting.

Questions for discussion:

1. How will you approach the patient?
2. How will you investigate the patient?
3. What could be the cause of the patient's symptoms?
4. How you will manage that?
5. What are the possible complications?

Checklist

History	Items	Done	Not done	Not applicable
General	Introduce himself/herself to the patient			
	Patient personal data (name, age, gender, nationality)			
	Chief complaint			
	Duration			
Pain	Onset			
	Site			
	Character			
	Radiation/shifting			
	Aggravating/relieving			
	Severity			
	Progression			
	Frequency			
Mass	Onset			
	Site			
	How did the patient notice it?			
	Any change since it was first noticed?			
	Other masses			
Bleeding per rectum	Onset			
	Amount			
	Relation to defecation			
	Fresh blood, clotted or melena			
	Another bleeding site			
Associated symptoms	Pain			
	Fever			
	Nausea			
	Vomiting			
	Diarrhea			
	Constipation			
	Abdominal distention			
	Jaundice			
Constitutional symptoms	Weight loss			
	Decrease appetite			
	Night sweating			

(continued)

History	Items	Done	Not done	Not applicable
Symptoms of metastases	Back pain			
	Cough			
	Shortness of breath			
	Abdominal distention			
Risk factors	Diet			
	Smoking			
	Family history of colon cancer (if yes, at what age and the degree of relationship)			
	Family history of IBD			
	Personal history of IBD			
Differential diagnosis	Urinary symptoms			
	Gynecological symptoms in female			
PMH	Previous similar attack			
	Previous investigation or colonoscopy			
	Previous admission			
	Chronic illnesses			
PSH	Previous surgery			
Family history	Of similar complain			
Social history	Occupation			
	Habits (smoking, alcohol, drugs)			
Other	Medication			
	Allergy			
	Transfusion			
Systemic review				
Physical examination				
General principle	Patient position			
	Exposure			
	Privacy			
	Wash hands			
General examination	Appearance			
	Body built			
	Color			
	Distress/decubitus			
	Environment			
Vital signs	BP, HR, Temperature, RR, SPO_2			
Hand signs	leukonychia, koilonychia, pallor			
Eyes	Jaundice, pallor			
Neck	Lymphadenopathy			
Chest	Respiratory and CVS examination			
Abdomen: Inspection	Distention			
	Asymmetry			
	Dilated veins			
	Striae			
	Visible peristalsis			
	Scars			
Palpation	Superficial then deep palpation			
	Tenderness			
	Palpable masses			
	Organomegaly			

History	Items	Done	Not done	Not applicable
Percussion	Shifting dullness			
	Fluid thrill			
Auscultation	Bowel sounds			
	Bruit, venous hum			
Groin and hernial orifices examination				
DRE and proctoscopy:				
If there is any palpable mass in the anorectal	Amount of the circumference involved			
	Site (anterior, posterior, and lateral)			
	Consistency			
	Distance from the anal verge			
Back tenderness				
Extraintestinal manifestations	Erythema nodosum			
	Arthritis			
	Sacroiliitis			
	Ankylosing spondylitis			
Differential diagnosis	According to the given scenario.			
Investigations				
General laboratory test	CBC with differential			
	Electrolytes			
	Liver function test			
	Blood grouping			
	Coagulation profile (PT, INR, aPTT)			
	RFT			
	CPR/ESR			
	Blood culture			
Specific tests	Tumor marker (CEA)			
	Fecal calprotectin			
	Serology (ANCA, PANCA, ASCA)			
	Stool analysis			
	Toxin A and B for *Clostridium Difficile*			
Imaging	X-ray			
	CT abdomen/CT staging			
	MRI pelvis			
	Endorectal ultrasound			
Endoscopy	Colonoscopy			
Biopsy	Biopsy/polypectomy			
Provisional diagnosis	According to the given scenario			
Management (depend on the diagnosis):				
IBD (fulminant colitis, toxic colitis, toxic megacolon)	Admission			
	NPO			
	IV fluid			
	Antibiotics			
	IV steroid			
	Antipyretic			
	Prophylaxis (DVT and stress ulcer)			
	If the patient did not improve or has toxic megacolon; surgical management			
	Consent			
	Stoma marking			
	Total colectomy with end ileostomy			

(continued)

History	Items	Done	Not done	Not applicable
IBD (elective surgery)	Admission			
	NPO			
	Bowel preparation			
	Prophylactic (antibiotic, DVT, stress ulcer)			
	Stress does of steroid if indicated			
	Consent			
	Stoma marking			
	Surgery (total proctocolectomy with end ileostomy, total proctocolectomy with IPAA)			
Non complicated diverticulitis	Admission/outpatient			
	NPO if required			
	IV fluid			
	Analgesia			
	DVT and stress ulcer prophylaxis			
	IV antibiotics			
	Elective colonoscopy after 4–6 weeks			
	Surgical management if indicated			
Complicated diverticulitis	Admission			
	NPO			
	IV fluid			
	Analgesia			
	DVT and stress ulcer prophylaxis			
	IV antibiotics			
	CT guided drainage if Hinchey I or II then elective resection			
	Hartmann's procedure if Hinchey III or IV			
Ischemic colitis	Bowel rest			
	Aggressive fluid resuscitation			
	Empirical antibiotics			
	Serial abdominal X-ray to follow dilatation			
	Surgery if indicated			
Clostridium Difficile colitis	Stop antibiotics			
	Metronidazole 500 mg TID for 14 days or Vancomycin tablet 125 mg QID for 10 days			
	Surgery when indicated			
Colonic volvulus	Admission			
	NPO			
	IV fluid			
	IV antibiotics			
	NGT			
	Foley's catheter			
	Analgesia			
	Endoscopic detorsion if the sigmoid volvulus			
	Stoma marking			
	Exploration if cecal or if there is peritonitis or failed endoscopy			
	Resection/fixation			
	Primary anastomosis or stoma			

History	Items	Done	Not done	Not applicable
Management of lower GI bleeding	Assure patency of the airway			
	Oxygenation and ventilation			
	Insert two large cannulas			
	Draw blood for investigations			
	Start IV fluid and blood transfusion			
	Rule out local cause			
	Rule out upper GI cause (NG aspirate)			
	Localization: Colonoscopy, tagged RBCs scan, angiography			
	Manage according to the cause			
Colon cancer	Admission			
	Multidisciplinary team discussion			
	CEA level			
	Staging			
	Complete colonic evaluation (colonoscopy or CT colonography)			
	o Prepare the patient for OR			
	o Anesthesia consultation			
	o ICU consultation			
	o Prepare blood stand by			
	o Consent			
	o NPO			
	o IV fluid			
	o Prophylactic antibiotic			
	o DVT and stress ulcer prophylaxis			
	o Colonic preparation			
	o Stoma marking			
	o Ureteric stent			
	o Resection (according to the site)			
	o Reconstruction			
	Adjuvant treatment as needed			
Rectal carcinoma	MRI pelvis			
	Endorectal ultrasound			
	CEA			
	Staging			
	Multidisciplinary team discussion			
	If the decision is resection:			
	o Prepare the patient for OR			
	o Anesthesia consultation			
	o ICU consultation			
	o Prepare blood stand by			
	o Consent			
	o NPO			
	o IV fluid			
	o Prophylactic antibiotic			
	o Ureteric stent			
	o Colonic preparation			
	o Stoma marking			
	o Surgery (APR vs LAR)			

(continued)

History	Items	Done	Not done	Not applicable
Metastatic colorectal tumor	If the decision is neoadjuvant chemoradiation:			
	o Refer to oncology and radiotherapy			
	o Re-evaluation			
	o Re-staging			
	o Prepare for operation			
	o Surgery (LAR vs APR)			
Postoperative care				
Early postoperative	Admission to HDU or ICU			
	Early mobilization and DVT prophylaxis			
	Enteral nutrition as early as possible			
	Analgesia			
	Stress ulcer prophylaxis			
	CBC and LFT daily			
	Electrolyte assessment			
	Monitor drain output and the nature of the fluid			
	Monitor the stoma itself and its output			
First outpatient visit	Clinical assessment			
	Remove sutures			
	Review the final pathology report			
	Arrange for multidisciplinary discussion if the case is cancer			
	Refer to oncology if adjuvant treatment is required			
Long term follow-up (for cancer)	History and physical examination and CEA level every 3 months for 2 years then every 6 months for the next 3 years			
	Annual CT CAP			
	Colonoscopy after 1 year (6 months if not completed preoperatively) then every 3 years if normal			

11.2.1 Answer Key

Case No. 1:

A 49-year-old male patient presented to the outpatient clinic due to blackish discoloration of stool and fatigue for 3 months.

Questions for discussion:

1. **How will you approach the patient?**
   Starting by obtaining a relevant history and performing a physical examination

   He is a 49-year-old male patient who presented to the surgery clinic due to melena for 3 months. It was on and off, increasing in frequency over the last month. It is associated with mild right-sided abdominal pain, generalized fatigability, dyspnea, and shortness of breath with exertion. He lost about 15 kg of his weight over the last 2 months. He has no history of hematemesis or bleeding from other sites.

   He is not on any anticoagulant or antiplatelet. His mother died of colon cancer when she was 59 years old. He is not known to have any chronic medical illness and has no previous surgical history.

   On examination:

   He is underweight, pale.

Table 11.3 Blood test for case 1

Test	Result	Normal value
WBC (k/ul)	7	4.8–10.8
HB (g/dl)	7	12.6–16.5
PLT (K/ul)	150	130–400
ALT (U/l)	120	10–130
AST (U/l)	31	10–34
Total bilirubin (mg/dl)	0.7	0–0.8
Direct bilirubin (mg/dl)	0.2	0–0.3
Albumin (g/dl)	3.6	2.4–4
Creatinine (mg/dl)	1	0.7–1.2
PT (seconds)	12	10–13
INR	1	1

Vital signs were stable.

The abdomen was soft with mild tenderness with deep palpation over the right iliac fossa.

DRE reveals no palpable masses but there was a black stool on the examiner's gloved finger.

2. **What will you do next?**

   Start investigation by sending for CBC, blood grouping, coagulation profile, LFT, RFT, and colonoscopy

   Blood test: Table 11.3

   Colonoscopy shows fungating mass at the cecum with ulceration and minimal bleeding. The rest of the colon was normal. Biopsy was taken and showed poorly differentiated adenocarcinoma.

3. **What will be your next step?**

   CT CAP for staging and CEA level

   CT shows soft tissue density narrowing the lumen of the cecum with enlarged multiple pericolic lymph nodes. No signs of extracolonic extension or signs of liver or pulmonary or peritoneal metastasis

   CEA is 345 ng/ml.

4. **How will you manage the patient?**
   - Multidisciplinary team discussion
   - Break the bad news to the patient.
   - Inform the patient about the management plan.
   - This patient needs right hemicolectomy.

5. **How will you prepare the patient for operation?**
   - Admission
   - Consent
   - NPO
   - IV fluid
   - DVT and stress ulcer prophylaxis
   - Prophylactic antibiotic
   - Bowel preparation (not necessarily for right-side colon surgery)
   - Confirm the availability of blood intraoperative if needed
   - Anesthesia consultation
   - ICU consultation if required
   - Instruct the patient to take shower the night before surgery
   - Stoma marking
   - Hair removal

6. **The patient underwent an uneventful right hemicolectomy with ileocolic anastomosis and discharge home after few days of hospitalization. How will you follow the patient post-operatively (short term)?**
   - **Early post-operative:**
     - NPO and resume the diet gradually once possible.
     - Monitor the vital signs.
     - Encourage mobilization.
     - Consider early removal of foley's catheter and NGT.
     - Encourage use of incentive spirometry.
     - Analgesia, antibiotic as indicated, stress ulcer and DVT prophylaxis
   - **Before discharge that:**
     - The patient has no significant complaint.
     - Tolerating oral diet
     - Check the wound status.
   - **First outpatient visit:**
     - Clinical assessment
     - Examine the wound and remove the sutures.
     - Review the final pathology result.
     - Discuss with a multidisciplinary team when the pathology is cancer.
     - Genetic counseling if indicated

7. **The final pathology report shows poor differentiated adenocarcinoma of the cecum, 5 × 6 cm in its greatest dimensions, that invade through but not beyond the muscularis propria with lymphovascular and perineural invasion. Four out of 13 lymph nodes were positive for metastasis. What further management should you over the patient?**
   - Multidisciplinary team approach
   - Inform the patient about the final result and the management plan and long-term follow-up.
   - He will need a referral to oncology to start adjuvant chemotherapy.
8. **How will you follow the patient (long term)?**
   - History, physical examination, and CEA every 3 months for 2 years and then every 6 months for the next 3 years.
   - Annual CT CAP
   - Colonoscopy after 1 year (6 months if was not completed preoperative) and then every 3 years if normal
9. **After 2 years of follow-up, you discover a single liver lesion about 2 × 2 cm at segment II. How will you manage that?**
   - Multidisciplinary team approach
   - Rule out local recurrence.
   - Refer to hepatobiliary surgery for assessment and management.

Case No. 2:

A 52-year-old female patient presented to the emergency department complaining of left-sided abdominal pain for 2 days

Questions for discussion:

1. **How will you approach the patient?**
   By taking a relevant history and performing a physical examination. The patient is a 52-year-old female patient who presented to the emergency department complaining of 2 days history of left lower dull aching abdominal pain that was not radiated or shifted elsewhere. It was associated with undocumented fever and multiple attacks of vomiting. She has a history of chronic constipation and weight loss. No history of lower or upper GI bleeding. No family or personal history of malignancy. No urinary or gynecological symptoms. She is diabetic on insulin and previous surgical history of appendectomy 30 years ago.

   On physical examination

   She was an underweight mid-aged female, looks sick.

   Her vital signs (BP: 123/78, PR: 114 bpm, Temperature: 38.9)

   Abdomen is soft with localized tenderness at the left iliac fossa
2. **What is your differential diagnosis?**
   - Diverticulitis
   - Infectious colitis
   - Inflammatory bowel disease
   - Clostridium difficile colitis
   - Colonic Neoplasm
   - Pelvic inflammatory disease
   - UTI
3. **How will you investigate that?**
   Blood investigation, urine analysis, erect CXR, CT abdomen with IV and oral contrast

   Blood investigation: Table 11.4

   Urine analysis and CXR are normal

   CT scan shows pericolic fat stranding around the sigmoid colon with thickening of that segment of the colon. There is a large area of fluid collection that was located retroperitoneally, about 5 × 6 cm with foci of air seen inside the collection. There is no pneumoperitoneum.

Table 11.4 Blood test for Case 2

Test	Result	Normal value
WBC (k/ul)	23	4.8–10.8
HB (g/dl)	10	12.6–16.5
PLT (K/ul)	158	130–400
ALT (U/l)	126	10–130
AST (U/l)	31	10–34
Total bilirubin (mg/dl)	1	0–0.8
Direct bilirubin (mg/dl)	0.2	0–0.3
Albumin (g/dl)	3.6	2.4–4
Creatinine (mg/dl)	1	0.7–1.2
PT (seconds)	12	10–13
INR	1	1
Glucose (mg/dl)	443	90–110

4. **What is your most likely diagnosis?**
   Complicated diverticulitis Hinchey II
5. **How will you manage that?**
   - Admission
   - NPO
   - IV fluid
   - IV antibiotics
   - Analgesia, antiemetic
   - DVT and stress ulcer prophylaxis
   - CT guided percutaneous drainage of the collection
6. **How will you follow the response to your management?**
   Follow-up CT scan
7. **The follow-up CT scan shows resolution of the collection with residual mass at the descending colon-sigmoid junction with multiple abnormal pericolic mesenteric lymph nodes. What will you do?**
   Colonoscopy and biopsy
   Colonoscopy shows a non-obstructing, ulcerated mass at the posterior wall of the sigmoid colon about 40 cm from the anal verge. The rest of the colon was normal. Biopsy was taken.
8. **The biopsy shows adenocarcinoma of the colon, what will you do?**
   - Staging CT CAP
   - CEA level
   - Multidisciplinary team approach
   - Break the bad news to the patient.
   - Inform her about the plan of the management.
9. **Staging CT scan is negative, and the CEA is 339 ng/ml. What is the clinical stage for this patient?**
   Stage III
10. **How will you manage the patient?**
    Left hemicolectomy with sigmoidectomy
11. **How will you prepare her for OR?**
    - Consent
    - NPO
    - IV fluid
    - DVT and stress ulcer prophylaxis
    - Prophylactic antibiotic
    - Bowel preparation
    - Confirm the availability of blood intraoperative if needed
    - Anesthesia consultation
    - ICU consultation if required
    - Ureteric stent
    - Instruct the patient to take shower the night before surgery.
    - Stoma marking
    - Hair removal
12. **She underwent a left hemicolectomy with colorectal anastomosis and the final pathology report shows a T4 poorly differentiated adenocarcinoma of the colon measuring 5 × 2 cm in its greater dimensions. Lymphovascular and perineural invasion are seen. Seven out of 13 lymph nodes harvested were positive for malignancy. What further management you should consider for this patient?**
    - Multidisciplinary team approach
    - Inform the patient about the final result and the management plan and long-term follow-up.
    - She will need a referral to oncology to start adjuvant chemotherapy.

Case No. 3:

A 77-year-old male patient presented to the emergency department complaining of abdominal pain and constipation for 4 days.

Questions for discussion:

1. **How will you approach the patient?**
   By taking a history and performing a physical examination

   The patient is a 77-year-old male patient known to have Alzheimer's disease and was brought by his son due to colicky lower abdominal pain for the last 4 days that was started gradually. It is associated with nausea and vomiting multiple times. He has a history of constipation for 4 days and his usual bowel habit is mostly constipation.

   There is no history of weight loss, no family or personal history of malignancy.

   On examination:

   He was conscious but disoriented, looks dehydrated.

   Vital signs: BP: 110/78 P: 99 bpm, Temperature: 37.4 °C

Table 11.5 Blood test for Case 3

Test	Result	Normal value
WBC (k/ul)	13	4.8–10.8
HB (g/dl)	14	12.6–16.5
PLT (K/ul)	329	130–400
ALT (U/l)	126	10–130
AST (U/l)	31	10–34
Total bilirubin (mg/dl)	0.7	0–0.8
Direct bilirubin (mg/dl)	0.2	0–0.3
Albumin (g/dl)	3.6	2.4–4
Creatinine (mg/dl)	1	0.7–1.2
PT (seconds)	12	10–13
INR	1	1
K (mEq/l)	3.2	3.5–5.1
Na (mEq/l)	135	135–145
Mg (mEq/l)	1.4	1.4–2.1

Abdomen is hugely distended, soft with mild tenderness all over but no peritonitis or rigidity. Tympanic on percussion

DRE: reveals empty rectum

2. **What will you do next?**

   Blood test, CXR erect, AXR erect and supine

   Blood test: Table 11.5

   CXR: unremarkable

   AXR: shows dilated loop of colon arising from the left iliac fossa with a demonstration of coffee bean sign.

3. **How will you manage the patient?**
   - Admission
   - NGT/foley's catheter
   - IV fluid
   - Correct electrolytes imbalance
   - IV antibiotics
   - Analgesia and antiemetic
   - DVT prophylaxis
   - Prepare for endoscopic detorsion
4. **The endoscopic detorsion of the colon was successful. What will be your definitive management?**

   Resection of the sigmoid colon with primary anastomosis
5. **The patient underwent uneventful sigmoid resection with primary colorectal anastomosis. Seven days post-operative he has discharge from the wound that is brown in color and has a bad smell. What will you do?**
   - Open few stitches to drain the collection
   - Send wound swab for culture and sensitivity.
   - Monitor the output.
   - Replace fluid deficit.
6. **How to confirm the most likely diagnosis?**

   CT abdomen with IV and rectal contrast to rule out a deep collection, anastomotic leak and define the anatomy of the fistula if present
7. **How to manage that?**
   - Control sepsis
   - Nutrition (enteral if the patient tolerated or parenteral)
   - Monitor the output
   - Wound care
   - Most likely the fistula will close spontaneously within few weeks. If did not close, surgical management by taking down the fistula and reform the anastomosis.

Case No. 4:

A 44-year-old male patient presented to the outpatient clinic complaining of bleeding per rectum for 1 month.

Questions for discussion:

1. **How will you approach the patient?**

   By taking a history and perform a physical examination

   The patient is a 44-year-old male patient who is complaining of multiple times of fresh bleeding per rectum, that starts with defection and continues for sometimes after that. It is associated with tenesmus and decrease stool caliber. He has no history of abdominal or anal pain. No history of any anal swelling or any other bleeding site.

   He lost about 18 kg of his weight in 1 month.

   No family or personal history of malignancy.

   He is not known to have any chronic medical illnesses and he is not on any regular medications.

   On examination

   He was conscious, oriented.

   Vital signs within the normal range

   The abdomen is not distended, soft, with no tenderness, organomegaly, or ascites

   DRE reveals a normal anal tone, no palpable masses.

Table 11.6 Blood test for Case 4

Test	Result	Normal value
WBC (k/ul)	10	4.8–10.8
HB (g/dl)	14	12.6–16.5
PLT (K/ul)	229	130–400
ALT (U/l)	126	10–130
AST (U/l)	31	10–34
Total bilirubin (mg/dl)	0.6	0–0.8
Direct bilirubin (mg/dl)	0.2	0–0.3
Albumin (g/dl)	3.6	2.4–4
Creatinine (mg/dl)	1	0.7–1.2
PT (seconds)	12	10–13
INR	1	1
K (mEq/l)	3.6	3.5–5.1
Na (mEq/l)	135	135–145
Mg (mEq/l)	1.4	1.4–2.1

Proctoscopy shows mass at the anterior wall of the rectum that easily bleed when touched.

2. **How will you confirm the most likely diagnosis?**
   Blood investigation, MRI pelvis, and colonoscopy
   Blood test: Table 11.6
   MRI pelvis shows hyperintense mass at the anterior wall of the rectum 6 cm from the anal rim. It is about 4 cm long and 1 cm thick and extends to the muscular layer. Multiple abnormal pelvic lymph nodes are noted.
   The colonoscopy shows an ulcerated mass at the anterior wall of the rectum at the level of the lower rectum. The rest of the colon is free.
   Biopsy was taken and shows moderately differentiated adenocarcinoma.
3. **What will you do?**
   Staging CT CAP: negative
   CEA level: 200 ng/ml
4. **How will you manage this patient?**
   - Multidisciplinary team approach
   - Break the bad news to the patient.
   - Inform the patient about the management plan.
   - Neoadjuvant chemoradiation followed by surgery
5. **The patient completed his neoadjuvant chemoradiation and referred back to surgery. What will you do?**
   - Repeat pelvic MRI
   - Re-staging
   - Prepare for operation (low anterior resection + diverting loop ileostomy) with the possibility of APR if necessary.
6. **Intraoperative you could not achieve distal 1 cm free margin without compromising the anal sphincter. What will you do?**
   Abdominoperineal resection with permanent end colostomy
7. **What are the possible complications?**
   - General: DVT, PE, atelectasis, pneumonia, MI
   - Specific: bleeding, infection, collection, anastomotic leak, injury to the ureter, autonomic nerves injury recurrence and metachronous metastasis and stoma complications

Case No. 5:
A 23-year-old female patient presented to the clinic asking for screening as she noticed multiple cases of colorectal cancer in her family.

Questions for discussion:

1. **How will you approach the patient?**
   Start with history and physical examination
   She is a 23-year-old female patient who has no active complaint. Her mother diagnosed with colon cancer at age of 50 years and her brother recently discovered to have multiple colonic polyps with a degree of dysplasia detected by histological examination.
   She is otherwise healthy with no PSH.
   Physical examination was normal.
2. **What will you do next?**
   Screening colonoscopy
   Genetic testing
   Screening colonoscopy shows diffuse colonic polyposis affecting the entire colon. Multiple biopsies were taken but did not show any malignancy (low-grade adenomas).
   Genetic testing was positive for APC mutation.
3. **How will you manage this patient?**
   Total proctocolectomy with ileorectal anastomosis or IPAA
4. **What further screening is required for such a patient?**
   Upper GI endoscopy

5. **She underwent an uneventful total proctocolectomy with ileal pouch-anal anastomosis. Two years later she presented to the ER with a picture of bowel obstruction. What could be the cause?**
   - Adhesions
   - Desmoid tumor
   - Hernia
6. **CT abdomen reveals the presence of intrabdominal mass near the root of the mesentery that causing obstruction to the small bowel. How will you manage that?**
   Non-resective procedure like bypass or ileostomy

Case No. 6:

A 35-year-old male patient presented to the emergency department complaining of constipation, abdominal distention, and vomiting

Questions for discussion:

1. **How will you approach the patient?**
   A 35-year-old male patient presented to the emergency department complaining of colicky abdominal pain that was started gradually 3 days ago and is associated with abdominal distention, nausea, and vomiting more than four times. It is also associated with constipation for the same period of time. His usual bowel habit is alternating between diarrhea and constipation. He had one attack of bloody diarrhea last month.

   He has history of weight loss despite normal appetite.

   He is not known to have any chronic illnesses and his PSH is positive for incision and drainage of perianal abscess twice during the last year.

   On examination:

   He looks dehydrated, cachectic

   Vital signs BP: 118/70, PR: 98 bpm, Temperature: 37.1

   Abdomen: distended, soft with mild tenderness during deep palpation over the left side of the abdomen

   Bowel sound is hyperactive

   DRE: scars of the two previous procedures. No bleeding or masses.

Table 11.7 Blood test for Case 6

Test	Result	Normal value
WBC (k/ul)	9	4.8–10.8
HB (g/dl)	13	12.6–16.5
PLT (K/ul)	229	130–400
ALT (U/l)	126	10–130
AST (U/l)	31	10–34
Total bilirubin (mg/dl)	0.7	0–0.8
Direct bilirubin (mg/dl)	0.3	0–0.3
Albumin (g/dl)	2	2.4–4
Creatinine (mg/dl)	1	0.7–1.2
PT (seconds)	12	10–13
INR	1	1
ESR (mm/h)	33	<15
CRP (mg/dl)	69	<3
K (mEq/l)	3.1	3.5–5.1
Na (mEq/l)	135	135–145
Mg (mEq/l)	1.4	1.4–2.1

2. **How will you investigate the patient?**
   Blood test: Table 11.7

   CT abdomen: there is a segmental narrowing of the descending colon causing large bowel obstruction.
3. **What could be the cause of the patient's symptoms?**
   Stricture or neoplasm secondary to IBD
4. **How you will manage that?**
   Surgical exploration

   Resection of the diseased segment to rule out malignancy or IBD
5. **What are the possible complications?**
   Bleeding, infection, leak, fistula, collection, recurrence, adhesion

References

1. Yesenia RK, Galandiuk S. The management of chronic ulcerative colitis. In: Cameron J, Cameron A, editors. Current surgical therapy. 13th ed. Canada: Elsevier; 2019.
2. Althumairi A, Efron JE. The management of toxic megacolon. In: Cameron J, Cameron A, editors. Current surgical therapy. 12th ed. Canada: Elsevier; 2016.
3. Kwaan MR, Stewart DB, Dunn KB. Colon, rectum, and anus. In: Brunicardi F, editor. Schwartz's principles of surgery. 11th ed. United States: McGraw-Hill Education; 2019.

4. Atallah CI, Efron JE, Fang SH. The management of chronic ulcerative colitis. In: Cameron J, Cameron A, editors. Current surgical therapy. 12th ed. Canada: Elsevier; 2016.
5. Fleshman JW, Peters WR. The management of Crohn's colitis. In: Cameron J, Cameron A, editors. Current surgical therapy. 12th ed. Canada: Elsevier; 2016.
6. Le Leannec IC, Wick E. Management of Crohn's colitis. In: Cameron J, Cameron A, editors. Current surgical therapy. 13th ed. Canada: Elsevier; 2019.
7. Althumairi AA, Gearhart SL. The management of diverticular disease of the colon. In: Cameron J, Cameron A, editors. Current surgical therapy. 12th ed. Canada: Elsevier; 2016.
8. Netz U, Galandiuk S. The management of ischemic colitis. In: Cameron J, Cameron A, editors. Current surgical therapy. 12th ed. Canada: Elsevier; 2016.
9. Stanley DJ, Dart BW. The management of clostridium difficile colitis. In: Cameron J, Cameron A, editors. Current surgical therapy. 12th ed. Canada: Elsevier; 2016.
10. Fabrizio AC, Wick EC. The management of large bowel obstruction. In: Cameron J, Cameron A, editors. Current surgical therapy. 12th ed. Canada: Elsevier; 2016.
11. Herline A, Geiger TM. The management of colonic volvulus. In: Cameron J, Cameron A, editors. Current surgical therapy. 12th ed. Canada: Elsevier; 2016.
12. Kovler ML, Hackam DJ. Appendicitis. In: Cameron J, Cameron A, editors. Current surgical therapy. 13th ed. Canada: Elsevier; 2019.
13. Kelley SR. Surgery for the polyposis syndromes. In: Cameron J, Cameron A, editors. Current surgical therapy. 12th ed. Canada: Elsevier; 2016.
14. Lightner AL, Mathis KL. The management of colonic polyps. In: Cameron J, Cameron A, editors. Current surgical therapy. 12th ed. Canada: Elsevier; 2016.
15. Mahmoud NN, Bleier JIS, Aarons CB, Paulson EC, Shanmugan S, Fry RD. Colon and rectum. In: Mattox CTRDBBMEK, editor. Sabiston textbook of surgery. 20th ed. Elsevier; 2016.
16. Kleiman DA, Guillem JG. The management of rectal cancer. In: Cameron J, Cameron A, editors. Current surgical therapy. 12th ed. Canada: Elsevier; 2016.
17. Azad N, Myzak CM. Neoadjuvant and adjuvant therapy for colorectal cancer. In: Cameron J, Cameron A, editors. Current surgical therapy. 12th ed. Canada: Elsevier; 2016.
18. Anandam JL, Choti MA. The management of colon cancer. In: Cameron J, Cameron A, editors. Current surgical therapy. 12th ed. Canada: Elsevier; 2016.
19. Tavakkoli A, Ashley SW. Acute gastrointestinal hemorrhage. In: Mattox CTRDBBMEK, editor. Sabiston textbook of surgery. 20th ed. Elsevier; 2016.
20. Husain F, Konder I, Lin E. Open lateral to medial. In: Wexner SD, JWF, editors. Master techniques in general surgery. Colorectal surgery. 9th ed. United States: Lippincott Williams and Wilkins; 2013.
21. Fleshman JW, Mutch MG. Open left and sigmoid colectomy. In: Wexner SD, JWF, editors. Master techniques in general surgery. Colorectal surgery. 9th ed. United States: Lippincott Williams and Wilkins; 2013.
22. Nogueras JJ. Open low anterior resection. In: Wexner SD, JWF, editors. Master techniques in general surgery. Colorectal surgery. 9th ed. United States: Lippincott Williams and Wilkins; 2013.
23. Rothenberger DA, Meaux GBM. Open abdominoperineal resection. In: Wexner SD, JWF, editors. Master techniques in general surgery. Colorectal surgery. 9th ed. United States: Lippincott Williams and Wilkins; 2013.

12 Surgical Aspects of Anal Diseases for Clinical Board Exams

12.1 Part I: Knowledge

> Our ability to achieve success depends on the strength of our wings gained through knowledge and experience. The greater our knowledge and experience, the higher we can fly.
> –Catherine Pulsifer

The Presenting Complaint Might Be Any of the Following:

- Anal pain
- Lower gastrointestinal bleeding
- Anal mass
- Refer to Table 12.1

Table 12.1 Differential diagnosis

Pain	Bleeding	Mass
Abscess Fissure Thrombosed hemorrhoid Prolapsed hemorrhoid	Hemorrhoid Fissure Anal neoplasm Colonic cause	Hemorrhoid Condyloma Abscess Neoplasm Rectal prolapse

History:

- Introduce yourself to the patient.
- Name, age, occupation, gender, nationality.
- Chief complaint and duration.
- History of presenting illness:
  – **Analysis of the chief complaint**

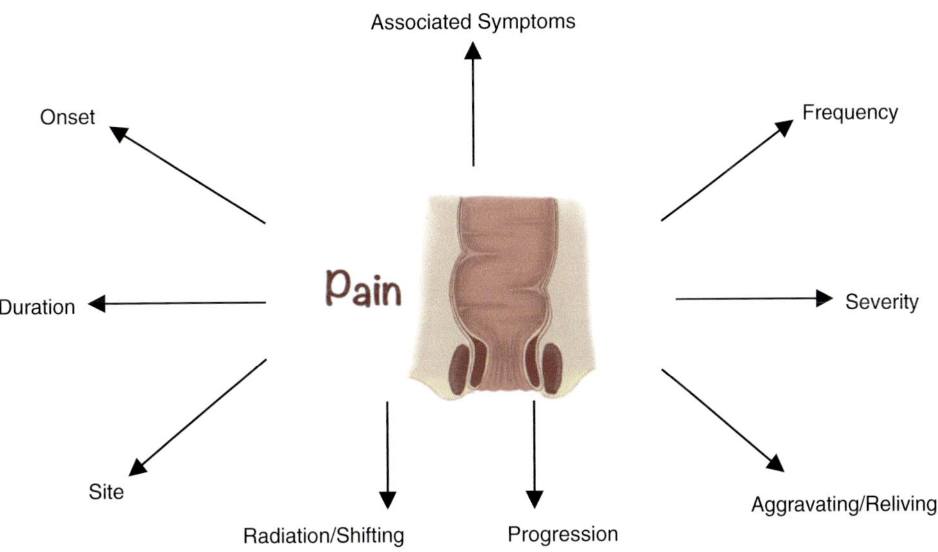

H. Alotaibi, *Study Surgery*, https://doi.org/10.1007/978-981-16-2305-9_12

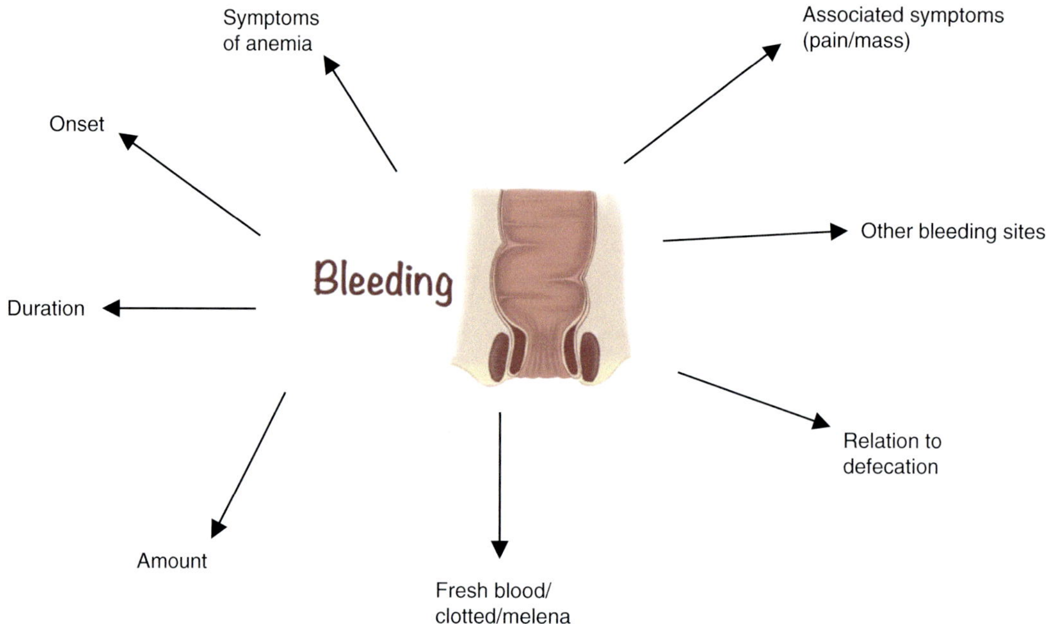
Symptoms of anemia
Associated symptoms (pain/mass)
Onset
Other bleeding sites
Bleeding
Duration
Relation to defecation
Amount
Fresh blood/ clotted/melena

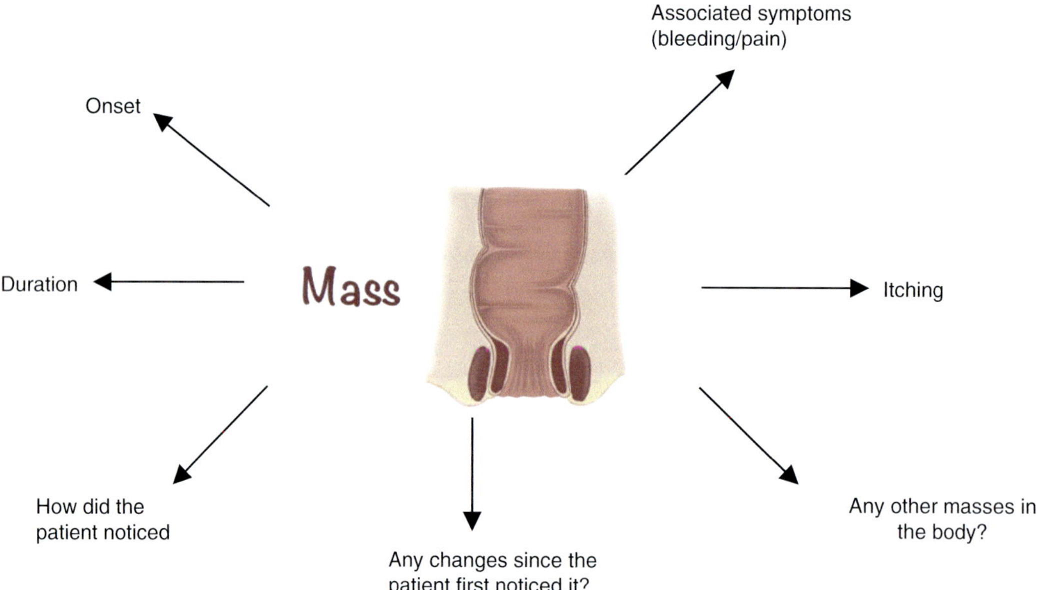
Associated symptoms (bleeding/pain)
Onset
Duration
Mass
Itching
How did the patient noticed
Any changes since the patient first noticed it?
Any other masses in the body?

- **Associated Symptoms**
  Pain, fever, nausea, vomiting, diarrhea, change in bowel habits, tenesmus, hematemesis, abdominal distention, incontinence, discharge
- **Constitutional Symptoms:**
  Weight loss, decrease appetite, night sweating, fever
- **Symptoms of Metastasis**
  Back pain, abdominal distention, cough, shortness of breath
- **Risk Factors:**
  Family history of similar complaint or malignancy (colon, breast, endometrial, and melanoma cancers)
  Personal history of cancer
  History of inflammatory bowel disease
  Smoking
- **Previous Similar Attack**, previous admission, previous investigation, or colonoscopy (if yes, when was it done and what was the finding?)
- **Systemic Review of Related System** (GIT)
  Dysphagia, heart burn, hematemesis, melena, history of bleeding, ecchymosis

- PMH.
- PSH.
- Family history.
- Social history.
- Medication, transfusion, allergy.
- Systemic review:
  - **CNS:** headache, eye and hearing symptoms, epilepsy, numbness, paralysis
  - **CVS:** chest pain, orthopnea, paroxysmal nocturnal dyspnea, lower limb edema, palpitation
  - **Respiratory system:** cough, fever, chest pain, hemoptysis
  - **Renal:** dysuria, flank pain, hematuria
  - **MSK:** weakness, arthritis, skin erythema

Physical Examination:
- Introduce yourself to the patient.
- Ask permission for examination.
- Assure privacy.
- Position: left lateral position with the left lower limb extended and the right hip is flexed.
- Exposure.
- Handwashing.

General Examination:

Appearance: ill, well, dehydrated
Body built: cachectic, obese
Color: pale, jaundice
Distress
Environment and connection to monitors, fluids
Vital signs: BP, HR, temperature, RR, SPO_2
Hands:

- Pallor
- Palmer erythema
- Koilonychia (iron deficiency anemia)
- Leukonychia (hypoalbuminemia)
- Pulse rate and its characteristics (rhythm, volume, etc.)

Eye:

- Jaundice
- Pallor

Mouth:

- Jaundice in mucus membrane, below the tongue, aphthous ulcers

Neck:

- Lymphadenopathy

Chest:

- Respiratory and CVS examination

Abdomen:

- Inspection:
- Distention
- Asymmetry
- Visible veins
- Scars/striae
- Dilated veins (caput medusa)
- Hernial orifices
- Stretch marks

- Visible peristalsis
- Palpations:
- Superficial then deep palpation
- Look for any tenderness
- Palpable masses
- Ascites
- Cough impulse at hernial orifices
- Organomegaly
- Percussion:
- Shifting dullness
- Fluid thrill
- Organomegaly
- Auscultation:
- Bowel sounds
- Bruit, venous hum

Groin:

DRE:

- Any obvious pathology (hemorrhoids, fissure, fistula).
- Hemorrhoid: external versus internal (determine the grade), any thrombosis or ulceration.
- Fissure (posterior, anterior, lateral).
- Fistula (external opening, distance from the anal verge, position "clock position").
- Abscess: tenderness, fluctuation, erythema, discharge.
- Introduce the finger (sometimes this may be impossible due to severity of the pain) and assess the tone, any palpable mass (if yes, estimate the distance and assess if it is circumferential or not).

Proctoscopy:

- For the presence of internal hemorrhoids.
- Internal opening of fistula.
- If there is any mass, clarify the position, distance, appearance, and circumference.

Lower limbs: edema, swelling, skin rash, weakness

If IBD or polyposis syndromes are suspected, look for extraintestinal manifestation.

Back: for tenderness

12.1.1 Management of Hemorrhoids

- Hemorrhoids are specialized vascular cushions located in the submucosal space in the anal canal.
- They contribute about 15–20% of anal resting pressure.
- They are located in the left lateral, right anterior, and right posterior positions.
- Internal hemorrhoids located above the dentate line and are covered with columnar mucosa and transitional epithelium.
- External hemorrhoids located distal to the dentate line and are covered with anoderm or skin.
- Clinical presentation include bleeding, mucoid discharge, itching, and prolapse. Pain typically is not associated with hemorrhoids unless there is an acute thrombosis.
- Grade I and grade II hemorrhoid can be managed by conservative treatment, change lifestyle, high fiber diet, drinking enough water, warm sitz bath, and topical over the counter therapies.
- For patients who fail conservative management, there are several types of procedures that may be used [1].

Office-Based Procedures:

I. **Rubber Band Ligation (RBL):**
   - Most commonly used office-based procedure.
   - For grade I, II, and III hemorrhoids.
   - Does not require anesthesia.
   - Position: left lateral or prone.
   - Procedure:
   - Using anoscopy, visualize the hemorrhoids and address the largest one first.
   - Place the rubber band 2 cm above the dentate line (above the level of somatic pain sensation).
   - Deploy the band.
   - It is successful in more than 99% of cases.
   - The results with rubber band ligation have been excellent with patient satisfaction of 80–91% in large series, but probably only

60–70% of patients have been completely cured of symptoms by one treatment session.
- It requires multiple sessions to address all the hemorrhoid cushions.
- It is contraindicated in patient using anticoagulant.
- Antiplatelet should be stopped for 1 week before the procedure.
- Complications include pain, urine retention, minor bleeding (delayed hemorrhage may also occur, usually 7–10 days post procedure as the banded tissue sloughs), vasovagal symptoms, and thrombosis of the adjacent hemorrhoids (secondary thrombosis of external hemorrhoids may occur in 2–11% of patients). Severe pain after placement indicates low level of placement (below the dentate line) and should be removed immediately. Pelvic sepsis is rare but serious complications and require urgent exploration and debridement of necrotic tissue [1, 2].

II. **Sclerotherapy:**
- For grade I and II hemorrhoids.
- Agent: 5% phenol, hypertonic saline, or ethanolamine.
- Procedure: inject above the dentate line into the submucosa of each hemorrhoid.
- One session treatment.
- Can be used in patient on anticoagulant.
- The long-term result is inferior to the RBL.
- Incorrect injection into the muscle or mucosa causes pain and slough of the mucosa [1].

III. **Infrared Coagulation:**
- Grade I and II.
- All three hemorrhoids can be addressed in the same session.
- Procedure: infrared coagulator tip is placed at the apex of the hemorrhoid and 1–1.5 s pulse is applied, 3–4 applications to each hemorrhoid.
- It is better tolerated by the patient and cause less pain than RBL.

IV. **HET System:**
- It is a new modality to treat the hemorrhoids in the office.
- It is for grade I and II hemorrhoids.
- It is applied to the apex of the hemorrhoid, which is clamped between the specialized anoscope, and bipolar energy applied.
- All three hemorrhoids can be managed in one setting [1].

Operative Treatment:

I. **Ferguson Hemorrhoidectomy (Closed Technique):**
- The most common surgical hemorrhoid procedure
- Procedure:
- Under spinal anesthesia with the patient in prone position.
- A V-shaped incision is made on the perianal skin toward the anal canal, and the hemorrhoid is elevated initially of the external sphincter and subsequently of the internal sphincter muscle as the dissection proceeds into the anal canal.
- Once the sphincter muscles have been identified clearly, the skin incision is then continued onto the mucosa.
- The apex of hemorrhoid with vascular pedicle is then clamped, and the hemorrhoid is excised, and the pedicle is suture ligated.
- The defect is then closed in a running locked fashion in the anal canal and simple running fashion on the perianal skin [1].

II. **Milligan Morgan Hemorrhoidectomy (Open):**
- Similar to the Ferguson hemorrhoidectomy, with dissection of the hemorrhoid off the sphincter muscle in the perianal skin and in the anal canal.
- The wounds are left open to heal by secondary intention.
- Outcomes between the techniques are similar, although wound healing is longer in the open technique [1].

III. **Modification of the Excisional Technique:**
- Energy device is used to excise the hemorrhoid.
- This is faster, less pain.
- Care must be taken to avoid damage to underlying sphincter muscles and avoidance of excessive removal of anoderm, which can result in anal stenosis [1].

IV. **Stapled Hemorrhoidopexy:**
- Grade II to grade IV.
- This technique uses a specialized circular stapler, which removes a circumferential area of mucosa and submucosa proximal to the hemorrhoids.
- It does not remove hemorrhoidal tissue but rather disrupts the vascular supply and puts the hemorrhoids back into their normal position.
- It has the advantages of no external wound and less pain in compare to excisional hemorrhoidectomy.
- It does not address external hemorrhoids.
- It has similar complication related to excisional hemorrhoidectomy.
- Long-term recurrence rate is slightly higher [1].

V. **Doppler-Guided Hemorrhoidal Artery Ligation:**
- For grade II to III hemorrhoids.
- Selective ligation of the hemorrhoidal artery will decrease the arterial inflow to the hemorrhoid.
- 90% of patient had symptoms improvement with this technique, with less postoperative pain than in other surgical technique because ligation is above the dentate line [1].
- Procedure:
- Special anoscope is placed into the anal canal.
- The vessels are localized using the attached Doppler.
- A Z-stitch or figure-of-8 stitch is placed at 2 cm above the anorectal junction.
- For patient with larger (grade III or IV) hemorrhoids, the addition of mucopexy, also called a recto-anal repair, has been advocated [1].

Management of External Hemorrhoids:
- For patients with symptomatic internal hemorrhoid who also have external hemorrhoid, excisional hemorrhoidectomy is preferred.
- Thrombosed hemorrhoids:
- If the patients present less than 72 h from the onset of symptoms, they may benefit from excision of the thrombus.
- If the patients present after 3–4 days, excision will not typically improve the symptoms, and those patients can benefit from symptomatic treatment with analgesics, fiber supplementation, and sitz baths [1].

Management of Acute Hemorrhoidal Disease:
- Acute hemorrhoidal disease (strangulated or prolapsed hemorrhoid that cannot be reduced) can be treated by urgent hemorrhoidectomy using Ferguson technique.
- Care must be taken to leave normal anoderm between suture lines to avoid postoperative anal stenosis [1].

12.1.2 Management of Anal Fissure

- Patient commonly present with severe pain during or after defecation and or bright blood per rectum.
- The patients usually describe the pain as a tearing pain with bowel movement and blood on the toilet paper when wiping.
- The diagnosis is suggested by history and physical examination.
- 75–90% of times located in the posterior midline, the anterior midline fissures make up the reminder.
- Anterior anal fissures are seen commonly in women and are associated with natural defect in the external sphincter muscle.
- Fissures not located in the midline should prompt a workup for other disease processes including Crohn's disease, cancer, tuberculosis, and sexually transmitted disease.
- Acute anal fissure: less than 6–8 weeks of symptoms.
- Chronic anal fissure characterized by fibrosis and skin tag at the distal end of the fissure

and/or hypertrophied papilla at the proximal end [3].

- **Management:**
  - **Acute Anal Fissure:**
    50% of patient will respond to the following:
    - Stool softener
    - Fiber supplementation
    - Symptomatic control
    - Sitz bath
    - Topical anti-inflammatory
  - **Chronic Anal Fissure:**
    Medical Therapy:
    - Fiber, pain control, and chemically induced relaxation of internal anal sphincter by topical therapy such as nitric oxide donor (e.g., glyceryl trinitrate GTN) or calcium channel blocker (nifedipine or diltiazem).
    - Botulinum toxin (Botox injection) is another way to induce internal sphincter relaxation.
    - If the anal fissure did not improve with medical therapy, examination under anesthesia (EUA) along with definitive surgical treatment is needed [3].

    Surgical Therapy:
    - The gold standard is lateral internal sphincterotomy (LIS).
    - Complete long-term healing rate exceed 90%.
    - LIS can be performed via either open or closed technique cutting 60% of the muscle.
    - The main complication associated with LIS is incontinence.
    - Tailoring the sphincterotomy to the length of the fissure rather than performing a complete sphincterotomy to the dentate line has helped to minimize the risk of incontinence.
    - Surgeon may consider fissurectomy with or without advancement flap as an alternative to sphincterotomy in patients who have low resting anal pressure. It is considered in patients who did not improve with lateral internal sphincterotomy and have high risk of incontinence [3].
  - **Recurrent Anal Fissure:**
    Recurrence after medical treatment is common, but recurrence after LIS is rare and should prompt further investigation.
    In patients with recurrent fissures, biopsy of the fissure edge should be considered to rule out other disease. Transrectal ultrasound, and anal manometry should be considered before undertaking further surgical intervention.
    If the resting anal pressure is high, repeat LIS on the contralateral side.
    If the pressure is low or there is sphincter defect, do fissurectomy with advancement flap [3].

12.1.3 Management of Anorectal Abscess

- The anal glands empty into the rectum through 10–15 crypts of Morgagni located at the dentate line (Fig. 12.1).
- When the drainage is blocked, pressure builds as the sepsis increases.
- The suppurative can extend to inter-sphincteric, submucosal, ischiorectal, post anal, or supra-levator space [4].
- **Locations** (Fig. 12.2):
  - **Inter-sphincteric abscesses:** located at the site of the anal glands tracks craniocaudally between the sphincter layers.
  - **Submucosal abscesses:** represents the least extensive suppurative process, located just beneath the mucosa above the dentate line.
  - **Perianal abscesses:** descend through the inter-sphincteric space to the subcutaneous tissue around the anus and below the sphincter complex.
  - **Ischiorectal abscesses:** extend from the inter-sphincteric space through or above the external sphincter to the ischiorectal space. This space encircles the external

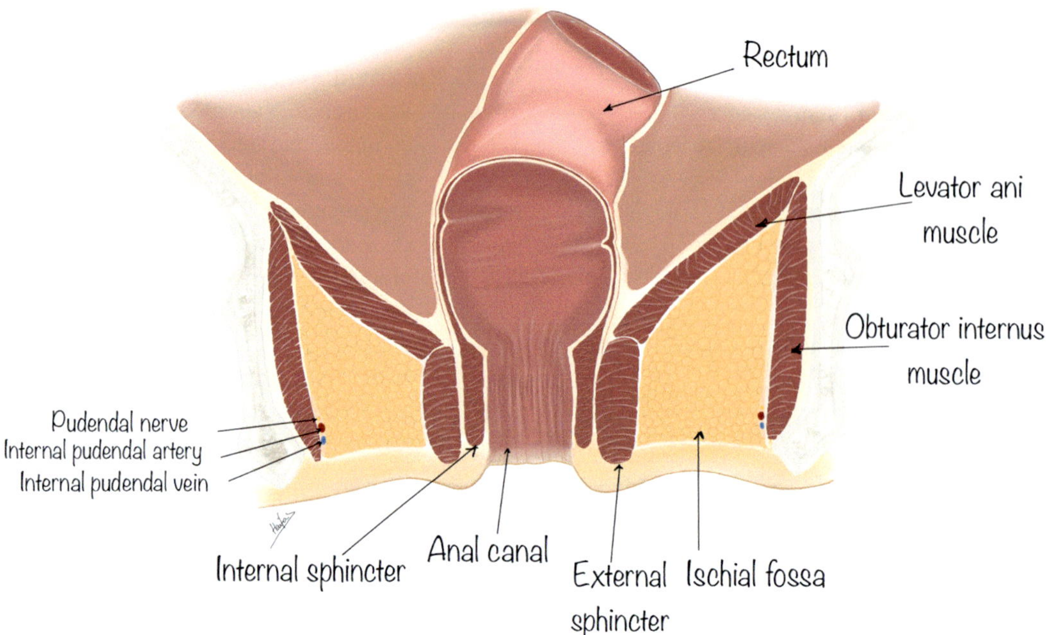

Fig. 12.1 Anatomy of the anal canal

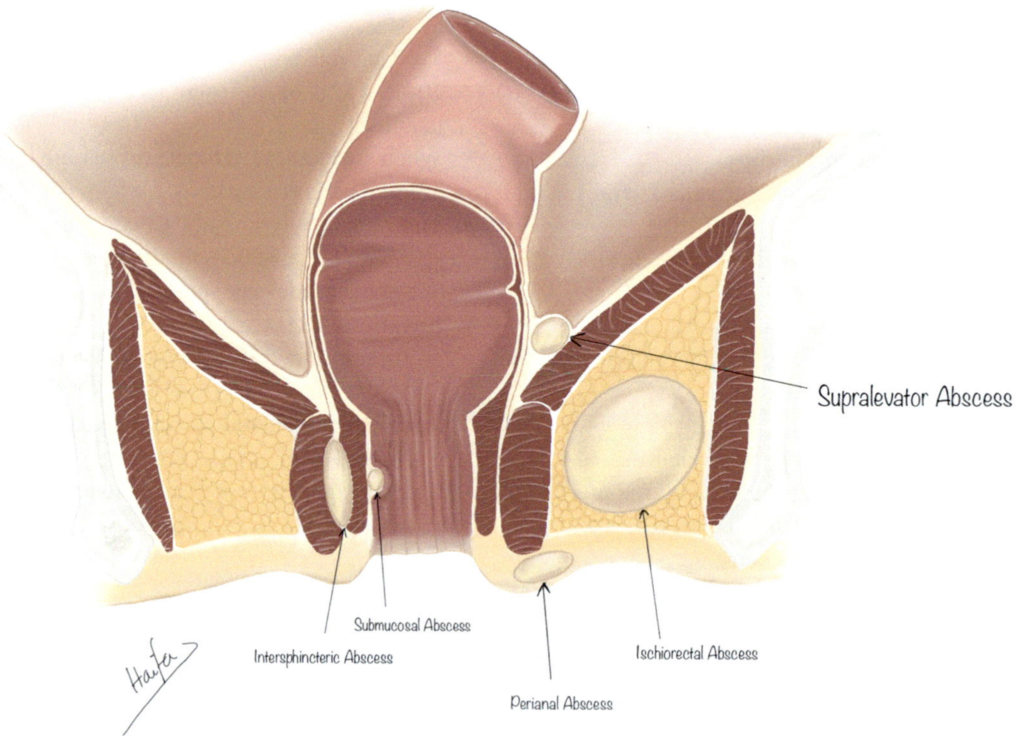

Fig. 12.2 Common locations of anorectal abscess

sphincter caudal to the levators and medial to the ischial tuberosities.
  - **Post anal space:** located posteriorly, between the levators (cranially) and the external sphincter (caudally).
  - **Supra-levators abscesses:** located above the levators and caused by either cranial extension of cryptoglandular sepsis or caudal extension of an intra-abdominal process such as diverticular disease [4].
- **Clinical Presentation:**
  - Anal pain independent of defecation.
  - Associated with fever and swelling.
  - Medical history of IBD or immunocompromised patient may be present.
  - Anorectal examination reveals an indurated bulge with fluctuance and cellulitis near the anal verge.
  - Inter-sphincteric abscess may show no external finding but severe tenderness on DRE.
  - Abscess limited to post anal space may have localized tenderness posterior to the anal verge but without apparent induration.
  - Ischiorectal abscess typically have gluteal findings of induration, tenderness, and fluctuance without tenderness on DRE.
  - Supra-levators abscess may have no anorectal finding and require further evaluation by pelvic imaging.
  - Patient who cannot tolerate DRE should undergo examination under anesthesia (EUA) [4].
- **Management:**
  - Surgical drainage is the definitive treatment of anorectal abscess.
  - Preoperative antibiotics with gram negative coverage is required. Most patients do not require antibiotic therapy post drainage. However, patients with large area of cellulitis, signs of systemic sepsis or shock, and immunocompromised patient and patients with prosthetic heart valve, prior bacterial endocarditis, congenital heart disease, and heart transplant with valvular disease need antibiotic treatment.
  - Send swab for culture and sensitivity.
  - Special considerations:

    For large ischiorectal abscess, ipsilateral counter incision can establish adequate drainage.

    Packing is usually not necessary.

    Drainage of post anal space abscess: radial incision is made from posterior anal verge toward the coccyx, subcutaneous tissue is divided, and the underlying fiber of the external sphincter muscle is separated with hemostatic clamp. The anococcygeal ligament is then divided to access the post anal space. If a horse show abscess is present, elliptical counter-incision is made over the involved ischiorectal fossa. Penrose drain can be looped between incisions to maintain patency.

    Inter-sphincteric abscess are addressed transanally. Mucosa overlying the bulge is divided vertically. Fine tip hemostat is inserted into the suppurative inter-sphincteric space. The internal sphincter can be divided over the hemostat with electrocautery, and this generally does not compromise fecal continence.

    The source of the supra-levators abscess determines the management. Descending abdominal or pelvic abscess typically are addressed using CT-guided percutaneous drainage. Ascending cryptoglandular abscess travels either through inter-sphincteric space (treated with transrectal or transanal drainage) or through the levators from ischiorectal fossa (should be drained via skin incision) [4].
- **Necrotizing Perianal Skin Infection:**
  - Destructive life-threatening infection.
  - Rapid development of severe anorectal pain that is out of proportion to findings on examination is the classic presentation.
  - Risk factors include diabetes, chronic renal failure, obesity, smoking, underlying neu-

rological disease such as dementia, or spinal cord injury.
- Tender, irregular red, violaceous or black macules, and blister are early signs of this serious infection.
- Septic shock and electrolyte disturbance may develop later.
- Management:
    Urgent debridement is necessary.
    Empiric coverage of antibiotics.
    Hyperbaric oxygen therapy can be used as adjunct treatment modality.
    Fecal diversion may be necessary in some patient [4].

12.1.4 Management of Fistula-in-Ano

- Fistulas are classified by their route between an internal opening in the anal canal and the external opening on perineal skin.
- **Types** (Fig. 12.3):
  - **Superficial fistula:** subcutaneous tract that does not involve the sphincter complex.
  - **Inter-sphincteric fistula:** the tract remains in the inter-sphincteric space.
  - **Trans-sphincteric:** the fistula tract passes from the inter-sphincteric plane through the external sphincter muscle.
  - **Supra-sphincteric:** upward extension of the fistula tract in the inter-sphincteric plane. The tract then passes above the level of the puborectalis muscle and continues downward through the ischiorectal fossa to the perianal area.
  - **Extra-sphincteric:** there is a tract that passes from the skin of the perineum through the ischiorectal fossa and the levator muscle before entering the rectal wall.
- Each of these fistulas can be categorized further into simple and complex fistula.
- **Clinical Presentation:**
  - Intermittent anal pain, pruritis, drainage that is mucoid, bloody or feculent, or occasionally blood per rectum.
  - Cyclic discomfort and swelling that is relieved after spontaneous drainage is common.
  - Previous episode of perianal abscess may be reported.
  - Examination can easily identify the external opening, and a palpable cord may be present and suggest the path of the tract. The internal opening occasionally can be palpated on DRE as a nodule,
  - Anoscopy can show the internal opening.
- **Principles of Surgical Management:**

1. Define the Fistula Anatomy:
   - It is established most often by EUA.
   - Goodsall's rule (Fig. 12.4) predicts that an external opening posterior to the transverse line across the anus drain to the posterior

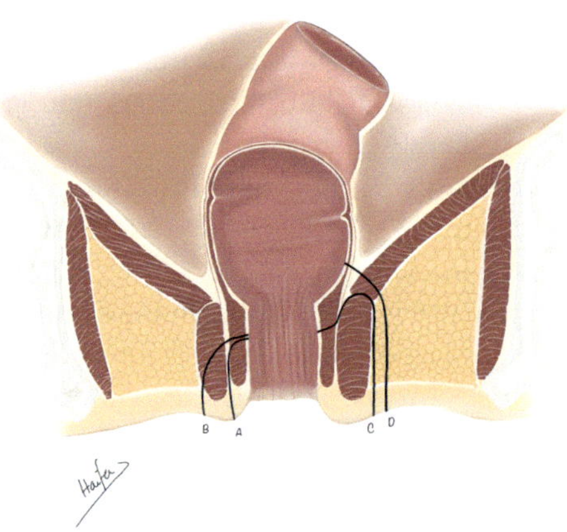

Fig. 12.3 Perianal fistula: (**a**) inter-sphincteric; (**b**) trans-sphincteric; (**c**) supra-sphincteric; (**d**) extra-sphincteric

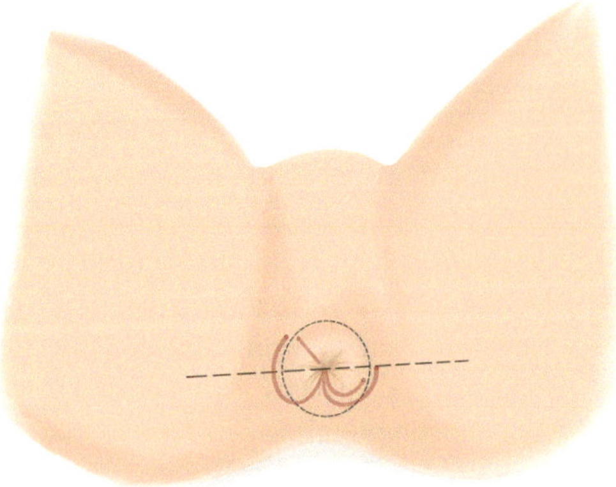

Fig. 12.4 Goodsall's rule; a fistula with the external opening anterior to an imaginary transverse line across the anus has its internal opening at the same radial position, and for an external opening posterior to this line, the internal opening is in the midline posteriorly with a horse-shoe track

midline internal opening; those that open anterior to the line have short, radial courses to the internal opening.
   - When the fistula is recurrent, thought to be complex, or if the anatomy could not be identified on EUA, imaging (transanal ultrasound or MRI) can help identify sites of persistent infection and define the anatomy.
2. Ensure the Resolution of Sepsis:
   - Staged approach with placement of seton initially then definitive procedure when the internal opening is less than 5 mm; the tract is simple, narrow, and without associated cavity.
3. Assess and Preserve Anal Sphincter Function:
   - Preservation of continence is always a priority when choosing the proper management strategy.
   - Division of the internal sphincter is well tolerated; division of the distal third of the internal sphincter is considered safe in healthy male individual.
   - **Options of Surgical Management:**

A. Fistulotomy:
   - Can be done at the time of abscess management or as a second stage procedure.
   - It is appropriate only in low-risk patient with superficial, low inter-sphincteric, or low trans-sphincteric fistula.
   - Wound edges can be left to heal with secondary intention or marsupialization of the wound edges to accelerate wound healing.
   - Success rate is generally more than 90%.

B. Seton:
   - A noncutting seton allows for drainage of sepsis and promote fibrosis and maturation of the fistula tract; often in a preparation for a second stage procedure.
   - The seton should not be tight.
   - The second stage procedure is usually performed 6–10 weeks later.

C. Ligation of Inter-sphincteric Fistula Tract (LIFT Procedure):
   - It is most commonly used for trans-sphincteric fistula after a mature tract developed.
   - The inter-sphincteric plane is entered, and the fistula tract is isolated, ligated, and then sharply divided.

D. Endorectal Advancement Flap:
   - It is considered as the gold standard sphincter-preserving operation.
   - It is used as a second stage procedure for high fistula tract, supra-sphincteric tracts, or in high-risk patients.
   - The flap is created by distal to proximal dissection with electrocautery including mucosa and submucosa and few fibers from the internal sphincter.

E. Fibrin Sealant and Collagen Plug

- **Fistula-in-Ano and Crohn's Disease:**
  - Usually high, complex fistulas
  - The treatment strategy is mainly conservative because of poor wound healing, high recurrence rate, increase vulnerability to incontinence related to frequent diarrhea, and poor rectal compliance.
  - The initial surgical goal is to treat sepsis, and this is usually addressed with loose seton and widening of the external opening.
  - Fistulotomy may be appropriate in patient with simple, low fistula but only in highly selected patient.
  - Prolonged wound healing (3–6 months) is expected
  - Endorectal advancement flap and LIFT procedures have been successful in patient without proctitis.
  - If sepsis cannot be controlled with local therapy, fecal diversion should be considered. Proctectomy is undertaken in refractory cases [4].

12.1.5 Management of Anal Canal Tumors

Surgical Anatomy:

- Arterial supply to the anal canal derives from superior, middle, inferior rectal arteries.
- The three main arcades, right anterior, right posterior, left lateral, originate primary from the superior rectal artery (Fig. 12.1).

- The upper anal canal drains by middle rectal vein then into the systemic circulation via internal iliac vein.
- The inferior anal canal drains by inferior rectal vein which communicates first with the pudendal vein before draining into the internal iliac vein.
- Lymphatic drainage varies based on the level:
  - Below the dentate line to the inguinal lymph nodes
  - Above the dentate line to the mesorectal, lateral pelvic, inferior mesenteric nodes
- Microscopy of the anal canal divided into three zones of mucosa:
  - Glandular: proximal to the dentate line.
  - Transitional: immediately proximal to the dentate line. It may contain mucin-producing cells, endocrine cells and melanocytes.
  - Non-keratinized squamous: distal to the dentate. It is absent of the epidermal appendages and merge with the epidermis of the perianal skin. The junction is called anal verge [5].

1. **Squamous Neoplasm:**
   - 93% of anal squamous cell carcinoma (SCC) is associated with human papilloma virous infection (HPV).
   - **Condyloma Acuminatum (Anal Warts):**
     - It is one of the manifestations of HPV infection.
     - Individuals with anal warts at increased risk of developing anogenital and head and neck cancers for 10 years or more after the diagnosis of anal warts.
     - The key histological features of condyloma are a verrucous architecture.
     - Its management depend on number and the extent of the disease:
       Large (1–2 cm) should be referred to surgeon.
       Topical therapies include antimitotic agents (podophyllotoxin), inducer of local cytokines (imiquimod cream), or antimetabolites (5-fluorouracil).
       Surgical therapies include cryotherapy, argon plasma beam, excision, or fulguration.
     - Regardless of the treatment modality, the recurrence is about 20–50%.
   - **Anal Intraepithelial Neoplasm (AIN):**
     - It is necessary but not obligate precursor to invasive anal SCC and divided into three grades:
       Grade I: low-grade dysplasia
       Grade II: moderate-grade dysplasia
       Grade III: high-grade dysplasia (Bowen's disease)
     - It is strongly associated with HPV (types 6, 11, 15, 18).
     - Bowen's disease (AIN III/SCC in situ):
       Symptoms include pruritis, bleeding, and mass.
       Characterized by erythematous, occasionally brown/red pigmented, scaly, or crusted plaques that sometimes have a moist or nodular surface.
       The standard treatment is wide local excision. Before resection, ensure clear margins and identify multifocal disease, biopsy should be taken from four quadrants at the dentate line, anal verge, and the perianal skin for frozen section.
       Recurrence rate up to 30% [5].
   - **Squamous Cell Carcinoma (SCC):**
     - Clinical presentation: slow-growing intra-anal or perianal mass, bleeding is common, and pain.
     - The diagnosis of SCC often is delayed because the non-specific symptoms.
     - Once the diagnosis is suspected, a disease-specific history should be performed. Risk factors include sexual history. Signs of advanced disease such as groin pain indicate regional involvement of inguinal lymph nodes.
     - Stage the tumor using TNM staging system (CT chest, CT/MRI abdomen and pelvis, PET scan may be considered for T2–T4 tumors or nodal disease) [5].

- Management:
  Nigro protocol:
  - Continuous infusion of 5-flurouracil (5- FU) at 1000 mg/m^2/day over treatment days 1–4 and 29–32.
  - Mitomycin (15 mg/m^2) on day 1.
  - 3000-rad full-pelvis dose radiation calculated to the mid-plane of the pelvis, delivered in 15 treatments of 200 rad each over a 3 weeks period.

  If the groin lymph node is positive, indicates the need for radiation therapy.
  Treatment for metastatic disease (most commonly liver and lung) is cisplatin and 5-FU.
- Role of surgery:
  Reserved for recurrent or persistent disease after chemoradiation.
  For most recurrent or persistent disease, APR will be the only appropriate surgical therapy.
- Role of inguinal lymphadenectomy:
  It should not be done prophylactically or after a good response to initial chemoradiation.
  It should be reserved for those who have either recurrent or persistent disease in the groin.
- Posttreatment surveillance:
  DRE, anoscopy, inguinal examination every 3–6 months for 5 years
  Annual CT CAP for patient with T3-4, N1 [5]

2. **Adenocarcinoma:**
   - Accounts for about 10% of all anal canal cancers.
   - It originates from the columnar epithelium in the upper zone of the anal canal or from the glandular cells of the anal transition zone.
   - The treatment is similar to rectal adenocarcinoma. The operative management is abdominoperineal resection (APR) [5].
3. **Paget's Disease**
   - May represent a true primary lesion arising form apocrine gland or represents synchronous or metachronous lesions in patients with internal malignancy.
   - Treatment of localized Paget's disease is surgical.
   - Recurrence rates between 30 and 70% [5].
4. **Melanoma:**
   - About 4% of anal canal tumors.
   - Frequently not pigmented and does not have macroscopically suspicious appearance.
   - The prognosis is poor.
   - Surgery is the treatment of choice because anal melanoma does not respond to chemoradiation.
   - Extent of surgical resection (APR vs. wide local excision) does not seem to significantly affect the outcome [5].
5. **Neuroendocrine Tumor:**
   - Originates from neuroendocrine cells in the anal transition zone.
   - Because lesions are often small, treatment is typically local excision.
   - Definitive or neoadjuvant chemoradiation may be indicated for high-grade neuroendocrine neoplasms [5].
6. **Mesenchymal Tumor:**
   - Most commonly GIST, but others like anorectal leiomyosarcoma or rhabdomyosarcoma angiosarcoma, and schwannoma have been reported.
   - Treatment: need multidisciplinary team approach. The curative surgical approach is wide local excision which may require APR to achieve negative margins. Neoadjuvant chemotherapy or radiotherapy is required in some cases [5].
7. **Lymphoma:** anal canal lymphoma is rare. The treatment is chemoradiation [5].

12.1.6 Anal Canal Operations

Preoperative Preparation:

- Admission.
- Consent.
- Nothing per oral (NPO).
- IV fluid.
- DVT and stress ulcer prophylaxis.
- Prophylactic antibiotic.
- Bowel preparation (if APR will be done).

- Sodium phosphate enema to clear the distal rectum (for anal surgery).
- Confirm the availability of blood intraoperative if needed.
- Anesthesia consultation.
- ICU consultation if required.
- Urology consultation for insertion of ureteric stent if APR is indicated.
- Instruct the patient to take shower the night before surgery.
- Stoma marking (if APR will be done).
- Hair removal.

Informed Consent:

- **Consent for Hemorrhoidectomy:**
  - *Describe the procedure for the patient*: examination under anesthesia (EUA) + excision of (internal/ external/ both) hemorrhoids under (general/ spinal) anesthesia (with/ without) closure of the wound.
  - *Mention if there is any other alternative* like office-based procedure, stapled hemorrhoidectomy, and other treatment modality.
  - *Mention all the possible complications*: bleeding, urine retention, surgical site infection, recurrence, injury to the sphincter muscles (which would lead to temporary or permanent incontinence), and anal stenosis.
- **Consent for Lateral Internal Sphincterotomy:**
  - *Describe the procedure for the patient*: EUA + partial division of the internal sphincter with or without debridement of the fissure to facilitate its healing.
  - *Mention if there is any alternative* like medical management and Botox injection.
  - *Mention all the possible complications*: bleeding, infection, recurrence, incontinence (temporary or permanent), and pain.

Closed Hemorrhoidectomy (Ferguson):

- Under general anesthesia/spinal anesthesia.
- Position: lithotomy, modified Sims' position, or prone jack-knife position.
- Prepare the whole perianal area (from symphysis pubis superior, to upper thighs laterally, and distally to the anus downward).
- Patient is draped in sterile fashion.
- Time out: confirm that correct patient, correct procedure, correct site, and all the required instruments are available.
- EUA: careful digital examination of the anal canal and distal rectum. Anoscopy to clearly inspect the hemorrhoidal tissue and anal canal with assessment of size, degree of prolapse, and any fragility or bleeding.
- Incision: V-shape incision.
- Details of the procedure:
  - A V-shape incision is made on the perianal skin toward the anal canal with preservation of the intervening anoderm.
  - Elevate the hemorrhoid off the external sphincter initially.
  - Then, elevated it off the internal sphincter muscle as the dissection proceed into the anal canal.
  - Once the sphincter has been identified clearly, the skin incision is then continued onto the mucosa.
  - The apex of the hemorrhoid with the vascular pedicle is then clamped.
  - Excise the hemorrhoid.
  - The pedicle is suture ligated.
  - The defect then is closed in running locked fashion in the anal canal and continued in simple running fashion on the perianal skin [1].

Open Hemorrhoidectomy (Milligan Morgan):

- The technique is similar to Ferguson, but the wounds are left open to heal by secondary intention.
- The intervening anoderm must be preserved [1].

Open Lateral Internal Sphincterotomy:

- Under general anesthesia/spinal anesthesia.
- Position: prone jack-knife position with buttocks retracted by tape to provide good exposure. Other positions like lithotomy or Sims' position can be used.
- Prepare the whole perianal area (from symphysis pubis, to upper thighs laterally, and distally to the anus).
- Patient is draped in sterile fashion.

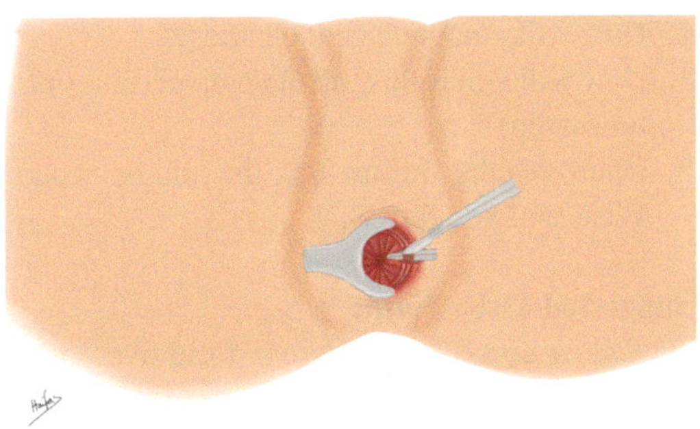

Fig. 12.5 Open lateral internal sphincterotomy

- Time out: confirm that correct patient, correct procedure, correct site, and all the required instruments are available.
- EUA: careful digital examination of the anal canal and distal rectum. Anoscopy to clearly inspect the anal canal. Confirm the fissure and hypertonic/spastic sphincter.
- Incision: small incision over the inter-sphincteric groove.
- Details of the procedure:
  - Insert a 35 Hill-Ferguson retractor with identification of the internal sphincter and inter-sphincteric groove.
  - Incision of the perianal skin overlying the inter-sphincteric groove (1.5–2 cm incision).
  - Isolation of the internal sphincter using a fine curved hemostat up to the level of the dentate line and division under direct vision (tailored LIS by dividing the internal sphincter up to the level of the proximal extent of the fissure) (Fig. 12.5).
  - Fissure debridement and excision of a sentinel tag and hypertrophic papilla.
  - Close the sphincterotomy site with interrupted absorbable suture [3].

Postoperative Management:

- Analgesia.
- The patient should be informed that the pain typically resolves within a week.
- Sitz bath.
- High fiber diet and/or fiber supplements.
- The patient can return to normal function within 2 weeks [3].

Complications:

- Urine retention
- Abscess
- Bleeding
- Recurrence
- Incontinence
- Stenosis [3]

12.2 Part II: Practice

Practice makes perfect. After a long time of practicing, our work will become natural, skillful, swift, and steady.
–Bruce Lee

12.2.1 Case Scenarios for Practice

Tips:

- Practice with a friend and try to mimic the real exam!
- Do not forget to set the timer!
- The clinical data is provided in the answer key section.
- Some twist points are suggested after some cases and can be used to change the scenario to a more difficult one.

Case No. 1:
A 28-year-old male patient presented to the emergency department complaining of perianal pain for 3 days.

Questions for Discussion:

1. How will you approach the patient?
2. What will you do next?
3. How will you manage that?
4. What further investigation will you ask for?
5. What will be your management of his condition?

Suggested Twist Point:
Despite what you did, you could not control the sepsis and perianal infection. What would you do?

Case No. 2:
A 45-year-old female patient presented to the colorectal clinic complaining of anal mass for 3 months.

Question for Discussion:
1. How will you approach the patient?
2. What is your differential diagnosis?
3. How will you investigate the patient?
4. How will you manage the patient?
5. How will you follow up the patient (long-term follow-up)?
6. Upon regular follow-up, the tumor recurs. What will you do?

Suggested Twist Point:
On follow-up CT scan, there is focal liver lesion on segment VI. What will you do?

Checklist

History	Items	Done	Not done	NA
General	Introduce himself/herself to the patient			
	Patient personal data (name, age, sex occupation, nationality)			
	Chief complaint			
	Duration			
Pain	Onset			
	Site			
	Character			
	Radiation/shifting			
	Aggravating/relieving			
	Severity			
	Progression			
	Frequency			
Mass	Onset			
	Site			
	How did the patient notice it?			
	Any change since it was first noticed?			
	other masses			
Bleeding per rectum	Onset			
	Amount			
	Relation to defecation			
	Fresh blood, clotted, or melena			
	Another bleeding site			
Associated symptoms	Pain (abdominal/anal)			
	Fever			
	Incontinence			
	Perianal/anal discharge			
	Pruritis			
	Nausea			
	Vomiting			
	Diarrhea			
	Constipation			
	Abdominal distention			
	Jaundice			

History	Items	Done	Not done	NA
Constitutional symptoms	Weight loss			
	Decrease appetite			
	Night sweating			
Symptoms of metastases	Back pain			
	Cough			
	Shortness of breath			
	Abdominal distention			
Risk factors	Smoking			
	Sexual history			
	Family history of colon cancer (if yes, at what age and the degree of relationship)			
	Family history of inflammatory bowel disease (IBD)			
	Personal history of IBD			
PMH	Previous similar attack			
	Previous investigation or colonoscopy			
	Previous admission			
	Chronic illnesses			
PSH	Previous surgery			
Family history	Of similar complaint			
Social history	Occupation			
	Habits (smoking, alcohol, drugs)			
Other	Medication			
	Allergy			
	Transfusion			
Systemic review				
Physical examination				
General principle	Patient position			
	Exposure			
	Privacy			
	Wash hands			
General examination	Appearance			
	Body built			
	Color			
	Distress/decubitus			
	Environment			
Vital signs	Bp, HR, temperature, RR, SPO_2			
Hand signs	Leukonychia, koilonychia, pallor			
Eyes	Jaundice, pallor			
Mouth	Aphthous ulcer			
Neck	Lymphadenopathy			
Chest	Respiratory and CVS examination			
Abdomen: Inspection	Distention			
	Asymmetry			
	Dilated veins			
	Striae			
	Visible peristalsis			
	Scars			
	Cough impulse			

(continued)

History	Items	Done	Not done	NA
Palpation	Superficial then deep palpation			
	Tenderness			
	Palpable masses			
	Organomegaly			
	Cough impulse at hernial orifices			
Percussion	Shifting dullness			
	Fluid thrill			
	Organomegaly			
Auscultation	Bowel sounds			
	Bruit, venous hum			
Groin				
DRE and proctoscopy:				
Inspection	Obvious pathology (hemorrhoid, fissure, fistula)			
Hemorrhoids	Type (external, internal, or mixed)			
	Determine the grade of the internal hemorrhoid			
	ulceration			
	thrombosis			
Fissure	The location of the fissure (anterior, posterior, lateral)			
	Skin tag or hypertrophic papilla			
	Anal tone			
Fistula	External opening			
	Distance from the anal verge			
	Position			
	Presence of discharge			
Abscess	Hotness			
	Induration			
	Fluctuation			
	Tenderness			
If there is any palpable mass in the anorectal	Amount of the circumference involved			
	Site (anterior, posterior and lateral)			
	Consistency			
	Distance from the anal verge			
Back tenderness				
Extraintestinal manifestations	Erythema nodosum			
	Arthritis			
	Sacroiliitis			
	Ankylosing spondylitis			
Differential diagnosis	According to the given scenario			
Investigations				
General laboratory test	CBC with differential			
	Electrolytes			
	Liver function test			
	Blood grouping			
	Coagulation profile (PT, INR, aPTT)			
	RFT			
	CPR/ESR			

History	Items	Done	Not done	NA
Specific tests	Tumor marker (CEA)			
	Fecal calprotectin			
	Serology (ANCA, PANCA, ASCA)			
	Stool analysis			
Imaging	CT abdomen/pelvis			
	MRI pelvis			
	CT staging			
	Endorectal ultrasound			
Endoscopy	Colonoscopy			
Biopsy	Biopsy/polypectomy			
Provisional diagnosis	According to the given scenario			
Management (depends on the diagnosis):				
Hemorrhoids	Lifestyle modification			
	High fiber diet			
	Encourage drinking water			
	Avoid constipation			
	Over the counter topical cream			
	Antipyretic if not responding to initial treatment, office-based procedure, for example, RBL and sclerotherapy			
	For grade III and IV or complicated disease surgical hemorrhoidectomy			
Fissure	Lifestyle modification			
	High fiber diet			
	Encourage drinking water			
	Avoid constipation			
	Sitz bath			
	Topical anti-inflammatory			
	Topical GTN or calcium channel blocker			
	Botox injection			
	Lateral internal sphincterotomy (if not responding to medical management)			
	Advancement flap (in case of recurrence with weak anal tone or sphincter defect)			
Abscess	Admission			
	NPO if required			
	IV fluid			
	Analgesia			
	IV antibiotics			
	Consent			
	Incision and drainage			
	Postoperative wound care			
Fistula-in-ano	Define the fistula anatomy (EUA if simple fistula or MRI if recurrent or complicated fistula)			
	Resolve any sepsis			
	Assess the anal sphincter function			
	Surgical management			

(continued)

History	Items	Done	Not done	NA
Anal cancer SCC	Admission			
	Multidisciplinary team discussion			
	Staging			
	Nigro protocol			
	5-FU			
	Mitomycin			
	Radiation therapy to the perianal area			
	Radiation to the groin if positive inguinal lymph nodes			
	Surgery if recurrent or persistent			
	• Consent			
	• NPO			
	• IV fluid			
	• Prophylactic antibiotic			
	• DVT and stress ulcer prophylaxis			
	• Colonic preparation			
	• Stoma marking			
	• Ureteric stent			
	• APR			
	Adjuvant treatment as needed			
Anal adenocarcinoma	MRI pelvis			
	Endorectal ultrasound			
	CEA			
	Staging			
	Multidisciplinary team discussion			
	Prepare the patient for OR			
	Anesthesia consultation			
	ICU consultation			
	Prepare blood standby			
	Consent			
	NPO			
	IV fluid			
	Prophylactic antibiotic			
	Ureteric stent			
	Colonic preparation			
	Stoma marking			
	Surgery APR			
Postoperative care				
Early postoperative (anal cancer)	Admission to HDU or ICU when needed			
	Early mobilization and DVT prophylaxis			
	Enteral nutrition as early as possible			
	Analgesia			
	Stress ulcer prophylaxis			
	CBC and LFT daily			
	Electrolyte assessment			
	Monitor drain output and the nature of the fluid			
	Monitor the stoma itself and its output (if any)			

History	Items	Done	Not done	NA
First outpatient visit	Clinical assessment			
	Remove sutures			
	Review the final pathology report			
	Arrange for multidisciplinary discussion if the case is cancer			
	Refer to oncology if adjuvant treatment is required			
Long-term follow-up (for adenocarcinoma)	History and physical examination and CEA level every 3 months for 2 years, then every 6 months for the next 3 years			
	Annual CT CAP			
	Colonoscopy after 1 year (6 months if not completed preoperatively), then every 3 years if normal			
Long-term follow-up for SCC	DRE, anoscopy, inguinal examination every 3–6 months for 5 years			
	Annual CT CAP for a patient with T3-4 or N1			

12.2.2 Answers Key

Case No. 1:

A 28-year-old male patient presented to the emergency department complaining of perianal pain for 3 days.

Questions for Discussion:

1. **How will you approach the patient?**

   By history and physical examination.

   The patient is a 28-year-old male patient presented to the emergency department complaining of perianal pain for 3 days. It was started gradually, throbbing in nature, associated with fever. He has multiple attacks of similar complaint, and multiple incision and drainage procedures were done for him. However, he has not been investigated for the underlying cause.

   He has history of alternating bowel habit, weight loss, and joints pain.

   No family history of similar complaint or colorectal malignancy.

   He has no history of contact with sick patient.

   He is a smoker.

   Examination reveals an underweight man who looks sick and in pain.

   Vital signs: BP: 120/77 mmHg, temperature: 38.4, PR: 111 bpm

   Abdomen: unremarkable.

   DRE: shows multiple scars, large area of induration at 3 O'clock position with a small area of fluctuation and abscess, about 2 cm from the anal verge with hotness and tenderness. There is discharging opening at 7 O'clock position "near a scar of previous incision and drainage" but no signs of inflammation at this area.

2. **What will you do next?**
   - Admission.
   - NPO.
   - IV fluid.
   - IV antibiotics.
   - Blood investigation.
   - Prepare for surgery.
3. **How will you manage that?**
   - EUA and drainage of the abscess.
   - Investigate the cause after treating the sepsis.
4. **What further investigations will you ask for?**
   - Inflammatory marker.
   - Serology (ANCA, PANCA, ASCA).
   - Fecal calprotectin.
   - Colonoscopy and biopsy.
   - Pelvic MRI

     Further investigations confirm the diagnosis of Crohn's disease.

     Pelvic MRI shows supra-sphincteric branching fistula with multiple blind ends.

5. **What will be your management of his condition?**
   Draining seton for the fistulae.
   Referral to a gastroenterologist to start medical management and induce remission.

Suggested Twist Point:

Despite what you did, you could not control the sepsis and perianal infection. What would you do? If sepsis cannot be controlled with local therapy, fecal diversion should be considered. Proctectomy is indicated in refractory cases.

Case No. 2:

A 45-year-old female patient presented to the colorectal clinic complaining of anal mass for 3 months.

Question for Discussion:

1. **How will you approach the patient?**
   By history and physical examination.
   The patient is a 45-year-old female patient who presented to the clinic complaining of anal mass for 3 months. It started gradually as a small lesion, then increased in size over time. It is associated with itching of the perianal area. The lesion itself is not painful, but she also noticed pain at the groin area, and when she checked, she noticed a small swelling. No history of bleeding per rectum and abdominal pain.
   She is divorced, and her ex-husband was diagnosed with HPV.
   She is a smoker otherwise healthy woman.
   On examination:
   She is conscious, alert.
   Vital signs are stable.
   Abdominal examination is normal.
   There are multiple right inguinal palpable lymph nodes.
   DRE: there is a hard fungating mass at 3 O'clock position of the anal canal just below the dentate line about 3*4 cm.
2. **What is your differential diagnosis?**
   Anal cancer (SCC)
   Condyloma acuminatum
   Warts
   Hemorrhoids
3. **How will you investigate the patient?**
   Blood investigation.
   Colonoscopy.
   Biopsy from this anal lesion.
   Blood investigation and colonoscopy are normal.
   Biopsy shows moderate differentiated squamous cell carcinoma.
4. **How will you manage the patient?**
   Staging
   Multidisciplinary team approach
   Nigro protocol (5 FU-mitomycin-radiation therapy) + radiation to the groin
5. **How will you follow the patient (long term)?**
   DRE, anoscopy, inguinal examination every 3–6 months for 5 years
   Annual CT CAP.
6. **Upon regular follow-up, the tumor recurs. What will you do?**
   Restaging
   Multidisciplinary team discussion
   Salvage surgery (APR)

Suggested Twist Point:

On follow-up CT scan, there is a focal liver lesion on segment VI. What will you do?

Discuss in a multidisciplinary team.
PET scan.
Refer to oncology for systemic treatment and hepatobiliary surgery for possible resection.

References

1. Blumetti J. The management of hemorrhoids. In: Cameron JL, Cameron AM, editors. Current surgical therapy. 12th ed. Toronto: Elsevier; 2016.
2. Beck DE. Hemorrhoids. In: David E, SDW B, Rafferty JF, editors. Gordon and Nivatvongs' principles and practice of surgery for the colon, rectum, and anus. 4th ed. New York: Thieme Medical Publisher; 2019.
3. Mitchem JB. The management of anal fissures. In: Cameron JL, Cameron AM, editors. Current surgical therapy. 12th ed. Toronto: Elsevier; 2016.
4. Christante DH. The management of anorectal abscess and fistula. In: Cameron JL, Cameron AM, editors. Current surgical therapy. 12th ed. Toronto: Elsevier; 2016.
5. Winner M, Ahuja N. The management of tumors of the anal region. In: Cameron JL, Cameron AM, editors. Current surgical therapy. 12th ed. Toronto: Elsevier; 2016.

Surgical Aspects of Trauma for Clinical Board Exams

13

13.1 Part I: Knowledge

Unless you try to do something beyond what you have already mastered, you will never grow.
—Ronald E. Osborn

13.1.1 Approach to Trauma Patient

- Wear your personal protective equipment (gown, gloves, and goggles)
- Follow the Advanced Trauma Life Support (ATLS) protocol
- Start with the primary survey

A. Airway and Cervical Collar

- All patients with blunt trauma require cervical spine immobilization by applying a hard cervical collar.
- For penetrating neck wounds, cervical collars are not recommended.
- Conscious patients who have a normal voice:
  - Unlikely to require early airway intervention.
  - Exceptions:
    Penetrating injuries to the neck with an expanding hematoma
    Evidence of chemical or thermal injury to the mouth, nares, or hypopharynx
    Extensive subcutaneous air in the neck
    Complex maxillofacial trauma
    Airway bleeding
  - In these cases, preemptive intubation should be performed before airway access becomes challenging.
- Patients who have an abnormal voice, abnormal breathing sounds, tachypnea, or altered mental status:
  - Require further airway evaluation.
  - Suctioning.
  - In the comatose patient, chin lift or jaw thrust.
  - An oral airway or a nasal airway is also helpful in maintaining airway patency.
  - Establishing a definitive airway (i.e., endotracheal intubation) is indicated in:
    Patients with apnea.
    Inability to protect the airway due to altered mental status.
    Impending airway compromise due to inhalation injury, hematoma, facial bleeding, soft tissue swelling, or aspiration.
    Inability to maintain oxygenation.
  - Because all patients are presumed to have cervical spine injuries, manual in-line cervical immobilization is essential.
  - Correct endotracheal placement is verified with:
    Direct laryngoscopy.
    Capnography.
    Audible bilateral breath sounds.
    Chest film [1].
  - Rapid sequence intubation (RSI):
    Preparation and equipment:
    - Universal precautions.

H. Alotaibi, *Study Surgery*, https://doi.org/10.1007/978-981-16-2305-9_13

- Airway equipment: laryngoscope of choice, endotracheal tubes, backup equipment (backup laryngoscope, elastic bougie, LMAs, needle cricothyrotomy kit, and surgical airway kit), oxygen source, and suction device.
- Medications (hypnotics, muscle relaxants, and pressors).
- Electrical defibrillator.
- Additional experienced assistants present, and discussion with trauma team leader regarding the timing.

Intravenous access:
- Essential for the administration of RSI agents and volume resuscitation.

Monitoring:
- ECG monitoring, recurrent blood pressure monitoring, pulse oximeter, and in-line capnography.

Positioning:
- Sniff positioning if possible: 8 to 10 cm head elevation with pads under the occiput and atlanto-occipital extension.
- Manual in-line stabilization needed to prevent neck extension in patients at risk for cervical spine injury.

Preoxygenation:
- Administration of 100% oxygen by sealed face mask, with or without assisted ventilation to prevent hypoxia during the period of RSI-associated apnea.
- Cricoid pressure (Sellick's maneuver).
- All trauma patients should be considered to have full stomach and risk of aspiration should be reduced.
- Compression of the esophagus against the cervical spine to reduce the risk of regurgitation and aspiration.

Administration of induction agents:
- Etomidate: 0.2–0.3 mg/kg.
- Ketamine: 2 mg/kg.
- Midazolam (the drug of choice): 0.05–0.15 mg/kg.

Administration of paralytic agents:
- Succinylcholine: 1.2–1.5 mg/kg.
- Rocuronium: 1.0–1.2 mg/kg.

Placement of the endotracheal tube:
- Select device based on patient's injuries and airway examination.
- Typical tube position: 21 cm at the incisors (women) and 23 cm (men); [age ÷ 2] + 12 cm (children).

Manual ventilation and confirmation of physiologic response:
- Confirmation of tube as described above [1, 2].

- Patients in whom intubation attempts have failed or are precluded from intubation due to extensive facial injuries require the operative establishment of an airway.
  - Cricothyroidotomy is performed through a generous vertical incision, with a sharp division of the subcutaneous tissues. Visualization may be improved by having an assistant retract laterally on the neck incision using retractors. The cricothyroid membrane is verified by digital palpation and opened in a horizontal direction (Fig. 13.1).
  - A 6.0 endotracheal tube is then advanced through the cricothyroid opening and sutured into place.

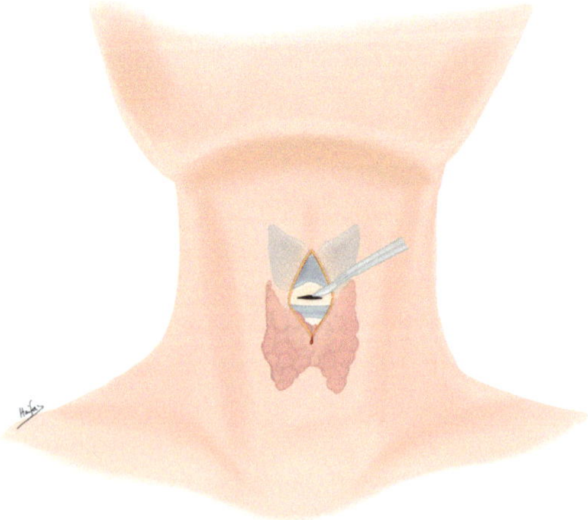

Fig. 13.1 Cricothyroidotomy; notice that the skin incision is longitudinal and the membrane incision is transverse

- Cricothyroidotomy is relatively contraindicated in patient < 11 years old due to the risk of subglottic stenosis.
- Emergent tracheostomy is indicated in patients with laryngotracheal separation or laryngeal fractures.
- If the trachea is completely transected, a nonpenetrating clamp should be placed on the distal aspect to prevent tracheal retraction into the mediastinum; this is particularly important before endotracheal tube placement [1].

B. Breathing and Ventilation

- All injured patients should receive oxygen and be monitored by pulse oximetry.
- **Tension pneumothorax:**
  - Manifestations: respiratory distress and hypotension combined with any of the following physical signs:
    - Tracheal deviation away from the affected side
    - Lack of or decreased breath sounds on the affected side
    - Subcutaneous emphysema on the affected side
  - Patients may or may not have distended neck veins.
  - Immediate needle thoracostomy decompression with a 14-gauge needle may be indicated in the field; tube thoracostomy in the midaxillary line should be performed immediately in the ED before a chest radiograph is obtained.
  - The location for needle decompression is the fifth intercostal space in the anterior axillary line [1, 3].
- **Open pneumothorax or "sucking chest wound":**
  - Full-thickness injury to the chest wall.
  - Free communication between the pleural space and the atmosphere.
  - Temporary management of this injury includes covering the wound with an occlusive dressing taped on three sides.
  - Definitive treatment: closure of the chest wall defect and tube thoracostomy remote from the wound [1, 3].
- **Flail chest:**
  - Three or more contiguous ribs are fractured in at least two locations.
  - Paradoxical movement of this free-floating segment of the chest wall is usually evident in patients with spontaneous ventilation due to the negative intrapleural pressure of inspiration.
  - Pulmonary contusions often progress during the first 12 h.
  - Resultant hypoventilation and hypoxemia may require intubation and mechanical ventilation.
  - Close monitoring and frequent clinical reevaluation are warranted [1, 3].
- **Major air leak:**
  - Occurs from tracheobronchial injuries.
  - Type I: within 2 cm of the carina. These may not be associated with a pneumothorax due to the envelopment in the mediastinal pleura.
  - Type II: more distal injuries within the tracheobronchial tree and, hence, manifest with a pneumothorax.
  - Bronchoscopy confirms the extent of the injury and its location and directs management [1, 3].
- **A massive hemothorax:**
  - Defined as >1500 mL of blood or, in the pediatric population, >25% of the patient's blood volume in the pleural space.
  - After blunt trauma, a hemothorax is usually due to multiple rib fractures with severe injury to the intercostal vessels, but occasionally bleeding is from lacerated lung parenchyma.
  - After penetrating trauma, a great vessel or pulmonary hilar vessel injury should be presumed.
  - In either scenario, a massive hemothorax is an indication for operative intervention [1, 3].

C. Circulation

- Hypotension is assumed to be caused by hemorrhage until proven otherwise.
- Patients with rapid, massive blood loss may have paradoxical bradycardia.

- The goal of fluid resuscitation is to reestablish tissue perfusion.
- Fluid resuscitation usually begins with isotonic crystalloid, typically Ringer's lactate.
- For persistent hypotension, activate a massive transfusion protocol (MTP).
- Consider tranexamic acid if <3 h and patient has massive bleeding.
- Intravenous (IV) access for fluid resuscitation and medication administration is obtained with two peripheral catheters, 16-gauge or larger in adults.
- For patients whose peripheral access is difficult, use intraosseous (IO) routes. The needle should be removed once alternative access is established to prevent potential osteomyelitis.
- Saphenous vein cut downs at the ankle: the vein found 1 cm anterior and 1 cm superior to the medial malleolus.
- Blood should be drawn simultaneously for a bedside hemoglobin level and routine trauma laboratory tests (CBC, ABG, cross match, renal function test, coagulation profile, and pregnancy test in females).
- Base deficit measurement is critical; a base deficit of >8 mmol/L implies ongoing cellular shock. Serum lactate also is used to monitor the patient's physiologic response to resuscitation.
- Control of any visible hemorrhage.
- For bleeding of the extremities, apply tourniquets for hemorrhage control if needed.
- Fracture reduction with stabilization via splints will limit bleeding both externally and into the subcutaneous tissues.
- Scalp lacerations tend to bleed profusely and can be temporarily controlled with skin staples or a full-thickness continuous running stitch.
- Focus assessment sonography of trauma should be performed (FAST scan).
- Persistent hemodynamic instability and positive FAST scan is an indication for emergency laparotomy.
- In patients arriving in shock with a high risk of pelvic fracture (e.g., auto-pedestrian accident), the pelvis should be presumptively stabilized with a sheet or binder [1].
- **Cardiac tamponade:**
  - It occurs most commonly after penetrating thoracic wounds, although occasionally blunt rupture of the heart, particularly the atrial appendage, is seen. Acutely, <100 mL of pericardial blood may cause pericardial tamponade.
  - Diagnosis of hemopericardium is best achieved by ultrasound of the pericardium.
  - In patients with any hemodynamic disturbance, a pericardial drain can be placed using ultrasound guidance.
  - Removing as little as 15–20 mL of blood will often temporarily stabilize the patient's hemodynamic status.
  - Patients with a persistent SBP <60 mmHg warrant resuscitative thoracotomy (RT) with the pericardium's opening for rapid decompression and control of bleeding [1].
- **Resuscitative thoracotomy:**

A. *Indications*:

I. **Salvageable postinjury cardiac arrest:**
  - Patients sustaining witnessed penetrating trauma to the torso with <15 min of prehospital CPR.
  - Patients sustaining witnessed blunt trauma with <10 min of prehospital CPR.
  - Patients sustaining witnessed penetrating trauma to the neck or extremities with <5 min of prehospital CPR.

II. **Persistent severe postinjury hypotension (SBP ≤60 mmHg) due to:**
  - Cardiac tamponade.
  - Hemorrhage—intrathoracic, intraabdominal, extremity, and cervical.
  - Air embolism.

B. *Contraindications*:
  - Penetrating trauma: CPR >15 min and no signs of life (pupillary response, respiratory effort, and motor activity).
  - Blunt trauma: CPR >10 min and no signs of life or asystole without associated tamponade.

C. *Procedure*:
  - **Incision:** Left anterolateral thoracotomy at the fourth or fifth intercostal margin, just below the nipple in a male or the inframammary fold in a female. The incision

should begin at the lateral border of the left sternocostal junction inferior to the nipple and is continued to the latissimus dorsi muscle.

- **Exposure:** The intercostal muscles are then cut with a scalpel, Mayo scissors, or Metzenbaum scissors. The incision should course the superior margin of the rib to avoid injuring the intercostal neurovascular bundle. Care should be taken to prevent lacerating the lung or heart while entering the thoracic cavity. A Finochietto retractor is then placed to spread the ribs.
- **Extension**: The incision can be extended to the right hemithorax across the sternum; if needed, it can be accomplished quickly with a Lebsche knife. Both of the internal mammary arteries then must be ligated.
- **Cardiac tamponade:** The pericardium should be opened routinely because one cannot visually rule out cardiac tamponade. The pericardium is incised anteriorly and opened parallel to the left phrenic nerve. The excision should extend superiorly to the aortic root and then inferiorly to the apex of the heart. Blood clots should be removed, and the heart should be thoroughly examined for injury.
- **Cardiac bleeding**: Should be controlled immediately with digital pressure while preparing for better temporizing measures. Inserting a Foley catheter, blowing up the balloon, and using gentle traction also can achieve temporary control of hemorrhage.
- **Aorta cross-clamping:** To expose the descending aorta, the lung is elevated anteriorly and superiorly. At this point, the inferior pulmonary ligament should be taken down for improved exposure and access to the aorta. Palpating the nasogastric or orogastric tube may help to differentiate the aorta from the esophagus. After the esophagus is separated anteriorly and the prevertebral fascia is separated posteriorly, the left hand should encircle the aorta while a clamp is applied with the right hand.
- **Bimanual internal cardiac massage:** Should begin immediately if there is true cardiac arrest. The preferred method is a hinged clapping motion with the wrists apposed and ventricular compression proceeding from the apex to the heart's base, which is best accomplished by cupping the left hand and placing it over the right ventricle. The fingers of the right hand are held tightly together to form a flat surface supporting the left ventricle.
- **Control of pulmonary hemorrhage:** Occasionally, bleeding from the lung can be controlled with either a Duval clamp or a vascular clamp. If simple clamping does not achieve hemostasis, several other methods are available. Occluding flow of the pulmonary hilum has the advantage of achieving complete inflow control, which can be accomplished by mobilizing the inferior pulmonary ligament and simply twisting the lung on the hilum [1, 4].

D. Disability:

- The Glasgow Coma Scale (GCS) score should be determined for all injured patients.
- It is calculated by adding the best motor response scores, best verbal response, and the best eye response.
- Scores range from 3 (the lowest) to 15 (normal).
- Scores of 13–15 indicate mild head injury, 9–12 moderate injury, and ≤8 severe injury.
- An abnormal mental status should prompt an immediate reevaluation of the patient's ABCs and consideration of central nervous system injury.
- Patients with neurogenic shock have hypotension with relative bradycardia and are often first recognized due to paralysis, decreased rectal tone, or priapism.
- Patients with high spinal cord disruption are at greatest risk for neurogenic shock. Treatment consists of volume loading and a dopamine infusion, both inotropic and chronotropic, as well as a vasoconstrictor [1].

E. Exposure:

- Seriously injured patients must have all of their clothing removed to avoid overlooking limb- or life-threatening injuries, but warmed blankets should be placed immediately to prevent hypothermia [1].

- **Adjunct to the primary survey:**
  - Chest and pelvic X-ray
  - FAST
  - Foley's catheter
  - NGT [1]
- **Secondary survey:**
  - Obtain a complete history (focus on AMPLE history: allergy, medications, past medical history, last meal, and the event that led to the trauma)
  - Perform head to toe examination
  - Log roll and examine the back
  - DRE
- Pan CT.
- At any point, if the patient deteriorates, re-evaluate following the approach ABCDE [1].

13.1.2 Management of Traumatic Brain Injury (TBI)

- In addition to the standard history, the use of antiplatelet or anticoagulant medications should be asked about specifically.
- A focused neurologic examination including brainstem reflexes, motor function in all extremities, and a Glasgow Coma Score should be obtained.
- The GCS ranges from 3 to 15 and can be divided into mild (13–15), moderate (9–12), and severe (3–8) TBI.
- The head CT should be evaluated for the presence of intracranial blood, midline shift, mass effect, herniation, and skull fractures [5].
- The initial treatment of patients with TBI should focus on three objectives:
  - **Hypotension and hypoxia:**

    SBP lower than 110 or 120 mmHg may be associated with worse outcomes.

    All patients with TBI should have continuous oxygen saturation monitoring in addition to supplemental oxygen.

    Persistent hypoxia and a GCS of 8 or less are both indications for intubation.
  - **Preventing herniation:**

    Clinical signs of elevated intracranial pressure (ICP) include hypertension, bradycardia, and irregular respirations (Cushing's triad). Progression to transtentorial uncal herniation results in loss of consciousness, ipsilateral pupillary dilation, and contralateral hemiparesis.

    Initial management:
    - Hypoventilation (short-term management).
    - Mannitol: 1 g/kg.
    - Hypertonic saline: Bolus doses of 250 mL of 7.5%, 75 mL of 10%, and 30 mL of 23.4% have all shown similar efficacy at reversing transtentorial herniation.

    If surgical decompression is indicated, the patient should be transferred expeditiously to the operating room or an institution with a neurosurgeon.
  - **Antiplatelet and anticoagulant reversal:**

    Reversal of anticoagulants or antiplatelet agents is indicated in the setting of intracranial hemorrhage (ICH) [5].
- **Epidural hematoma (EDH):**
  - It is often arterial injuries in the setting of skull fractures but can result from venous or sinus injuries.
  - On head CT, EDHs have a biconvex or lens shape created by the blood pushing the dura away from the skull.
  - Because of strong dural attachments at the cranial sutures, EDHs typically do not cross suture lines.
  - Acute EDH should be evacuated surgically in a GCS setting of 8 or less, anisocoria, or a volume larger than 30 cm^3.
  - Nonoperative management should be considered only in patients without focal neurologic deficits, GCS higher than 8, hematoma volume smaller than 30 cm^3, hematoma thickness less than 15 mm, and a midline shift less than 5 mm.
  - These patients must be watched closely in an ICU setting with serial neurologic examinations and repeat head CT [5].

- **Subdural hematoma (SDH):**
  - SDHs usually are caused by bleeding from torn bridging veins in the subdural space and frequently are associated with parenchymal lesions.
  - On head CT, they classically appear as crescent-shaped collections that cross sutures lines and layer along the falx.
  - An acute SDH should be evacuated, regardless of the patient's GCS, if the hematoma is more than 10 mm thick or a midline shift greater than 5 mm.
  - Other indications for surgical evacuation in patient with SDH and GCS ≤8:
    - The patient's GCS has dropped by 2 or more points since the time of injury.
    - The patient has anisocoria or fixed pupils.
    - The ICP is greater than 20 mm Hg.
  - Patients with a GCS of 8 or less who do not meet the criteria for surgery can be managed nonoperatively but must have an ICP monitor, close observation in an ICU setting, and serial head CT [5].
- **Open and depressed skull fractures:**
  - All open fractures should receive antibiotics with appropriate gram-negative coverage to prevent meningitis.
  - All open fractures with evidence of dural injury (e.g., CSF leakage and visible brain matter), depression greater than 10 mm, significant ICH, pneumocephalus, gross wound contamination, or frontal sinus involvement should be repaired surgically because of the risk of infection [5].

13.1.3 Management of Chest Trauma

- **Rib fractures and flail chest:**
  - Lower rib fractures (ninth to eleventh) should direct attention to possible abdominal solid organ injury (left side spleen, kidney, right side liver, and kidney).
  - Upper rib fractures (first to third) are associated with injuries to the head, neck, spinal cord, and great vessels.
  - Flail chest is a specific rib fracture pattern defined by three or more adjacent ribs with fractures in two or more places.
  - Flail chest represents the most severe form of chest wall injury after blunt trauma, with more than 80% of patients needing ICU admission and more than 50% requiring mechanical ventilation.
  - It is important to note that such paradoxical motion is eliminated during positive pressure ventilation (PPV), which may lead to initial oversight of the injury, especially in intubated patients before arrival in the trauma bay.
  - The treatment of rib fractures and flail chest is nonoperative in the vast majority of cases. Patients usually can be managed successfully with aggressive pain control, early and effective pulmonary toilet, and supportive care.
- **Sternal Fractures:**
  - History, physical examination, basic imaging, and electrocardiography at the time of initial evaluation are adequate to rule out associated injuries.
  - Cardiac biomarkers generally are not useful for the management of suspected cardiac contusion.
  - Operative repair of sternal fractures is sometimes indicated for significant displacement and overlap.
- **Clavicle fractures and dislocations:**
  - Distal clavicle fractures managed operatively because of high risk of nonunion.
  - Acromioclavicular dislocation (or "shoulder separation") often is managed nonoperatively, concomitant coracoclavicular disruption, and may require operative reduction.
  - Sternoclavicular dislocation indicates a high force injury.
- **Pneumothorax:**
  - Occult pneumothorax (not apparent on initial CXR but later seen on CT) can be observed safely with interval CXRs and this strategy can be extended to patients who are undergoing positive pressure ven-

tilation (according to the American Association for the Surgery of Trauma [AAST] recommendation).

- **Hemothorax**
  - Depending on the quantity of blood, upright AP CXR may reveal blunting of the costophrenic angle or complete opacification of the hemothorax. In general, the minimum amount of blood needed to produce plain X-ray findings is 200–500 mL.
  - The management of occult hemothorax is not clear.
  - Generally, hemothoraces less than 1.5 cm in maximal cross-sectional diameter on CT can be observed safely.
  - Retained hemothorax is defined as a residual hemothorax despite attempted evacuation by tube thoracostomy.
  - The diagnosis should be suspected when there is a persistent opacity on CXR after tube thoracostomy and is best confirmed by noncontrast chest CT.
  - Management depend on the amount of the retained blood: <300 ml observe, 300–900 ml: VATS and >900 ml (especially when associated with diaphragm injury) most likely will need thoracotomy.
  - Fibrinolytics, additional tube thoracostomies, and image-guided procedures are often ineffective in this setting and, therefore, are discouraged for treatment of retained hemothorax [3].

13.1.4 Management of Liver Injury

- All trauma patients should have an initial evaluation according to Advanced Trauma Life Support (ATLS) protocols.
- For unstable patients, a focused assessment with sonography for trauma (FAST) should be performed as part of the primary survey.
- For unstable victims with equivocal FAST results (patients whose body habitus precludes appropriate sonographic interpretation), diagnostic peritoneal lavage (DPL) can be performed. If 10 mL of blood are aspirated before any infusion or if more than 100,000 red blood cells (RBCs) per μL are detected in the peritoneal lavage, the DPL is considered positive and transfer to the operating room should follow.
- For patients who are hemodynamically stable and in which there is a suspicion for intraabdominal injury, CT scan with intravenous contrast should be performed.
- Grading of the injuries should be done using trauma liver injury scale that was published by The American Association for the Surgery of Trauma (AAST).

Nonoperative Management:

- **Blunt trauma:**
  - Except for grade VI lacerations, patients with any grade of liver injury have the potential to be managed with a nonoperative approach.
  - ICU admission.
  - Frequent clinical assessment.
  - A regular check for hemoglobin, hematocrit, and INR levels.
  - Transfer to a nonmonitored setting usually can be done after 24 h for patients with grade I and II liver injuries; those with higher-grade injuries will require longer monitoring periods, ranging from 2 to 3 days.
  - Chemical deep venous thrombosis (DVT) prophylaxis should be held initially.
  - Because the risk for this complication is high, trauma patients have mechanical DVT prophylaxis devices.
  - Once the patient shows evidence of recovery and the patient's hemoglobin remains stable, starting anticoagulation should be considered.
  - Selective embolization can be used as an adjunct to nonoperative management because arterial bleeding within the liver parenchyma can be controlled.
  - Failure of nonoperative management can occur and is marked by hemodynamic instability. Any deterioration requires immediate

assessment, balanced resuscitation, and ultimately hemostatic intervention.
  - Risk factors for nonoperative management failure include injury to the spleen and kidney, positive FAST, hemoperitoneum over 300 mL, and need for transfusion.
  - If the patient becomes unstable or if active bleeding cannot be controlled with interventional procedures, operative intervention is warranted.
- **Penetrating trauma:**
  - For highly selected patients treated at specialized trauma centers, who are seen with right upper quadrant wounds and isolated liver injuries, a nonoperative approach can be considered.
  - Suppose the patient is hemodynamically stable, has a reliable physical examination, and has a CT scan showing no other injury, the patient is a candidate for nonoperative management.
  - Treatment approaches are the same as those for nonpenetrating liver injury. They involve repeat imaging as deemed necessary, laboratory follow-up, admission to a monitored bed, use of mechanical DVT prophylaxis only, and bed rest [6].

Operative Management:
- **Preoperative considerations:**
  - Calling an experienced hepatobiliary surgeon for assistance when there is a concern for a complex injury.
  - The operating room should be warmed, and a balanced resuscitation with warm products should continue.
  - Massive transfusion protocol should be activated immediately.
  - Rapid infusers and fluid warmers should remain available and be used as indicated.
  - If there is no evidence of enteric spillage and immediately available, a cell saver unit can be set up and used.
  - Two Yankauer suction tips also should be ready for immediate use.
  - A self-retaining retractor such as a Thompson, Omni, or Bookwalter retractor should be available to optimize exposure.
  - An argon beam coagulator and topical hemostatic agents should be requested and available for use.
  - Preoperative antibiotics with gram-negative and anaerobic coverage should be started and redosed according to blood loss and case length.
  - Continuous communication with anesthesia providers.
- **Initial operative approach:**
  - The patient should be prepared widely from chin to knees.
  - A wide laparotomy incision from the xiphoid process to the symphysis pubis.
  - When vascular control of the suprahepatic inferior vena cava (IVC) is needed, the celiotomy extension to a sternotomy or right thoracotomy is indicated.
  - Once the peritoneum is opened, massive bleeding may be encountered as the tamponade effect exerted by the abdominal cavity is released.
  - It is crucial to alert the anesthesia providers to enter the abdomen.
  - The abdomen should be packed with laparotomy pads in all four quadrants.
  - It is important to place laparotomy pads on the liver's anterior and posterior surface, as this may create a tamponade that minimizes bleeding from the liver parenchyma.
  - Care must be taken to avoid compressing the IVC with packing, which will compromise venous return to the heart.
  - While the pads are in place, the self-retaining retractor should be placed, and resuscitation should continue [6].
- **Blunt trauma:**
  - *Minor injuries:*

    Direct compression for 5–10 min can usually control it. If unsuccessful, topical agents, electrocautery, and the argon beam coagulator can be used. Fibrin glue, hemostatic fabric, and topical collagen can be applied to the compromised surface.

    Clear inspection for possible bile leaks should be done. If there is no evidence of bleeding or bile leak, no further treatment is needed.

If compression is unsuccessful, suture hepatorrhaphy can be performed. Transcapsular #0 chromic sutures with blunt-nosed needles should be performed.

Care should be taken to minimize necrosis of viable liver by placing sutures close to the edge of the injury [6].

– *Moderate-to-severe injuries:*

Deep liver lacerations should be explored to identify defects in the bile system and vascular structures. With 5-0 prolene suture, figure-of-eight stitches are placed to control spillage and bleeding.

A tongue of vascularized omentum can be prepared, packed into the laceration, and secured with transcapsular sutures.

Larger vascular branches deep within the laceration, the finger fracture technique should be the initial approach. Expansion of the wound allows identifying the larger branches that are usually on the deep aspect of the wound. Suture ligation and clips are then used to control the bleeding. Omental packing also can be performed.

If there is massive bleeding after the release of hepatic packing, a different approach should be taken. Packing should be reestablished immediately.

The liver's vascular inflow should be controlled rapidly by performing Pringle's maneuver. The surgeon's left index finger should be placed through Winslow's foramen and compression applied between the thumb and index finger, which will control the hepatic artery and the portal vein. The gastrohepatic ligament should be opened with electrocautery, careful not to injure a replaced or accessory left hepatic artery. A vascular clamp, Penrose drain, or Rummel's tourniquet can be applied. Pringle's maneuver can be applied for 20 min, followed by 5 min of reperfusion.

Once the inflow has been controlled, the liver must be mobilized to identify the injury.

The injury should be evaluated carefully. If intrahepatic vessels are identified as sources, suture ligation or clipping should be performed. Any visualized bile ducts should be ligated.

Consideration of adjunctive percutaneous embolization may be beneficial.

Extrahepatic suture ligation of the right or left hepatic artery can be used as an attempt to control bleeding. If the right hepatic artery is ligated, consideration should be given to performing cholecystectomy immediately or at a later date.

Common hepatic artery ligation is the ultimate damage control maneuver; however, it carries a high risk for liver and biliary duct ischemia.

In cases where there is devascularization of a segment or lobe of the liver, a hepatectomy can be performed; it usually occurs in a nonanatomic distribution and may involve central vessels.

After mobilization, the surgeon can pack the liver more effectively. The abdomen then can be closed with a temporary dressing, and the patient is transported to the ICU for close monitoring, resuscitation, and warming. Angiography is an important adjunct and the patient may be taken to interventional radiology after packing the liver for selective angioembolization to control arterial bleeding. The patient should return to the operating room within 24–72 h, and the packs removed. Once the decision to close the abdomen has been made, a thorough evaluation for the presence of bile and identification of additional injuries should be performed. The surgeon should consider leaving closed suction drains [6].

- **Penetrating injury:**
  – With the use of a Penrose drain and a red rubber catheter, a balloon can be created to tamponade deep wounds. The red rubber

catheter is prepared by cutting holes in the distal portion of the catheter. The catheter is then advanced through the Penrose drain and secured to the catheter with silk ties. The device is then inserted into the wound and, using saline, the balloon is inflated.
  - Mobilizing the liver and packing it with laparotomy pads assist in further controlling any additional injuries. A temporary abdominal closure system can be used, and the patient is then transported to the ICU for further resuscitation and treatment. Within 24–72 h, the patient should be taken back to the operating room, and the balloon deflated.
  - Extrahepatic biliary and vascular structures are injured more frequently with penetrating injuries. Before performing any repair to these structures, Kocher's maneuver should be performed to have better exposure of the portal structures and avoid further injury.
  - If the portal vein is injured, primary repair should be attempted with a lateral venorrhaphy technique and 5-0 Prolene sutures. If the patient is in critical condition and the portal vein is not amenable to primary repair, ligation can be performed.
  - If any of the arteries are injured, primary repair should be attempted. The right and left hepatic arteries can be isolated and ligated. The common hepatic artery also can be ligated, especially if the portal vein remains intact.
  - If there is a minor injury of the extrahepatic bile duct injury, primary repair or placement of a T-tube should be attempted. If there is extensive injury, closed suction drains should be placed, and plans should be made to perform a Roux-en-Y biliary-enteric anastomosis at a later time [6].
- **Retrohepatic caval injury:**
  - It is very difficult to manage and carries significant mortality.
  - If a hematoma is seen when mobilizing the triangular ligament, the dissection should stop. Perihepatic packing with laparotomy pads and intraparenchymal packing with omentum should be used. Resuscitation is continued in the ICU and, if indicated, adjunctive radiologic techniques can be considered.
  - Otherwise, vascular liver isolation should be considered in an attempt to repair the injured structures [6].

Complications of Liver Trauma:

- Abscess:
  - Treatment includes intravenous antibiotics with gram-negative and anaerobic coverage.
  - Source control with imaging-guided percutaneous drainage.
  - Surgical drainage if the patient did not improve.
- Pseudoaneurysm:
  - If CT scan of the abdomen reveals a pseudoaneurysm, angiographic evaluation and embolization should be performed.
  - If the abnormality is found at the common hepatic artery level, stent placement or open ligation and bypass should be considered.
- Bile leaks:
  - Liver function test (LFT) should be performed.
  - CT scan should be obtained, and if a fluid collection is identified, percutaneous drainage should follow.
  - Monitoring of output after drainage is necessary.
  - If drainage decreases and eventually stops, no further treatment is necessary.
  - If the drainage is greater than 50 mL/day for 14 days, further assessment should be pursued; cholangiographic evaluation of the biliary tree should be performed with ERCP or MRCP.
  - Sphincterotomy and stent placement can be performed in an attempt to minimize the bile leak.
  - PTC and percutaneous biliary drainage can also be attempted for treatment if cannulation of Oddi's sphincter is difficult.

- Hemobilia:
  - They usually result from arteriobiliary fistulae; therefore, hepatic angiography, embolization, and resuscitation in the ICU are the pillars of treatment.
- Necrosis
- Rebleeding [6]

13.1.5 Management of Splenic Injury

- All trauma patients should have an initial evaluation according to Advanced Trauma Life Support (ATLS) protocols.
- For unstable patients, a focused assessment with sonography for trauma (FAST) should be performed as part of the primary survey.
- Patient with hemodynamic instability and positive FAST scan should be taken for emergency laparotomy.
- Stable patient can be further evaluated by CT scan.
- Grading of the injuries should be done using trauma spleen injury scale that was published by The American Association for the Surgery of Trauma (AAST) [7].

Nonoperative Management:

- **Blunt trauma:**
  - It is appropriate only in the hemodynamically stable patient without signs of peritonitis.
  - Patients are admitted for serial hemoglobin measurements (every 6–8 h) and a period of bed rest proportional to the severity of the injury.
  - Overall length of inpatient observation is congruent to the severity of the injury, with a rough guideline being the grade of injury plus 1 for the total length of stay (days).
  - Early initiation (defined as within 48 h) of pharmacologic venous thromboembolism (VTE) prophylaxis does not appear to affect the failure rate or the need for transfusion.
  - Risk factors for failure include:

    Age older than 40 years

    High injury severity score, grade III, or higher splenic injury (particularly grades IV and V)

    The need for transfusion of blood product
  - An adjunct for splenic injury is selective arterial embolization, which is typically performed through percutaneous femoral access.
  - The presence of a contrast blush, pseudoaneurysm, or extravasation as an indication for embolization in any grade of splenic injury.
  - The most current EAST guidelines do not recommend routine follow-up imaging.
- **Penetrating injury:**
  - Most penetrating abdominal injuries require operative exploration [7].

Operative Management:

- Indicated for patients who initially are seen with hemodynamic instability, peritonitis, associated injuries that require laparotomy, or after the failure of nonoperative management.
- When operative management is indicated, the standard treatment is trauma laparotomy, exploration, and splenectomy.
- The majority of the minor splenic injuries that in the past were managed with splenorrhaphy are now managed successfully with nonoperative management.
- Minor splenic injuries identified at the time of trauma laparotomy in an otherwise hemodynamically stable patient may be repaired.

Vaccination:

- Patients who have undergone a splenectomy require vaccination against *Streptococcus pneumoniae*, *Neisseria meningitidis*, and *Haemophilus influenzae type B*.
- The optimal timing for vaccination appears to be 2 weeks after splenectomy.
- Vaccines require periodic boosters to ensure adequate titers, and thus coordination with the patient's primary physician is important.
- Daily antibiotic prophylaxis is no longer recommended for adults after splenectomy [7].

13.1.6 Management of Pancreatic and Duodenal Injury

- A high index of suspicion is necessary to make the diagnosis.
- Certain injury patterns should prompt suspicion for the potential of pancreatic or duodenal trauma. Significant blunt force to the epigastrium, as may be seen after sudden abdominal compression with a bicycle handlebar or a seatbelt during rapid deceleration, should trigger concern for this injury.
- FAST contributes little to the diagnosis of pancreaticoduodenal injury because of the retroperitoneal location of these structures.
- On CT, injury to the pancreas is suggested by parenchymal laceration, intrapancreatic or retroperitoneal hematoma, peripancreatic fluid, phlegmon, or fluid between the pancreas and splenic vein. Bowel wall thickening, extraluminal gas, and contrast extravasation on CT suggest duodenal injury.
- ERCP is sensitive and specific for delineating pancreatic duct injury.
- MRCP is a noninvasive means of determining duct integrity; it is useful for evaluating the anatomy and integrity of the pancreatic duct but rarely is used in the acute setting.
- Analysis of serum amylase and lipase also can be helpful in the diagnosis of pancreatic and duodenal.
- In the patient with indications for emergent laparotomy, the diagnosis of injury to the pancreas and duodenum should be made during surgery.
- Findings suggestive of injury during exploration include central retroperitoneal hematoma, bile staining, or air in the surrounding tissue planes.
- Control of hemorrhage and contamination are priorities and should come before any effort to definitively address an injury to the pancreas or duodenum [8].

Duodenal Injury:

- Duodenal injuries can be identified on CT.
- When suspected during exploration, complete exposure and mobilization of the duodenum are required. The Cattell-Braasch maneuver facilitates the exposure of the second, third, and fourth portions of the duodenum by mobilizing the ascending colon and small bowel's posterior parietal attachments medially while rotating the viscera en bloc to the midline.
- The American Association for the Surgery of Trauma-Organ Injury Scale (AAST-OIS) classifies injury to the duodenum based on a grading scale from I to V.
- Duodenal hematoma, when diagnosed by CT and in the absence of any other indications for surgery, supportive care consisting of IV hydration, nasogastric decompression, and parenteral nutrition, is usually a successful treatment approach. Most duodenal hematomas will resolve spontaneously within 3 to 4 weeks.
- Failure to improve is an indication to repeat imaging to reevaluate the obstructive process, and operative intervention may be necessary.
- If the diagnosis of significant duodenal hematoma is made during laparotomy, the serosa should be incised carefully over the hematoma to allow for the contained blood's evacuation. The resulting partial-thickness defect should be repaired primarily. Closed-suction drainage and nasojejunal feeding are recommended.
- The majority of all full-thickness injuries to the duodenum can be repaired primarily with careful alignment of edges. Repair consists of debridement of devitalized tissue and a two-layer closure of the defect. The closure generally should be oriented in a transverse direction, and the omentum should be used to buttress the repair.
- Pyloric exclusion is generally reserved for protecting the most complex repairs of the duodenum or combined injuries to both the duodenum and pancreas.
- Large proximal and distal duodenal injuries may be repaired by resection and primary duodenoduodenostomy.
- Duodenal injuries that involve the ampulla, common bile duct, or pancreas are more complex. If the ampulla is injured, it may be repaired primarily or reimplanted into the

duodenum or Roux loop of the jejunum. Any injury that cannot be reconstructed may necessitate pancreaticoduodenectomy.

- Injuries to the distal common bile duct also complicate the management of duodenal trauma. Exploration of the posterior pancreatic head enhances visualization of the injury. Smaller injuries to the common bile duct (less than 50% of the circumference) can be repaired over a stent. Larger defects or involvement of the intrapancreatic or intraduodenal common bile duct requires reimplantation of the duct or pancreaticoduodenectomy [8].

Pancreatic Injury:

- The diagnosis of pancreatic injury can be made by imaging in the emergency room or during laparotomy in the operating room.
- The AAST classifies injury to the pancreas based on a grading scale from I to V.
- CT is the preferred imaging modality, findings suggestive for pancreatic injury like transverse mesocolon hematoma, fluid in the lesser sac, duodenal hematoma or injury, and chance fracture. Diagnostic findings like parenchymal laceration or hematoma, disruption of the head of the pancreas, or diffuse swelling suggest posttraumatic pancreatitis.
- Low-grade pancreatic injuries identified on CT scan can usually be treated safely with a nonoperative approach. Endoscopic transpapillary pancreatic duct stenting may be used.
- During exploration, full exposure and careful inspection of the pancreas are key to injury identification.
- Dissection of the lesser sac through the greater and lesser omentum to inspect the pancreas.
- The Cattell-Braasch maneuver is used for visualizing the pancreatic head, and the Mattox maneuver is used to visualize the tail of the pancreas.
- Exposure of the pancreas is incomplete without mobilizing the superior and inferior borders, making sure that the pancreas' posterior aspect is palpated for defects.
- The degree of injury helps to determine which management approach would be most appropriate. When grades I and II injuries to the pancreas are discovered at laparotomy, most can be treated with simple hemostasis and closed suction drainage.
- Ductal injuries at or distal to the neck of the pancreas are best treated definitively with distal pancreatectomy.
- Ductal injuries proximal to the neck of the pancreas, wide external drainage is recommended when there has not been complete destruction or massive devascularization of the pancreatic head.
- High-grade injuries to the pancreas (grades IV and V) thankfully are rare but may require pancreaticoduodenectomy [8].

13.1.7 Management of Bowel Injury

- The finding of tachycardia or abdominal tenderness may suggest the presence of hollow viscus injury.
- Laboratory abnormalities, including elevations in the white blood cell (WBC) count, amylase, and lactic acid, may point to the presence of hollow viscus injury but are relatively nonspecific.
- In hemodynamically stable patients with blunt trauma, CT is the most commonly used diagnostic modality.
- Findings of free intraperitoneal fluid without solid organ injury, pneumoperitoneum, bowel wall thickening, oral or rectal contrast extravasation, mesenteric hematoma, or vascular blush are predictive of small bowel or large bowel injury [9].

Management of Small Bowel Injuries:

- Grade I small bowel injury (partial thickness or contusion/bruising): the seromuscular layers are reapproximated in a single layer with 3-0 nonabsorbable Lembert suture.
- Small full-thickness (grade II) and larger full-thickness (grade III) injuries: repaired with limited debridement and closure. Closure can be performed in either one or two layers. Transverse closure is preferred to avoid luminal narrowing.

- Full-thickness injuries that are closely opposed should be converted to a single defect and primarily repaired.
- If multiple perforations are present within the same segment, they are best treated with resection and anastomosis.
- For more extensive wounds and wounds associated with devascularization (grades IV and V), resection with anastomosis.
- Mesenteric injuries may be encountered without an associated small bowel injury. This segment of the small bowel should be inspected closely for vascular compromise. If the bowel is viable with adequate blood flow, the mesentery defect should be reapproximated to prevent an internal hernia.
- Do not explore small nonexpanding mesenteric hematomas except when the mesenteric border of the small bowel wall is obscured by it. Bowel wall injury or perforation has to be excluded. Expanding hematomas should be opened and bleeding vessels oversewn [9].

Management of Colonic Injuries:

- Partial-thickness lacerations or serosal tears (grade I) can be repaired with interrupted nonabsorbable Lembert sutures.
- Full-thickness lacerations (grade II) may be closed in one or two layers; however, we prefer the latter.
- Destructive colonic injuries are defined as wounds that completely transect the colon (grade IV) or involve tissue loss and devascularized segments.
- In right-sided injuries (grades III to V), the majority receive a total right colectomy with reconstruction using an ileocolostomy.
- Complex left-sided injuries undergo resection with colocolostomy.
- Destructive colonic injuries with comorbid medical conditions or transfusion requirements greater than 6 units of blood were at significantly higher risk for suture line breakdown. It is highly recommended that these patients receive an ostomy.
- Colostomy reversal should be done in a timely manner. It usually is performed around 3 to 6 months after hospital discharge.
- Before closure, a contrast enema is obtained to rule out the presence of a distal stricture [9].

13.1.8 Management of Rectal Injuries

- Injuries are classified as intraperitoneal or extraperitoneal.
- Injuries to the anterior and lateral surface of the upper two-thirds of the anterior portion are classified as intraperitoneal.
- The extraperitoneal rectum comprises the posterior aspect, which is adherent to the presacral soft tissues along the curvature of the sacrum, and the lower one-thirds of the anterior portion.
- **Diagnosis:**
  - Recognition of rectal injuries requires that the surgeon maintains a high index of suspicion.
  - Digital rectal examination (DRE) is an essential tool to assess for blood within the rectal vault.
  - Proctosigmoidoscopy may reveal a rectal injury location, but visualization often is impaired by the presence of blood or stool.
  - CT may be a useful adjunct in the stable patient to identify the missile tract and evaluate for concomitant intraabdominal injury. CT cystography may also help the preoperative diagnosis of an associated bladder injury if hematuria is detected during Foley catheter insertion [10].
- **Management:**
  - **Intraperitoneal injuries:**

    Management strategies for intraperitoneal rectal injuries are similar to those used for colon wounds.

    Nondestructive injuries without devitalization of tissue and not requiring significant debridement (grades I to III) can be repaired primarily.

    If there is significant tissue loss or vascular compromise, resection of the injured segment is appropriate. Primary anastomosis without diverting colostomy is appropriate in the presence of hemodynamic stability.

Suppose there is evidence of shock (prolonged hypotension, and transfusion requirement greater than 6 units of packed red blood cells) or multiple associated injuries, an end colostomy with the closure of the rectal stump is advised [10].

- **Proximal extraperitoneal injuries:**

  Injuries involving the extraperitoneal rectum proximal to the peritoneal reflection usually can be repaired with limited mobilization of the mesorectum.

  Primary repair should be attempted using the two-layer technique described previously without the need for proximal diversion or presacral drainage.

  Diverting colostomy should be based on the patient's physiologic status, the suspicion of a more distal injury, and the complexity of the surgical repair required.

  Destructive rectal injuries not amenable to immediate primary repair should be treated with Hartmann's procedure [10].

- **Distal extraperitoneal injuries:**

  Diversion is accomplished via a loop sigmoid colostomy, making sure that the sigmoid colon is mobilized sufficiently to avoid tension and that the posterior wall of the loop is maintained above the level of the skin.

  Wounds to the posterior portion of the distal extraperitoneal rectum, manage by proximal diversion with presacral drainage.

  For injuries to the anterior portion of the distal extraperitoneal rectum, managed by placement of presacral drain, and injuries are treated primarily with proximal diversion.

  Presacral drainage is performed by making a curvilinear incision between the coccyx and anus, followed by bluntly dissecting through Waldeyer's fascia to gain entry to the presacral space. A 1-inch Penrose drain is placed within the space and gradually withdrawn between postoperative days 5 and 7 [10].

Anorectal Injuries:

- A simple laceration to the anal mucosa can be repaired primarily, but complex lesions involving the distal perineum and rectum may require diverting colostomy.
- In the case of foreign body insertion, it is crucial to perform rigid sigmoidoscopy to evaluate the patient for proximal rectal injury.
- If extensive tissue debridement is required, overlapping sphincteroplasty is the repair of choice, as simple apposition of muscle is associated with a failure rate of 40%.
- In the case of a complex injury to the pelvic floor with a significant soft-tissue defect, referral to a colorectal specialist for transposition of the gluteus or gracilis muscle creating a new sphincter is advised.
- In the event of complete destruction of the sphincter complex, abdominoperineal resection may be the most viable option [10].

13.1.9 Management of Urinary Injuries

Renal Injuries:

- **Penetrating renal injury:**
  - Parenchymal injuries: treated with hemostatic and reconstructive techniques similar to those used for injuries of the liver and spleen.
  - The collecting system should be closed separately, and the renal capsule should be preserved to close over the repair of the collecting system.
  - Renal vascular: may be deceptive due to tamponade by Gerota's fascia, which results in delayed hemorrhage.
  - Arterial reconstruction using graft interposition should be attempted within 5 h of the injury for renal preservation.
  - For destructive parenchymal or irreparable renovascular injuries, nephrectomy may be the only option; a normal contralateral kidney must be palpated.

- **Blunt renal trauma:**
  - Operative intervention is limited to renovascular injuries and destructive parenchymal injuries that result in hypotension.
  - The success rate for renal artery repair is limited. Still, an attempt is reasonable if the injury is <5 h old or if the patient has a solitary kidney or bilateral injuries.
  - Image-guided endoluminal stent placement is possible when the injuries are recognized by CT scanning.
  - Reconstruction after blunt renal injuries may be difficult.
  - If repair is not possible within this timeframe, leaving the kidney in situ does not necessarily lead to the late sequelae of hypertension or abscess formation.
  - During laparotomy for blunt trauma, expanding or pulsatile perinephric hematomas should be explored. If necessary, emergent vascular control can be obtained by placing a curved vascular clamp across the hilum from an inferior approach [1].

Ureter Injuries:

- It may occur in patients with pelvic fractures and penetrating trauma.
- If an injury is suspected during exploration but is not clearly identified, methylene blue or indigo carmine is administered IV with observation for extravasation.
- Injuries are repaired using 5-0 absorbable monofilament, and mobilization of the kidney may reduce tension on the anastomosis.
- Distal ureteral injuries can be treated by reimplantation facilitated with a psoas hitch and/or Boari flap.
- In damage control circumstances, the ureter can be ligated on both sides of the injury, and a nephrostomy tube placed [1].

Bladder Injuries:

- Intraperitoneal ruptures:
  - Ruptures or lacerations of the intraperitoneal bladder are operatively closed with a running, single-layer, 3-0 absorbable monofilament suture.
  - Laparoscopic repair is becoming common in patients not requiring laparotomy for other injuries.
- Extraperitoneal ruptures:
  - Treated nonoperatively with bladder decompression for 2 weeks [1].

Urethral Injuries:

- Managed by bridging the defect with a Foley catheter, with or without direct suture repair.
- Strictures are not uncommon but can be managed electively [1].

13.1.10 Penetrating Abdominal Trauma

- The presence of abdominal rigidity and hemodynamic compromise is an indication for prompt surgical exploration.
- **Gunshot wounds:**
  - Laparotomy is warranted for gunshot or shotgun wounds that penetrate the peritoneal cavity because most have significant internal injuries.
  - The exception is penetrating trauma isolated to the right upper quadrant; in hemodynamically stable patients with trajectory confined to the liver by CT scan, nonoperative observation may be reasonable.
  - In obese patients, if the gunshot wound is thought to be tangential through the subcutaneous tissues, CT scan can delineate the track and exclude peritoneal violation.
  - Laparoscopy is another option to assess peritoneal penetration for tangential wounds; it should not be done in unstable patients.
  - Gunshot wounds to the back or flank are more difficult to evaluate because of the injured abdominal organs' retroperitoneal location. A triple-contrast CT scan can delineate the bullet's trajectory and identify peritoneal violation or retroperitoneal entry and associated injuries [1, 11].
- **Stab wounds:**
  - Anterior abdominal stab wounds (from the costal margin to inguinal ligament and bilateral midaxillary lines) should be

explored under local anesthesia in the ED to determine if the fascia has been violated.
  - Injuries that do not penetrate the peritoneal cavity do not require further evaluation, and the patient may be discharged from the ED.
  - Patients with fascial penetration must be further evaluated for intraabdominal injury because there is up to a 50% chance of requiring laparotomy.
  - Patients with stab wounds to the right upper quadrant can undergo CT scanning to determine trajectory and confinement to the liver for potential nonoperative care.
  - Those with stab wounds to the flank and back should undergo contrasted CT to assess the potential risk of retroperitoneal injuries of the colon, duodenum, and urinary tract [1, 11].
- **Thoracoabdominal injury**:
  - Penetrating thoracoabdominal wounds may cause occult injury to the diaphragm. Patients with gunshot or stab wounds to the left lower chest should be evaluated with diagnostic laparoscopy or DPL to exclude diaphragmatic injury.
  - In general, penetrating right diaphragm injury is ignored unless there is a major underlying liver injury with a risk of biliopleural fistula [1, 11].

13.1.11 Management of Vascular Injuries

- **Principles:**
  - Initial control of vascular injuries is accomplished digitally by applying enough direct pressure.
  - Sharp dissection is used to define the injury and mobilize sufficient length for proximal and distal control.
  - Fogarty thromboembolectomy should be done proximally and distally to optimize collateral blood flow.
  - Heparinized saline (50 units/mL) is then injected into the injured vessel's proximal and distal ends to prevent small clot formation on the exposed intima and media.
  - Ragged edges of the injury site should be debrided using sharp dissection.
  - Intravascular shunts are used when there are multiple life-threatening injuries or the arterial injury is anticipated to require saphenous vein interposition reconstruction [1].
- **Options for the treatment of vascular injuries:**
  - Observation.
  - Ligation.
  - Lateral suture repair.
  - End-to-end primary anastomosis.
  - Interposition grafts:
    - Autogenous vein.
    - Polytetrafluoroethylene graft.
    - Dacron graft.
  - Transpositions.
  - Extra-anatomic bypass.
  - Endovascular:
    - Stents.
    - Embolization [1].
- **Arterial injuries:**
  - Arterial repair should always be done for the aorta, carotid, innominate, brachial, superior mesenteric, proper hepatic, renal, iliac, femoral, and popliteal arteries.
  - Named arteries that usually tolerate ligation include the right or left hepatic artery and the celiac artery.
  - In the lower extremities, at least one artery with distal runoff should be salvaged [1].
- **Venous injuries:**
  - Venous repair should be performed for injuries of the superior vena cava, the inferior vena cava proximal to the renal veins, and the portal vein. However, the portal vein may be ligated in extreme cases.
  - The SMV should be repaired optimally, but >80% of patients will survive following ligation.
  - The left renal vein can usually be ligated adjacent to the IVC due to collateral decompression [1].
- **Types of operative repair for a vascular injury:**
  - It is based on the extent and location of the injury.
  - Lateral suture repair is preferred for arterial injuries with minimal loss of tissue.

  - End-to-end primary anastomosis is performed if the vessel can be repaired without tension.
  - Arterial defects of 1–2 cm often can be bridged by mobilizing the severed ends of the vessel after ligating small branches.
  - Interposition grafts are used when end-to-end anastomosis cannot be accomplished without tension despite mobilization.
  - For vessels <6 mm in diameter (e.g., internal carotid, brachial, superficial femoral, and popliteal arteries), autogenous greater saphenous vein (GSV) from the contralateral groin should be used.
  - When GSV is not available, autologous options include the cephalic and basilic veins.
  - Larger arteries (e.g., subclavian, innominate, aorta, and common iliac) are bridged by PTFE grafts.
  - Transposition procedures can be used when an artery has a bifurcation, and one vessel can be ligated safely.
  - Venous injuries should be repaired when technically feasible [1].
- **Extremities vascular injuries:**
  - Immediate stabilization of fractures or unstable joints is done in the ED using Hare traction, knee immobilizers, or plaster splints.
  - Vascular injuries, either isolated or in combination with fractures, require emergent repair.
  - On-table angiography in the OR facilitates rapid intervention and is warranted in patients with evidence of limb threat on arrival.
  - *Subclavian or axillary artery repairs*:

    Six-millimeter PTFE graft or RSVG are used depending on the location.

    Because associated injuries of the brachial plexus are common, a thorough neurologic examination of the extremity is mandated before operative intervention.
  - *Brachial artery injury*:

    Approached via a medial upper extremity longitudinal incision and proximal control may be obtained at the axillary artery. An S-shaped extension through the antecubital fossa provides access to the distal brachial artery.

    The injured vessel segment is excised, and an end-to-end interposition RSVG graft is performed.

    Upper extremity fasciotomy is rarely required because of the rich collateral perfusion via the profunda.
  - *Superficial femoral artery injuries:*

    External fixation of the femur is typically performed, followed by end-to-end RSVG of the injured SFA segment.

    Close monitoring for calf compartment syndrome is mandatory.
  - *Popliteal artery injuries:*

    Preferred access to the popliteal space for an acute injury is the medial, one-incision approach with a detachment of the semitendinosus, semimembranosus, and gracilis muscles.

    Another option is a medial approach with two incisions using a longer RSVG, but this requires interval ligation of the popliteal artery and geniculate branches.

    If the patient has an associated popliteal vein injury, this should be repaired first with a PTFE interposition graft while the artery is shunted.

    For an isolated popliteal artery injury, RSVG is performed with an end-to-end anastomosis.

    Four-compartment fasciotomies are warranted in patients with combined arterial and venous injury.
  - Once the vessel is repaired and restoration of arterial flow is documented, completion angiography should be done in the OR if there is no palpable distal pulse.
  - Rarely, immediate amputation may be considered due to the severity of orthopedic and neurovascular injuries [1].

13.1.12 Penetrating Neck Injury

- Zones:
  - Zone I: from the thoracic inlet to the cricoid cartilage.

- Zone II: between cricoid cartilage and angle of mandible.
- Zone III: from the angle of the mandible to skull base.

- Regardless of the anatomic location, a stable neck injury can be evaluated with selective diagnostic studies.
- Priorities:
  - Emergency airway control.
  - Prompt control of active bleeding.
  - Urgent operative treatment of major injuries not causing airway compromise or life-threatening bleeding.
  - Timely diagnostic intervention for patient not requiring emergent or urgent operation.
  - Whether to explore or observe the stable patient.
  - Optimal exposure for patient requiring operation.
  - Care of specific injuries [1, 12, 13].

1. **Airway:**
   - If the airway is compromised, intubate.
   - Orotracheal, if no excessive bleeding in the airway.
   - Nasal route, when there is excessive bleeding, and use fiber optic.
   - Cricothyroidotomy is rarely needed; however, use it if you suspect airway rupture.
   - If the patient has significant hemoptysis, airway tracheal fistula, inflate the balloon below the suspected fistula [1, 12, 13].
2. **Bleeding:**
   - Direct pressure by gloved finger and take the patient to OR.
3. **Urgent operation:**
   - Patients who should go to OR without imaging:
     - Large hematoma.
     - Continuous oozing.
     - Cervical crepitus.
     - Hoarseness.
     - Pulsatile hematoma.
     - Large wound with severe injury to soft tissue that needs reapproximation [1, 12, 13].
4. **Urgent diagnostic investigations:**
   - If the patient has no hard signs and no emergent or urgent indication for OR, do a diagnostic study to exclude subtle injury.
   - Those patients may have soft signs:
     - History of bleeding.
     - Mild neck swelling.
     - Bruit.
     - Hoarseness.
     - Dysphagia.
     - Blood streak sputum.
   - Investigations:
     - History and physical examination of the oral cavity and chest examination.
     - CXR.
     - CTA.
     - Endoscopy or bronchoscopy as indicated [1, 12, 13].
5. **Exploration versus observation in a stable patient without hard signs or instability:**
   - Depend on the diagnostic investigation findings.
6. **Operative exposure:**
   - An ipsilateral incision along the anterior border of the sternocleidomastoid.
   - The incision is extended through platysma into deeper planes.
   - Retract trachea, thyroid anteriorly, and retract neurovascular bundle and esophagus posteriorly: This will expose the tracheoesophageal groove and allow the operator to dissect anteriorly or posteriorly as determined by operative findings.
   - When zone III injury require repair of the internal carotid artery at the base of the skull, the mandible can be detached posterior to angle and subluxated anteriorly to facilitate the primary repair.
   - When the injury involves zone I structures in the thoracic outlet, an incision can be extended into a median sternotomy, which will give exposure to the thymus, trachea, innominate artery, left common carotid artery, subclavian artery and vein, innominate vein, and superior vena cava.
   - When injury involved subclavian vessel as they pass laterally, an incision can be extended along the medial half of the clavicle and then over the cephalic vein [1, 12, 13].
7. **Repair of specific injury:**
   - **Venous injury:**
     - Injury to small veins including the external jugular can be ligated.

- Internal jugular vein: Can be repaired primarily with running nonabsorbable fine suture.
- When there is a large through and through wound to IJV, then the vein should be ligated [1, 12, 13].

- **Thoracic duct injury:**
  - If an obvious injury is present (whitish drainage), ligate it.
  - If no obvious leak (e.g., the patient has not eaten recently), it will present as a leak through the drain later, treat it conservatively [1, 12, 13].
- **Arterial injury:**
  - Carotid artery:
    Control active bleeding with digital pressure.
    Get proximal and distal control.
    Keep pressure till distal control is obtained.
    Minimal injury: simple lateral repair by #5-0 nonabsorbable suture.
    If extensive injury, resect the segment. If the gab is 1 cm or less, end-to-end anastomosis can be performed.
    Larger segment: reverse saphenous graft.
    Local instillation of heparin proximally and distally.
    Temporary shunt if a repair cannot be obtained within 30 min [1, 12, 13].
  - External carotid in zone II:
    Branches of external carotid can be ligated safely.
  - Disruption of bifurcation:
    The intact external carotid can be anastomosed to the internal carotid artery distal to the injury area and ligate distal external carotid stump.
    Primary repair of the carotid in a patient with a neurological deficit is controversial [1, 12, 13].
- **Esophageal injury:**
  - Expose the esophagus.
  - Surround it with a Penrose drain.
  - Unilateral stab wound: Repair primary in two layers with absorbable suture for the inner layer and nonabsorbable suture for the outer layer.
  - Bilateral injury:
    The esophagus can be rotated to facilitate the bilateral repair.
    Extend ipsilateral wound repair the contralateral from inside.
  - It is essential to identify all the wounds.
  - After closure, drain must be left in place.
  - If suspected is fistula, send for amylase.
  - If fistula confirmed, NGT feeding and fistula mostly will close in 3 weeks.
  - Leave NGT in place for feeding [1, 12, 13].
- **Tracheal injury:**
  - Perforation of the posterior wall: repair it primarily with absorbable 3-0.
  - You must exclude esophageal injury.
  - Perforation of the anterior wall: apply the suture above the superior ring and below the inferior ring.
  - Significant injury requires formal tracheostomy.
  - High tracheostomy (at the second tracheal ring) is prevented even if the injury is more distal: to avoid erosion to the innominate artery [1, 12, 13].
- **Nerves:**
  - Recurrent laryngeal nerve:
    Gunshot: unlikely to be repairable, so leave it alone.
    Stab wound: repair primarily with fine suture.
  - Vagus Nerve:
    Should be repaired with #5-0 nonabsorbable suture.
    If partially injured, leave it alone [1, 12, 13].

13.1.13 Trauma Operations

Preoperative Preparation:

- Start preparation.
- Inform the OR and the anesthesia team that you have an emergency case.
- Prepare blood and blood products.
- Inform the blood bank to initiate MTP if needed.
- Ask the OR to prepare: cell saver, blood warmer, rapid infusion, increase OR

temperature, laparotomy, thoracotomy, and vascular set.
- Ask for help if specific injuries are expected (vascular surgeon, obstetrician, or orthopedic surgeon).
- Inform the ICU if postop ICU bed.
- Consent.

Damage Control Operation:
- Indicated when the patient in the lethal triad of acidosis, hypothermia, coagulopathy, and hypotension. Aim: control bleeding and contamination.
- Position: supine.
- Under general anesthesia and endotracheal intubation.
- Time-out: confirm correct patient, procedure, and ensure the availability of the needed instruments and blood products.
- Prepping from the chin to the knees, draping in a usual sterile fashion.
- Incision: from xiphoid till symphysis pubis.
- Coordinate with the anesthesiologist that you are opening the abdomen as the hemodynamic may deteriorate due to loss of tamponade effect.
- Pack the four quadrants after the evacuation of blood and clots (around the liver, spleen, and in the pelvis).
- Give time for anesthesia to resuscitate.
- Remove the packs serially from the least to the most suspected area of injury.
- Damage control for specific organs:
- **Liver:**
  - If there is a visible bleeding vessel, clamp and ligate.
  - If there is diffuse bleeding from a small hole, control it with balloon tamponade.
  - If bleeding persists, take Penrose drain and cut to the required length, secure both ends with suture to a red rubber catheter passing within, insert it into the track, and inflate the catheter with saline until the bleeding stopped.
  - If the injury is deep, ill-defined, or uncontrollable bleeding, perform Pringle maneuver, and if the time permits, do hepatorrhaphy with #0 chromic and blunt needle.
  - If you fail to control the bleeding, targeted packing with an abdominal sponge is placed around the liver. The sponge should be adjacent to retrohepatic vena cava to prevent compression and decrease venous return.
  - Nonbleeding contained hematoma around the retrohepatic vena cava should be packed and left unopened.
- **Spleen:** splenectomy.
- **Kidney:**
  - Small, nonpulsatile, and nonexpanding hematoma should be left alone.
  - If there is active bleeding, nephrectomy after assurance is made that the contralateral kidney is normal in size and not injured.
- **Vascular structures:**
  - Small bleeding vessels can be clamped and ligated.
  - IMA, hypogastric vessels, and infrarenal IVC can be ligated.
  - Injuries to SMA, portal vein, suprarenal IVC, and iliac vessels can be either repaired or temporary shunt.
  - Abdominal aorta should be repaired.
  - Intact pelvic hematoma should be left alone.
  - Pelvic hematoma overlying iliac vessels or if it is actively bleeding or expanding, open and control the bleeding.
- **Pancreas:**
  - Priority is to control any bleeding.
  - Secondly, control the duct leak by packing and inserting of closed suction drain.
- **Hollow viscus injury:**
  - The aim is to control the contamination.
  - Small and simple laceration: repair if the tissue is healthy.
  - Destructive injury: divide by intestinal stapler and leave it.
  - Duodenal injury that cannot be resected: suture repair and reinforce with a loop of the small bowel (Thal patch) in addition to wide drainage [14].

Abdominal Closure in DCS:
It should be closed temporarily to prevent abdominal compartment and preserve the fascia after resuscitation and definitive closure.

- Methods:
  - Towel clips.
  - Bogota bag.
  - Negative pressure dressing [14].

Damage Control Vascular Surgery:

- If there is suspicion of extremity vascular injury:
  - Field's tourniquet and dressing should be left in place and not removed until the patient is in OR, anesthetized, resuscitated, and proximal control replaced.
  - The injury site is cleaned and draped broadly for proximal and distal control in addition to the uninvolved lower extremity for the possible use of great saphenous vein for repair.
  - The wound is explored to confirm a vascular injury.
  - Proximal and distal control is obtained sometimes with separate incisions.
  - Certain vessels such as the external carotid artery, internal jaguar vein, infrageniculate, forearm arteries, and veins can be ligated better than repaired.
  - Most other vessels should be shunted during damage control surgery unless small (< 50 % circumference), and the surgeon can apply rapid suture for repair.
  - If the decision is made to shunt, the injured ends of the transacted vessels are left alone and not derided until definitive surgery.
  - Shutting tube is selected (pediatric feeding tube or IV line); shunt dipped in heparin solution before use.
- Before applying the shunt:
  - The surgeon should perform three maneuvers:

    Test for back bleeding in the distal artery; if inadequate, balloon embolectomy should be performed.

    Instill 20 mL of heparinized saline 20 IU/mL into both proximal and distal limbs of transacted vessel.

    Distal fasciotomy precedes shunt placement in all cases when the flow cannot be restored within 2 h.

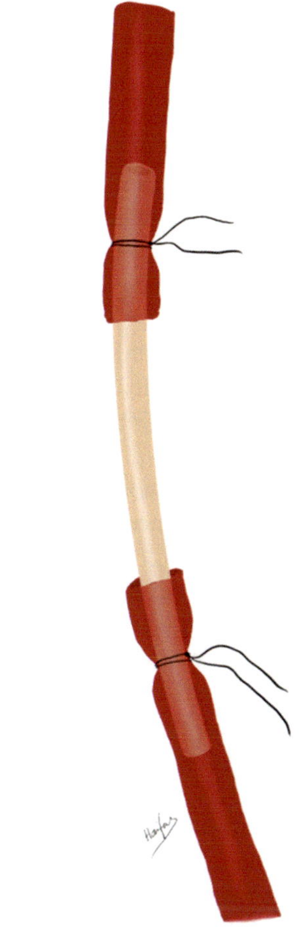

Fig. 13.2 Vascular shunt

- Shunt placement:
  - An appropriate diameter is selected and cut into a length adequate for securing proximal and distal vessel ends.
  - Blood flow is reestablished as each end of the shunt is placed within the vessels.
  - #0 silk ties are used to secure the shunt within the ends of the vessel.
  - Shunt longer than 5–6 cm should be secured using silk ligature at the middle of the shunt to the surrounding tissue (Fig. 13.2).
  - Assess the distal perfusion with Doppler or pulse oximetry.
  - Cover the repaired or shunted vessels.
  - Definitive repair typically is performed 24 h after DCS once ICU resuscitation is complete [14].

Pelvic Fracture (Damage Control):
Unless laparotomy is required for other indications, the surgeon should use a step-wise approach to pelvic extravasation control.

A. Pelvic binder or sheet wrap:
Circumferentially incorporating and compressing the space between the anterior superior iliac spine and femoral greater trochanter.
B. Pelvic external fixation.
C. Resuscitative endovascular balloon occlusion of the aorta with angioembolization.
D. Extraperitoneal packing (via space of Retzius into space of Bogors).
   – A lower abdominal incision is made and carried down to the peritoneum, which is left intact.
   – Perivesical blood is evacuated.
   – The bladder is pressed posteriorly.
   – Three laparotomy sponges are introduced into each side of the perivesical space between the pelvic sidewall and bladder and downward toward the sacrum.

After Damage Control Surgery in ICU:
- If the lactic acidosis, hypotension, and coagulopathy worsen despite vigorous resuscitation, there is a probability of ongoing hemorrhage, contamination, or gangrenous necrosis, which could warrant early return to OR.
- Monitor for abdominal compartment syndrome.

Definitive Surgery:
- Regardless of what happens in DCS, always presume missed injury.
- It is essential to perform meticulous and comprehensive reexploration.
- Unpack the abdominal pack gently (underwater).
- If the hemorrhage recurs, repack.
- If all gauzes are removed, do radiograph as usually sponge count in first surgery is inaccurate and should not be trusted.
- If there is a shunt and fracture, fix the fracture before replacing the shunt with definitive repair [14].

Emergency Splenectomy:
- Indicated in a patient with hemodynamic instability, peritonitis, or other injuries that require an operation, or patient with failed initial nonoperative management.
- Anesthesia: GA with endotracheal intubation.
- Position: supine.
- Prepping and draping (standard trauma laparotomy prepping: chin to mid-thigh).
- Time-out.
- NGT to decompress the stomach.
- Generous midline laparotomy from the Xiphoid till the symphysis pubis.
- On entering the abdomen: blood clots should be evacuated.
- Four quadrants packing to control bleeding.
- Packs are removed sequentially to identify and address the source.
- Mobilize the spleen.
- Retract the left costal margin.
- Medial traction of the spleen by the surgeon left hand.
- Splenorenal and splenophrenic ligaments are avascular and can be divided with Mets scissor and blunt dissection.
- The spleen and tail of the pancreas are mobilized to the midline (plane to be developed anterior to the kidney).
- Place packs posteriorly.
- The gastrosplenic ligament should be divided between clamps and tied (tied close to the spleen) to avoid the stomach's injury.
- The splenocolic ligament is dissected to free the lower pole.
- Ligate and divide the hilar vessels, take care not to injure the tail of the pancreas (Fig. 13.3).
- Traditionally ligate artery and vein separately.
- Inspect the left upper quadrant and the abdominal diaphragm.
- Hemostasis.
- Complete exploration if not done before.
- If an injury to the pancreas is suspected, insert a closed suction drain.
- Close the abdomen in layers.

Possible Complications:
- Pancreatic leak.

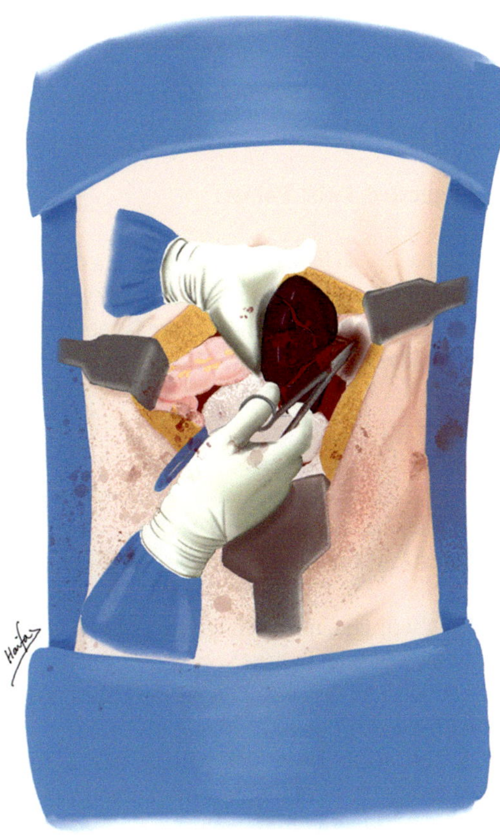

Fig. 13.3 Emergency splenectomy (lateral-to-medial approach)

- Bleeding.
- Collection.
- Post splenectomy sepsis.
- Stomach injury [1, 13].

Emergency Nephrectomy:

- Indication for renal exploration:
  Absolute indications:
- Persistent life-threatening hemorrhage believed to be from renal injury.
- Grade V injury (pedicle avulsion).
- Expanding, pulsatile, or uncontrolled retroperitoneal hemorrhage.
- Ureteropelvic junction avulsion.
- **Operative steps:**
  - Midline incision, transperitoneal approach.
  - After exploration, packing, and control of hemorrhage and resuscitation.
  - Right-side nephrectomy: right medial visceral rotation (Cattell Braasch).
  - Left-side nephrectomy: left medial visceral rotation (Mattox).
  - Incise the Gerota's Fascia along its lateral aspect to:
  - Avoid dissecting the kidney in the subcapsular plane.
  - Avoid ureteric injury.
  - Preserve perinephric fat for reconstruction.
  - Significant renal vein injury may require ligation, and partial laceration may be repaired via #5-0 proline after careful dissection and control.
  - Injury to the left renal vein can be ligated solely, provided gonadal and adrenal collateral have been preserved.
  - The right renal vein lacks collateral outflow, and nephrectomy is indicated if repair is not possible.
  - Renal artery thrombosis in a stable patient and normal contralateral kidney can be managed expectantly.
  - Injury to renal artery in unstable patient: nephrectomy if the contralateral kidney is present and not damaged.
  - If in a stable patient:
    Sharp debridement.
    Suture ligation of the bleeding vessel.
  - Water-tight repair of the collecting system.
  - Hemostasis.
  - Closure [14].

Complications:

- Early:
  - Urine extravasation.
  - Sepsis and abscess.
  - Adynamic ileus.
  - Decrease renal function.
  - Urinoma.
- Late:
  - Delayed bleeding
  - A-V fistula.
  - Pseudoaneurysm.
  - HTN.

13.2 Part II: Practice

> Always realize that you can get better. Your best work has not been done yet. Practice! Practice! Practice!
> —Les Brown

13.2.1 Case Scenarios for Practice

Tips:

- Practice with a friend and try to mimic the real exam!
  Do not forget to set the timer!
- The clinical data are provided in the answer key section.
- Some twist points are suggested after some cases and can be used to change the scenario to a more difficult one.

Case No. 1:
A 23-year-old male patient was brought to the emergency department by the EMS due to a road traffic accident (RTA).

Questions for discussion:

1. How will you approach the patient?
2. What will you do next?
3. What will you do intraoperatively?
4. The intraoperative finding as described above. What will you do next?
5. A few days later, he has a persistent leak from the drain. What will you do?
6. The laboratory tests confirm the diagnosis. How will you manage this?
7. What further management will he need?

Suggested Twist Points:

- Intraoperatively, the patient is unstable, acidotic, and hypothermic. What will you do?

Case No. 2:
A 33-year-old female patient involved in RTA and brought to the emergency department.

Questions for discussion:

1. How will you approach the patient?
2. What will you do next?
3. Describe what you will do?
4. The intraoperative finding as described. What will you do?
5. On the next day, the drain output is bile. What will you do?

Suggested Twist Points:

- On the second look operation, there is a devascularized segment of the liver. What will you do?
- On the initial exploration, there is retroperitoneal hematoma at zone I. How will you manage it?

Case No. 3:
A 44-year-old male policeman, a victim of a gunshot wound to the abdomen.

Questions for discussion:

1. How will you approach the patient?
2. What will you do next?
3. The intraoperative finding as described. What will you do?
4. A few days later, the patient has a foul-smelling, large amount of discharge from the wound. What will you do?
5. How will you manage that?

Suggested twist points:

- There is intraperitoneal urinary bladder rupture. How will you manage it?
- There is intraperitoneal rectal injury. How will you manage it?

Case No. 4:
A 35-year-old male patient brought to the emergency due to severe RTA.

Questions for discussion:

1. How will you approach the patient?
2. What will you do next?
3. How will you manage the patient?
4. The patient was improving on nonoperative management. How will you follow the patient?
5. What will you do?

Suggested twists points:

- The patient failed to respond to nonoperative management. How will you manage that?

Checklist

Assessment	Items	Done	Not done	NA
General	Personal protective equipment			
	Follow the ATLS protocol			
Airway	Airway assessment and apply C collar			
	Talk to the patient			
	Suction any secretions			
	Remove any foreign body			
	Chin left/jaw thrust			
	Oropharyngeal/nasopharyngeal			
	Definitive airway (endotracheal intubation and cricothyroidotomy)			
	Assess the GCS before intubation			
	Confirm the position of the tube			
Breathing	Look, listen, and feel			
	Oxygen supplementation			
	Needle decompression if tension pneumothorax			
	Chest X-ray			
	Chest tube for pneumothorax or hemothorax			
	Three-sided dressing if open pneumothorax			
Circulation	Assess the BP and pulse rate			
	Control any external bleeding			
	Inert two large cannulas			
	Draw blood for investigation			
	Tranexamic acid when indicated			
	Initiate massive transfusion protocol when needed			
	Start fluid resuscitation with 1 L of RL			
	Give blood if required			
	Search for any internal bleeding (FAST and pelvic X-ray)			
	Apply pelvic binder if unstable pelvis			
	Splint any extremities fracture			
Disability	Assess the GCS			
	Pupil examination			
	Look for any signs of lateralization			
Exposure	Undress the patient			
	Look for any obvious wounds or deformity			
	Log roll and examine the back			
	DRE			
	Cover the patient to avoid hypothermia			
Adjunct to primary survey	NGT			
	Foley's catheter			
	X-rays			
Secondary survey	History			
	Head to toe examination			
	Assess the lab result			
	Further imaging as indicated, for example, Pan CT			
	Consult other specialties as indicated			

(continued)

Assessment	Items	Done	Not done	NA
Splenic and liver injury that can be treated conservatively	Admission to ICU			
	Bed rest			
	IV fluid and blood transfusion as indicated			
	Stress ulcer prophylaxis and antibiotics			
	Mechanical DVT prophylaxis			
	Serial Hb and coagulation profile assessment			
	Angioembolization if needed			
If the patient requires an emergent or urgent operation	Inform the operating room			
	Inform the anesthesia team			
	Inform the blood bank to prepare blood and blood product			
	Ask the OR team to prepare cell saver, blood warmer, rapid infuser, warmer, and adjust the OR temperature			
	Thoracotomy, laparotomy, and vascular sets to be ready			
	Ask for help if expecting specific injuries, for example, vascular surgeon, obstetrician, or orthopedic surgeon			
	Inform the ICU to prepare postoperative bed			
	Consent			
Intraoperative (laparotomy)	Supine position and the arms 90°			
	Prepping and draping from chin to knees			
	Generous midline laparotomy			
	Coordinate with the anesthesia team to catch up with resuscitation			
	Evacuate any blood and clots			
	Pack the four quadrants			
	Resuscitate			
	Withdraw the packs gradually			
	Proper exploration (GIT, diaphragms, retroperitoneal, pancreas, liver, biliary, spleen, and pelvis)			
	Decide whether definitive surgery or damage control surgery is appropriate			
Damage control surgery	Spleen: splenectomy			
	Kidney: nephrectomy if actively bleeding Check the contralateral kidney			
	Vessels: ligate, if cannot be, repair, or temporary shunt			
	Pancreas: control the bleeding and wide suction drainage			
	Hollow viscus: control the contamination (repair or resect and leave the two ends)			
	Liver: pack			
	Pelvic fracture with significant hematoma: extraperitoneal packing			
	Temporary closure			
	Shift the patient to ICU			
	Monitor for compartment syndrome or other indication for an immediate return to OR			
	Return to OR after 24–48 h for definitive repair			

Assessment	Items	Done	Not done	NA
Penetrating abdominal injury	Approach using the ATLS protocol			
	Laparotomy if unstable or there is peritonitis, evisceration, and a gunshot wound to the anterior abdominal wall			
	Local wound exploration if stab wound to the anterior abdominal wall			
	CT if an injury to the RUQ, flank, and back			
	Laparoscopy or DPL if a thoracoabdominal wound			
Postoperative complications management	Drain any collection			
	If there is pseudoaneurysm: embolization			
	Bile or pancreatic leak: ERCP and sphincterotomy+/- stent			
	Enterocutaneous fistula to be managed conservatively initially			
	Do not forget vaccination 2 weeks postsplenectomy			
Penetrating neck injury (initial assessment)	Control the airway			
	Control any active bleeding			
	Urgent operation if a major injury			
	Diagnostic intervention, if not urgent operation is required (CXR, CTA, endoscopy, or bronchoscopy)			
	Decide whether to observe or explore			
Intraoperative management of penetrating neck injury	Ipsilateral incision along the anterior border of sternocleidomastoid muscle			
	Retract the trachea and thyroid anteriorly			
	Retract the neurovascular bundle and esophagus posteriorly			
	Detach the angle of the mandible posteriorly if zone III injury			
	Extend the incision to median sternotomy if zone I injury			
	Extend the incision to the medial half of the clavicle if subclavian vessels injury			
	Venous injury: repair or ligate			
	Thoracic duct: ligate if obvious injury or drain it			
	Carotid artery: proximal and distal control, repair primarily, resect, and anastomose if small segment or shunt			
	Injury to branches of external carotid: can be ligated			
	Esophageal: repair in two layers and drain it and NGT for feeding			
	Tracheal injury; and posterior injury: repair primarily Anterior injury: apply suture above the superior ring and below the inferior ring			
	Vagus nerve: repair			
	RLN: repair if stab wound			

13.2.2 Answer Key

Case No. 1:
A 23-year-old male patient brought to the emergency department by the EMS due to a road traffic accident (RTA).

Questions for discussion:

1. **How will you approach the patient?**
   Following the ATLS protocol.
   Airway and C collar: the patient was lethargic but conscious and able to talk freely, and the C collar applied.
   Breathing: oxygen via nasal cannula was provided, air entry was equal, and his SPO_2 is 94%.
   Circulation: BP: 87/56 mmHg, and PR: 132 bpm. Two large cannulas were inserted, and blood was drawn for investigation, and resuscitation was started with fluid and blood products. There are no signs of external bleeding. FAST scan is positive for fluid. The abdomen is soft, slightly distended, and tender, mainly over the left side with guarding.
   Despite resuscitation, the patient is not responding.
   GCS: 14/15 and no signs of lateralization.
   Exposure reveals no abnormality.
   CXR and PXR: unremarkable.
   Foleys catheter (brought clear urine) and NGT were inserted.
   AMPLE history: The patient is not allergic, not on regular medication, not known to have chronic illnesses, and the last meal was 4 h prior to the presentation to the ER. He was the driver, and another car hits his car from his left side. The vehicle did not roll over, and no other victims died from the accident.
2. **What will you do next?**
   Take the patient for emergency laparotomy exploration.
3. **What will you do intraoperatively?**
   Position: supine.
   Under general anesthesia and endotracheal intubation.
   Time-out: confirm correct patient, procedure, and ensure the availability of the needed instruments and blood.
   Prepping from the chin to the knees, draping in a usual sterile fashion.
   Incision: from xiphoid till symphysis pubis.
   Coordinate with anesthesia team that you are opening the abdomen, and the hemodynamic may deteriorate due to loss of tamponade effect.
   Pack the four quadrants after the evacuation of blood and clots (around the liver, spleen, and in the pelvis).
   Give time for anesthesia team to resuscitate.
   Apply retractors.
   Remove the packs serially from the least to the most suspected area of injury.
   The hemodynamic improves with packing and resuscitation. The bleeding source was a ruptured spleen.
4. **The intraoperative finding as described above. What will you do next?**
   Emergency splenectomy and intraabdominal drain is inserted.
   Proper exploration for other injuries (abdominal esophagus, stomach, duodenum, pancreas, small and large bowel, rectum, liver, and retroperitoneum) revealed no other injuries.
5. **A few days later, he has a persistent leak from the drain. What will you do?**
   Send fluid for amylase.
   The fluid was positive for amylase (>3 times the serum level).
6. **The laboratory tests confirm the diagnosis. How will you manage this?**
   - NPO.
   - IV fluid.
   - Nasojejunal feeding/TPN.
   - Octreotide.
   - Antibiotic if indicated.
   - Monitor the drain output.
   - Wound care.
   - Most of the pancreatic fistula will close spontaneously.
   - ERCP sphincterotomy +/- pancreatic stent if not closed.
7. **What further management will he need?**

Vaccination for encapsulated bacteria 2 weeks postsurgery.

Suggested twist points:

- **Intraoperative, the patient is unstable, acidotic, and hypothermic. What will you do?**
  - Splenectomy.
  - Packing and temporary closure second look after 24–48 h.

Case No. 2:

A 33-year-old female patient involved in RTA and brought to the emergency department.

Questions for discussion:

1. **How will you approach the patient?**

   Following the ATLS protocol.

   Airway and C collar: the patient was anxious but conscious and able to talk freely, and the C collar applied.

   Breathing: oxygen via nasal cannula was provided, air entry was equal, and his SPO_2 is 92%.

   Circulation: BP: 69/46 mmHg and PR: 136 bpm. Two large cannulas were inserted, and blood was drawn for investigation. Resuscitation was started with fluid and blood products, and the blood bank is contacted to initiate massive transfusion protocol. There are no signs of external bleeding. FAST scan is positive for fluid. The abdomen is soft, distended, and tender.

   Despite resuscitation, the patient is not responding.

   GCS: 14/15 and signs of lateralization.

   Exposure reveals no abnormality.

   CXR and PXR: unremarkable.

   Foleys catheter (brought a little amount of clear urine) and NGT were inserted.

   AMPLE history: the patient is allergic to eggs, not on regular medication, not known to have chronic illnesses, and the last meal was 8 h prior to the presentation to the ER. He was the driver, unrestrained, and involved in front collision. He could not remember a lot due to transient loss of consciousness.
2. **What will you do next?**

   Take the patient for emergency laparotomy exploration.
3. **Describe what you will do?**
   - Position: supine.
   - Under general anesthesia and endotracheal intubation.
   - Time-out: confirm correct patient, procedure, and ensure the availability of the needed instruments and blood.
   - Prepping from the chin to the knees, and draping in a usual sterile fashion.
   - Incision: from xiphoid till symphysis pubis.
   - Coordinate with anesthesia team that you are opening the abdomen, and the hemodynamic may deteriorate due to loss of tamponade effect.
   - Pack the four quadrants after the evacuation of blood and clots (around the liver, spleen, and in the pelvis).
   - Give time for anesthesia to resuscitate.
   - Apply retractors.
   - Remove the packs serially from the least to the most suspected area of injury.

The bleeding was coming from deep laceration in the liver. Once you removed the packs, the bleeding recurs. The patient received 6 units of PRBCs, and his intraoperative ABG result is showing severe metabolic acidosis. His temperature is 35.6°C.

4. **The intraoperative finding as described. What will you do?**

   Pack again, insert drains, and temporarily close the abdomen and shift the patient to the ICU for further resuscitation +/- angioembolization.
5. **On the next day, the drain output is bile. What will you do?**

   If the patient's hemodynamics improves, take her back to the OR and do the definitive repair. ERCP with sphincterotomy is another option, but the patient is going for surgery anyhow, and better to visualize the area of injury to repair it.

   Suggested twist points:

- **On the second look operation, there is a devascularized segment of the liver. What will you do?**
  Nonanatomical hepatic resection.
- **On the initial exploration, there is retroperitoneal hematoma at zone I. How will you manage it?**
  Exploration.

Case No. 3:
A 44-year-old male policeman, a victim of a gunshot wound to the abdomen.

Questions for discussion:

1. **How will you approach the patient?**
   Following the ATLS protocol.
   Airway: The patient is conscious and able to talk freely.
   Breathing: Oxygen via nasal cannula was provided, air entry was equal, and his SPO_2 is 99%.
   Circulation: BP: 98/76 mmHg and PR: 116 bpm. Two large cannulas were inserted, and blood was drawn for investigation, and resuscitation was started with fluid. There are no signs of external bleeding. FAST scan is negative. The abdomen is soft and tender all over, with entry wound at the left iliac fossa and no exit wound. The abdominal X-ray shows a bullet inside the abdomen. The blood pressure improves with 1 L of RL.
   GCS: 15/15 and signs of lateralization.
   Exposure reveals no abnormality.
   CXR and PXR: unremarkable.
   Foleys catheter and NGT were inserted.
   AMPLE history: The patient is not allergic, not on regular medication, not known to have chronic illnesses, and the last meal was 5 h prior to the presentation to the ER. He was following one suspect when he received a gunshot to his abdomen from a long distance.
   Secondary survey reveals no other injuries.
2. **What will you do next?**
   Take the patient to OR for urgent laparotomy exploration.
   There were multiple through and through injuries involving a 50 cm segment of the small bowel. No other injuries and the bullet was found near the right psoas muscle.
3. **The intraoperative finding as described. What will you do?**
   Resection and anastomosis of the small bowel.
   Exclude ureteric injury.
4. **A few days later, the patient has a foul-smelling, large amount of discharge from the wound. What will you do?**
   Open the wound.
   Drainage the collection.
   Antibiotic.
   Swab for culture and sensitivity.
   CT abdomen to rule out an intraabdominal collection.
   Wound care.
   CT: No intraabdominal collection. There is an enterocutaneous fistula, connecting the anastomotic site to the anterior abdominal wall.
5. **How will you manage that?**
   Parenteral nutrition if the patient has high output fistula.
   Antibiotic.
   Protect the wound from the effluent.
   Fluid and electrolytes replacement.
   Most of the time, the fistula will close spontaneously.
   If did not close, operative management.
   Suggested twist points:

- **There is intraperitoneal urinary bladder rupture. How will you manage it?**
  Primary repair.
- **There is intraperitoneal rectal injury. How will you manage it?**
  Primary repair or resect and primary anastomosis ± diverting stoma.

Case No. 4:
A 35-year-old male patient brought to the emergency due to severe RTA.

Questions for discussion:

1. **How will you approach the patient?**
   Following the ATLS protocol.
   Airway: The patient is not responding, and the EMS provider applied the C collar. The

GCS is 8/15. The airway is secured with endotracheal intubation following rapid sequence intubation protocol.

Breathing: There is an asymmetry of the chest with an obvious expansion of the left side. Absent air entry on the left side, the neck veins are distended, and the trachea is shifted to the right side. SPO_2 is 85%.

Needle decompression followed by chest tube insertion.

Circulation: Initial BP: 85/69 mmHg and PR: 118 bpm, which improved after decompression of the chest (the latest BP: 109/78 mmHg and PR: 98 bpm). Two large cannulas were inserted, blood was drawn for investigation, and resuscitation was started with fluid. There are no signs of external bleeding. FAST scan is positive. The abdomen is soft and tender over the left side.

GCS: 8/15 before intubation and no signs of lateralization.

Exposure reveals swelling of the right leg with palpable click on examination. The distal pulses are intact.

CXR: Confirms the position of the tube and the lung expanded.

PXR: Unremarkable.

Foleys catheter and NGT were inserted.

AMPLE history: The patient is not known to have allergic history, not on regular medication, not known to have chronic illnesses, and the last meal was 3 h prior to the presentation to the ER. He was the front passenger, unrestrained, the car rolled over multiple times, and the driver dies immediately in the scene.

2. **How will you manage the patient?**
   Secondary survey and Pan CT scan.

   Secondary survey reveals no additional significant injuries.

   CT head: Small epidural hematoma with no midline shift.

   Chest CT: The chest tube is in place, and there is left-side pneumothorax with lower lobe contusion.

   CT abdomen: Grade 4 splenic injury but no active extravasation of contrast.

   X-ray of the right leg showed a tibial fracture.
3. **What will you do next?**
   ICU admission.
   Bed rest.
   IV fluid and blood transfusion as indicated.
   Mechanical DVT prophylaxis.
   Antibiotics.
   Stress ulcer prophylaxis.

   Serial monitoring of Hb level and coagulation profile.

   Consultation for the orthopedic and neurosurgeon.
4. **The patient was improving on nonoperative management. How will you follow the patient?**
   Follow-up CT scan after 72 h.

   CT follow-up shows pseudoaneurysm of the splenic artery.
5. **What will you do?**
   Angiography and stenting.
   Suggested twists points:

- **The patient failed to respond to nonoperative management. How will you manage that?**
  Operative exploration and splenectomy.

References

1. Burlew CC, Moore EE. Trauma. In: Brunicardi FC, editor. Schwartz's principles of surgery. 11th ed. New York: McGraw-Hill Education; 2019.
2. Klinger K, Mackersie RC. Airway management in the trauma patient. In: Cameron JL, Cameron AM, editors. Current surgical therapy. 12th ed. Toronto: Elsevier; 2016.
3. Moore SM, Jurkovich GJ. Chest wall, pneumothorax, and hemothorax. In: Cameron JL, Cameron AM, editors. Current surgical therapy. 12th ed. Toronto: Elsevier; 2016.
4. Menaker J. Emergency department thoracotomy. In: Cameron JL, Cameron AM, editors. Current surgical therapy. 12th ed. Toronto: Elsevier; 2016.
5. Sims C. The management of traumatic brain injury. In: Cameron JL, Cameron AM, editors. Current surgical therapy. 12th ed. Toronto: Elsevier; 2016.
6. Rueda M. The management of liver injuries. In: Cameron JL, Cameron AM, editors. Current surgical therapy. 12th ed. Toronto: Elsevier; 2016.
7. Waltz P, Peitzman AB. Injury to the Spleen. In: Cameron JL, Cameron AM, editors. Current surgical therapy. 12th ed. Toronto: Elsevier; 2016.

8. Rotondo MF. Pancreatic and duodenal injuries. In: Cameron JL, Cameron AM, editors. Current surgical therapy. 12th ed. Toronto: Elsevier; 2016.
9. Mason LL III. Injuries to the small and large bowel. In: Cameron JL, Cameron AM, editors. Current surgical therapy. 12th ed. Toronto: Elsevier; 2016.
10. Ryan ML. The management of rectal injuries. In: Cameron JL, Cameron AM, editors. Current surgical therapy. 12th ed. Toronto: Elsevier; 2016.
11. Ayoung-Chee P. Penetrating abdominal trauma. In: Cameron JL, Cameron AM, editors. Current surgical therapy. 12th ed. Toronto: Elsevier; 2016.
12. Lucas CE. Penetrating neck trauma. In: Cameron JL, Cameron AM, editors. Current surgical therapy. 12th ed. Toronto: Elsevier; 2016.
13. Martin RS, Meredith JW. Management of acute trauma. In: Townsend CM, Beauchamp RD, Evers BM, Mattox KL, editors. Sabiston textbook of surgery. 20th ed. St. Louis, MI: Elsevier; 2016.
14. Aurelio Rodriguez DE. Damage control operation. In: Cameron JL, Cameron AM, editors. Current surgical therapy. 12th ed. Toronto: Elsevier; 2016.

14 Surgical Aspects of Skin and Soft Tissue Diseases for Clinical Board Exams

14.1 Part I: Knowledge

If you want the answer—ask the question.
–Lorii Myers

The Chief Complaint Could Be One of the Following:

- Pigmented skin lesion.
- Lump (extremities, groin, abdomen).
- Abdominal pain and distention in case of complicated hernias.
- Refer to Table 14.1 for differential diagnosis.

History:

- Introduce yourself to the patient.

Table 14.1 Differential diagnosis

Pigmented skin lesion	Extremities mass	Groin mass
Naevus Seborrheic keratosis Melanoma Basal cell carcinoma Squamous cell carcinoma	Lipoma Abscess Sarcoma Osteoma	Inguinal hernia Femoral hernia Lipoma of the cord Varicocele Hydrocele Lymph node

- Name, age, occupation, gender, nationality.
- Chief complaint and duration.
- History of Presenting Illness:

a. **Analysis of the chief complaint:**

H. Alotaibi, *Study Surgery*, https://doi.org/10.1007/978-981-16-2305-9_14

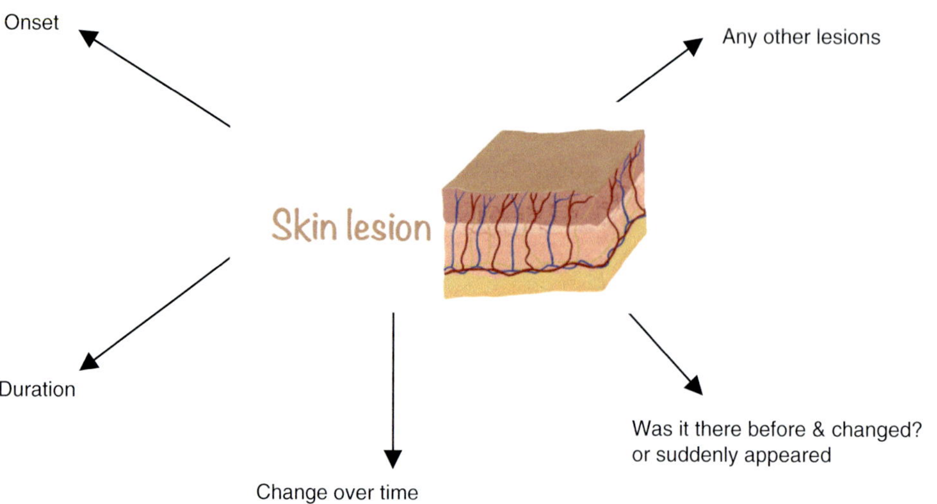
Onset
Any other lesions
Skin lesion
Duration
Change over time
Was it there before & changed?
or suddenly appeared

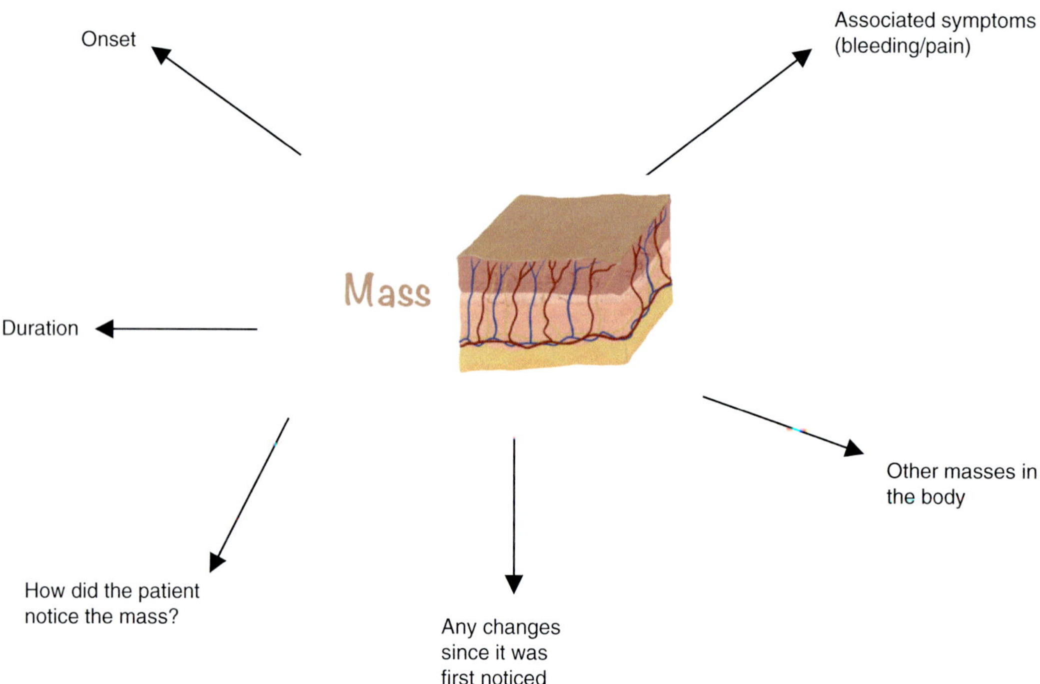
Onset
Associated symptoms
(bleeding/pain)
Mass
Duration
Other masses in
the body
How did the patient
notice the mass?
Any changes
since it was
first noticed

b. **Associated symptoms:**
   Itching, bleeding, pain, constipation, abdominal distention, nausea, vomiting
c. **Constitutional symptoms:**
   Weight loss, decrease appetite, night sweating, fever.
d. **Symptoms of metastasis**
   Back pain, abdominal distention, cough, shortness of breath
e. **Risk factors:**
   - **Risk factors for melanoma:**
     Sun exposure
     Tanning bed use
     Immunosuppression
     Personal history of cancer
     Family history of similar complaints
   - **Risk factors for sarcoma:**
     History of long-standing edema
     History of radiation
     Immunosuppression
     Personal history of cancer
     Family history of similar complaints
     History of radiation
   - **Risk factors for hernias:**
     Chronic cough
     Lifting heavy objects
     Chronic constipation and straining
     Previous abdominal surgery
f. **Differential Diagnosis:**
   - Recent history of trauma
   - History of radiation
g. **Symptoms of metastasis:** abdominal pain, distention, cough, SOB, jaundice
h. **Previous similar attack**, previous biopsy
i. **Systemic review of related system**:
   Skin rash, erythema, discharge

- PMH.
- PSH.
- Family history.
- Social history.
- Medication, transfusion, allergy.
- Systemic review:
  - **CNS:** headache, eye/hearing symptoms, epilepsy, numbness, paralysis
  - **CVS:** chest pain, orthopnea, paroxysmal nocturnal dyspnea, lower limb edema, palpitation
  - **Respiratory:** cough, fever, chest pain, hemoptysis
  - **Renal:** Dysuria, flank pain, hematuria
  - **MSK:** weakness, arthritis, skin erythema

Physical Examination:

- Introduce yourself to the patient.
- Ask permission for examination.
- Assure privacy.
- Position.
- Exposure.
- Handwashing.

General Examination:

Appearance: ill, well, dehydrated
Body built: cachectic, obese
Color: pale, jaundice
Distress
Environment and connection to monitors, fluids
Vital signs: BP, HR, Temperature, RR, SPO_2

- **Local Examination of the Lesion:**
  - Site
  - Size
  - Border
  - Color
  - Surface
  - Symmetry (pigmented skin lesion)
  - fixed to underlying structure or not
  - Tenderness
  - Hotness
  - Skin over it (erythema in case of strangulated hernia
- Examine the lymph node basin.
- Examine the entire skin and mucosal surface including nail bed for any other lesion.
- **Lymph nodes:** cervical, axillary, inguinal, popliteal.
- **Chest**: respiratory and CVS examination.
- **Abdomen**: distention, tenderness, ascites, organomegaly, bowel sound, hernial orifices.
- If the patient has hernia, determine the site, type, check reducibility, assess the defect, and look for any signs of strangulation or incarcerations.
- **DRE.**
- **Back**: for any tenderness.

14.1.1 Approach to Patient with Suspected Melanoma

- **History and physical examination as described above**
- **Investigations**:
  - CBC, coagulation profile, blood group
  - LFT, RFT, LDH
  - Biopsy:
    Excisional:
    - For small lesions.
    - Under local anesthesia.
    - Full thickness specimen (extend to subcutaneous).
    - With narrow margin (1–3 mm).
    - Close the defect by suture.
    - Orient the specimen.
    - Incision should be oriented in fusiform or such a way to easily allow subsequent wide local excision if necessary.
    - Longitudinal orientation in extremities; in another organ, orient the incision with least tension and best cosmetic outcome in the event that wide local excision is needed.

    Incisional:
    - Punch biopsy (simplest incisional biopsy): used for large lesion
    - Technique:
      - Anesthetized the area.
      - Should be performed through the thickest area of the lesion.
      - Using a disposable instrument is twisted to narrow 2–8 mm of skin and subconscious.
      - Thickness at least 4 mm.
      - Close the defect by one or two simple sutures.
  - Do not do shave biopsy if you are suspecting melanoma [1].
- **Histological Subtype:**
  - Superficial spreading: the most common type
  - Acral lentiginous
  - Lintigo maligna: better prognosis
  - Nodular melanoma: poor prognosis
- **Berslow Thickness:**
  - Thin ≤ 1 mm
  - Intermediate >1–4 mm
  - Thick > 4 mm
- **Clark's Level:**
  - **Level 1** is also called melanoma in situ—the melanoma cells are only in the outer layer of the skin (the epidermis).
  - **Level 2** means there are melanoma cells in the layer directly under the epidermis. This is known as the papillary dermis (superficial dermis).
  - **Level 3** means the melanoma cells are touching the next layer down known as the reticular dermis (deep dermis).
  - **Level 4** means the melanoma has spread into the reticular dermis.
  - **Level 5** means the melanoma has grown into the layer of fat under the skin (subcutaneous fat) (Fig. 14.1).
- **Ulceration:**
  - Present
  - Absent
- **Staging:**
  - T1: ≤ 1 mm
  - T2: > 1–2 mm
  - T3: > 2–4 mm
  - T4: > 4 mm [1]
- **Imaging** [2]:
  - Imaging to evaluate specific signs or symptoms suggestive of possible metastases is recommended in all stages.

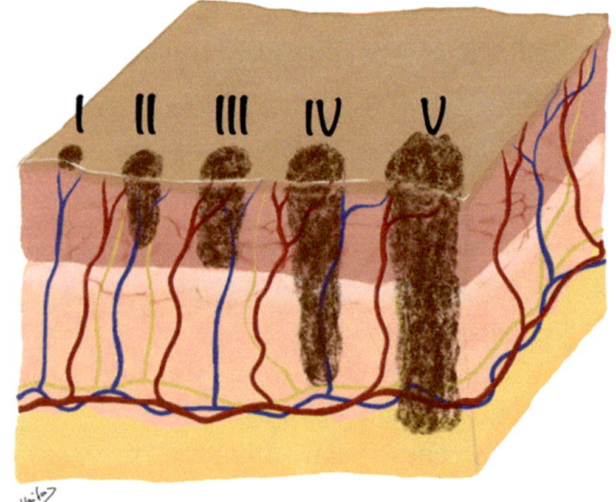

Fig. 14.1 Clark's level

- Stage-specific recommendations for routine imaging during workup:
  Stage 0, IA, IB, II
  - Routine cross-sectional imaging with or without brain imaging is not recommended.

  Stage I/II:
  - Consider nodal basin ultrasound prior to SLNB for melanoma patients with an equivocal regional lymph node physical exam.
  - Abnormalities or suspicious lesions on nodal basin US should be confirmed histologically. Nodal basin ultrasound is not a substitute for SLNB. Negative nodal basin ultrasound is not a substitute for biopsy of clinically suspicious lymph nodes.

  Stage IIIA (sentinel node positive)
  - Consider cross-sectional imaging for baseline staging.

  Stage IIIB/C/D
  - Cross-sectional with or without brain imaging for baseline staging.

  True scar recurrence (persistent disease)
  - Imaging workup should be appropriate to primary tumor characteristics (see above recommendations for stage 0, IA, IB, II).

  Stage IV or recurrence with distant metastatic disease
  - Cross-sectional and brain imaging

  Local satellite/in-transit recurrence; nodal recurrence
  - Cross-sectional with or without brain imaging to assess extent of disease [2]

- **Clinical Staging:**
  - Follow the AJCC guideline for staging
  - Stage 0: in situ
  - Stage III: when any lymph node is positive
  - Stage IV: when any metastasis positive [1]
- **Management:**

Principles:

- Multidisciplinary team discussion.
- Consider sentinel lymph node biopsy (SLNB) in stage IB and II.
- Tissue should be sent for permanent section histopathology with immunohistochemical stains for melanoma markers (e.g., S-100, HMB-45, and Melan-1). Immediate frozen section histology should be avoided because even expert pathologists have difficulty in diagnosing micrometastatic melanoma in the SLN on frozen sections.
- Once you have positive SLNB or clinically positive node, staging is indicated.
- If positive SLNB:
  - Active nodal basin surveillance
  - Or completion lymph node dissection
- If clinically positive lymph node, do FNA. If positive, therapeutic lymph node dissection is indicated [1].

Management of Melanoma Itself:

- Wide local incision
- Margins depend on the Berslow thickness:
  - In situ: 0.5 cm margin
  - 1–2 mm: 1 cm margin
  - >2 mm: 2 cm margin
- **Adjuvant Radiation:**
  - When close margin for invasion melanoma, where re-resection is not feasible
- **Follow-up** [2]:
  - **Common follow-up:**
    History and physical examination (with emphasis on nodes and skin) at least annually.
    Patient education in regular skin and lymph node self-examination.
    Patient education in principles of sun safety, including sun avoidance during peak hours, use of sun-protective clothing/hat/eyewear, and regular application of broad-spectrum sunscreen to exposed skin when outdoors, particularly in individuals with sun sensitivity/light complexion.
    In patients with an equivocal lymph node exam, short-term follow-up and/or additional imaging (ultrasound [preferred] or CT) should be considered, with imaging-directed biopsy as warranted.

Regional lymph node ultrasound in patients with a positive SLNB who did not undergo CLND should be considered where expertise is available.

It would be appropriate for the frequency of clinical exam and ultrasound surveillance to be consistent with the two prospective randomized trials (MSLT-II and DeCOG):

- Every 4 months during the first 2 years
- Then every 6 months during years 3 through 5

Follow-up schedule is influenced by risk of recurrence and new primary melanoma, which depends on patient/family history of melanoma, mole count, and/or presence of atypical moles/dysplastic nevi.

Consider genetic counseling referral for p16/CDKN2A mutation testing in the presence of three or more invasive cutaneous melanomas, or a mix of invasive melanoma, pancreatic cancer, and/or astrocytoma diagnoses in an individual or family.

Multigene panel testing is also recommended for patients with invasive cutaneous melanoma who have a first-degree relative diagnosed with pancreatic

Testing for other genes that can harbor melanoma-predisposing mutations may be warranted.

- **Stage 0:**

  History and physical examination (with emphasis on skin) at least annually.

  Routine blood tests are not recommended.

  Routine imaging to screen for asymptomatic recurrence or metastatic disease is not recommended.

- **Stage IA-IIA:**

  History and physical examination (with emphasis on nodes and skin) every 6–12 months for 5 years, then annually as clinically indicated.

  Routine blood tests are not recommended.

  Routine imaging to screen for asymptomatic recurrence or metastatic disease is not recommended.

  Imaging as indicated to investigate specific signs or symptom.

- **Stage IIB-IV:**

  History and physical examination (with emphasis on nodes and skin) every 3–6 months for 2 years, then every 3–12 months for 3 years, then annually as clinically indicated.

  Routine blood tests are not recommended.

  - Imaging as indicated to investigate specific signs or symptoms.
  - Consider imaging every 3–12 months for 2 years, then every 6–12 months for another 3 years (unless otherwise mandated by clinical trial participation) to screen for recurrence or metastatic disease.

  Routine imaging to screen for asymptomatic recurrence or metastatic disease is not recommended after 3–5 years, depending on risk of relapse [2].

14.1.2 Approach to Patient with Suspected Sarcoma of the Extremities

- History and physical examination as described before
- Investigations:
  - Blood Investigations:

    CBC

    Electrolytes

    Coagulation profile

    Blood grouping

    LFT

    RFT

    LDH
  - Imaging:

    MRI

    CT chest (for staging if the diagnosis is confirmed)

- Biopsy:
  Place biopsy along future resection axis with minimal dissection and careful attention to hemostasis.
  Core needle is preferred.
  Incisional biopsy if core needle biopsy is not possible or nondiagnostic.
  Excisional biopsy if easily accessible and <3 cm. It should not be performed for the hand and the foot.

- The pathological assessment should comment on the histological subtype and the histological grade.
- Staging:
  - If intermediate or high grade, do staging CT chest.
  - CT abdomen is indicated if the subtype is myxoid or round cell.
  - Brain imaging is indicated if the subtype is alveolar, angiosarcoma, or clear cell.
- All the cases should be discussed in a multidisciplinary team meeting.
- Preoperative Preparation:
  - Admit the patient.
  - NPO.
  - IV fluid.
  - IV medications (stress ulcer prophylaxis, antibiotic prophylaxis if indicated).
  - DVT prophylaxis.
  - Consent for wide local excision ± re-resection ± amputation.
  - Surgical site marking.
  - Consult plastic surgeon if expecting large defect [3].
- Management:
  A. Low-grade tumor: functional sparing complete excision with 1–2 cm free margins.
    - If the margins are negative, no adjuvant treatment is required.
    - If the margins are positive, consider radiation therapy postoperative.

  B. High-grade tumors:
    - Tumor ≤ 5 cm: functional sparing excision. Further treatment depends on the margins:
      - ≥1 cm: no adjuvant treatment is required.
      - <1 cm or positive margins: consider radiation therapy.
    - Tumor > 5–10 cm: consider neoadjuvant chemotherapy if synovial sarcoma, round cell, or pleomorphic sarcoma followed by functional sparing excision. Further treatment depends on the margins:
      - ≥1 cm: consider adjuvant radiation therapy
      - <1 cm or positive margins: radiation therapy
    - Tumor ≥ 10 cm: consider neoadjuvant chemotherapy followed by functional sparing excision followed by radiation therapy regardless the margins.
    - Ewing sarcoma or rhabdomyosarcoma: neoadjuvant chemotherapy followed by excision and radiation therapy [3].
- Postoperative follow-up:
  - First postoperative visit:
    Clinical assessment.
    Check the wound and remove sutures.
    Review the final pathology report.
    Discuss in a multidisciplinary team meeting to decide if further treatment is required.
  - Long-term follow-up
    History and physical examination every 3–6 months for 2–3 years
    History and physical examination every 6 months for 3 years
    Then, annually
    CT chest abdomen and pelvis to be done on regular interval
    Base line MRI at 3 months then as indicated

14.1.3 Approach to Patient with Suspected Retroperitoneal Sarcoma

- History and physical examination
- Workup:
  - Imaging:
    Chest/abdominal/pelvic CT ± abdominal/pelvic MRI
    PET/CT
  - Biopsy:
    Proof of the histologic subtype by biopsy is necessary for patients before

receiving preoperative chemotherapy or radiation therapy.

Biopsy should be considered if there is suspicion of malignancies other than sarcoma.

Image-guided (CT or ultrasound) core needle biopsy is preferred over open surgical biopsy.

If a retroperitoneal sarcoma is encountered unexpectedly when a laparotomy is performed for some other reason, a core needle biopsy should be done to establish the diagnosis as well as the histopathologic type and grade of tumor. Then, the optimal subsequent resection could be performed.

 – Staging

- Management:

  A. Resectable disease:
     - Resection to obtain oncological appropriate margins
     - Or preoperative chemotherapy or radiotherapy followed by surgery ± intraoperative radiation therapy (RT)
     - Postsurgery treatment:
       – Postoperative RT should not be administered routinely to patients with negative margin resection (R0) or microscopically positive margins (R1 resection) due to risk of morbidity.
       – Highly selected candidates for postoperative RT: patients with pathologic findings of high-grade disease, extremely large tumors, close surgical margins, or high risk of recurrence.

  B. Unresectable (stage IV) Disease:
     - Unresectable tumors are defined as those that involve vital structures or tumors whose removal would cause unacceptable morbidity.
     - Biopsy is recommended before any treatment for a patient with unresectable or metastatic disease.
     - Patients with unresectable or stage IV disease could be treated with chemotherapy, chemoradiation, or RT in an attempt to downstage tumors.
     - Follow-up imaging is recommended to assess treatment response.
     - Patients whose tumors become resectable following primary treatment should be managed as resectable disease.
     - If no response, asymptomatic patients can be observed, whereas symptomatic patients can be treated with palliative therapy [3].

- Follow-up:
  – History and physical examination with imaging (chest/abdominal/pelvic CT or MRI) every 3–6 months for 2–3 years, then every 6 months for the next 2 years, and then annually.

14.1.4 Approach to Patient with Suspected Hernia

- History and physical examination
- Workup:
  – Blood investigation:
    CBC
    Electrolytes
    Coagulation profile
    RFT
  – Imaging
    Ultrasound
    CT scan

Ventral Hernias:

- The evaluation of abdominal wall hernias requires diligent physical examination. The anterior abdominal wall is evaluated with the patient in standing and supine positions, and a Valsalva maneuver is also useful to demonstrate the site and size of a hernia.
- Imaging modalities may play a greater role in the diagnosis of more unusual hernias of the abdominal wall.

A. **Umbilical hernia:**

- Strangulation is unusual in most patients.
- Strangulation or rupture can occur in chronic ascitic conditions.

- Small asymptomatic umbilical hernias barely detectable on examination need not be repaired.
- Adults who have symptoms, a large hernia, incarceration, thinning of the overlying skin, or uncontrollable ascites should have a hernia repair.
- Spontaneous rupture of umbilical hernias in patients with ascites can result in peritonitis and death.
- Classically, repair was done using the vest over pants repair proposed by Mayo, which uses imbrication of the superior and inferior fascial edges.
- Small defects are closed primarily after separation of the sac from the overlying umbilicus and surrounding fascia.
- Defects larger than 3 cm are closed using prosthetic mesh [4].

B. **Epigastric hernia:**

- They are multiple in up to 20% of patients, and approximately 80% are in the midline.
- The defects are small and often produce pain out of proportion to their size because of incarceration of preperitoneal fat.
- Repair usually consists of excision of the incarcerated preperitoneal tissue and simple closure of the fascial defect, similar to that for umbilical hernias.
- Small defects can be repaired under local anesthesia.
- Epigastric hernias are better repaired anteriorly because the defect is small and fat that has herniated from within the peritoneal cavity is difficult to reduce.

C. **Incisional hernia:**

- Occur as a result of excessive tension and inadequate healing of a previous incision, which may be associated with surgical site infection.
- These hernias enlarge over time, leading to pain, bowel obstruction, incarceration, and strangulation.
- Large hernias can result in loss of abdominal domain, which occurs when the abdominal contents no longer reside in the abdominal cavity.
- Return of displaced viscera to the abdominal cavity during repair may lead to increased abdominal pressure, abdominal compartment syndrome, and acute respiratory failure. [4]
- Component separation:
  - **Posterior component separation**:
    The retrorectus space is bordered laterally by the linea semilunaris.
    In very large hernias, further advancement can be obtained by incising the posterior rectus sheath approximately 1 cm medial to the linea semilunaris.
    At this location, the posterior leaflet of the internal oblique and the transversus abdominis muscle are incised to gain access to the preperitoneum.
    This plane can be extended to the retroperitoneum and eventually to the psoas muscle if necessary (Fig. 14.2).
    Very large sheets of prosthetic mesh can be placed in this location with wide defect coverage [4].

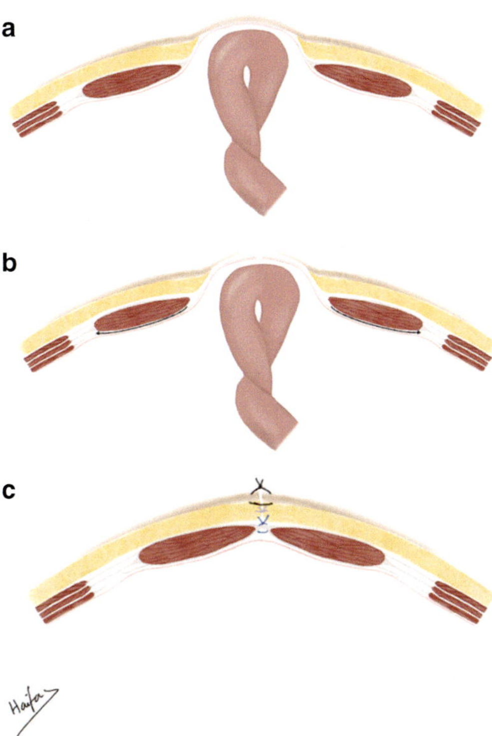

Fig. 14.2 Posterior component separation, (**a**) abdominal wall defect, (**b**) lateral relaxing incision on the lateral oblique aponeuroisis, (**c**) closure of the defect

- **Anterior component separation**:
  Separating the lateral muscle layers of the abdominal wall to allow their advancement.
  The procedure is performed by raising large subcutaneous flaps above the external oblique fascia.
  These flaps are carried laterally past the linea semilunaris.
  This lipocutaneous dissection itself can provide some advancement of the abdominal wall.
  Large perforating subcutaneous vessels can be preserved to prevent ischemic necrosis of the skin flaps.
  A relaxing incision is made 2 cm lateral to the linea semilunaris on the lateral external oblique aponeurosis from several centimeters above the costal margin to the pubis.
  The external oblique is then bluntly separated in the avascular plane, away from the internal oblique, allowing its advancement (Fig. 14.3).
  Additional release can be safely achieved by incising the posterior rectus sheath.
  These techniques, when applied to both sides of the abdominal wall, can yield up to 20 cm of mobilization.
  It is important that patients understand that a lateral bulge can occur after release of the external oblique aponeurosis.
  If a bioprosthetic is placed, it can be secured with an underlay or onlay technique [4].

Inguinal Hernia:

- Classified as direct or indirect.
- The sac of an indirect inguinal hernia passes from the internal inguinal ring obliquely toward the external inguinal ring and ultimately into the scrotum.
- The sac of a direct inguinal hernia protrudes outward and forward and is medial to the internal inguinal ring and inferior epigastric vessels [4].

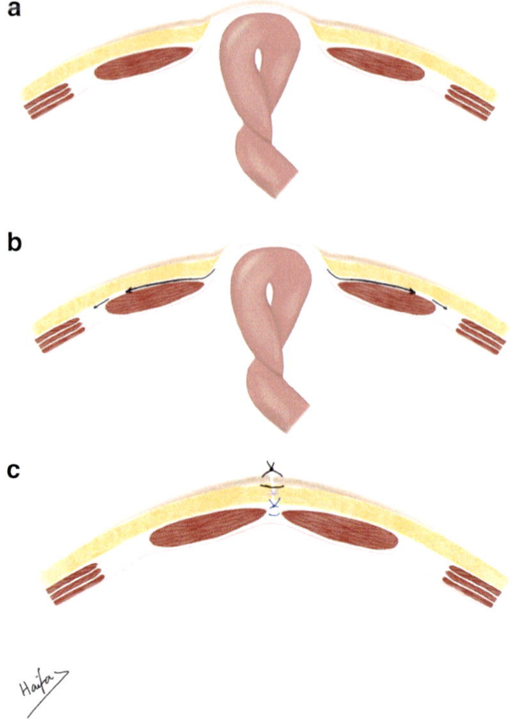

Fig. 14.3 Anterior component separation, (**a**) abdominal wall defect, (**b**) lateral relaxing incision on the lateral oblique aponeuroisis, (**c**) closure of the defect

- **Anatomy of the groin:**
  - **External oblique muscle and aponeurosis:**
    The most superficial of the lateral abdominal wall muscles.
    Its fibers are directed inferiorly and medially and lie deep to the subcutaneous tissues.
    The external oblique aponeurosis serves as the superficial boundary of the inguinal canal.
    The inguinal ligament (Poupart ligament) is the inferior edge of the external oblique aponeurosis and extends from the anterior superior iliac spine to the pubic tubercle, turning posteriorly to form a shelving edge.
    The lacunar ligament is the fan-shaped medial expansion of the inguinal ligament, which inserts into the pubis and

forms the medial border of the femoral space.

The external (superficial) inguinal ring is an ovoid opening of the external oblique aponeurosis that is positioned superiorly and slightly laterally to the pubic tubercle [4].

- **Internal oblique muscle and aponeurosis:**

  The internal oblique muscle forms the middle layer.

  The fibers of the internal oblique are directed superiorly and laterally in the upper abdomen.

  The internal oblique muscle serves as the cephalad (or superior) border of the inguinal canal.

  The medial aspect of the internal oblique aponeurosis fuses with fibers from the transversus abdominis aponeurosis to form a conjoined tendon which is present in only 5–10% of patients.

  The cremaster muscle fibers arise from the internal oblique, encompass the spermatic cord, and attach to the tunica vaginalis of the testis [4].

- **Transversus abdominis muscle and transversalis fascia:**

  The transversus abdominis muscle layer is oriented horizontally.

  The lower margin of the transversus abdominis arches along with the internal oblique muscle over the internal inguinal ring to form the transversus abdominis aponeurotic arch.

  The transversalis fascia is the connective tissue layer that underlies the abdominal wall musculature [4].

  The iliopubic tract:

  It is an aponeurotic band that is formed by the transversalis fascia and transversus abdominis aponeurosis and fascia.

  The iliopubic tract is located posterior to the inguinal ligament and crosses over the femoral vessels and inserts on the anterior superior iliac spine and inner lip of the wing of the ilium (Fig. 14.4).

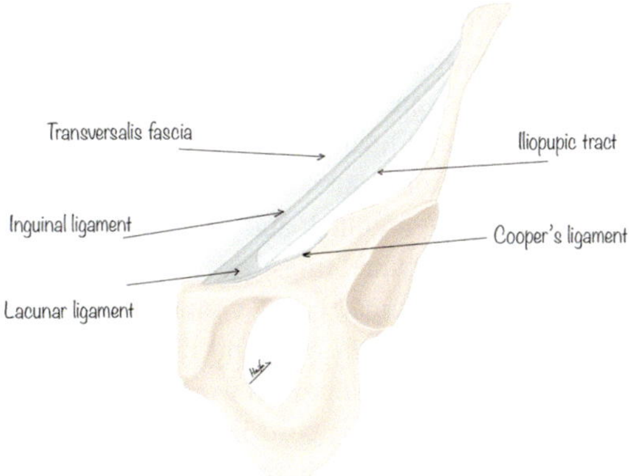

Fig. 14.4 Ligaments of the inguinal region

  The iliopubic tract is an extremely important structure in the repair of hernias from the anterior and posterior approaches.

  It composes the inferior margin of most anterior repairs.

  The portion of the iliopubic tract lateral to the internal inguinal ring serves as the inferior border below which staples or tacks are not placed during a laparoscopic repair because the femoral, lateral femoral cutaneous, and genitofemoral nerves are located inferior to the iliopubic tract [4].

- **Pectineal (Cooper) ligament:**

  The pectineal (Cooper) ligament is formed by the periosteum and aponeurotic tissues along the superior ramus of the pubis (Fig. 14.4).

  This structure is posterior to the iliopubic tract and forms the posterior border of the femoral canal.

  In approximately 75% of patients, there will be a vessel that crosses the lateral border of Cooper ligament that is a branch of the obturator artery. If this vessel is injured, troublesome bleeding can result.

  Cooper ligament is an important landmark for open and laparoscopic repairs and is a useful anchoring structure, particularly in laparoscopic repairs [4].

- **Inguinal canal:**

  The inguinal canal is about 4 cm in length and is located just cephalad to the inguinal ligament.

  The canal extends between the internal (deep) inguinal and external (superficial) inguinal rings.

  The inguinal canal contains the spermatic cord in men and the round ligament of the uterus in women.

  The spermatic cord is composed of the cremaster muscle fibers, testicular artery and accompanying veins, genital branch of the genitofemoral nerve, vas deferens, cremasteric vessels, lymphatics, and processus vaginalis.

  The cremasteric vessels are branches of the inferior epigastric vessels.

  The inguinal canal boundaries:

  - Superficial (anterior) wall: the external oblique aponeurosis
  - Superior wall: The internal oblique and transversus abdominis musculoaponeuroses
  - Inferior wall: the inguinal ligament and lacunar ligament
  - Posterior wall (floor): the aponeurosis of the transversus abdominis muscle and transversalis fascia. [4]

- **Hesselbach triangle:** The inferior epigastric vessels serve as its superolateral border, the rectus sheath as the medial border, and the inguinal ligament and pectineal ligament as the inferior border. Direct hernias occur within Hesselbach triangle, whereas indirect inguinal hernias arise lateral to the triangle.

  - **Cutaneous nerves:**

    The iliohypogastric and ilioinguinal nerves provide sensation to the skin of the groin, base of the penis, and ipsilateral upper medial thigh.

    The iliohypogastric and ilioinguinal nerves lie beneath the internal oblique muscle to a point just medial and superior to the anterior superior iliac spine, where they penetrate the internal oblique muscle and course beneath the external oblique aponeurosis.

    The main trunk of the iliohypogastric nerve runs on the anterior surface of the internal oblique muscle and aponeurosis medial and superior to the internal ring.

    The ilioinguinal nerve runs anterior to the spermatic cord in the inguinal canal and branches at the superficial inguinal ring.

    The genital branch of the genitofemoral nerve innervates the cremaster muscle and skin on the lateral side of the scrotum and labia.

    This nerve lies on the iliopubic tract and accompanies the cremaster vessels to form a neurovascular bundle [4].

  - **Femoral canal:**

    The boundaries of the femoral canal are the iliopubic tract anteriorly, Cooper ligament posteriorly, and femoral vein laterally. The pubic tubercle forms the apex of the femoral canal triangle.

    A femoral hernia occurs through this space and is medial to the femoral vessels [4].

- **Clinical Presentation:**
  - Most patient will present with bulge at the groin area.
  - Pain or vague discomfort in the region: groin hernias are usually not extremely painful unless incarceration or strangulation has occurred [4].
- **Management:**
- Nonoperative management:

  Patients with minimal symptoms, the clinician is often faced with balancing the risk for hernia-related complications, such as incarceration and bowel strangulation, with the potential for complications in the short and long term.

  Nonoperative management is not used for femoral hernias because of the high incidence of associated complications, particularly strangulation.

- Operative management:

Most surgeons recommend operation on discovery of a symptomatic inguinal hernia because the natural history of a groin hernia is that of progressive enlargement and weakening, with a small potential for incarceration and strangulation [4].

Femoral Hernia:

- A femoral hernia produces a mass or bulge below the inguinal ligament.
- A femoral hernia can be repaired by the standard Cooper ligament repair, a preperitoneal approach, or a laparoscopic approach.
- The incidence of strangulation in femoral hernias is high; therefore, all femoral hernias should be repaired, and incarcerated femoral hernias should have the hernia sac contents examined for viability. In patients with a compromised bowel, the Cooper ligament approach is the preferred technique because mesh is contraindicated. When the incarcerated contents of a femoral hernia cannot be reduced, dividing the lacunar ligament can be helpful [4].

Special Problems:

- Sliding Hernia:
  - A sliding hernia occurs when an internal organ composes a portion of the wall of the hernia sac.
  - The most common viscus involved is the colon or urinary bladder.
  - The sliding hernia contents are reduced into the peritoneal cavity, and any excess hernia sac is ligated and divided.
  - After reduction of the hernia, one of the techniques described earlier can be used for repair of the inguinal hernia [4].
- Recurrent Hernia:
  - The repair of recurrent inguinal hernias is challenging, and results are associated with a higher incidence of secondary recurrence.
  - Recurrent hernias almost always require placement of prosthetic mesh for successful repair.
  - Recurrences after anterior hernia repair using mesh are best managed by a laparoscopic or open posterior approach, with placement of a second prosthesis [4].
- Strangulated Hernia:
  - Repair of a suspected strangulated hernia is most easily done using a preperitoneal approach.
  - With this exposure, the hernia sac contents can be directly visualized, and their viability assessed through a single incision.
  - The constricting ring is identified and can be incised to reduce the entrapped viscus with minimal danger to the surrounding organs, blood vessels, and nerves.
  - If it is necessary to resect strangulated intestine, the peritoneum can be opened, and resection done without the need for a second incision [4].
- Bilateral Hernias:
  - The approach to repair of bilateral inguinal hernias is based on the extent of the hernia defect.
  - Simultaneous repair of bilateral hernias has a similar recurrence rate to unilateral repair, regardless of whether the open or laparoscopic technique is used.
  - The use of a giant prosthetic reinforcement of the visceral sac (Stoppa repair) or the laparoscopic repair is preferred for simultaneous repair of bilateral inguinal hernias [4].

14.1.5 Open Inguinal Hernia Repair:

Preoperative Preparation:

- Admission
- NPO
- IV fluid
- Prophylaxis (antibiotic, DVT as indicated)
- Bladder decompression before the operation
- Surgical site marking
- Hair removal
- Consent

Informed Consent:

Open Inguinal Hernia Repair:

Describe the procedure: under general or spinal anesthesia, the surgeon will repair (right/left) inguinal hernia using (tissue repair/prosthetic mesh) after examining the content of the hernia with possibility of only reduction of the content or resection of the nonviable bowel if the hernia is strangulated.

Mention if there are any other alternatives like nonoperative management or laparoscopic repair.

Mention the possible complications such as nerve orchitis, injury to the vas deference, chronic pain (nerve injury), urinary retention, recurrence, or wound infection.

Open Inguinal Hernia Repair:

Technique:

- Anesthesia: Can be performed under local-regional-or general anesthesia.
- Time out: confirm the correct patient, correct procedure, correct site. Confirm the availability of the required instruments and mesh.
- Prepping and draping in usual sterile fashion.
- Surgeon will stand on the same side of the hernia.
- Incision: oblique incision, parallel, and above inguinal ligament by 1 cm. The length of the incision is about 5–7 cm from the area of internal ring to the external ring (2 cm lateral to the pubic tubercle).
- Once the skin incision is made, it is carried down to the external oblique aponeurosis.
- Incise the external oblique aponeurosis along its fiber (place the finger into the superficial ring and incise the aponeurosis from medial to lateral).
- Cephalad and caudal flap are developed; cephalad to expose the conjoined tendon and caudal to the inguinal ligament.
- Apply self-retaining retractor.
- Identify the ilioinguinal nerve and preserve it.
- Mobilize the spermatic cord, elevate it off the pubic tubercle along with its cremasteric layer
- Apply Penrose drain.
- The spermatic cord must be elevated from 2 cm distal to pubic tubercle all the way to the internal ring [4].
- Open the cremasteric muscle in the line of its fibers.
- If you identify indirect hernial sac, retract it cephalad and laterally while mobilizing the cord medially.
- The sac can be opened and examined if necessary.
- Assess the integrity of the floor of the inguinal canal [4].

Repair Technique:

Tissue Repair:

a. **Iliopubic Tract Repair:**
   - Approximate transverse abdominus aponeurosis to the iliopubic tract with the use of interrupted sutures.
   - Repair begin at the pubic tubercle and extend laterally past the internal ring [4].
b. **Shouldice Repair:**
   - Multilayers repair of the posterior wall.
   - Reconstruct the posterior wall of the inguinal canal by super imposing running suture line progressing from deep to more superficial layers.
   - Initial suture line: transverse abdominus aponeurosis to iliopubic tract.
   - Next, the internal oblique and transverse abdominus to the inguinal ligament [4] (Fig. 14.5).
c. **Bassini Repair:**
   - Suture the transverse abdominus and internal oblique or the conjoined tendon if present to the inguinal ligament [4] (Fig. 14.6).
d. **Cooper Ligament Repair (MacVay):**
   - Suited for strangulated femoral hernia mainly but can be used for large indirect or direct hernia.

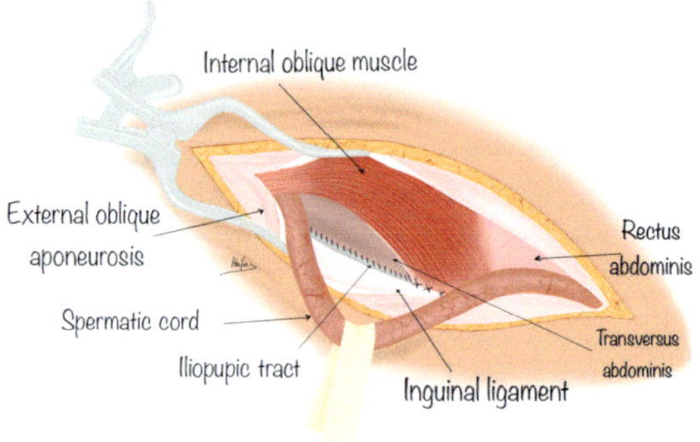

Fig. 14.5 Shouldice repair

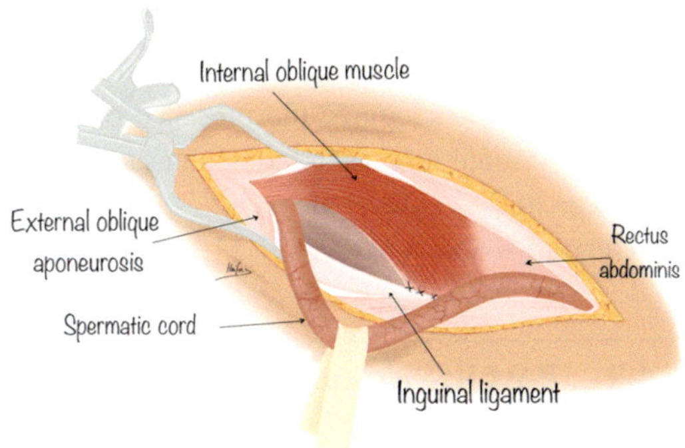

Fig. 14.6 Bassini repair

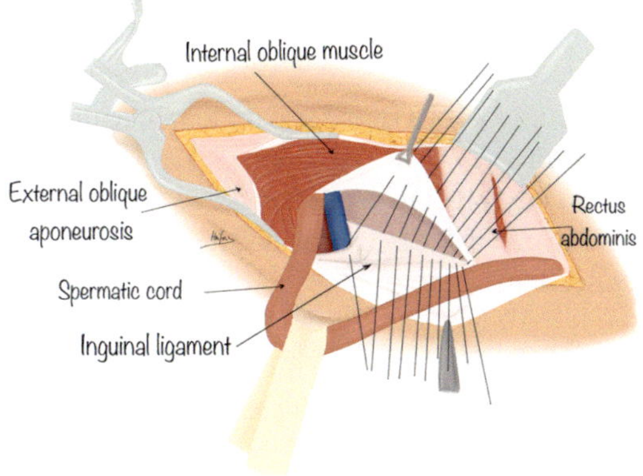

Fig. 14.7 MacVay repair

- An important principle of this repair is the need of relaxing incision.
- This incision is made by reflecting the external oblique aponeurosis cephalad and medial to exposes the anterior rectus sheath.
- The incision is made in curvilinear direction beginning 1 cm from above the pubic tubercle throughout the extent of the anterior sheath t near its lateral border.
- Interrupted nonabsorbable sutures are used to approximate the edge of the transverse abdominus aponeurosis to cooper ligament.
- When medial aspect of the femoral canal is reached, transition suture is placed to incorporate the cooper ligament and iliopubic tract.
- Lateral to this transition stitch, the transverse abdominus is secured to the iliopubic tract [4] (Fig. 14.7).

e. **Tension-Free Anterior Inguinal Hernia Repair:**
   - After careful dissection of inguinal canal, high ligation of an indirect hernial sac is performed.
   - The spermatic cord structures retracted inferiorly.
   - Sheet of polyproline mesh is fashioned to fit the inguinal canal about 6–8 cm width.
   - Slit is made in the lateral aspect of the mesh and the spermatic cord is placed between the two tails of the mesh.
   - The spermatic cord is placed between the two tails of the mesh.
   - The spermatic cord is retracted in cephalad direction.
   - Remove the Penrose drain.
   - Medial aspect of the mesh overlaps pubic bone by 2 cm.
   - The mesh is sutured to the aponeurotic tissue overlying the pubic tubercle medially. Suturing is continued superiorly along the transverse abdominus or conjoined tendon.
   - The inferolateral edge of the mesh is sutured to the iliopubic tract or shelving edge of the inguinal ligament to a point lateral the internal ring.
   - The tails created by the slit are sutured together around the spermatic cord.
   - It is important to protect ilioinguinal nerve and genital branch of genitofemoral nerve from entrapment.
   - Hemostasis.
   - Close the external oblique using #1-0 absorbable suture, taking care not to make the external ring too tight.
   - Close the scarp's fascia.
   - Close the skin.
   - Dressing.
   - In male patients, make sure testis in its place [4].

Postoperative Complications:

- **Nerve Injuries and Chronic Pain Syndromes:**
  - Nerve injuries are an infrequent and underrecognized complication of inguinal hernia repair.

- Injury can occur from traction, electrocautery, transection, and entrapment.
- The nerves most commonly affected during open hernia repair are the ilioinguinal, genital branch of the genitofemoral, and iliohypogastric nerves.
- During laparoscopic repair, the lateral femoral cutaneous and genitofemoral nerves are most often affected.
- Transient neuralgias involving sensory nerves can occur and are usually self-limited and resolve within a few weeks after surgery.
- Persistent neuralgias usually result in pain and hyperesthesia in the area of distribution.
- Symptoms are often reproduced by palpation over the point of entrapment or hyperextension of the hip and may be relieved by flexion of the thigh.
- Transection of a sensory nerve usually results in an area of numbness corresponding to the distribution of the involved nerve.
- Early symptoms are treated with anti-inflammatory agents, analgesics, and local anesthetic nerve blocks.
- Patients with nerve entrapment syndromes are best treated by repeated exploration with neurectomy and mesh removal through an anterior approach.
- Laparoscopic nerve injuries are minimized by not placing any tacks or staples below the lateral portion of the iliopubic tract. If nerve entrapment occurs, patients undergo reoperation to remove the offending tack or staple [4].

• **Ischemic Orchitis and Testicular Atrophy:**
  - Ischemic orchitis usually occurs from thrombosis of the small veins of the pampiniform plexus within the spermatic cord.
  - It is treated with anti-inflammatory agents and analgesics. Orchiectomy is rarely necessary.
• **Injury to the Vas Deferens and Viscera:**
  - Injury to the vas deferens and intra-abdominal viscera is unusual.
  - Most of these injuries occur in patients with sliding inguinal hernias when there is failure to recognize the presence of intra-abdominal viscera in the hernia sac.
• **Surgical Site Infection**
• **Hernial Recurrence** [4]

14.2 Part II: Practice

What you practice, is what you'll do.
–Benny Urquidez

14.2.1 Case Scenarios for Practice

Tips:

• Practice with a friend and try to mimic the real exam!
• Do not forget to set the timer!
• The clinical data is provided in the answer key section.

Case No.1:

A 53-year-old male patient presented to the clinic due to abnormal pigmented lesion in his left thigh for 1 month.

Questions for Discussion:

1. How will you approach the patient?
2. What will you do next?
3. What are the histological features that you should look for?
4. What further work up you need to do?
5. How will you manage the patient?
6. How will you follow up the patient?

Case No.2:

A 65-year-old female patient was referred from urology clinic due to retroperitoneal mass that was discovered during workup for hydronephrosis?

Questions for Discussion:

1. How will you approach the patient?
2. What will you do next?
3. How will you manage the patient?
4. How will follow up the patient?

Case No. 3:

A 39-year-old male patient presented to the emergency department complaining of painful swelling at the right lower abdomen for 1 day.

Questions for Discussion:

1. How will you approach the patient?
2. What will you do next?
3. How will you manage the patient?
4. Intraoperative findings as described. What will you do?
5. How will repair the defect?
6. The patient presents to the clinic for follow-up, and he is complaining of severe pain around the surgical site since postoperative despite multiple analgesics. How will you manage that?

Checklist

History	Items	Done	Not done	NA
General	Introduce himself/herself to the patient			
	Patient personal data (name, age, gender, nationality)			
	Chief complaint			
	Duration			
Mass	Onset			
	Site			
	How did the patient notice it?			
	Any change since it was first noticed?			
	Other masses			
Pigmented skin lesion	Onset			
	Changes over time			
	Was it there before and recently changed?			
	Any other lesion			
Associated symptoms	Pain			
	Itching (skin lesion or mass)			
	Bleeding (skin lesion or mass)			
	Nausea (hernia)			
	Diarrhea (hernia)			
	Constipation (hernia)			
Constitutional symptoms	Weight loss			
	Decrease appetite			
	Night sweating			
Symptoms of metastases	Back pain			
	Cough			
	Shortness of breath			
	Abdominal distention			
Risk factors	Sun exposure (melanoma)			
	Tanning bed use (melanoma)			
	Immunosuppression (sarcoma)			
	Personal history of cancer (melanoma and sarcoma)			
	Family history of similar complain (melanoma and sarcoma)			
	Chronic cough (hernia)			
	Lifting heavy object (hernia)			
	Chronic constipation and straining (hernia)			
	Previous abdominal surgery (hernia)			
	History of long-standing lymphedema (sarcoma)			
	History of radiation (sarcoma)			
	Personal history of malignancy			

(continued)

History	Items	Done	Not done	NA
Differential diagnosis	Recent history of trauma			
PMH	Previous similar attack			
	Previous investigation			
	Previous admission			
	Chronic illnesses			
PSH	Previous surgery			
Family history	Of cancers or similar complain			
Social history	Occupation			
	Habits (smoking, alcohol, drugs)			
Other	Medication			
	Allergy			
	Transfusion			
Systemic review				
Physical examination				
General principle	Patient position			
	Exposure			
	Privacy			
	Wash hands			
General examination	Appearance			
	Body built			
	Color			
	Distress/decubitus			
	Environment			
Vital signs	Bp, HR, temperature, RR, SPO_2			
Chest	Respiratory and CVS examination			
Abdomen (in case of suspected hernia)	Scars			
	Distention			
	Tenderness			
	Ascites			
	Hernia examination (site, signs of strangulation, reducibility, cough impulse)			
	Organomegaly			
	Bowel sound			
	DRE			
Skin lesion or mass	Site			
	Size			
	Shape			
	Border			
	Symmetry			
	fixation to underlying tissue			
	Hotness			
	Tenderness			
	Examine the entire skin and mucus membranes for similar lesions			
Lymph node	The draining lymph nodes basin			
Back	For tenderness			
Lower limb for any edema				
Differential diagnosis	According to the given scenario.			
Investigations				

History	Items	Done	Not done	NA
General laboratory test	CBC with differential			
	Electrolytes			
	Liver function test			
	LDH			
	Coagulation profile (PT, INR, aPTT)			
	Blood grouping			
	RFT			
Imaging	Ultrasound abdomen (hernia)			
	CT abdomen/MRI (hernia/ retroperitoneal sarcoma			
	Extremity MRI (sarcoma)			
	CT chest, abdomen, brain (when indicated for staging)			
	PET scan			
Biopsy	Punch biopsy for melanoma			
	Core needle biopsy/ incisional/ Excisional (sarcoma)			
Provisional diagnosis	According to the given scenario			
Management (depend on the diagnosis)				
Melanoma	Staging			
	Multidisciplinary team			
	Break the bad news to the patient			
	Admission			
	Prepare for OR			
	Consent			
	Surgical site marking			
	Wide local excision			
	Sentinel lymph node biopsy if clinically negative			
	Lymph node dissection if positive lymph nodes			
	Margin size depends on the Berslow thickness			
	Closure			
	Adjuvant radiation therapy when indicated			
Sarcoma of the extremities	Staging			
	Multidisciplinary team discussion			
	Break the bad news			
	Neoadjuvant chemotherapy if high grade tumors			
	Admission			
	Prepare for OR			
	Consent			
	Surgical site marking			
	Functional sparing complete excision with 1–2 cm margins			
	Adjuvant radiation therapy if indicated			
Retroperitoneal sarcoma (resectable)	Staging			
	Multidisciplinary team discussion			
	Break the bad news			
	Neoadjuvant chemotherapy or radiotherapy if indicated			
	Admission			
	Prepare for surgery			
	Surgical resection			
	Intra- or postoperative radiation therapy as indicated			

(continued)

History	Items	Done	Not done	NA
Hernias	Admission			
	Preoperative preparation			
	Consent			
	Surgical site marking			
	Repair			
Postoperative care				
Early postoperative	Admission to HDU or ICU if indicated			
	Early mobilization and DVT prophylaxis			
	Enteral nutrition when possible			
	Analgesia			
	Stress ulcer prophylaxis			
	Laboratory test as needed			
	Wound care			
First outpatient visit	Clinical assessment			
	Remove sutures			
	Review the final pathology report			
	Arrange for multidisciplinary discussion if the case is cancer			
	Refer to oncology or radiotherapy if adjuvant treatment is required			
Long-term follow-up (melanoma)	Every 3–6 months history and physical examination for 2–3 years then every 12 months for three years then annually			
	Imaging ass indicated			
	Consider genetic counselling if personal or family history of pancreatic cancer or astrocytoma is positive			
Long-term follow-up Extremities sarcoma	Every 3–6 months history and physical examination for 2–3 years then every 6–12 months for 3 years then annually			
	CT chest, abdomen, and pelvis on regular interval			
	Baseline MRI at 3 months then as indicated			
Long-term follow-up for retroperitoneal sarcoma	Every 3–6 months history and physical examination for 2–3 years then every 6–12 months for 3 years then annually			
	CT chest, abdomen and pelvis on regular interval			

14.2.2 Answer Key

Case No. 1:

A 53-year-old male patient presented to the clinic due to an abnormal pigmented lesion in his left thigh for 1 month.

Questions for Discussion:

1. **How will you approach the patient?**

   By obtaining a relevant history and performing a physical examination.

   The patient is a 53-year-old male patient who has pigmented lesion on his left thigh. It was not there before and appeared gradually as a dark brown lesion. It is increasing in size since that and associated with itching and no other similar lesions in the body.

   He was spending his summer vacation in one of the coastal cities of East Asia. He has no personal history of similar complaints. He is not smoker and otherwise healthy man.

   On examination:

   Conscious, looking well white man.

   Vital signs within normal limits.

   The entire skin and mucus membrane are examined and reveals only a single dark brown

lesion at the medial side on the middle part of his left thigh. It is about 2 × 1 cm, irregular shape, ill-defined edges with some areas of it raised above the skin level. There are scratch marks around the lesion with area of ulceration at the center of it.
The left inguinal lymph nodes are palpable.

2. **What will you do next?**
LFT and LDH: normal
Punch biopsy of the lesion: invasive melanoma. Berslow thickness is 5 mm
FNA from the lesion: positive for malignant cells
3. **What are the histological features that you should look for?**
   - **Presence of ulceration:** positive
   - **Presence of macroscopic satellite lesions:** negative
   - **Dermal mitotic rate per mm^2: 2/mm^2**
   - **Lymphovascular/angiolymphatic invasion:** present
   - **Histologic subtype (if desmoplastic, specify pure or mixed):** nodular melanoma
   - **Neurotropism/perineural invasion:** positive
4. **What further workup you need to do?**
Staging CT: negative for metastasis.
5. **How will you manage the patient?**
Wide local excision to achieve 2 cm negative margin
Therapeutic inguinal lymphadenectomy
6. **What are the indications of pelvic dissection?**
   - If the PET/CT or pelvic CT scan reveals iliac and/or obturator lymph node involvement
   - If a positive Cloquet's lymph node is found on intraoperative frozen section
   - Clinically positive inguinal-femoral nodes or if three or more inguinofemoral nodes are involved
7. **How will you follow up the patient?**
   - History and physical examination every 3–6 months for 2 years
   - History and physical examination every 12 months
   - Then annually, as clinically indicated
   - Imaging as indicated
   - Consider genetic counseling
   - If there is a family history or personal history of pancreatic cancer or astrocytoma

Case No. 2:
A 65-year-old female patient was referred from the urology clinic due to a retroperitoneal mass that was discovered during workup for hydronephrosis.

Questions for Discussion:

1. **How will you approach the patient?**
The patient is a 65-year-old female patient who has been evaluated by her urologist for right flank pain and hydronephrosis. Her CT KUB shows a large, cystic, nonenhancing mass on the right side of the abdomen, closely related to the right psoas muscle with secondary compression of the right ureter and resultant right-sided hydronephrosis.
Apart from her right flank pain, she has no other significant symptoms. No significant GI symptoms. She has no history of weight loss, fever, or night sweating. She has no chest pain, shortness of breath or cough and no family or personal history of malignancy. She is not a smoker. She is diabetic on oral hypoglycemic medication. PSH is negative
On examination:
She looks well.
Vital signs: normal.
Abdominal examination is not conclusive.
2. **What will you do next?**
Basic labs including RFT are normal.
MRI of the abdomen with contrast: 18 × 16.4 × 19 cm, high T2 signal intensity lesion in the right retroperitoneum. On T1 fat saturated sequences, it appeared hypointense with thin internal mildly enhancing septations. Right-sided hydronephrosis was observed.
3. **How will you manage the patient?**
   - Staging CT CAP: negative for metastasis.
   - Discuss in a multidisciplinary team meeting.
   - Inform the patient and discuss the plan with her.

- Prepare the patient for surgery.
- Excision of the tumor: the patient underwent uneventful excision of the tumor and right nephrectomy. The final pathology is myxoid liposarcoma. The resection margins are negative (R0).

4. **How will follow up the patient?**
History and physical examination with imaging (chest/abdominal/pelvic CT or MRI) every 3– 6 months for 2–3 years, then every 6 months for the next 2 years, and then annually.

Case No. 3:

A 39-year-old male patient presented to the emergency department complaining of painful swelling at the right lower abdomen for 1 day.

Questions for Discussion:

1. **How will you approach the patient?**
The patient is a 39-year-old male patient who presented to the emergency department due to a painful bulge at the right inguinal area. He has this swelling for 3 years and usually is reduced when he lied down, but after he performed heavy exercise at the gym yesterday, it did not and was associated with severe pain, nausea, and vomiting multiple times. He has no fever, abdominal distention, or constipation.
PMH and PSH are unremarkable.
On examination:
The patient appears ill.
Vital signs: BP: 98/67 mmHg, PR: 119 bpm, temperature: 36.9°C.
Abdomen is not distended with obvious right inguinal hernia. The skin over the hernia is erythematous. On palpation, it is soft, except over the hernia, which is significantly tender with guarding. Bowel sound is normal.
PR: normal color soft stool in the rectum.
2. **What will you do next?**
Blood investigation:
Chest and abdomen X-ray: no signs of bowel obstruction
3. **How will you manage the patient?**
Prepare the patient for urgent exploration of the hernial content and repair,
with the possibility of bowel resection ± stoma formation.
Intraoperative: through an inguinal incision, the hernial sac was identified (indirect hernia) with gangrenous bowel inside it.
4. **Intraoperative findings as described. What will you do?**
Divide the inguinal ligament, resect the dead bowel, and primary anastomosis if the patient condition is suitable.
5. **How will you repair the defect?**
Tissue repair without mesh.
6. **The patient presents to the clinic for follow up, and he is complaining of severe pain around the surgical site since postoperative despite multiple analgesics. How will you manage that?**
Nerve block.
If the pain continues, it can be managed by triple neurectomy.

References

1. Kimbrough CW, McMasters KM. Melanoma and cutaneous malignant neoplasms. In: Townsend CM, Beauchamp RD, Evers BM, Mattox KL, editors. Sabiston textbook of surgery. 20th ed. St. Louis, MI: Elsevier; 2016.
2. Referenced with permission from the NCCN Clinical Practice Guidelines in Oncology (NCCN Guidelines®) for Melanoma: cutaneous V.2.2021. © National Comprehensive Cancer Network, Inc. All rights reserved. Accessed [March 18]. To view the most recent and complete version of the guideline, go online to NCCN.org. NCCN makes no warranties of any kind whatsoever regarding their content, use or application and disclaims any responsibility for their application or use in any way.
3. Gonzalez RJ, Pollock RE. Soft tissue sarcomas. In: Brunicardi FC, editor. Schwartz's principles of surgery. 11th ed. New York: McGraw-Hill Education; 2019.
4. Malangoni MA. Hernias. In: Townsend CM, Beauchamp RD, Evers BM, Mattox KL, editors. Sabiston textbook of surgery. 20th ed. St. Louis, MI: Elsevier; 2016.

15 Surgical Aspects of Vascular Diseases for Clinical Board Exams

15.1 Part I: Knowledge

> The greatest enemy of progress is the illusion of knowledge.
> –John Young

15.1.1 Approach to Patient with Vascular Complaint

The Chief Complaint Could be one of the Following:

- Limb pain
- Abdominal pain (abdominal aortic diseases)
- Ulcer, discharge, and discoloration

History:

- Introduce him/herself to the patient.
- Name, age, occupation, sex, nationality.
- Chief complaint and duration.
- History of presenting illness:

H. Alotaibi, *Study Surgery*, https://doi.org/10.1007/978-981-16-2305-9_15

– **Analysis of the chief complaint**

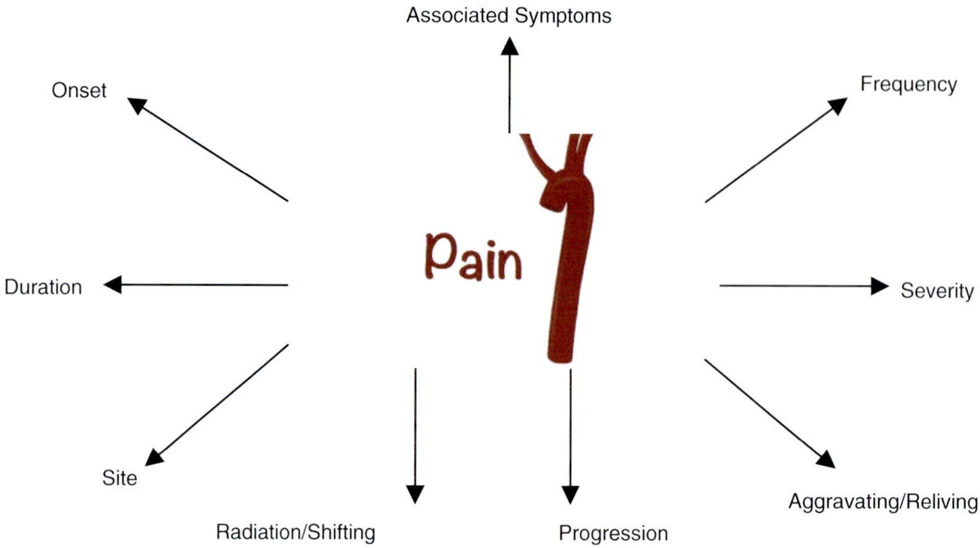

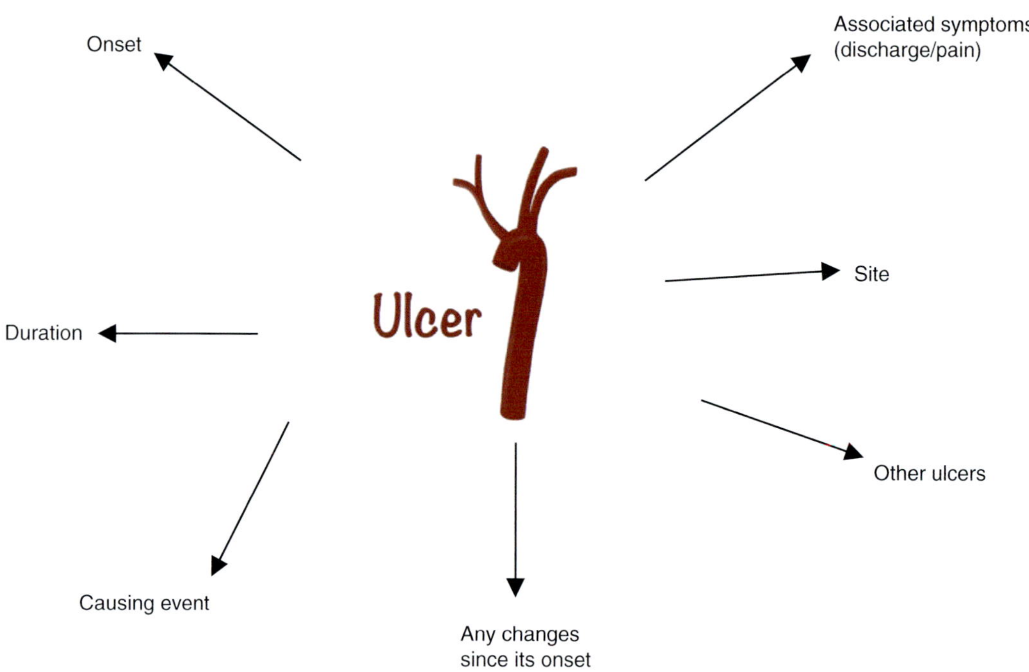

- **Associated Symptoms**
  Rest pain, fever, discharge, discoloration, ulcer, numbness, coldness, paralysis, claudication, postprandial abdominal pain, weight loss
- **Risk Factors:**
  Smoking
  Diabetes mellitus
  Hypertension
  History of trauma
  Cardiac disease (MI, valvular disease, and atrial fibrillation)
  Prior vascular intervention
  Prior cardiac surgery
  History of hyperlipidemia
- **Differential Diagnosis:**
  Prolong immobilization (DVT).
  In case the patient presented with abdominal pain, ask about other symptoms that suggest Gastrointestinal tract (GIT) or Genito-urinary (GU) causes rather than vascular-like vomiting, change bowel habit, jaundice, dysuria, hematuria.
- **Previous Similar Attack**: previous admission, previous investigation, or angiography (if yes, when was it done, and what was the finding?)
- **Systemic Review of the Related System (vascular)**
  Chest pain, palpitation, and lower limb swelling
- **Past Medical History (PMH)**
- **Past Surgical History (PSH)**
- **Family History**
- **Social History**
- **Medication, Transfusion, Allergy**
- **Systemic Review**
  CNS: Headache, eye and hearing symptoms, epilepsy, numbness, paralysis
  GIT: Abdominal pain, jaundice, vomiting, diarrhea, constipation
  Respiratory: Cough, fever, chest pain, hemoptysis
  Renal: Dysuria, flank pain, hematuria
  MSK: weakness, arthritis, skin erythema

Physical Examination:

- Introduce himself/herself to the patient.
- Ask permission for examination.
- Assure privacy.
- Position: supine.
- Exposure: nipple to mid-thigh for abdominal examination.
- Exposure: expose both sides for limb examination.
- Handwashing.

General Examination:
Appearance: ill, well
Body built: cachectic, obese
Color: Pale, jaundice
Distress
Environment: connection to monitors, fluids
Vital signs: BP, HR, Temperature, RR, SPO_2

Hands:

- Pallor
- Pulse rate and its characteristics: rhythm, volume, regularity, radioradial delay, radiofemoral delay

Eye:

- Pallor
- Arcus senilis
- Xanthelasmata and xanthomata around the eyes

Neck:

- Jugular venous pressure
- Carotid artery pulsation and auscultate for any bruit
- Thoracic outlet obstruction

Chest:

- Respiratory system
- Cardiovascular examination

Upper Extremities:

- Pulses (axillary, brachial, radial)

Abdominal Examination:

- Palpation: for any pulsatile masses
- Auscultation: for any bruit

Lower Limb:

- **Inspection:**
  - Scars
  - Pallor
  - Color when supine and with the elevation of the limb
  - Venous filling
  - Nail changes
  - Edema
  - Erythema
  - Loss of hair
  - Skin shining
  - Ulcer
  - Discoloration
  - Fissures or wounds
  - Discharge
  - Inspect between the toes for any fungal infection
- **Palpation:**
  - Skin temperature
  - Capillary refilling time
  - Palpate the lower limb arterial pulse:

    Arterial anatomy of the lower limb (Fig. 15.1).

    Palpate the pulses starting from proximal to distal.

    Compare the abnormal to the normal.

    The femoral pulse: it is usually palpable midway between the anterior superior iliac spine and the pubic tubercle.

    The popliteal artery:

    - Palpate the popliteal fossa with the knee flexed to 45° and the foot supported on the examination table to relax the calf muscles.
    - Palpation of the popliteal artery is a bimanual technique. Both thumbs are placed on the tibial tuberosity anteriorly, and the fingers are placed into the popliteal fossa between the two heads of the gastrocnemius muscle.
    - The popliteal artery is palpated by compressing it against the posterior aspect of the tibia just below the knee.

    The posterior tibial pulse: detected by palpation 2 cm posterior to the medial malleolus.

    The dorsalis pedis: detected 1 cm lateral to the hallucis longus extensor tendon, which dorsiflexes the great toe and is clearly visible on the dorsum of the foot.

    Check the capillary refill [1].

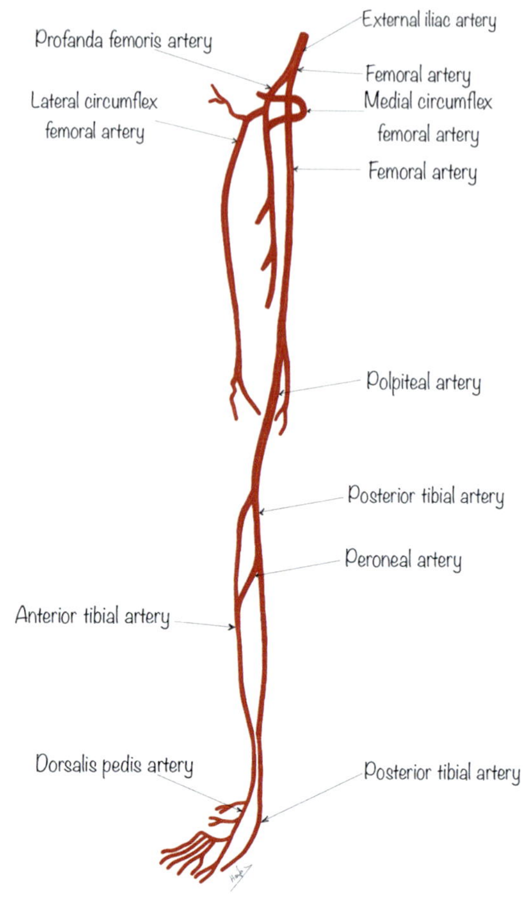

Fig. 15.1 Arterial anatomy of the lower limb

- **Foot Examination:**
  - If there is any ulcer, inspect for the following:
    - Number of ulcers
    - Shape
    - Size
    - Edges
    - Floor
    - Discharge
    - Skin around it
  - Palpate for the following:
    - Hotness
    - Tenderness
    - The base of the ulcer
    - Fluctuation
    - Edema
  - Palpate the draining lymph nodes.
  - Neurological examination (sensory and motor).

Special Tests:

- Doppler (handheld): to assess the pulse.
- Ankle-brachial pressure index (ABPI):
  - Technique:
    - Blood pressure is measured in both upper extremities using the highest systolic blood pressure as the denominator for the ankle-brachial index (ABI).
    - The ankle pressure is determined by placing a blood pressure cuff above the ankle and measuring the return to flow of the posterior tibial and dorsalis pedis arteries using a pencil Doppler probe over each artery.
    - The ratio of the systolic pressure in each vessel divided by the highest arm systolic pressure can be used to express the ABI in both the posterior tibial and dorsalis pedis arteries [1].
  - Interpretation (Table 15.1):
  - Any ABPI value >1.2 should be interpreted with caution, as calcification and hardening of the arteries may cause a falsely high ABPI [1].

- Examine the footwear in case of diabetic foot.

Table 15.1 Interpretation of ankle-brachial pressure index (ABPI)

Severity	ABPI
Normal	>0.9
Mild peripheral arterial disease (PAD)	0.8–0.9
Moderate PAD	0.5–0.8
Severe PAD	<0.5

Investigations:

- Blood tests:
  - CBC
  - Coagulation profile
  - Blood grouping
  - RFT
  - D-dimer
  - Lipid profile
  - Blood sugar
- Imaging:
  - Plain X-ray
  - Duplex ultrasound
  - CT angiography
  - MRA
  - Conventional angiography (diagnostic)

15.1.2 Management of Acute Limb Ischemia (ALI)

- ALI is defined as a sudden decrease in limb perfusion that threatens its viability.
- The most common etiologies of ALI include:
  - Embolism (most common).
  - The original source may be because of AF, post-MI mural thrombus, abdominal aortic aneurysm, or prosthetic heart valves.
  - Thrombosis in a native vessel or graft thrombosis.
  - Trauma (less common).
- Presenting symptoms in ALI are pain and loss of sensory or motor function.
- The abruptness and time of onset of the pain, its location and intensity, and change in severity over time should all be taken into consideration. The duration and intensity of the pain and presence of motor or sensory changes are very important in clinical deci-

sion-making and the urgency of revascularization [1, 2].

- **Clinical Manifestation:**
  - The "six Ps":
    - **P**ain
    - **P**allor
    - **P**ulselessness
    - **P**aresthesia
    - **P**erishingly cold
    - **P**aralysis
  - Pain is the usual symptom that causes a patient to present to the emergency room.

    Typically, a patient will complain of foot and calf pain.

    Pulses are absent, and there may be a diminution of sensation. Inability to move the affected muscle group is a sign of very severe ischemia and necessitates urgent revascularization.

    Classes (Table 15.2).

- The finding of palpable contralateral pulses and the absence of ipsilateral pulses in the acutely ischemic leg are suggestive of an embolus, irrespective of the presence of Doppler signals [1, 2].

- **Work Up:**
  - Ideally, patients with acute ischemia should be investigated with imaging, especially if there is an antecedent vascular reconstruction; however, the clinical condition and access to resources must guide further investigations.
  - Unnecessary delays can result in amputation.
  - CT angiography, arteriography, if it can be performed in a timely fashion, is an excellent modality for localizing obstructions and deciding which type of intervention (endovascular, embolectomy, or bypass) patients will benefit more from [1, 2].
- **Management:**
  - **Principles:**

    Patients with an ischemic lower extremity should be immediately anticoagulated. This will prevent propagation of the clot into unaffected vascular beds.

    Intravenous fluid should be started, and a Foley's catheter should be inserted to monitor urine output.

    Baseline labs should be obtained, and creatinine levels are noted. A hypercoagulable workup should be performed prior to initiation of heparin if there is sufficient suspicion.

    Conservative management can be considered in patients with Rutherford 1 and 2a.

    There is no clear superiority for thrombolysis over surgery in terms of 30-day limb salvage or mortality.

    Urgent surgical intervention is mandatory in patients with Rutherford 2b [1, 2].
  - **Endovascular Treatment**

    Available options: thrombolytic, clot removal

    Thrombolysis:

    - Preferable to open surgery as first-line treatment in patients with ALI (classes I and IIa).
    - Advantages of thrombolytic therapy over balloon embolectomy include the reduced endothelial trauma and potential for more gradual and complete clot lysis in branch vessels usually too small to access by embolectomy balloons.

Table 15.2 Categories of acute limb ischemia (Rutherford's classification) [1]

Category	Description	Sensory loss	Motor loss	Arterial Doppler	Venous Doppler
I	Viable	None	None	Audible	Audible
IIa	Marginally threatened	Minimal	None	Inaudible	Audible
IIb	Immediately threatened	More than one toe	Mild, moderate	Inaudible	Audible
III	Irreversible damaged	Profound	Paralysis	Inaudible	Inaudible

- Irreversible damage to muscle tissue starts after 3 h of ischemia and is nearly complete at 6 h.
- When the musculature and microvasculature are severely damaged, amputation rather than attempts at revascularization may be the most prudent course to prevent the washout of toxic by-products from the ischemic limb into the systemic circulation.
- Patients with small-vessel occlusion are poor candidates for surgery because they lack distal target vessels to use for bypass.
- The major contraindications of thrombolysis are recent stroke, primary intracranial malignancy, brain metastases, or intracranial surgical intervention.
- Relative contraindications for the performance of thrombolysis include renal insufficiency, allergy to contrast material, cardiac thrombus, diabetic retinopathy, coagulopathy, and recent arterial puncture or surgery [1, 2].

Embolectomy/thrombectomy:

- Percutaneous mechanical thrombectomy and thromboaspiration may extend the applicability of this intervention to patients with more advanced degrees of ALI (class IIb) and contraindications to thrombolysis.
- Several thrombectomy devices have received FDA approval for acute lower extremity arterial thrombosis.
- The utility of these thrombectomy devices is that they can be used as standalone therapy when there are contraindications for thrombolytic therapy. Additionally, these thrombectomy devices can be used in conjunction with thrombolytic agents for pharmacomechanical thrombectomy to enhance clot lysis and to limit the doses and time required for thrombolysis [1, 2].

– **Surgical Treatment:**

Embolectomy:

- The abdomen, contralateral groin, and entire lower extremity are prepped in the field.
- The groin is opened through a vertical incision, exposing the CFA and its bifurcation.
- Frequently, the location of the embolus at the femoral bifurcation is readily apparent by the presence of a palpable proximal femoral pulse, which disappears distally.
- The artery is clamped and opened transversely over the bifurcation.
- Thrombus is extracted by passing a Fogarty balloon embolectomy catheter.
- Good back-bleeding and antegrade bleeding suggest that the entire clot has been removed.
- Embolic material often forms a cast of the vessel and is sent for culture and histologic examination.
- Completion angiography is advisable to ascertain the adequacy of clot removal.
- The artery is then closed and the patient is fully anticoagulated.
- When an embolus lodge in the popliteal artery: A femoral approach is preferred because the larger diameter of the femoral artery results in decreased likelihood of arterial compromise when the arteriotomy is closed. Alternatively, approach it through a popliteal approach [1, 2].

Bypass Graft:

- Indicated when an in situ thrombosis develops on top of preexisting atheroma because, frequently, embolectomy catheters will not pass through these occlusions.
- Angiography is useful to determine the extent of the occlusion to search for inflow and distal outflow vessels, and to decide whether thrombolysis or surgery will be the better intervention.

- If there are good distal vessels and the saphenous vein is suitable, surgical bypass is recommended because it is fast, durable, and reliable.
- In the absence of a good distal target and saphenous vein, or in a patient at high risk for surgery, lysis is recommended [1, 2].

Bypass Graft Thrombectomy:

- Bypass thrombectomy is more likely to succeed with prosthetic bypasses.
- Bypass graft revision or replacement is more appropriate for acute vein graft failures because they are less likely to respond to thrombolysis and require some type of revision, such as valve lysis, interposition, or extension.
- Thrombectomy of autogenous grafts is prone to failure unless an anatomic cause for failure, such as a retained valve or unligated side branch is found and corrected.
- The performance of a fasciotomy to circumvent reperfusion injury/compartment syndrome is an important consideration [1, 2].

- **Complications Related to Treatment for Acute Limb Ischemia:**
  - **Bleeding:**

    Hemorrhagic stroke from a thrombolysis procedure has been reported to be 1–2.3%, with 50% of hemorrhagic complications occurring during the thrombolytic procedure.

    Gastrointestinal bleeding is reported in 5–10% of cases.

    Hemorrhage requiring transfusion can occur in approximately 25% of patients undergoing thrombolysis [1, 2].
  - **Reperfusion Syndrome:**

    Directly relates to the severity and extent of the ischemia.

    Patients with a saddle embolus of the aortic bifurcation and severely ischemic limbs may develop the full-blown "reperfusion syndrome," whereas patients with minimal muscle ischemia who are re-perfused in a timely fashion essentially develop no effects.

    Many patients with ALI have severe underlying cardiac disease and are unable to tolerate even short ischemic periods [1, 2].
  - **Compartment Syndrome:**

    Occurs after prolonged ischemia is followed by reperfusion.

    The capillaries leak fluid into the interstitial space in the muscles, which are enclosed within a nondistensible fascial envelope. When the pressure inside the compartment exceeds the capillary perfusion pressure, nutrient flow ceases and progressive ischemia occurs, even in the presence of peripheral pulses.

    Every patient who has sustained an ischemic event and is re-perfused should be monitored for compartment syndrome, which is characterized by excessive pain in the compartment, pain on passive stretching of the compartment, and sensory loss due to nerve compression of the nerves coursing through the compartment.

    The most commonly affected compartment is the anterior compartment in the leg.

    Numbness in the web space between the first and second toes is diagnostic due to compression of the deep peroneal nerve.

    Compartment pressure is measured by inserting an arterial line into the compartment and recording the pressure.

    Pressures greater than 20 mmHg are an indication for fasciotomy.

    Laboratory evidence of rhabdomyolysis is seen in 20% of cases. The myoglobin from damaged muscle precipitates in kidney tubules and causes acute tubular necrosis. Alkalinization of urine increases the solubility of myoglobin, thus preventing it from crystallizing in the tubules.

    In addition to alkalinization, therapy consists of forced saline diuresis and removal of the source of dead muscle that is releasing the myoglobin [1, 2].

15.1.3 Management of Chronic Limb Ischemia

- Chronic limb ischemia is typically caused by atherosclerosis.
- **Risk Factors**
  - Modifiable:
    Smoking
    Diabetes mellitus
    Hypertension
    Hyperlipidemia
    Renal failure
    Obesity
    physical inactivity
  - Non-modifiable:
    Increasing age
    Family history
- **Clinical Manifestation:**
  - Depends on its severity.
  - **Intermittent claudication:** a cramping pain in the calf, thigh, or buttock after walking a fixed distance (the "claudication distance"), relieved by rest within minutes.
  - **Critical limb ischemia:** the advanced form of chronic limb ischemia. Its clinical presentation is:
    Ischemic rest pain for greater than 2-week duration
    Presence of ischemic ulcer or gangrene [3]
- **Classification:** (Tables 15.3 and 15.4)
- To assess the severity of the disease and the anatomical location of the lesions, further imaging should be done, initially by duplex ultrasound, then by **CT angiography** or MR angiography as an alternative.
- Patient should have a **cardiovascular risk assessment**. This includes blood pressure, blood glucose, lipid profile, and ECG [3].
- **Management**
  - Risk Factor Modification:
    Smoking cessation.
    Lifestyles change and regular exercise.
    Weight reduction.
    Lipid lowering medication.
    Antiplatelet therapy.
    Optimize diabetes and blood pressure control.
  - Claudicant patient should start **supervised exercise program** to improve the walking distance and claudication distance, and should be used as first-line therapy in any patient without critical limb ischemia.
  - Patient with critical limb ischemia or disabling claudication should be offered revascularization [3].

15.1.4 Management of Diabetic Foot

- Approximately, 1 in 4 patients with diabetes will develop a foot complication during their lifetime.
- Risk factors include poor glycemic control, impaired immune function, peripheral neuropathy, and vascular insufficiency.
- It is important to determine whether a diabetic ulcer is complicated by infection.
- **Microbiology:**
  - An acute, superficial infection, *Staphylococcus aureus* and beta-hemolytic

Table 15.3 Rutherford classification of chronic limb ischemia [3]

Stage 0	Asymptomatic
Stage 1	Intermittent claudication
Stage 2	Moderate claudication
Stage 3	Severe claudication
Stage 4	Rest pain
Stage 5	Ischemic ulceration not exceeding ulcer of the digits of the foot
Stage 6	Severe ischemic ulcers or frank gangrene

Table 15.4 Fontaine classification for chronic limb ischemia [3]

Stage 1	Asymptomatic
Stage 2	Mild claudication
	IIa: intermittent claudication after more than 200 m of pain-free walking
	IIb: intermittent claudication after less than 200 m of walking
Stage 3	Rest pain
Stage 4	Ischemic ulcers or gangrene

streptococci are implicated most commonly.
  - In patients with chronic wounds at risk for loss of limb, aerobic Gram-negative and anaerobic organisms likely are accountable [4].
- **Clinical Presentation:**
  - Many of diabetic wound manifest with signs of local and systemic inflammation (pain, purulent drainage, fever, or frank shock).
  - Sensory neuropathies can minimize much of the pain associated with these wounds, even in the context of a severe, necrotizing infection.
  - The latter typically harbors additional physical examination findings, such as cutaneous blistering, gas formation, skin discoloration, and malodorous discharge [4].
- **Diagnosis:**
  - **Principles:**
    Determine the extent of involvement (superficial or deep).
    Appreciate patient-specific risk factors.
    Identify the causative organism.
  - The diagnosis is based on clinical examination findings (erythema, warmth, or purulent drainage) and a detailed history (fever, chills, and labile blood glucose).
  - The wound should be irrigated copiously, and all necrotic tissue and foreign bodies should be removed.
  - Wounds lacking purulence and erythema in a patient without systemic signs of infection can be presumed to be "uninfected."
  - The presence of fever, hypotension, or bacteremia should alert the physician to a severe infection or an immunocompromised host.
  - The wound base should be probed to evaluate for sinus tracts or exposed bone.
  - Factors that raise the suspicion for the presence of osteomyelitis include an ulcer greater than 2 cm^2 or 3 mm deep, the presence of a "sausage toe," an erythrocyte sedimentation rate greater than 70 mm/h, a nonhealing ulcer after appropriate conservative management, and radiographic evidence of bony destruction below the ulcer.
  - If the diagnosis is uncertain, magnetic resonance imaging (MRI), which is highly sensitive and specific, should be obtained.
  - Deep cultures should be sent when there is concern for a multidrug-resistant organism.
  - To quantify the extent of baseline vascular disease, a thorough pulse examination should be performed. In addition, obtaining ABI can provide valuable information regarding the patient's burden of arterial insufficiency. It is critical that any significant arterial disease be mitigated to facilitate an appropriate response to local wound therapy [4].
- **Treatment:**
  - Multidisciplinary team approach.
  - Early debridement is an important component in the treatment plan.
  - The wound bed should be washed out thoroughly and all necrotic tissue removed.
  - Abscess cavities should be incised and drained completely.
  - Digital ulcers and gangrene are managed with amputation with or without extension to include the metatarsal head.
  - If multiple toes are infected, a more extensive procedure such as a transmetatarsal amputation may be required to clear all of the affected tissue and avoid a chronically nonhealing wound. Delayed, definitive closure often is used.
  - Correction of underlying vascular disease should be pursued to achieve an appropriate recovery or as a primary strategy in patients with critical limb ischemia (i.e., ABI or toe-brachial index (TBI) <0.4).
  - These interventions should be attempted only once the acute infection has been addressed with local debridement and antibiotic therapy.
  - Restoration of perfusion is best achieved via revascularization of the tibial or pedal vessels, as the peroneal artery has no direct branches below the ankle. It is important to note that although direct flow to the plantar

arch is not always required to relieve claudication or rest pain, it is preferred to meet the high metabolic demands of a healing diabetic ulcer.
- The decision to utilize either endovascular therapies or more conventional open techniques depends on the patient's overall condition as well as the characteristics of the target lesions.
- The small-vessel disease most common in diabetic patients typically is not amenable to percutaneous intervention.
- The defect present after debridement can be substantial and prove difficult to cover with the remaining local soft tissue. Negative-pressure, vacuum-assisted dressings can lead to a reduction in the defect size and assist in primary closure or subsequent tissue transfer [4].

15.1.5 Management of Abdominal Aortic Aneurysm (AAA)

- Definition: a 1.5-fold increase in the normal aortic diameter or an aortic diameter greater than 3 cm. Individuals at highest risk include older patients, white patients, males, those with a family history of aneurysms, and those with cardiovascular risk factors and concomitant cardiovascular and peripheral vascular disease.
- The risk of rupture is increased in patients with chronic obstructive pulmonary disease (COPD), hypertension, family history of AAA, and rapid AAA expansion and most notably with aneurysm size.
- **Asymptomatic Aneurysm:**
  - Rupture risk correlates directly with aneurysm size and is very low for aneurysms smaller than 5 cm in diameter.
  - Other predictors of rupture include female gender, family history of AAA, smoking status, hypertension, and COPD.
  - Current clinical data support aneurysm repair at a threshold size of 5.5 cm in male patients and 5.0 cm in female patients [5, 6].
  - Screening:

    Once an aneurysm has been detected, the Society for Vascular Surgery Clinical Practice Council recommends further screening intervals as follows, based on aneurysm size (maximum external aortic diameter) and associated risk of rupture:

    <2.6 cm: no further screening recommended

    2.6–2.9 cm: re-examination at 5 years

    3–3.4 cm: re-examination at 3 years

    3.5–4.4 cm: re-examination at 12 months

    4.5–5.4 cm: re-examination at 6 months [7]
- **Ruptured AAA:**
  - Mortality of 80–90%.
  - Two-thirds of these individuals die before reaching a hospital and many more before reaching the operating room.
  - The classic triad of symptoms and findings for ruptured AAA: hypotension, abdominal or back pain, and a pulsatile abdominal mass.
  - Aneurysms can produce other symptoms like duodenal obstruction, gastrointestinal hemorrhage with erosion into the gastrointestinal tract, femoral neuropathy, dysuria, congestive heart failure with an aortocaval fistula, and many others.
  - With rupture (rather than slow expansion), pain is typically severe and unrelenting.
  - **Initial Management:**

    Patients who die before reaching medical attention, most often experience free rupture of the aneurysm into the peritoneal cavity with profound hypotension followed by death.

    Those who reach medical attention likely have achieved some degree of tamponade.

    One of the goals of early management is to minimize further hemorrhage through permissive hypotension.

    Large-bore venous access should be obtained. Fluid resuscitation should be gauged to produce systolic blood pressures in the 80–100 mmHg range with the goal of maintaining consciousness and preventing myocardial and renal ischemia.

Intubation should be avoided in patients who can protect their airway until aortic control is imminent because the drugs associated with intubation result in the interruption of sympathetic tone, which can hasten cardiopulmonary collapse.

Patients who are unstable should be taken directly to the operating room, even if the diagnosis is not confirmed.

If there is time and an accessible scanner and expertise, an ultrasound can be obtained in the emergency room so that the presence of abdominal aortic aneurysm can be confirmed.

If a patient is stable at the time of presentation or has achieved stability after resuscitation, a CT scan should be performed and can suggests rupture or impending rupture, whereas a retroperitoneal hematoma or contrast extravasation confirms that rupture has occurred [6].

– **Intraoperative Principles:**

Permissive hypotension is maintained until proximal aortic control is obtained.

The operating room should be warm to prevent hypothermia.

For open surgery, the timing of intubation is critical; patients should not be intubated until they are completely prepped and draped, and the surgical team is ready for incision.

Nasogastric tube placement is necessary for open operations because the tube aids in identification of the esophagus if supra-celiac aortic control is required [6].

– **Open Surgery Versus Endovascular Aortic Repair (EVAR):**

The superiority of EVAR versus open repair has been difficult to demonstrate.

The endovascular repair has some advantages like the ability to intervene without a general anesthetic and the aneurysm can be repaired without relieving abdominal tamponade, and thus stability is maintained throughout the intervention. Fluid shifts, temperature changes, and the ileus associated with a laparotomy can be avoided.

In practice, more stable patients may be offered EVAR and those with less stability treated with open repair.

Patients with more favorable anatomy likely will be offered EVAR, and those with more complex anatomy will be subject to open repair.

Centers that have appropriate imaging, endovascular teams, a broad array of grafts, as well as surgeons with significant experience are well positioned to achieve favorable outcomes with EVAR. Alternatively, in centers without this expertise, open repair may remain a better alternative [6].

– **Open Repair:**

If open repair is planned, in most circumstances, after laparotomy, rapid control of the supra-celiac aorta should be gained.

This is particularly important in an unstable patient or if there is a large retroperitoneal hematoma that extends to the base of the mesentery.

Control at this level is lifesaving but results in visceral ischemia, and thus the clamp should be moved distally as soon as possible.

Care must be taken when dissecting the proximal and distal necks. A large hematoma can obscure adjacent anatomy, leading to injuries to the vena cava, renal vein, duodenum, and the mesentery of the left colon [6].

The surgeon should attempt to perform the simplest and most efficient adequate repair, thereby minimizing the physiologic insult.

Tube grafts are preferred over anastomoses to the iliac or femoral vessels [6].

- **Endovascular Aneurysm Repair:**
  EVAR is initiated through bilateral groin access.
  Proximal aortic occlusion should be performed through the side contralateral to that chosen for placement of the main body of the graft.
  An angiogram can be performed with the aortic balloon inflated to delineate the renal arteries and identify the landing zone.
  Immediately before deployment of the graft, the aortic occlusion balloon is withdrawn to prevent entanglement in the graft's fixation mechanism.
  The balloon can be reintroduced into the center of the graft via the ipsilateral limb if necessary.
  Angiogram is then performed to confirm a complete seal [6].
  Endoleaks:
  - Type I: occurs when there is an incomplete seal between the stent-graft device and the native vessel, either at the proximal (type Ia) or distal (type Ib) attachment site, resulting in continued blood flow into the aneurysm sac and concomitant sac growth.
  - Type II: results from persistent retrograde blood flow into the aneurysm sac secondary to branch vessels of the infrarenal abdominal aorta, usually the inferior mesenteric artery or patent lumbar arteries.
  - Type III: results from a defect or misalignment between the components of endografts.
  - Type IV: occurs soon after some EVAR procedures due to the porosity of certain graft materials.
  - Type V (endotension): It is thought to occur when increased graft permeability allows pressure to be transmitted through the aneurysm sac [1].

- **Complications of Aortic Aneurysm Repair:**
  - General: MI, renal failure, respiratory failure, and coagulopathy
  - Lower extremities ischemia
  - Abdominal compartment syndrome
  - Ischemic colitis
  - Graft infection
  - Groin access complications, for example, femoral pseudoaneurysm, groin, or retroperitoneal hemorrhage [6]

15.1.6 Management of Venous and Lymphatic Disorder

Deep Venous Thrombosis:

- The triad of stasis, hypercoagulable state, and vessel injury is present in most surgical patients.
- The diagnosis of DVT requires a high index of suspicion.
- Homan's sign, which refers to pain in the calf on dorsiflexion of the foot.
- Major venous thrombosis involving the iliofemoral venous system results in a massively swollen leg, with pitting edema pain, and blanching, a condition known as phlegmasia alba dolens.
- With further progression of disease, there may be such massive edema that arterial inflow can be compromised. This condition results in a painful blue leg, a condition called phlegmasia cerulea dolens.
- With this evolution of the condition, venous gangrene can develop unless flow is restored.
- Diagnostic tests:
  - Venography
  - Impedance plethysmography
  - Fibrin and fibrinogen assays
  - Duplex ultrasound: The current test of choice for the diagnosis of DVT
  - Magnetic resonance venous imaging

- Treatment:
  - Anticoagulation
    A minimum treatment time of 3 months.
    If the patient has a known hypercoagulable state or has experienced episodes of venous thrombosis, however, lifetime anticoagulation is required in the absence of contraindications.
    The accepted INR range is 2.0 to 3.0.
  - Thrombolysis:
    In the patient with phlegmasia, for whom thrombolysis is advocated for relief of significant venous obstruction.
  - Endovascular reconstruction:
    Recanalization of the occluded iliac vein is performed endovascularly. Balloon dilation of the lesion is then performed, and a stent is placed across the dilated segment.
    Endovascular iliac therapy has evolved to become first-line therapy for iliac occlusions.
  - Vena Cava filter
    The most worrisome and potentially lethal complication of DVT is pulmonary embolism.
    The symptoms of pulmonary embolism, ranging from dyspnea, chest pain, and hypoxia to acute cor pulmonale, are nonspecific and require a high index of suspicion.
    The gold standard remains pulmonary angiography, but increasingly, this has been displaced by computed tomography angiography.
    Indications of vena cava filter:
    - Recurrent thromboembolism despite adequate anticoagulation.
    - Deep venous thrombosis in a patient with contraindications to anticoagulation.
    - Chronic pulmonary embolism and resultant pulmonary hypertension.
    - Complications of anticoagulation.
    - Propagating iliofemoral venous thrombus in anticoagulation [8].

Primary Venous Insufficiency:

- There are three main anatomic categories of primary venous insufficiency: telangiectasias, reticular veins, and varicose veins.
- Risk factors: advancing age, female gender, multiparity, heredity, history of trauma to the extremity, obesity and positive family history.
- **Symptoms:**
  - The patient with symptomatic varicose veins commonly reports heaviness, discomfort, and extremity fatigue.
  - The pain is characteristically dull, does not usually occur during recumbency or early in the morning, and is exacerbated in the afternoon, especially after periods of prolonged standing. Swelling is commonly described.
  - Pruritus occurs from excess hemosiderin deposition and tends to be located at the distal calf or in areas of phlebitic varicose branch segments.
  - Patients may report cramping pain that occurs during or after exercise and is relieved with rest and leg elevation. This syndrome is termed venous claudication and is a clinical manifestation of venous outflow obstruction, secondary venous insufficiency.
  - Predominant causes of venous claudication include a prior deep venous thrombosis (DVT) and May-Thurner syndrome [8].
- **Physical Examination:**
  - The venous examination includes assessment of the patient in the standing and supine positions.
  - Inspection: location of varicosities, hyperpigmentation in the distal calf or gaiter distribution, secondary to hemosiderin deposition, and lipodermatosclerosis.
  - Venous ulcers are not generally painful and appear at the medial malleolus, not in the mid to distal foot [8].
- **Diagnostic Evaluation:**
  - The handheld Doppler instrument can confirm an impression of saphenous reflux

- Duplex imaging (the first and best modality to assess for the normal function and presence of venous insufficiency of the lower extremities).
- Venography.
- Magnetic resonance venous imaging [8].

- **Treatment**:
  - Nonoperative management:
    - Patients are instructed to put the stockings on as soon as the day begins; swelling with standing will make stocking placement difficult.
    - Care must be taken with patients who have concomitant arterial insufficiency because the compression stockings may exacerbate arterial outflow to the foot.
    - Ankle-brachial index of less than 0.7 contraindicates the use of 20 to 30 mmHg compression stockings.
    - Lower extremity elevation for two brief periods during the day.
    - Patients who exhibit venous stasis ulceration will require local wound care.
  - Treatment options for telangiectasias (spider veins and reticular veins):
    - Injection sclerotherapy
    - Transdermal laser treatment
  - Surgery for axial venous incompetence:
    - Vein stripping
    - Percutaneous vein ablation [8].

Lymphedema:

- Lymphedema is the result of an inability of the existing lymphatic system to accommodate the protein and fluid entering the interstitial compartment at the tissue level.
- **Classification:**
  - Primary: congenital, lymphedema praecox, or lymphedema tarda.
  - Secondary: resection or ablation of regional lymph nodes by surgery, radiation therapy, tumor invasion, direct trauma, or less commonly, an infectious process [9].
- **Stages:**

I. **Stage I:**

- Impaired lymphatic drainage results in protein-rich fluid accumulation in the interstitial compartment.
- Manifested as soft pitting edema.

II. **Stage II:**

- The clinical condition is further exacerbated by accumulation of fibroblasts, adipocytes, and perhaps most important, macrophages in the affected tissues, which culminates in a local inflammatory response.
- Tissue edema is more pronounced. It is nonpitting type and has a spongy consistency.

III. **Stage III:**

- The affected tissues sustain further injury as a result of both the local inflammatory response and recurrent infectious episodes that typically result from minimal subclinical breaks in the skin.
- Excessive subcutaneous fibrosis and scarring with associated severe skin changes characteristic of lymphostatic elephantiasis [9].
- **Diagnosis:**
  - For patients with suspected secondary forms of lymphedema, computed tomography and magnetic resonance imaging are valuable and indeed essential for exclusion of underlying oncologic disease states.
  - For patients with edema of unknown cause and a suspicion for lymphedema, lymphoscintigraphy is the diagnostic test of choice.
- **Treatment:**
- Combination of limb elevation, a high-quality compression garment, complex decongestive physical therapy, and compression pump therapy.
- Operative treatment may be considered for patients with advanced complicated lymphedema for whom management with nonoperative means has failed [9].

15.1.7 Vascular Operations

Preoperative Preparation:

- Admission.
- Consent.
- Nothing per oral (NPO).
- IV fluid.
- DVT and stress ulcer prophylaxis.
- Prophylactic antibiotic.
- Confirm the availability of blood products intraoperatively if needed.
- Anesthesia consultation.
- ICU consultation if required.
- Instruct the patient to take shower the night before surgery.
- Hair removal (should be done on table to minimize risk of graft infection).
- Surgical site marking.

Informed Consent:
Consent for open Lower Limb Thrombectomy/ Embolectomy:

- *Describe the procedure for the patient:* under local anesthesia, the surgeon will remove the clot/thrombus from the right/left lower limb artery and close the arteriotomy.
- *Mention if there is any alternative:* like endovascular thrombolysis or embolectomy. Amputation in case of failure of the treatment and progression of the ischemia to irreversible damage.
- *Mention the possible complications:* bleeding, reperfusion syndrome, compartment syndrome, infection, or failure to clear the vessels.

Consent for Lower Limb Amputations:

- *Describe the procedure for the patient:* under spinal/general anesthesia, the surgeon will do toe amputation/transmetatarsal/below-knee/ above-knee amputation with or without primary closure of the wound.
- *Mention if there is any alternative.*
- *Mention the possible complications*: bleeding, infection, DVT, poor wound healing, phantom limb pain, or stump osteomyelitis.

Lower Extremity Thrombectomy/ Embolectomy:
Procedure:

- The patient is on intravenous heparin at a continuous infusion and given a dose of intravenous antibiotics.
- Under local anesthesia.
- Time out: confirm correct patient, procedure, site and availability of any special instruments.
- Position: supine, the lower extremity is prepped from the umbilicus down to the toes bilaterally.
- Incision: is made in the groin over the common femoral artery of the ischemic limb.
- The common femoral artery as well as the superficial femoral artery and profunda femoris artery are carefully dissected and encircled with vessel loops, taking care not to injure the crossing lateral circumflex vein, which is found at the crux of the femoral artery bifurcation.
- With the patient on heparin, proximal and distal control is obtained by clamping the common femoral artery, the superficial femoral, and the profunda femoris artery.
- A transverse arteriotomy is made in the common femoral artery near the femoral bifurcation.
- A Fogarty embolectomy catheter is passed first distally. Usually for the lower extremity, a Fogarty embolectomy catheter is advanced with markers of 10 cm marked on the catheter. The catheter is passed down the superficial femoral artery as far as it can go, and the balloon is carefully inflated with gentle back-tension retrieving the clot (Fig. 15.2).
- A similar maneuver is performed after cannulating the profunda femoris artery. These steps are repeated until there is no retrieval of clot after two passages through both arteries.
- The thromboembolectomy is performed through the proximal portion of the common femoral artery using the same techniques.
- At this point, the transverse arteriotomy is closed with interrupted 6-0 polypropylene sutures. Prior to the completion of the anasto-

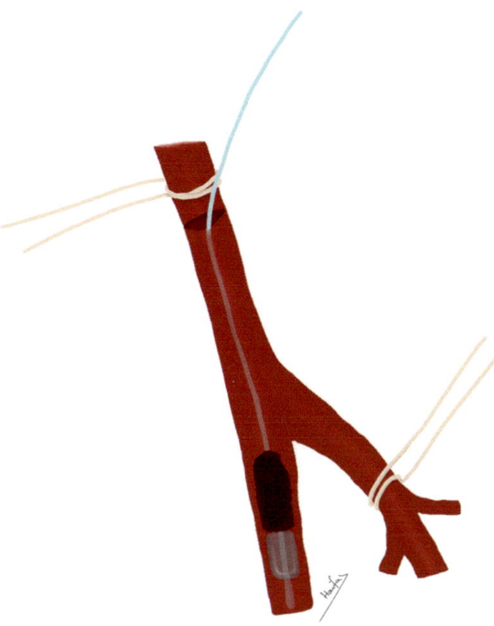

Fig. 15.2 The Fogarty catheter is passed down the artery as far as it can go, and the balloon is carefully inflated with gentle back-tension retrieving the clot

mosis, it is flushed proximally and distally, the anastomosis completed, and then the clamps removed sequentially.

- The clamps are first removed from the common femoral artery, the profunda femoris artery, and then the superficial femoral artery, restoring flow to the lower extremity.
- A completion angiogram is performed to delineate the adequacy of the thromboembolectomy.
- If this is inadequate or if there is residual clot in the tibial vessels, the next approach is to cut down on the below-knee popliteal artery through a medial incision.
- The incision is made just below the knee in the soft part of the medial aspect of the leg approximately 2 cm posterior to the posterior edge of the tibia. In making the incision, it is important to be careful of the greater saphenous vein traveling along this course.
- The incision is carried down to the level of the superficial fascia, which is incised. The gastrocnemius muscle is retracted posteriorly, and the vascular fossa is identified.
- With careful dissection in this avascular plane, the below-knee popliteal artery is carefully identified as well as its paired popliteal veins. The artery is carefully dissected from the popliteal veins and encircled with vessel loops.
- A thromboembolectomy is performed using the Fogarty catheter as described above in a similar manner through transverse arteriotomy and repaired in a similar manner.
- A completion angiogram is performed, confirming the adequacy of the thromboembolectomy.
- Any residual clot of significance should be retrieved through repeat of the above-outlined steps.
- Hemostasis, and closure [10].

Fasciotomy: Lower Extremity (leg)
Procedure:

- Under general anesthesia and endotracheal intubation.
- Time out: confirm correct patient, procedure, site and availability of any special instruments.
- The patient is in a supine position.
- Most fasciotomies are performed through two incisions: one incision is medial and one incision lateral. The lateral incision is approximately 5–7 cm in length, about 2 cm posterior to the posterior aspect of the tibia carried down through the subcutaneous tissue.
- Both the anterior and the lateral fascial compartments and the septum separating these two are identified (Fig. 15.3).
- The anterior compartment is then incised using electrocautery, and the whole length of the compartment is decompressed using scissors incising the fascial band, both proximally and distally.
- A similar technique is utilized for decompression of the lateral compartment, taking care to limit the amount of fascial incising proximally because of the location of the superficial peroneal nerve just beyond the head of the fibula on the lateral aspect of the leg.
- The posterior compartments, the deep and superficial, are approached through a medial

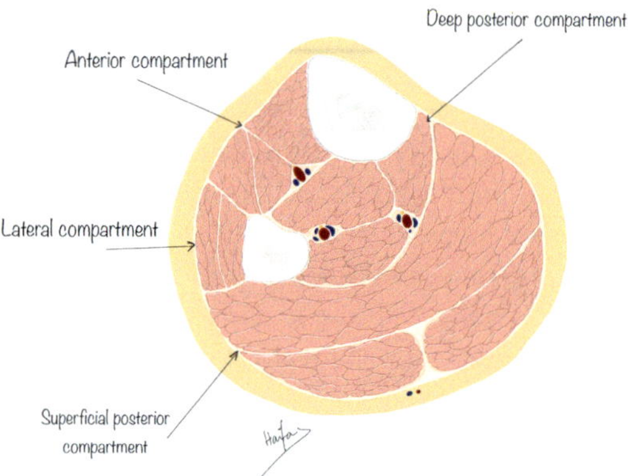

Fig. 15.3 The leg four compartments

incision. The incision is approximately 5–7 cm in length and approximately 2 cm beyond the posterior aspect of the tibia in the soft part of the leg. Through this longitudinal incision, frequently the saphenous vein will be identified, and care should be taken to preserve this if possible (Fig. 15.4).

- The superficial fascia is incised, retracting the gastrocnemius muscle posteriorly.
- The deep compartment is then decompressed by taking down the attachments of the soleus muscle to the posterior aspect of the tibia using electrocautery. This should be done carefully because of the proximity of the posterior tibial and peroneal vessels just below the fascial band. This is incised to the length of approximately 5 cm.
- Hemostasis is obtained and most fasciotomy sites are packed open with a moist gauze.
- After approximately 3 days, the patient may be returned to the operating room for primary closure, split-thickness skin graft, or these wounds may be allowed to close secondarily [11].

Toe Amputation
Procedure:

- The local anesthetic is given if desired using 1% lidocaine without epinephrine on either side of the web spaces of the desired toe amputation site. Or, if an ankle block or a spinal has been administered, this should be tested.

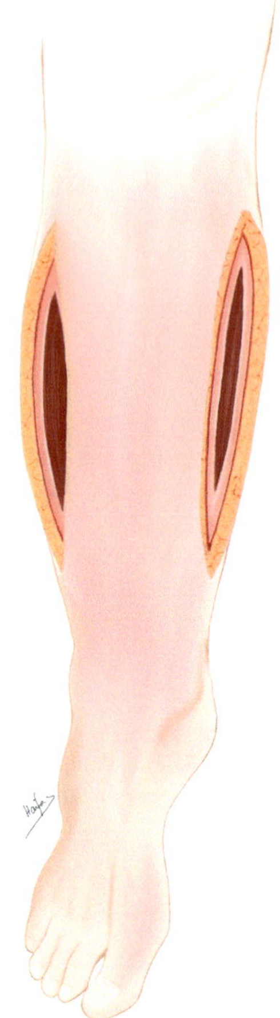

Fig. 15.4 Two-incision leg fasciotomy

- If the toe amputation is to be either the second, third, or fourth toe, an elliptical incision is made with the apices of the incision on the dorsum and plantar aspect of the foot and the toe amputated either at the proximal phalanx site or proximal to the metatarsal head (Fig. 15.5).
- The incision is carried down to the level of the bony tissue. Hemostasis is obtained at the digital vessels and the bone transected using a bone cutter. If the level of amputation requires resection of the metatarsal head, the joint space is entered, and the metatarsal head resected back using rongeurs.

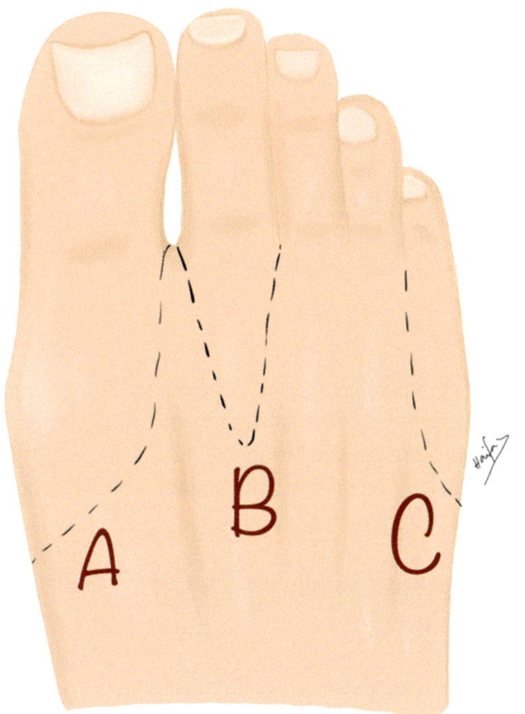

Fig. 15.5 Incisions for toe amputation, A: for big toe, B: for the 2nd, 3rd, and 4th toes, C: for the 5th toe

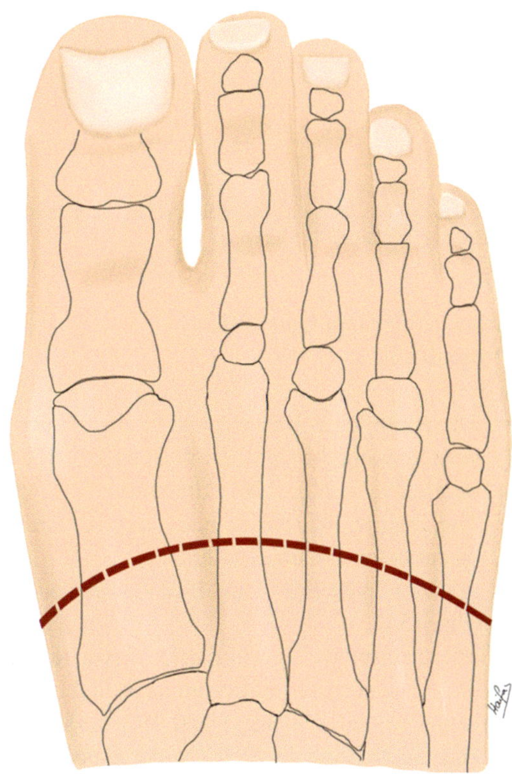

Fig. 15.6 The incision for transmetatarsal amputation

- The ligaments and tendons are transected back as far proximally as possible.
- The wound is irrigated with saline solution. If it is dry gangrene or a clean wound, it may be closed primarily with interrupted vertical mattress 3-0 nylon sutures. If it is infected or a wet gangrene amputation site, it is packed open with a moist saline-soaked gauze.
- If the toe amputation is of either the first or second toe, a racquet-shaped incision is utilized as opposed to an elliptical incision and the amputation performed as described above [12].

Transmetatarsal Amputation
Procedure:

- An incision is made on the dorsal surface of the foot at the mid-metatarsal level (Fig. 15.6).
- Extend the incision to create a plantar flap, which should be as long as possible while preserving only viable tissue.
- The dorsal incision is carried down to the bone, dividing the extensor tendon as proximally as possible.
- Metatarsal bones are divided with a saw, just proximal to the plantar foot incision.
- Remaining tendons are pulled taut and divided as proximally as possible with a scalpel.
- The plantar flap is then cut to the appropriate size so that it can be rotated anteriorly without tension.
- The subcutaneous tissue is approximated with interrupted absorbable suture.
- The skin is closed with interrupted monofilament suture, being careful not to tie the sutures too tightly.
- A bulky protective dressing is applied [13].

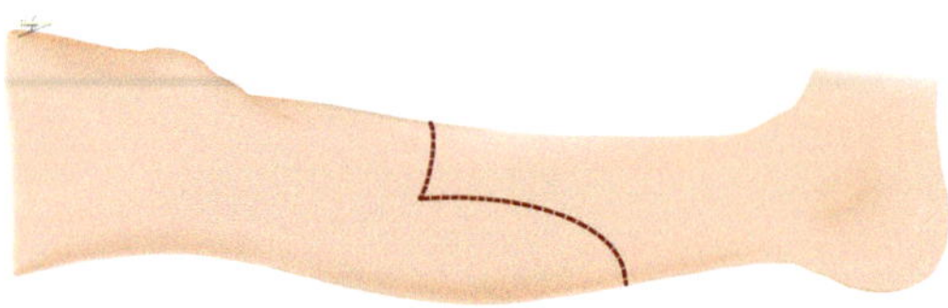

Fig. 15.7 The Incision for below-knee amputation, notice long posterior flap incision

Below-Knee Amputation (BKA)

Procedure:

- The entire leg is prepped and draped. If possible, any open or infected wounds should be covered with an occlusive dressing.
- The anterior incision is made approximately 10 cm below the tibial tuberosity.
- A long posterior flap incision is made (Fig. 15.7).
- The anterior incision is carried down to the tibia. The anterior vessels are identified in the lateral wound. The artery and vein are identified, ligated, and divided. The nerve is placed under tension and divided.
- The musculature of the leg is divided with cautery and the fibula is exposed. It must be exposed about 5 cm above the skin incision.
- The musculature of the medial leg is divided with cautery. The posterior tibial and peroneal vessels are identified, ligated, and divided.
- The tibia is then exposed, and the periosteum is elevated. The tibia is divided transversely 1–2 cm above the anterior skin incision. The fibula is then divided 1–2 cm above the point of transection of the tibia.
- A small bevel of anterior tibia should be sawed off at a 45° angle.
- The flail leg is then placed on mild traction. The tibial nerve is placed on mild tension, ligated, divided, and allowed to retract.
- An amputation knife is then used to create the posterior flap of gastrocnemius and soleus muscles. Long smooth strokes are used, and the flap is tapered.
- A rasp or saw is used to smooth the surface of the tibia.

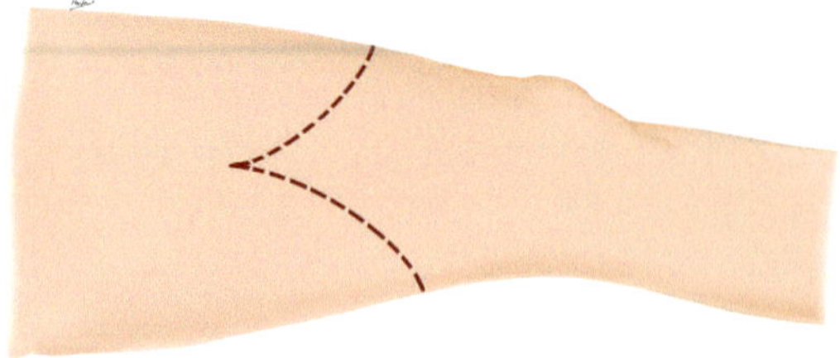

Fig. 15.8 The fish-mouth incision for above-knee amputation

- The posterior flap is rotated anteriorly and interrupted absorbable suture is used to close the subcutaneous tissue.
- Interrupted monofilament suture or staples are used to close the skin [14].

Above-Knee Amputation (AKA)

Procedure:

- A wide fish-mouth or circumferential incision is made in the skin (Fig. 15.8).
- The greater saphenous vein is identified, ligated, and divided.
- Muscles are cut using cautery and are allowed to retract upward.
- In the medial leg, the femoral artery and vein are identified. They are ligated and divided individually. The proximal end is suture ligated.
- The femur is exposed, and a periosteal elevator is used to expose bone about 10 cm above the incision.
- In the posterior thigh, the sciatic nerve is identified. This is placed on traction and ligated as high as possible. It is then divided and allowed to retract high into the thigh.
- The femur is divided about 10 cm above the skin incision.
- A rasp or the saw is used to round off the edges of the bone.
- The fascia is closed with interrupted absorbable suture.
- The skin is closed with interrupted monofilament suture or staples.
- A soft bulky dressing is applied [15].

15.2 Part II: Practice

The more you practice the better you'll be, the harder you train the great in you they'll see
–Alcurtis Turner

15.2.1 Case Scenarios for Practice

Tips:

- Practice with a friend and try to mimic the real exam!
- Do not forget to set the timer!
- The clinical data is provided in the answer key section.

Case No. 1:
A 65-year-old male patient presented to the emergency department complains of discharging wound at the sole of his right big toe for 1 week.

Questions for Discussion:

1. How will you approach the patient?
2. What further investigation will you ask for?
3. How will you manage the patient?
4. Despite what you did still the patient's condition deteriorated, and he is showing signs of septic shock. What will you do next?
5. The patient presented later with discharging sinus at the tip of the stump. What will you do?

Case No 2:
A 75-year-old female patient presented to the emergency department complaining of severe left leg pain for 6 h.

Questions for Discussion:

1. How will you approach the patient?
2. What is your most likely diagnosis?
3. What further investigations may you ask for?
4. How will manage the patient?
5. Few hour later, the patient complains of severe leg pain and swelling. What could be the cause?
6. How will you confirm that?
7. What will be your next step in management?

Case No. 3
A 45-year-old female patient presented to the emergency department complaining of sudden onset of severe left flank pain for 2 h.

Questions for Discussion:

1. How will you approach the patient?
2. What is your differential diagnosis?
3. How will you investigate the most likely diagnosis?
4. How will you manage the patient condition?
5. The patient underwent emergency laparotomy and open repair of her ruptured infrarenal AAA. Three days later, the patient complains of left-sided abdominal pain associated with bloody stool. What could be the cause?
6. How will you manage that?

Checklist

History	Items	Done	Not done	Not applicable
General	Introduce himself/herself to the patient			
	Patient personal data (name, age, sex, etc.)			
	Chief complaint			
	Duration			
Pain	Onset			
	Site			
	Character			
	Radiation/shifting			
	Aggravating/relieving			
	Severity			
	Progression			
	Frequency			
Ulcer	Onset			
	Site			
	Causing event			
	Any change since its onset?			
	Other ulcers			
Associated symptoms	Rest pain			
	Fever			
	Discharge			
	Discoloration			
	Wounds			
	Numbness			
	Coldness			
	Paralysis			
	Claudication			
	Postprandial abdominal pain			
	Weight loss			
Risk factors	Smoking			
	Diabetes mellitus (DM)			
	Hypertension (HTN)			
	History of trauma			
	Cardiac disease			
	Prior vascular intervention			
	Prior cardiac surgery			
	History of hyperlipidemia			
Differential diagnosis	History of prolong immobilization (DVT)			
	Other GIT symptoms			
	Other urinary symptoms			
PMH	Previous similar attack			
	Previous investigation angiography			
	Previous admission			
	Chronic illnesses			
PSH	Previous surgery			
Family history	Of similar complain			
Social history	Occupation			
	Habits (smoking, alcohol, drugs)			
Other	Medication			
	Allergy			
	Transfusion			

History	Items	Done	Not done	Not applicable
Systemic review				
Physical examination				
General principle	Patient position			
	Exposure			
	Privacy			
	Wash hands			
General examination	Appearance			
	Body built			
	Color			
	Distress/decubitus			
	Environment			
Vital signs	Bp, HR, temperature, RR, SPO_2			
Hand signs	Leukonychia, koilonychia, pallor			
Eyes	Jaundice, pallor			
Neck	Jagular venous pressure (JVP)			
	Carotid artery pulse and check for bruit			
	Thoracic outlet obstruction			
Chest	Respiratory and cardiovascular system (CVS) examination			
Abdomen	Palpable pulsatile abdominal mass			
	Bruit			
Lower limb: Inspection	Scar			
	Color: pallor, cyanosis or blackish			
	Nail changes			
	Edema			
	Erythema			
	Loss of hair			
	Skin shinning			
	Ulcers:			
	• Site			
	• Number			
	• Size			
	• Edges			
	• Floor			
	• Discharge			
	• Skin around it			
	Fissure			
	Callus			
	Interdigital toe infection			
	Discharges			
Palpation	Pulses: femoral			
	Popliteal			
	Posterior tibial			
	Dorsalis pedis			
	Capillary refill			
Palpate the ulcer and skin around it	Hotness			
	Tenderness			
	The base of the ulcer			
	Fluctuation			
	Edema			
Lymphatic examination				

(continued)

History	Items	Done	Not done	Not applicable
Neurological examination				
Doppler				
ABPI				
Footwear				
Differential diagnosis	According to the given scenario			
Investigations				
General laboratory test	CBC with differential			
	Electrolytes			
	Liver function test			
	Blood grouping			
	Coagulation profile (PT, INR, aPTT)			
	RFT			
	C-reactive protien (CRP)/ESR			
	Blood culture			
	Arterial blood gas (ABG)			
	Lactic acid			
	D-dimer			
Imaging	X-ray			
	ECG			
	Doppler/duplex ultrasound			
	MRI			
	CT/MRI angiography			
	Conventional angiogram			
Wound	Swab for culture			
Biopsy	From chronic nonhealing ulcer			
Provisional diagnosis	According to the given scenario			
Management (depends on the diagnosis):				
Management of acute limb ischemia	Admission			
	NPO			
	IV fluid			
	Antibiotics			
	IV heparin			
	Endovascular management (thrombolysis, embolectomy)			
	Surgical management (thrombectomy, embolectomy, bypass, or amputation)			
Compartment syndrome	Admission			
	NPO			
	IV fluid			
	Diuretics			
	Alkalization of the urine			
	Consent			
	Surgical site marking			
	Urgent operative management: fasciotomy			
	Delayed closure			

History	Items	Done	Not done	Not applicable
Management of infected diabetic foot	Admission			
	NPO if the patient needs surgical intervention			
	IV fluid			
	Glycemic control			
	IV antibiotics			
	Antipyretic			
	Stress ulcer and DVT prophylaxis			
	Drainage of any abscess			
	Debridement of any necrotic tissue			
	Daily dressing			
	Adjunct: vacuum dressing, hyperbaric oxygen therapy			
	Revascularization if needed			
	Surgical amputation when indicated			
Rupture AAA	Admission to ICU			
	NPO			
	IV fluid			
	Analgesia			
	Hemodynamic monitoring (permissive hypotension)			
	Stress ulcer prophylaxis			
	Endovascular management			
	Surgical management			
Postoperative care				
Early postoperative	Admission to high dependency unit (HDU) or ICU			
	Early mobilization and DVT prophylaxis			
	Resume feeding after full recovery			
	Analgesia			
	Stress ulcer prophylaxis			
	Laboratory investigation as needed			
	Electrolyte assessment			
	Monitor the wound and dressing regularly			
First outpatient visit	Clinical assessment			
	Remove sutures			
	Review the final pathology report if requested			
	Regular follow-up and referral to vascular surgery when indicated			

15.2.2 Answer Key

Case No.1:

A 65-year-old male patient presented to the emergency department complains of discharging wound at the sole of his right big toe for 1 week.

Questions for Discussion:

1. **How will you approach the patient?**
   By obtaining a relevant history and performing a physical examination.

The patient is a 65-year-old male patient who is complaining of right big toe wound after he stepped on a broken piece of glass. The wound is not healing since that and from 3 days, it starts to produce purulent discharge. It is associated with fever and pain.
No other ulcers in the body. No previous history of similar complaint. No history of rest pain, paresthesia or claudication.
The patient has diabetes for 30 years and his blood sugar became difficult to control since he got this wound.

No other chronic illnesses.
PSH is negative.
On examination:
The patient appears sick.
Vital signs: Bp: 132/78 mmHg, PR: 105 bpm, temperature: 39.1°C.
The right foot is swollen, with erythema extending from the sole of the foot to the dorsum. There is an irregular shape wound at the planter surface of the right big toe with necrotic tissue and pus discharge. The foot is warm and tender in comparison to the left-hand side.
The distal pulses are palpable on both side.

2. **What further investigation will you ask for?**
   CBC: shows leukocytosis (WBC: 19×10^9/L), Hb is 12 g/dl
   Foot X-ray shows no fracture or signs of osteomyelitis
3. **How will you manage the patient?**
   - Admission
   - IV antibiotics
   - IV antipyretic
   - DVT prophylaxis
   - Debridement and wound care
4. **Despite what you did, still the patient's condition deteriorated, and he is showing signs of septic shock. What will you do next?**
   - Resuscitate
   - Prepare the patient for toe amputation
   - NPO
   - Anesthesia consultation
   - Consent
   - Surgical site marking

   The patient underwent toe amputation, and his condition improved and discharged to home for outpatient follow-up.
5. **The patient presented later with discharging sinus at the tip of the stump. What will you do?**
   - Wound care
   - Antibiotics
   - MRI of the foot to rule out osteomyelitis of the stump

Case No 2:
A 75-year-old male patient presented to the emergency department complaining of severe left leg pain for 6 h.

Questions for Discussion:

1. **How will you approach the patient?**
   By obtaining a relevant history and performing a physical examination.
   The patient is a 72-year-old male patient who presented to the emergency department due to sudden onset of severe left leg pain. The pain is mainly at the calf region but the whole leg is painful even at rest. He has no ulcers or discharge. He has no history of trauma. He has no previous history of claudication.
   He is a known case of atrial fibrillation on an anticoagulant, but he is not compliant with his medication recently.
   PSH: laparotomy and small bowel resection due to embolic mesenteric ischemia before 1 year.
   Medication: warfarin
   On examination
   He is conscious, in pain
   Vital signs: BP: 130/90 PR: 118 bpm (irregular pulse)
   The left leg is pale, cold in comparison to the right, with absent pulses from the popliteal artery downward.
   Neurological examination revealed diminished sensation and intact motor response.
2. **What is your most likely diagnosis?**
   Acute limb ischemia (embolic).
3. **What further investigation may you ask for?**
   Angiography/CT angiography.
   CT shows complete occlusion of the popliteal artery.
4. **How will manage the patient?**
   Admission
   Heparinization
   Urgent embolectomy

5. **A few hours later, the patient complains of severe leg pain and swelling. What could be the cause?**
   Compartment syndrome.
6. **How will you confirm that?**
   Measure the compartmental pressure.
7. **What will be your next step in management?**
   Urgent 2-incisions fasciotomy to decompress the four compartments of the leg.

Case No. 3

A 45-year-old female patient presented to the emergency department complaining of sudden onset of severe left flank pain for 2 h

Questions for discussion:

1. **How will you approach the patient?**
   Check the stability of the patient.
   If unstable:
   Start with resuscitation following the ABC approach
   A: ensure the patency of the airway
   B: oxygen supplementation and assess the ventilation and oxygen saturation
   C: insert two large cannulas and start fluid and blood product administration
   Withdraw blood for investigation (CBC, electrolytes, LFT, RFT, coagulation profile, blood grouping and crossmatch, ABG).
   After achieving hemodynamic stability, obtain a relevant history and perform a physical examination.
   The patient is a 45-year-old female patient who presented to the emergency department due to sudden onset of left flank pain that was tearing in nature. The pain is not radiated or shifted, and no specific relieving factor. It is associated with dizziness and fainting one time at home. She has no other significant associated symptoms like vomiting, change in bowel habits, or urinary symptoms.
   She is smoker, otherwise healthy female.
   On examination:
   The patient looks ill, pale, and lethargic.
   Vital signs after initial fluid resuscitation BP: 87/59 P: 123 bpm, RR: 19.
   The abdomen is soft but tender at epigastric area with pulsatile abdominal mass 10 * 10 cm.
2. **What is your differential diagnosis?**
   - Rupture AAA
   - Pancreatic mass
   - Gastric mass
   - Abdominal wall lipoma
   - Divercation recti
   - Ventral hernia
3. **How will you investigate the most likely diagnosis?**
   Abdominal ultrasound: showed AAA of the infrarenal aorta.
4. **How will you manage the patient's condition?**
   - Admission to the ICU.
   - Analgesia.
   - Permissive hypotension.
   - Avoid stress.
   - Vascular surgery consultation.
   - Prepare for emergency repair (endovascular or open repair).
5. **The patient underwent emergency laparotomy and open repair of her ruptured infrarenal AAA. Three days later, the patient complains of left-sided abdominal pain associated with bloody stool. What could be the cause?**
   Ischemic colitis.
   Aortoenteric fistula.
   Colonoscopy was done and showed signs of ischemic colitis.
6. **How will you manage that?**
   Conservative management: bowel rest, IV antibiotics, IV fluid and improve her hemodynamic status.

References

1. Lin PH, Chen C, Veith FJ. Arterial disease. In: Brunicardi FC, editor. Schwartz's principles of surgery. 11th ed. New York: McGraw-Hill Education; 2019.
2. Patel MS. Peripheral arterial embolism. In: Cameron JL, Cameron AM, editors. Current surgical therapy. 12th ed. Toronto: Elsevier; 2016.

3. Pipinos II. Peripheral arterial disease. In: Townsend CM, Beauchamp RD, Evers BM, Mattox KL, editors. Sabiston textbook of surgery. 20th ed. St. Louis, MI: Elsevier; 2016.
4. Grimm JC, Hassoun HT. The diabetic foot. In: Cameron JL, Cameron AM, editors. Current surgical therapy. 12th ed. Toronto: Elsevier; 2016.
5. Lancaster RT. Open repair of abdominal aortic aneurysms. In: Cameron JL, Cameron AM, editors. Current surgical therapy. 12th ed. Toronto: Elsevier; 2016.
6. Phelan PJ. The management of ruptured abdominal aortic aneurysm. In: Cameron JL, Cameron AM, editors. Current surgical therapy. 12th ed. Toronto: Elsevier; 2016.
7. Tracci MC. The Aorta. In: Townsend CM, Beauchamp RD, Evers BM, Mattox KL, editors. Sabiston textbook of surgery. 20th ed. St. Louis, MI: Elsevier; 2016.
8. Freischlag JA. Venous disease. In: Townsend CM, Beauchamp RD, Evers BM, Mattox KL, editors. Sabiston textbook of surgery. 20th ed. St. Louis, MI: Elsevier; 2016.
9. Pipinos II. The lymphatics. In: Townsend CM, Beauchamp RD, Evers BM, Mattox KL, editors. Sabiston textbook of surgery. 20th ed. St. Louis, MI: Elsevier; 2016.
10. Eskandari MK. Lower extremity thrombectomy/embolectomy. In: Bell RH, editor. Northwestern handbook of surgical procedures. 11th ed. Austin, TX: Landes Bioscience; 2005.
11. Eskandari MK. Fasciotomy: lower extremity. In: Bell RH, editor. Northwestern handbook of surgical procedures. 11th ed. Austin, TX: Landes Bioscience; 2005.
12. Eskandari MK. Toe amputation. In: Bell RH, editor. Northwestern handbook of surgical procedures. 11th ed. Austin, TX: Landes Bioscience; 2005.
13. Schindler N. Transmetatarsal amputation. In: Bell RH, editor. Northwestern handbook of surgical procedures. 11th ed. Austin, TX: Landes Bioscience; 2005.
14. Schindler N. Below knee amputation (BKA). In: Bell RH, editor. Northwestern handbook of surgical procedures. 11th ed. Austin, TX: Landes Bioscience; 2005.
15. Schindler N. Above knee amputation (AKA). In: Bell RH, editor. Northwestern handbook of surgical procedures. 11th ed. Austin, TX: Landes Bioscience; 2005.

Surgical Aspects of Urological Diseases for Clinical Board Exams

16

16.1 Part I: Knowledge

> The larger the island of knowledge, the longer the shoreline of wonder.
> –Ralph W. Sockman

Common Urological Symptoms are as follows:

- Hematuria
- Hematospermia
- Loin pain
- Suprapubic pain
- Urinary incontinence
- Scrotal pain
- Scrotal swelling
- Urethral discharge
- Pneumaturia
- Lower urinary tract symptoms (LUTS)
  - Storage: Frequency, urgency, and nocturia
  - Voiding: Weak stream, postvoid dribbling, intermittency, hesitancy, straining, and dysuria

Differential diagnosis: Table 16.1

A) **History of Urological Complaints**
- Introduce yourself to the patient
- Personal data
- Chief complaint and duration
- History of presenting illness
- Analysis of the chief complaint
  - **Loin Pain**: Onset, site, severity, progression, duration, radiation, aggravating and relieving factors, and association with fever, nausea, and vomiting.
    NOTE: Pain at flanks commonly due to obstruction like in stones disease and it can radiate to lower abdomen and groin with presence of LUTS especially with stone passage.
  - The presence of obstructing clot as a cause of loin pain is not uncommon, and it can form due to bleeding from stone passage or cancer of upper urinary tract.
  - **Suprapubic Pain:** Onset, site, severity, progression, duration, radiation, aggravating, and relieving factors.
    NOTE: Suprapubic pain commonly reflects a pathology in the bladder when it is inflamed or distended without the ability to void.
  - **Hematuria:** Onset, duration, gross vs microscopic, timing, associated pain, presence of clots, and shape of clots.
    NOTE: Timing of hematuria is important in knowing the possible source (initial: prostate or urethra, terminal: bladder neck, total: bladder or upper tract).
  - **Hematospermia:** Most of the time it is a self-limited condition of nonspecific benign inflammatory condition. It necessitates further work up looking for sexually transmitted disease (STD)

H. Alotaibi, *Study Surgery*, https://doi.org/10.1007/978-981-16-2305-9_16

Table 16.1 Differential diagnosis

Hematuria	Hematospermia	Loin pain
Renal cell carcinoma Bladder cancer Urinary calculi Trauma UTI (pyelonephritis, cystitis) BPH Prostate cancer Exercise-induced TB Schistosomiasis Arteriovenous malformation Renal vein thrombosis Urethritis	Postprostate biopsy Prostate inflammation Seminal vesicle inflammation Prostate cancer Urethral tumor	Urinary calculi Hydronephrosis Pyelonephritis Pyeonephrosis Renal/ureteric tumors Renal cystic disease Blood clot Congenital anomaly Ureteric stricture Retroperitoneal fibrosis Gravid uterus
Suprapubic pain	**Urinary incontinence**	**Scrotal pain**
Cystitis Bladder stone Urinary retention Prostatitis	Pelvic floor weakness Detrusal overactivity Detrusal underactivity Spinal cord abnormality Upper motor neuron lesion Diabetes Prostate enlargement Ectopic ureter Vesicovaginal fistula	Testicular torsion Torsion of testicular appendage Epididymoorchitis Hydrocele Varicocele Testicular tumor Strangulated hernia Skin dermatitis Fournier's gangrene Herpes simplex
Scrotal swelling	**Urethral discharge**	**Pneumaturia**
Hydrocele Spermatocele Varicocele Hematocele Testicular tumor Testicular torsion Epididymoorchitis Inguinal hernia	Gonorrhea Chancroid Chancre Urethritis (non-STD) Prostatitis TB Urethral tumor	Enterovesical fistula Colovesical fistula Gas-forming infection Recent catheterization Recent instrumentation Urinary tract injury during laparoscopy
LUTS		
UTI BPH Prostate cancer Bladder stone Distal ureteric stone Bladder tumor Urethral stricture Interstitial cystitis Schistosomiasis Foreign body in the bladder		

or genitourinary malignancy when not resolved after several weeks.

- **Urinary Incontinence:** Total, urge, stress, mixed (urge and stress), or overflow.
- **Urethral Discharge:** Onset, duration, discharge nature, and sexual history.

  NOTE: Urethral discharge is a symptom of STD, urethral cancer is suspected if it is bloody.
- **Pneumaturia:** Passage of gas through urethra, it can be due to gas-forming infection, recent instrumentation, or fistula between gastrointestinal tract and urinary tract.

- **LUTS:** Indicate functional or mechanical bladder abnormality, which will affect the normal urination either in storage or voiding ability.
- **Scrotal Pain:** Onset, site, severity, progression, duration, radiation, aggravating and reliving factors, and association with fever, nausea, vomiting, swelling, and trauma.
  NOTE: Scrotal pain can be primary (inflammation, torsion, or any primary pathology) or referred (ureteric stone or hernia).
- **Scrotal Swelling:** When and how it was noticed, progression, disappearance, and association with fever, pain, and trauma [1, 2].

- Associated symptoms
- Constitutional symptoms
- Risk factors:
  - **Renal Cell Carcinoma:**
    Smoking, factory workers, survivor of Wilm's tumor, end-stage renal disease (ESRD), hypertension (HTN), family history of renal cell carcinoma (RCC), obesity, trichloroethylene exposure, urban living, and radiation exposure
  - **Bladder Cancer:**
    Smoking, aromatic amine exposure, analgesic (Phenacetin), schistosomiasis, recurrent urinary tract infection (UTI), bladder calculi, pelvic radiation, chronic catheterization, cyclophosphamide, blackfoot disease, and *Aristolochia fangchi*
  - **Prostate Cancer:**
    Family history, African descent, and advanced age > 65 years
  - **Testicular Cancer:** Cryptorchidism, gonadal dysgenesis, family history, infertility, history of testicular cancer, and intratubular germ cell neoplasia (ITGCN)
  - **Urolithiasis:**
    Low water intake, heat and sun exposure, obesity, family history, previous history, and sedentary jobs
  - **Fournier's Gangrene:**
    Diabetes mellitus (DM), surgery in the local area, alcohol, malnutrition, traumatic catheterization, old age, paraphimosis, immunosuppression, and obesity
  - **Retroperitoneal Fibrosis:**
    Male gender, peri-aortitis, methysergide, lymphoma, radiation beta blocker, gonorrhea, and tuberculosis (TB)
- Systemic review
- Past medical history
- Past surgical history
- Medications, allergy, and transfusion
- Family history
- Social history

B) **Physical Examination:**

- **Kidneys Examination:**
  - Inspect for any visible mass at upper abdomen.
  - Palpate the kidneys during deep inspiration by applying the left hand at costovertebral angle posteriorly and the right hand below the costal margin anteriorly, looking for tenderness and renal mass.
  - Palpate the ribs as flanks tenderness can be due to inflamed kidneys or radiculitis (nerve roots compression) as in bone spur, bone abnormalities, and Herpes zoster involving area, T11–L2.
  - Normal kidneys are difficult to palpate because of their locations in retroperitoneum and surrounded by ribs and diaphragm.
  - Right kidney located lower than the left kidney, and it is possible to palpate its lower pole especially in thin men, women, and children.
  - Percuss over the costovertebral angels looking for tenderness.
  - Auscultate the upper abdomen looking for renal artery bruit [2, 3].
- **Bladder Examination:**
  - Inspect suprapubic area for visible bladder distension, it can be seen when bladder is markedly distended in thin patient.

- Bladder can be felt and percussed when it is full of urine >150 mL.
- Palpate the suprapubic area for tenderness and possibly outlining the bladder if the patient is thin.
- Percuss starting from symphysis pubis toward the umbilicus for fluid dullness, in case of marked fullness, the upper level of dullness can reach above the umbilicus.
- Bimanual examination (under anesthesia) between abdomen and rectum in male or vagina in female, to assess bladder tumor extension [2, 3].

- **Male Genital Examination:**
  - Inspect the patient's genital region and the surrounding areas for hair distribution, rash, bruising, swelling, erythema, gangrene, and scars.
  - Retract the foreskin to check for phimosis (narrowing of the foreskin) or adhesions and describe any abnormalities on the glans (ulcers/discharge/scarring).
  - If you are unable to retract the foreskin, ask the patient to do this himself, be aware that a patient may be circumcised and comment on this to the examiner.
  - Open the urethral meatus to check patency. Replace the foreskin once examined to prevent paraphimosis (this is where the retracted foreskin obstructs venous return from the glans, thus resulting in painful swelling of the glans.
  - Examine each testicle individually. Use both thumbs and index fingers to gently palpate the whole testicle, your remaining fingers should be placed behind the testicle to immobilize it. Palpation involves a gentle rubbing motion between thumb and index finger.
  - If you are unable to locate a testicle, palpate along the path of the inguinal ligament for an undescended testicle.
  - If a mass is found, assess the size, shape, regularity, consistency, tenderness, ability to get above the mas, presence of cough impulse, and trans-illumination.
  - Palpate the epididymis for swelling or tenderness.
  - Phren's test: If testicular pain is relieved by elevating the testis, this is strongly suggestive of epididymitis.
  - Cremasteric reflex: Stroke or pinch the patient's medial thigh which leads to stimulation of the cremasteric reflex and elevates the testicle. Loss of cremasteric reflex may suggest testicular torsion.
  - Palpate for spermatic cord at the superior aspect of the testicle using your thumb and index finger. Palpate along the cord assessing for presence of vas deference, masses and tenderness.
  - Scrotum need to be assessed during standing and lying supine [2, 3].
- **Digital Rectal Examination:**
  - Position: Standing with bent over the bed or on knee-chest position
  - Inspect the anus after separating the buttocks for any pathology
  - Insert the index finger after lubrication into the anus, assess the anal tone which is likely to have the same tone as that of the urinary sphincter (lax or spastic)
  - Examine the prostate for size, shape, tenderness, and consistency
  - Advance the finger gently to the maximum extent and examine all the directions for any abnormalities (hemorrhoids, polyp, or mass)
  - Withdraw the finger and assess the stool on the gloves [2, 3]
- **Female Genital Examination:**
  - Position: Lithotomy with abducted thighs
  - Inspect external genitalia and introitus for abnormalities (erosions, atrophic changes, warts, and discharge) and

inspect the meatus for caruncles, redness, and mucosal prolapse
  - Ask the patient to perform Valsalva maneuver and assess for pelvic organ prolapse
  - Ask the patient to cough and look for urinary incontinence
  - Palpate the urethra for any mass or diverticulum [2, 3]
- **Neurological Assessment:**
  - Assess the integrity of sacral roots and nerves.
  - Check the sensation of the penis, scrotum, vagina, labia, and the perineum area.
  - Bulbocavernosus reflex assessed by placing index finger in the anal canal and squeeze the glans or clitoris or by pulling the Foley's catheter. Normally it reflexes by contraction of the anal canal [2, 3].

C) **Investigations:**
- **Urinalysis:**

Examining the color of the sample is helpful in knowing the abnormality if present. (Table 16.2)

Table 16.2 Urinalysis [2, 4]

Color	Interpretation
Yellow	Normal
Colorless	Diluted urine
Cloudy	Pyuria Phosphaturia
Red	Hematuria Hemoglobinuria Myoglobinuria Rifampin
Orange	Dehydration Pyridium
Green-blue	Indigo carmine Methylene blue Phenol
Brown	Urobilinogen Flagyl Nitrofurantoin Bleeding Sorbitol

  - Urine specific gravity (1.001–1.035), reflecting urine concentration. To assess hydration status and renal ability to concentrate urine.
  - Check urine pH. Average (5.5–6.5), acidic (4.5–5.5), and alkaline (6.5–8).
  - Hematuria is considered when more than three red blood cells (RBCs)/high power field (HPF) are present.
  - UTI is suggested when urine is positive for bacteriuria, leukocyte esterase, nitrite, and more than three white blood cells (WBCs)/HPF for male and five WBCs/HPF for female.
  - Proteinuria >20 mg/dL suggesting kidney disease (tubulointerstitial, renal vascular, or glomerular).
  - Cellular casts are indicative of renal disease, RBC casts indicate glomerular bleeding, and WBC casts indicate nephritis.
  - Stones crystals can be detected in the urine sample and help to determine the type of stone.
  - Glucose and ketones normally not detected in urine; their presence is suggestive for diabetes mellitus.
  - Urine has no bilirubin normally; its presence indicates hepatic or biliary disease [2, 4].
- **Urine Cytology:**
  - Used to examine exfoliated urothelial cells in urine for malignant abnormality
- Prostate-Specific Antigen **(PSA):**
  - Total PSA increases with prostate cancer > 4.0 ng/mL and can increase with benign prostatic hyperplasia (BPH), prostatitis, and bladder instrumentation.
  - Free PSA and PSA density can help to differentiate PSA elevation due to prostate cancer or benign conditions.
  - Free PSA of < 10% is associated with > 50% probability of prostate cancer diagnosis, when the free PSA percentage increase > 10% the probability of prostate cancer will decrease.

- PSA density measured by dividing total PSA level over the prostate volume (PSA/prostate volume).
- Result of PSA density ≥ 0.15 is suggesting prostate cancer [2, 4].

- Kidney, Ureter, and Bladder **(KUB) X-ray:**
  - Useful in identifying radio-opaque urinary stones and checking stents or drain position [5, 6]
- **Retrograde Urethrogram:**
- Used to assess urethra for strictures, injuries (extravasation), and fistulas [5, 6]
- **Cystogram:**
  - Used to assess bladder for capacity, wall shape, filling defects, injuries (extravasation), fistulas between bladder and vagina or bowel, and healing after bladder surgery.
  - Voiding cystourethrogarm (VCUG) helps in assessing reflux and ability of normal voiding [5, 6].
- **Retrograde Pyelogram:**
  - Useful in assessing ureters and collecting system for filling defects, strictures, injuries, and hydroureter or hydronephrosis [5, 6]
- **Intravenous Pyelogram (IVP):**
  - Used to give anatomical and functional information for the urinary tract. It is useful to assess for renal masses, filling defects, strictures, congenital anomalies, and injuries [5, 6].
- **Ultrasonography:**
  - Used to assess:

    Renal size and growth
    Hydronephrosis
    Renal masses
    Follow up of benign renal lesions
    Renal stones
    Renal vascularity by Doppler US
    Renal vein thrombosis
    Renal artery stenosis
    Ureteric jet by Doppler US (ureteric obstruction assessment)
    Perinephric fluid
    Bladder volume and postvoid residual
    Bladder wall thickness
    Bladder stones and masses
    Prostate enlargement
    Scrotal examination for benign and malignant lesions [7]
- **Computed Tomography Scan:**
  - Used to assess:

    Renal colic
    Hematuria
    Pyelonephritis and renal abscess
    Renal tumors
    Staging of renal cancer
    Urinary tract trauma
    Urine extravasation
    Bladder tumor
    Staging of bladder cancer
    Lymphadenopathy
    Prostatic abscess
    Staging of testicular cancer [5, 6]
- **Magnetic Resonance Imaging:**
  - Used to assess:

    Renal tumors
    Renal cancer staging
    Renal vein and inferior vena cava (IVC) tumor thrombus
    Renal vascular abnormalities [magnetic resonance angiogram (MRA)]
    Bladder cancer staging (adjacent structure invasion)
    Staging of prostate cancer and local extension
    Testicular assessment when other radiological tests not conclusive
    Undescended testis [5, 6]
- **Radioisotope Scan:**
  - MAG3 renogram used to assess the split function of the kidneys and renal obstruction if present.
  - Dimercaptosuccinic acid (DMSA) scan used to assess the split function of the kidneys and area of parenchymal scarring
  - Diethylenetriaminepentaacetic acid (DTPA) used to assess glomerular filtration rate (GFR) and renal obstruction [5, 6].
- **Urodynamic Study:**
  - Useful in assessing voiding physiology of bladder, urethral sphincter, and urethra and determine abnormality of emptying [5, 6]

D) **Management:**

1. **Urinary Stones:**
   - **Medical Management:**
     - **General recommendations:**
       Sufficient fluid intake, 2–3 liters/day
       Limited protein diet, 1.0 grams/kg/day
       Limited calcium intake, 1000–1200 mg/day
       Low sodium diet, < 2300 mg/day
       Low oxalate diet
     - **Hypercalciuria (> 200 mg/day):**
       Thiazide (Hydrochlorothiazide 25–50 mg daily or b.i.d.) in case of absorptive or renal leak hypercalciuria
       Parathyroidectomy in case of resorptive hypercalciuria (primary hyperparathyroidism)
       Cellulose sodium phosphate or orthophosphate in case of refractory response to thiazide (use with caution for side effects)
     - **Hyperuricosuria (> 600 mg/day)**
       Decrease purine diet
       Urine alkalinization (potassium citrate 20 mEq b.i.d. or t.i.d.)
       Allopurinol 300 mg/day if urinary alkalinization failed
     - **Hypocitraturia (< 300 mg/day)**
       Citrate in urine is potent stone inhibitor and can be corrected by potassium citrate.
     - **Hyperoxaluria (> 45 mg/day)**
       Primary hyperoxaluria is treated with pyridoxine 25–50 mg/day and might need combined liver and renal transplant to correct enzyme defect.
       Decrease oxalate diet if the cause is high dietary intake.
       Oral calcium supplements can bind to oxalate in gut and prevent its absorption.
     - **Hypomagnesiuria (< 50 mg/day)**
       Urinary magnesium is a stone-forming inhibitor.
       Magnesium oxide, 140 mg/q.i.d.
     - **Cystinuria (> 30 mg/day)**
       Urine alkalinization (potassium citrate)
       Increase cysteine solubility in urine by:
       - α-mercaptopropionylglycine (Thiola) first line
       - Penicillamine-D
       - Captopril
     - **Struvite Stone**
       Surgical treatment is the main management.
       Acetohydroxamic acid inhibits urease and restricted to severe cases with recurrence [8].
   - **Surgical Management**
     - **Conservative Treatment**
       Recommended before surgical intervention by giving chance for stone passage.
       When pain, nausea, and vomiting are controlled.
       Preserved kidney function.
       Stone is small <10 mm.
       Encourage well oral hydration.
       α-Blocker (Tamsulosin, 0.4 mg/day).
       Patient is instructed to observe for stone passage in urine and should be followed with radiological imaging [9].
     - **Indications for Immediate Intervention:**
       Associated pyelonephritis
       Solitary kidney
       Bilateral urinary stones
       Intractable symptoms (pain, nausea, or vomiting)
       Failure of conservative treatment
       Renal impairment
       Prolonged obstruction
       High-grade obstruction [9]
     - **Kidney Stones:**
       Less than 20 mm in size can be treated with extracorporeal shock wave lithotripsy (ESWL) or ureteroscopy.

Ureteroscopy is superior when the stone is located in the lower renal calyces because of high chance of failure through stone passage after ESWL.
Greater than 20 mm in size, percutaneous nephrolithotomy (PCNL) is recommended [9].
- **Ureteric Stones:** Ureteroscopy or ESWL [9]
- **Bladder Stones**
  Cystoscopy and stone removal
  Open surgical removal (Cystolithotomy) for larger stones
  Supra-pubic percutaneous endoscopic removal in case of patient with urinary diversion

2. **Benign Prostatic Hyperplasia (BPH):**
   - Medical Management
     - *Alpha-Blockers*
       Alpha-blockers inhibit alpha-1 receptors and cause relaxation to bladder neck and prostate smooth muscles.
       Terazosin, doxazosin, and alfuzosin are non-selective alpha-1 blockers.
       Tamsulosin is selective alpha-1A blocker and has faster and better improvement compared to others [10].
     - *5Alpha-Reductase Inhibitors*
       Finastride and dutasteride inhibit 5alpha-reductase which convert testosterone to dihydrotestosterone (DHT).
       It improves urinary symptoms by reducing prostate volume.
     - Combination of both medications showed good improvement in BPH symptoms compared to either agent alone [10].
   - Surgical Management
     - *Transurethral Needle Ablation*
       In office procedure
       Local anesthesia
       Use radiofrequency ablation
       Ideally for prostate size < 80 cc
       Contraindicated in patients with pacemakers, defibrillators, and pelvic implants
       Increased chance for re-treatment [11]
     - *Transurethral Microwave Thermotherapy*
       In office procedure
       Local anesthesia
       Not ideal for prostate with large middle lobe
       Ideally for prostate size 25–100 cc
       Contraindicated in patients with pacemakers, defibrillators, and pelvic implants
       Increased chance for retreatment [11]
     - *Urolift*
       Implants placed into the prostate to anchor the enlarged lobes to the capsule (lifting the lobes away from the urethra)
       Ideally for prostate size <80 cc
       Transurethral Incision of Prostate
       Incising the bladder neck and extend to verumontanum posterolaterally
       Ideal for small prostate <30 cc and patients with mild symptoms
       Can preserve normal ejaculation [11]
     - *Transurethral Resection of Prostate (TURP)*
       Gold standard procedure for BPH.
       Ideal for prostate < 80 cc.
       Monopolar or bipolar electrical current
       Spinal anesthesia is administered to monitor the patient's alertness for signs of dilutional hyponatremia [transurethral resection (TUR) syndrome] which might be happen, due to absorption of the irrigant fluid used during the procedure.
       TUR syndrome can be avoided by using bipolar electrode and isotonic solution.
       Intra- and post-operative bleeding is the most common complication [11].
     - *Transurethral Laser Therapy*
       (Holmium: Yttrium, Aluminum and Garnet) Ho:YAG, Neodymium (Nd):YAG, and Thulium (Tm):YAG lasers used.
       It works by either resecting or vaporizing the tissue.
       Laser therapy has low-risk of bleeding and good post-operative recovery and overall results.
       Ideal for very large prostate and replacing open prostatectomy [11].

– *Open Prostatectomy*
 Reserved for patients with large prostate >80 cc
 Ideal for cases with concomitant bladder stone or diverticulum [11]

3. **Testicular Torsion:**
   - Urgent surgical exploration (waiting for imaging is contraindicated).
   - Untwist the affected testis and wrap it in warm-soaked gauze, if viable to do orchidopexy.
   - If not viable to do orchidectomy.
   - The other normal testis should always fix by orchidopexy.
   - In case of torsion of the appendix testis, management is directed to reduce inflammation by ice packing, anti-inflammatory medications, and restricted movement. Surgery is rarely indicated.
4. **Fournier's Gangrene:**
   - Broad-spectrum empiric intravenous (IV) antibiotic.
   - Immediate aggressive surgical debridement.
   - Subcutaneous pocket in thigh can be made to place testicles.
   - Supra-pubic urinary catheterization.
   - Diverting colostomy, if rectal or anal involvement by infection.
   - Place Penrose drain at the debrided tissue to prevent fluid accumulation.
   - Re-debridement after 24 h.
   - Wet to dry dressing three times daily.
   - Hyperbaric oxygen may be of benefit.
   - Skin grafts or flaps may be necessary after healing [12].
5. **Renal Cell Carcinoma:**
   - Note:
     Use the American Joint Committee on Cancer for Staging
     Use the Memorial Sloan Kettering cancer center (MSKCC/Motze) risk classification for metastatic disease [13]
   - Management: Table 16.3

Table 16.3 Management according to the stage [13]

Staging	Treatment
T1a	• Partial nephrectomy (open, laparoscopic, or robotic) especially in patients with solitary kidney, bilateral tumors, familial renal cell cancer, or renal insufficiency • Radical nephrectomy should be reserved for cases where partial nephrectomy is not technically feasible • Nonsurgical options (i.e., active surveillance, cryoablation, and radiofrequency ablation) recommended in patients with significant comorbidities that interdict surgical intervention
T1b and T2	Radical nephrectomy
T3	Radical nephrectomy with excision of tumor thrombus in renal vein, inferior vena cava, and right atrium
Ipsilateral adrenal gland	Excision is indicated in upper pole kidney tumors or the presence of adrenal gland lesion
Lymph node dissection	Resection of the regional lymph nodes (within Gerota's fascia) is an integral part of radical nephrectomy
Metastatic disease	• Resectable primary tumors with solitary metastasis or multiple resectable lung metastases: These patients should undergo nephrectomy and resection of the metastatic lesion/s • Resectable primary and multiple non-resectable metastasis should undergo resection of the primary tumor then start systemic therapy • Systemic therapy: **Clear cell histology** with ***good or intermediate risk*** options include either sunitinib, bevacizumab, and interferon 2a or pazopanib. ***Poor risk*** systemic therapy is temsirolimus • **Nonclear cell histology** options of therapy include temsirolimus, sunitinib, or sorafenib
Non-resectable primary tumor	Systemic therapy according to their histological results and MSKCC risk group
Recurrent disease postprimary nephrectomy	• If resectable: Surgical resection should be attempted and No systemic therapy • If nonresectable: Treated as metastatic disease according to histological results and MSKCC Risk Score

6. **Urothelial Cell Carcinoma of Urinary Bladder:**

   Note: Use the American Joint Committee on Cancer for Staging

   - **Management of Non-Muscle Invasive Tumors:**
     - Transurethral resection of bladder tumor (TURBT)
     - Repeat TURBT after 4 weeks, if the resection was incomplete, the disease is high-grade Ta or T1, or if no muscle examination found
     - Post-operative instillation of intravesical chemotherapy (mitomycin C)
     - Provide further treatment according to risk stratification
     - Low risk: Solitary small <3 cm low-grade Ta tumor
     - Intermediate risk: Multifocal or large low-grade Ta tumors or recurrence at 3 months
     - High risk: High-grade Ta and all T1, clinically isolated syndrome (CIS)
     - Management of low risk: Surveillance cystoscopy (3–6 months) intervals
     - Management of intermediate risk: Intravesical [Bacillus Calmette-Guerin (BCG)] induction (weekly for 6 weeks), surveillance cystoscopy, and upper tract imaging every 2 years
     - Management of high risk: Intravesical BCG induction (weekly for 6 weeks) followed by maintenance therapy (3 weekly injections) at 3, 6, 12, 18, 24, 30, and 36 months from induction, closer surveillance cystoscopy, and upper tract imaging
     - Consider early cystectomy in recurrent Carcinoma in situ (CIS), T1, and high-grade disease with prior treatment of two induction courses of intravesical therapy [14]
   - **Management of Muscle Invasive Tumors:**
     - Clinical T2–T4a disease with negative lymph nodes: Neo-adjuvant cisplatin-based combination chemotherapy and radical cystectomy with extended lymphadenectomy.
     - Clinical T4b or positive locoregional lymph node disease: Cisplatin-based combination chemotherapy or chemoradiation.
     - If chemoradiation used: Observe if complete response and do radical cystectomy if partial response.
     - If chemotherapy used, consider chemoradiation or radical cystectomy. If complete response and if partial response, consider chemoradiation [15].
   - **Management of Metastatic Disease:** Chemotherapy is the mainstay treatment (cisplatin with gemcitabine if normal renal function and carboplatin with gemcitabine if abnormal renal function) [15].

7. **Prostate Adenocarcinoma:**

The management options for prostate adenocarcinoma depends on the stage (AJCC staging) and risk group (D'Amico risk groups for prostate cancer) [16].

- **Localized Disease (cT1-2 N0):**
  - Low risk: Therapy options depend on the following factors:

    If a patient is asymptomatic with life expectancy <5 years: No further intervention required until symptoms or clinical progression develops.

    If asymptomatic with life expectancy between 5 and 10 years: Active surveillance involves active monitoring of the course of disease with the expectation to intervene with curative intent if cancer progresses.

    If asymptomatic with life expectancy >10 years: Options include active surveillance, radical prostatectomy, external beam radiation, or brachytherapy [16].
  - Intermediate risk –Therapy options depend on the following:

    If life expectancy is <5 years, a patient will have no further intervention until he becomes symptomatic or develops clinical progression.

If life expectancy is between 5 and 10 years, options include active surveillance, radical prostatectomy with lymph node dissection, or external beam radiation with 6 months of androgen deprivation therapy.

If life expectancy is >10 years, options are radical prostatectomy with lymph node dissection or external beam radiation with 6 months of androgen deprivation therapy [16].

- High risk—Therapy options include external beam radiation (including pelvic lymph nodes with or without brachytherapy boost) with androgen deprivation therapy for 18 months or radical prostatectomy with lymph node dissection [16].

- **Locally Advanced Disease (cT3-4 or N1):**
  - External beam radiation (including pelvic lymph nodes and with or without brachytherapy boost) with androgen deprivation therapy for 2–3 years
  - Radical prostatectomy with lymph node dissection (only if no clinical evidence of lymph node involvement and no tumor fixation) [17]
- **Metastatic Disease:**
  - Castration-sensitive prostate cancer: Chemo-hormonal therapy with six cycles of docetaxel and androgen deprivation therapy.
  - Androgen deprivation therapy options include bilateral orchiectomy, luteinizing hormone-releasing hormone (LHRH) agonist, LHRH antagonists, and complete androgen blockade.
  - Castration-resistant prostate cancer:

    Treatment options for those who did not receive chemo-hormonal therapy include docetaxel with prednisone, abiraterone with prednisone, enzalutamide, and radium-223.

    Treatment options for those who have progressed on or after docetaxel include cabazitaxel with prednisone, abiraterone with prednisone, enzalutamide, and radium-223 [17].

8. **Testicular Cancer:**
   - Note: Use the American Joint Committee on Cancer for Staging
   - Obtain serum tumor markers [beta human chorionic gonadotropin (beta-hCG), alpha-fetoprotein (AFP), and lactate dehydrogenase (LDH)], chest X-ray (CXR), and CT abdomen and pelvis with oral and IV contrast
   - Offer sperm banking prior to treatment
   - Radical inguinal orchidectomy
   - Further management based on histological diagnosis and staging use AJCC TNM staging [18]
   - Treatment of Seminoma:
     - Stage IA or IB, if compliant and T1–T3 surveillance and if non-compliant or T4 to give chemotherapy two cycles of carboplatin or radiation to retroperitoneal lymph nodes (RPLN)
     - Stage IS, radiation to RPLN
     - Stage IIA or IIB, radiation to RPLN and ipsilateral iliac LN
     - Stage IIC or III, for good risk to receive chemotherapy BEP (bleomycin, etoposide, and cisplatin) three cycles or (etoposide and cisplatin) EP four cycles. For intermediate risk to receive BEP four cycles [18]
   - Treatment of non-Seminoma:
     - Stage IA or IB, if compliant and T1 observe and if no compliant or T2–T4, do unilateral retroperitoneal lymph node dissection (RPLND) or chemotherapy BEP two cycles
     - Stage IIA or IIB, bilateral RPLND or BEP three cycles or EP four cycles
     - Stage IS, BEP three cycles or EP four cycles
     - Stage IIC or III, chemotherapy for good risk BEP three cycles or EP four cycles and for intermediate and poor risk BEP four cycles [18]

Surgical Operations

Reduction of Testicular Torsion

- Incision: Make incision through the skin and then through dartos fascia in the median raphe of the scrotum
- Extend the incision onto the tunica vaginalis
- Open the tunica vaginalis
- Untwist the cord and then wrap the testis in warm saline sponges
- Check the color of testis, if it is dark, the testis is not viable, proceed with an orchidectomy by dividing the cord structures between clamps and ligating with sutures including a transfixing stitch
- If testis is viable, place two or three interrupted absorbable sutures in the cut edges of tunica vaginalis
- Place the testis in a dartos pouch or suture tunica albuginea to the scrotum with two or more sutures
- In all cases, open the contralateral scrotal sac and fix that testis as well
- Close the dartos layer with absorbable suture and approximate the skin with subcuticular suture
- Place a dry dressing with scrotal support [19]

Radical Orchidectomy:

- Incision is made at the beginning approximately 2 cm superior and lateral to the pubic tubercle, and extended laterally along a Langer's line for 5–7 cm.
- The incision is carried onto the external abdominal oblique aponeurosis.
- The external abdominal oblique aponeurosis is sharply opened over the inguinal canal extending medially to the external inguinal ring and laterally to a point overlying the level of the internal inguinal ring.
- The ilioinguinal nerve dissected free from its investing external spermatic fascia.
- Gentle blunt dissection circumscribing the spermatic cord.
- The cord should be secured with Penrose drain passed twice around and clamped with a hemostat.
- Push the testicle from hemi-scrotum toward the incision to facilitate delivery of the testicle.
- Blunt and/or electrocautery dissection to free the tunica vaginalis from its investing fascial layers.
- Gubernaculum should be incised by electrocautery.
- The delivered testicle within the tunica vaginalis is then free and attached only by spermatic cord.
- Ligate and divide the vas deferens separately from cord at this level with 2-0 permanent suture.
- The cord is doubly ligated and divided at this level with 0 permanent suture.
- Long tails of this permanent suture aid with identification of the cord stump during retroperitoneal lymphadenectomy.
- The surgical field is irrigated and meticulous hemostasis is obtained.
- The external abdominal oblique aponeurosis is approximated.
- The subcutaneous fascial tissue layers are approximated with absorbable suture.
- The skin is closed in a routine fashion [20].

Robotic-Assisted Laparoscopic Prostatectomy:

- A 12-mm vertical incision is made superior to the umbilicus, the abdomen is insufflated.
- Trocar is introduced through this incision for the robotic camera.
- The patient is marked approximately 15-cm superior to the symphysis pubis.
- The patient is marked approximately 7–8 cm left lateral to the reference mark, and an 8-mm robotic trocar is introduced under direct vision, second 8-mm robotic trocar is placed 7–8 cm lateral to the first robotic trocar (Accommodate robotic arms 2 and 3)
- Attention is then turned to the right side, 8-mm robotic trocar is placed under direct vision, approximately 7–8 cm lateral to the reference mark (Accommodate robotic arm 1)
- A 12-mm trocar is placed approximately 3–4 cm superomedial to the iliac crest.
- Lastly, a 5-mm assistant port is placed directly between the two previously placed right-sided ports.

- Incision is made in the peritoneum above pubic symphysis, the median umbilical ligaments and urachus are divided to develop the space of Retzius.
- The peritoneal incision is carried along lateral pelvis to the level of the vas deferens at the internal inguinal ring.
- The lateral attachments of the bladder are sharply developed, this allows the bladder to fall posteriorly and expose the prostate.
- Fatty tissue overlying the prostate excised.
- Control the dorsal vein complex by suturing for division later.
- Monopolar electrocautery scissors are used to dissect at the prostatovesical tissue.
- The foley catheter is deflated and withdrawn into urethra to expose the bladder trigone.
- The incision is carried through the posterior bladder neck.
- Both seminal vesicles are freed completely and the vas deferens is divided bilaterally.
- Dissect posteriorly between the prostate and Denonvillier's fascia and laterally between the prostatic fascia and the lateral pelvic fascia.
- The prostatic pedicle can then be identified posterolaterally and stapling device can control the pedicle.
- The dorsal vein complex should be divided sharply immediately proximal to the hemostatic sutures that was placed earlier.
- The urethra can be divided sharply with scissors at the level of prostatic apex.
- Then the surgical specimen is removed.
- Mucosal-to-mucosal vesicourethral anastomosis with a running suture carried out.
- Finally undock the robot and close the wound [21].

Open Supra-Pubic Prostatectomy:

- Patient on supine position and Pfannenstiel or lower midline incision may be used.
- Incise the anterior rectus fascia.
- Separate the rectus muscle bellies from the fascia with blunt finger dissection and electrocautery.
- Separate the rectus muscle bellies in the midline and retract them laterally.
- Use the electrocautery to open the underlying transversalis fascia.
- Develop the space of Retzius anterior to the bladder.
- Place self-retaining retractor.
- Open the bladder 2–3 cm superior to the bladder neck.
- Place stay sutures inferior and superior to the bladder incision that is made.
- Identify the ureteral orifices.
- Remove any vesical calculi if present.
- Identify and palpate the adenoma protruding at the bladder neck.
- Incise the bladder epithelium circumferentially around adenoma.
- The enucleation should be initiated by inserting the index finger into the prostatic fossa and cracking the anterior commissure.
- Blunt enucleation should be carried out.
- Sweep and roll finger laterally, working side-to-side, proximal and distal, until the lobes have been freed.
- The urethra should be divided sharply or blunt by pinching between two fingers just proximal to the distal apical adenoma.
- Grasp adenoma with forceps and remove it.
- Once the adenoma is removed, inspect the prostatic fossa and control sizeable bleeders with suture ligatures.
- Place figure of eight hemostatic sutures at the 5 and 7 o'clock positions.
- Place drains near the bladder neck.
- Close the bladder in two or three layers.
- Complete routine wound closure with absorbable suture, including approximation of the rectus muscle [22].

Radical Nephrectomy:

- Start the procedure by subcostal incision.
- Divide the anterior rectus sheath and the external oblique muscle.
- Divide or bluntly split the internal oblique and digitally separate the fibers of the transversus abdominis muscle.
- Incise the transversalis fascia.
- Sweep the peritoneum bluntly off the abdominal wall laterally and inferiorly to the iliac crest.

- Right kidney: Incise the white line of Toldt from the hepatic flexure to the common iliac artery and reflect the ascending colon medially.
- Left kidney: Incise white line of the Toldt from the splenic flexure to the common iliac artery and reflect the descending colon medially.
- Right kidney: Reflect the duodenum medially by means of Kocher maneuver.
- Left kidney: Divide the lienocolic and lienorenal ligaments to mobilize spleen and pancreas cranially.
- Right kidney: Use anteromedial surface of the inferior vena cava as a guide to identify the short right renal vein.
- The right renal artery is usually located deep to the right renal vein.
- Left kidney: Use the anterior surface of the aorta as a guide to identify the long left renal vein.
- The left renal artery is usually located cranial and deep to the renal vein.
- Double clamp the artery and vein separately and divide the vessels between the clamps.
- Tie the vessels with a 2-0 silk ligature.
- Dissect the adrenal gland from the upper pole of the kidney.
- Free the superior and postero-lateral attachments of kidney.
- Mobilize the lower pole of the kidney and divide the ureter.
- Irrigate the surgical site and secure hemostasis.
- Close the abdominal layers followed by wound closure. [23]

Partial Nephrectomy:

- Follow the same steps mentioned in radical nephrectomy till you identified the renal pedicles.
- Dissect the entire surface of the kidney free of the perirenal fat, with exception of the fat overlying the tumor.
- Administer intravenous mannitol.
- The renal pedicles will be clamped only during partial nephrectomy.
- Circumferentially score the renal cortex surrounding the tumor with electrocautery.
- Bluntly dissect it with small closed Metzenbaum scissors.
- Excise the tumor.
- Place a Nu-Knit pledget along each border of crater and place Nu-Knit bolster into the bottom of the crater.
- Close the defect with a horizontal mattress using 2-0 absorbable suture.
- The sutures should be placed through the pledgets and about 1–2 cm into renal parenchyma.
- Replace the perirenal fat and renal fascia around the kidney.
- Leave a close suction drain in the pararenal space.
- Close the abdominal layers and the wound [24].

16.2 Part II: Practice

Practice doesn't make perfect.
Practice reduces the imperfection.
–Toba Beta

16.2.1 Case Scenarios for Practice

Tips:

- Practice with a friend and try to mimic the real exam!
- Don't forget to set the timer!

Case No. 1

A 60-year-old male presented to urology clinic complaining of three episodes of hematuria in the last 2 months.

Questions for Discussion:

1. **How will you approach this patient?**
   Obtaining a history, physical examination, and initiating the work up aiming to assess him for the possibility of having urinary malignancy as the most common and serious cause of hematuria.

He is having **gross** and **painless** hematuria three times in the last 2 months, and it was **totally** present during urination. It was associated with **round** shape **clots**. He denies any lower urinary tract symptoms and no other urological complaints. There is no fever, weight loss, or anorexia. Other systemic review is unremarkable.

Patient has no history of UTI, urinary calculi or any urological diseases. He is known to have DM and HTN and negative for other chronic conditions including malignancies. There is no exposure to radiation nor being working in industrial jobs. He has negative past surgical history.

He is on atenolol and insulin with no history of allergy. There is no family history of similar conditions nor history of malignancy.

The patient is smoker (1 pack/day) for 30 years and working as teacher.

On Examination: He looks well, average body weight, not in distress and no pallor or jaundice. His vital signs within normal limits. There are no enlarged lymph nodes.

His abdomen is soft with no tenderness or palpable masses and the bladder is not distended.

He has normal genital exam and digital rectal examination reveal smooth mildly enlarged prostate without tenderness or nodules.

Initial Work-Up: Complete blood count (CBC) showing normal values and no drop in hemoglobin, his creatinine is 0.7 mg/dL, and electrolytes are normal.

Urine analysis showed 50 RBC/HPF and no picture of UTI.

Urine cytology showing malignant urothelial cells.

2. **What is your next step?**
   You need to assess the bladder by cystoscopy and the upper urinary tract by IVP or CT with IV contrast and if case of renal impairment magnetic resonance imaging (MRI) urogram or retrograde pyelography with non-contrast CT.

   CT urogram showed no filling defects or other abnormality.

   Cystoscopy showed papillary growth at the posterior bladder wall.
3. **What is your next step in management?**
   Patient need transurethral resection of bladder tumor (TURBT).

   Obtain:

   Informed consent.

   Pre-operative labs (CBC, coagulation profile, and blood group).

   Inform the patient for the need of post-operative intravesical single dose of chemotherapy (Mitomycin C).

   TURBT was done and the pathology examination showed 2 cm low-grade Ta bladder urothelial carcinoma.
4. **What is the risk stratification for this patient?**
   He has small <3 cm low-grade Ta tumor, so he is a low-risk patient.
5. **How will you follow this patient?**
   He will be followed by surveillance cystoscopy with 3–6 months intervals.

   During follow-up at 1 year, recurrence of multiple tumors was identified and TURBT was done (pathology showed T1 tumor, muscle specimen was present and free of involvement).
6. **What is your next step?**
   Patient now stratified as high risk and he needs intravesical BCG induction 2–4 weeks after TURBT to allow bladder healing followed by maintenance therapy, with closer surveillance by cystoscopy, urine cytology, and upper tract imaging.

Case No. 2

A 45-year-old lady came to emergency department complaining of left flank pain for 6 h.

Questions for Discussion

1. **How will you approach this patient?**
   Obtaining a history, physical examination, and initiate workup.

   Her pain at left flank is colicky and started insidiously, radiating to lower abdomen and left groin. The pain is markedly severe without any improvement when taking acetaminophen. It is associated with nausea, vomiting, and fever.

She has dysuria, frequency, and urgency the day before and no other urological symptoms. Systemic review unremarkable.

She had history of urinary calculi before which passed smoothly and also had history of UTI and was treated with oral antibiotic.

There are no other urological diseases, and she is not known to have chronic conditions. Her past surgical history is negative.

The patient is not on regular medications and has no allergy.

Her diet is high in salts and she is not having adequate water intake.

On Examination: She looks as if in pain and her vital signs are showing high temperature and tachycardia.

Abdomen is soft with left costovertebral angle tenderness and no palpable masses. The bladder is not distended.

2. **What is your next step?**

   Patient is highly suspected to have obstructed left kidney with picture of pyelonephritis. She should be investigated with CBC, renal function test, urine analysis, and culture and to obtain plain CT scan of abdomen and pelvis.

   CBC: WBC 13,000 per microliter Cr: 0.9 mg/dL

   Urine analysis: 4 RBC/HPF and 12 WBC/HPF

   Urine culture: Pending

   CT scan: Obstructing left ureteric stone (7 mm)

   Note: Make sure to check pregnancy test before proceeding with CT

3. **What is your next step in management?**

   She is having obstructed kidney with picture of pyelonephritis and she needs to be covered by empiric IV antibiotic and stabilized by IV fluid and analgesics followed by urgent relive of obstruction by inserting ureteral stent (J-J stent) or nephrostomy tube if not stable for anesthesia.

4. **What are the indications for immediate intervention in urinary stone disease?**
   - Associated pyelonephritis
   - Prolonged obstruction
   - Solitary kidney
   - High-grade obstruction
   - Bilateral urinary stones
   - Intractable symptoms (pain, nausea, or vomiting)
   - Failure of conservative treatment
   - Renal impairment

5. **How will you follow the patient after ureteral stent placement?**

   Following the urine culture result showed *Escherchia coli* growth which was treated by antibiotic and the patient improved in term of pain, nausea, vomiting, and temperature.

   After antibiotic course and repeated negative urine culture, she was discharged home.

6) **What is the next step in management?**
   - Patient needs definitive treatment for the ureteric stone, and options include ESWL or ureteroscopy with laser fragmentation.
   - Discuss both options with patient regarding possible complications, need for anesthesia, success rate, and need for further procedure.
   - Before any intervention, make sure to have negative urine culture and give prophylactic antibiotic.

Case No. 3

A 30-year-old male complaining of left-side scrotal pain and swelling for 10 days.

Questions for Discussion:

1. **How will you approach this patient?**

   Obtaining a history and performing a physical examination and initiate workup.

   His pain starts 10 days ago and progresses gradually, its severity is increasing and he limits his activity in the last 3 days. He has little improvement when he is lying down. The scrotal pain is followed by swelling that is getting larger and he cannot estimate the size.

His complaints are associated with low-grade fever and no other symptoms including urethral discharge or LUTS and there is no history of scrotal trauma and has no sexual activity. Other systemic review unremarkable.

Patient has no chronic medical conditions and his surgical history positive for left orchidopexy at age of 17 years. The patient is not on any medications. He is not married and working as registered nurse.

On examination: Has low-grade fever and other vital signs within normal.

Genital exam showed circumcised penis with swelling and redness of the left hemiscrotum, no other skin changes or urethral discharge. The left-sided scrotum is tender on palpation and the testis is difficult to be felt due to scrotal swelling and has positive trans illumination test.

Patient investigated with CBC (WBC 12,000 per microliter), urine analysis (within normal), and ultrasound (US) scrotum which showed enlarged left testis and epididymis with increased blood flow.

2. **What is your next step?**
   Patient has picture of Epididymo-orchitis and need to be started on:

   Antibiotic (Levofloxacin or Ofloxacin)

   Scrotal support

   Non-steroidal anti-inflammatory drugs (NSAIDs)

   Ice pack

   Patient return to the clinic after 2 weeks with pain resolved and scrotal swelling persist.

   You obtain US scrotum for re-assessment and it showed 1.5 cm hypoechoic mass in the left testis.

3. **What is your next step in management?**
   Patient is suspected to have testicular cancer and you have to recommend surgical excision (radical inguinal orchidectomy) and check tumor markers (AFP, beta-hCG, and LDH) before and after the surgery.

   The result came high for beta-hCG (20 mIU/mL) and others are normal.

   Always recommend for the patient to do sperm banking before going for surgery and chemotherapy.

   Patient who underwent left radical inguinal orchidectomy and the pathology examination showed pure seminoma limited to the testis without invasion to tunica vaginalis.

4. **What is your next step?**
   Mention that you will follow the tumor markers and stage the patient by CXR and CT abdomen/pelvis with oral and IV contrast.

   The result came as normalized beta-hCG and no evidence of lymph nodes or distant metastasis.

5. **What will you do next?**
   The patient is on stage IA seminoma and his treatment optionsinclude the following:

   Surveillance if he is compliant by obtaining history, physical examination, tumor markers, and CT abdomen/pelvis every 3 months for the first year and every 6 months for the second and third years and every 12 months for the fourth and fifth years.

   If non-compliant: chemotherapy two cycles of carboplatin or radiation to retroperitoneal lymph nodes (RPLN).

References

1. Breyer BN. Symptoms of disorders of the genitourinary tract. In: McAninch JW, Lue TF, editors. Smith & Tanagho's general urology. 19th ed. New York: McGraw-Hill Companies; 2020.
2. Gerber GS. Evaluation of the urologic patient , history, physical examination and urinalysis. In: Wein AJ, Kavoussi LR, Partin AW, Peters CA, editors. Campbell-Walsh urology. 11th ed. Philadelphia, PA: Elsevier; 2015.
3. Meng MV. Physical examination of the genitourinary tract. In: McAninch JW, Lue TF, editors. Smith & Tanagho's general urology. 19th ed. New York: McGraw-Hill Companies; 2020.
4. Odisho AY, Greene KL. Urologic laboratory examination. In: McAninch JW, Lue TF, editors. Smith & Tanagho's general urology. 19th ed. New York: McGraw-Hill Companies; 2020.
5. Daniela Franz SG, Hricak H. Radiology of the urinary tract. In: McAninch JW, Lue TF, editors. Smith & Tanagho's general urology. 19th ed. New York: McGraw-Hill Companies; 2020.

6. Bishoff JT. Urinary tract imaging: basic principles of computed tomography, magnetic resonance imaging, and plain film. In: Wein AJ, Kavoussi LR, Partin AW, Peters CA, editors. Campbell-Walsh urology. 11th ed. Philadelphia, PA: Elsevier; 2015.
7. Gilbert BR. Urinary tract imaging: basic principles of urologic ultrasonography. In: Wein AJ, Kavoussi LR, Partin AW, Peters CA, editors. Campbell-Walsh urology. 11th ed. Philadelphia, PA: Elsevier; 2015.
8. Lipkin ME, Preminger GM. Evaluation and medical management of urinary lithiasis. In: Wein AJ, Kavoussi LR, Partin AW, Peters CA, editors. Campbell-Walsh urology. 11th ed. Philadelphia, PA: Elsevier; 2015.
9. Matlaga BR, Lingeman JE. Surgical management of upper urinary tract calculi. In: Wein AJ, Kavoussi LR, Partin AW, Peters CA, editors. Campbell-Walsh urology. 11th ed. Philadelphia, PA: Elsevier; 2015.
10. McNicholas TA, Kirby RS. Evaluation and nonsurgical management of benign prostatic hyperplasia. In: Wein AJ, Kavoussi LR, Partin AW, Peters CA, editors. Campbell-Walsh urology. 11th ed. Philadelphia, PA: Elsevier; 2015.
11. Welliver C. Minimally invasive and endoscopic management of benign prostatic hyperplasia. In: Wein AJ, Kavoussi LR, Partin AW, Peters CA, editors. Campbell-Walsh urology. 11th ed. Philadelphia, PA: Elsevier; 2015.
12. Richard Edward Link. Cutaneous diseases of the external genitalia. In: Alan J. Wein, Louis R. Kavoussi, Alan W. Partin and Craig A. Peters, editor. Campbell-Walsh urology. 11th ed: Elsevier: Philadelphia, PA; 2015.
13. Campbell SC. Malignant renal tumors. In: Wein AJ, Kavoussi LR, Partin AW, Peters CA, editors. Campbell-Walsh urology. 11th ed. Philadelphia, PA: Elsevier; 2015.
14. Jones JS. Non-muscle-invasive bladder cancer (Ta, T1, and CIS). In: Wein AJ, Kavoussi LR, Partin AW, Peters CA, editors. Campbell-Walsh urology. 11th ed. Philadelphia, PA: Elsevier; 2015.
15. Guzzo TJ. Management of metastatic and invasive bladder cancer. In: Wein AJ, Kavoussi LR, Partin AW, Peters CA, editors. Campbell-Walsh urology. 11th ed. Philadelphia, PA: Elsevier; 2015.
16. Catalona WJ, Han M. Management of localized prostate cancer. In: Wein AJ, Kavoussi LR, Partin AW, Peters CA, editors. Campbell-Walsh urology. 11th ed. Philadelphia, PA: Elsevier; 2015.
17. Meng MV, Carroll PR. Treatment of locally advanced prostate cancer. In: Wein AJ, Kavoussi LR, Partin AW, Peters CA, editors. Campbell-Walsh urology. 11th ed. Philadelphia, PA: Elsevier; 2015.
18. Stephenson AH. Neoplasms of the testis. In: Wein AJ, Kavoussi LR, Partin AW, Peters CA, editors. Campbell-Walsh urology. 11th ed. Philadelphia, PA: Elsevier; 2015.
19. Corbett ST. Reduction of testicular tension. In: Smith OS, McGuire EJ, Preminger GM, editors. Hinman's atlas of urologic surgery. 3rd ed. Philadelphia, PA: Elsevier; 2012.
20. Elmajian DA. Radical orchiectomy. In: Smith OS, McGuire EJ, Preminger GM, editors. Hinman's atlas of urologic surgery. 3rd ed. Philadelphia, PA: Elsevier; 2012.
21. Smith JA. Robotic-assisted laparoscopic prostatectomy. In: Smith OS, McGuire EJ, Preminger GM, editors. Hinman's atlas of urologic surgery. 3rd ed. Philadelphia, PA: Elsevier; 2012.
22. Modder JK. Suprapubic prostatectomy. In: Smith OS, McGuire EJ, Preminger GM, editors. Hinman's atlas of urologic surgery. 3rd ed. Philadelphia, PA: Elsevier; 2012.
23. Blute ML. Radical nephrectomy. In: Smith OS, McGuire EJ, Preminger GM, editors. Hinman's atlas of urologic surgery. 3rd ed. Philadelphia, PA: Elsevier; 2012.
24. Blute ML. Partial nephrectomy. In: Smith OS, McGuire EJ, Preminger GM, editors. Hinman's atlas of urologic surgery. 3rd ed. Philadelphia, PA: Elsevier; 2012.

17 Communication Skills for Clinical Board Exams

17.1 Part I: Knowledge

> Communication is a skill that you can learn. It's like riding a bicycle or typing. If you're willing to work at it, you can rapidly improve the quality of every part of your life.
> Brian Tracy

17.1.1 Breaking Bad News

Use SPIKES Protocol:

- Step I: **S**etting up the interview
- Step II: Assessing the patient **P**erception
- Step III: Obtaining patient **I**nvitation
- Step IV: Giving **K**nowledge and information to the patient
- Step V: Addressing patient's **E**motions with empathic response
- Step IV: **S**trategy and **S**ummary

Step I: Setting up the Interview
The aim is to maximize privacy and avoid interruptions.

What?
- Make sure you have checked all the available information and have test results
- Decide general terminology to be used

Where?
- Arrange for some privacy

Who?
- Who should break the news, should other staff be there or significant others?

Starting off?
- Introduction and appropriate opening

Step II: Assessing the Patient Perception
Find out how much the patient knows, in particular how serious he/she thinks the illness is, and/or how much it will affect the future

For example, what did doctor X tell you when he sends you here?

Step III: Obtaining Patient Invitation
Finding out how much the patient wants to know

It is not "Do you want to know?"

It is "at what level do you want to know?"

For example,

You don't want to be bothered with the details, do you?

Would you like me to tell you the details of the diagnosis?

Step IV: Giving Knowledge and Information to the Patient
Four Crucial Headings:

- Diagnosis
- Treatment plan
- Prognosis
- Support

H. Alotaibi, *Study Surgery*, https://doi.org/10.1007/978-981-16-2305-9_17

Note:

- Start from the patient's starting point, having found out what the patient knows, reinforce those parts which are correct
- The warning shot, for example, "well, this situation does appear to be more serious than that"
- Give the information in small parts
- Use non-medical terms
- Check reception often and clarify, for example, "Do you follow what I'm saying?"
- Reinforce information often and clarify, for example, "could you just tell me what I have been saying to check I've explained it clearly?"
- Repeat important points
- Use diagrams, written messages
- Listen to the patient agenda, what their concerns, for example, patient may be worried about hair loss from a disease treatment not the potential risk of the disease

Step V: Addressing Patient Emotions with Empathic Responses

- Observe the patient and give them time
- Acknowledge any shock and ask them what are they thinking of or feeling?
- Allow silence, empathy allows the patient to express their feeling and worries and provide support
- Don't argue, allow expression of emotions without criticism

Step IV: Strategy and Summary

- Planning and follow through
- Make a plan or strategy and explain it
- Invite questions
- Tell them what happened next [1]

17.1.2 Consenting for a Procedure

1. Initiating session:
   Greets, introduces, and know the patient name and age
2. Identify reason for the visit
3. Information gathering:
   - Background of reasons for needing procedure
   - Past medical history (PMH) and past surgical history (PSH)
   - Drug history and allergy
   - Social history
   - Family history including surgical complications
4. Preparation for information giving:
   - Establish patient's starting knowledge of the procedure
   - Establish how much patient want to know about the procedure
5. Giving information:
   - Clarify name of the procedure, explain any basic anatomy or physiology that may need clarifying
   - Use visual aid
   - Explain the details of the procedure including the events that will occur before, during, and after the procedure
   - Explain the risk of the procedure
   - Explain the benefit of the procedure
   - Discuss the consequences of not having the procedure
   - State alternatives
   - Safety nets (the recovery timeline and signs of complications)
   - Check patient understanding
6. Closing the visit:
   - Invite further questions
   - Thank the patient [2]

17.1.3 Consultation

SBAR (Situation, Background, Assessment, Recommendation)
Situation:

- Introduce self, role, and the team/ward on which you are working
- Confirm that you are speaking to the correct person and ask their name if necessary
- State patient's name, hospital ID number, and location
- State the reason for the call

Background:
- State why the patient was admitted to or arrived at hospital and how long ago
- Notes previous medical history and any other relevant findings on the history
- Describe the course in the hospital or event prior to admission
- Give details of the current event

Assessment:
- State what you think the problem is and why you are concerned
- State the most recent observation and what change there have been from baseline
- Describe the examination finding
- State what investigations and interventions have been done so far

Recommendation:
- State what you would like to be done
- Ask if any further investigations or management needs to be done
- Thank the receipt of the call [3]

17.1.4 Dealing with Angry Patient

Examples for Reasons Why Patient/Relatives Become Angry?
- They have been left to wait longtime before being seen in clinic or emergency room (ER).
- An error has been made by medical and surgical team.
- Delay in diagnosis or treatment.
- Patient/relative expectation not met.

Steps
1. Recognize anger
2. Adjust communication
3. Understand anger
4. Respond to anger
5. Things to avoid

1. **Recognize that the Patient is Angry**
   You might see the following
   - Loud speak or shouting
   - Verbal abuse
   - Over sensitivity of what being said
   - Aggressive posturing, not wanting to sit down
   - Raise in pitch of voice
2. **Adjust your Style of Communication**

   Voice:

   - Try to keep a calm tone
   - Speak slowly and clearly
   - Don't raise the volume of your voice if the patient is shouting

   Body Language:

   - Adopt professional yet relaxed posture and take care not to appear like you don't care.

At this stage, pointing to the patient how they come across can be helpful.

For example, You are looking upset by all of this.

This will help the patient or relative to recognize their emotion.

3. **Try to Understand Why they are Angry**
   - Ask open questions to identify the focus of their angry
   - For example, Why are you feeling this way?
   - Is there anything else that happened that is making you angry?
   - Demonstrate active listening
   - Eye contact, nodding, and verbal response, for example, "mmm"
   - Give them space to speak
   - Avoid interrupting
4. **Respond to Anger**
   - Empathy
   - For example, "give everything you've told me; it is understandable you feel that way"
   - Apologize if any error has happened
   - If the patient is angry of medical error that happened
   - For example, "I'm sorry this mistake has occurred and caused you/your relative harm"

- If no error from medical team has happened, be careful about how you apologize
- For example, "I'm sorry that you are feeling so angry about what has happened"
- Thank the patient
- For example, "thank you for sharing how you feel with me. It is important I understand how you feel so we can work together to help you."
- Encourage questions/solutions
- For example, "What can I do to help you?"
- Closing the interview
- Thank the patient and formulate some action
- For example, organize meeting with relative nurse, specialist ... etc.
- Advise that you are going to pass the information to a senior if error has happened
- Organize follow-up meeting with the patient or relative if they wish to discuss the situation further

5. **Things to Avoid**
   - Suggesting a quick fix
   - Depending on the scenario but think carefully before coming up with rapid solution
   - Getting angry yourself
   - Being defensive [4]

17.2 Part II: Practice

There is only one rule for being a good talker—learn to listen.
Christopher Morley

17.2.1 Case Scenarios for Practice

Tips

- Practice with a friend and try to mimic the real exam!
- Don't forget to set the timer!
- No ideal answers for the cases as everyone have his/her own way of communication
- Read the steps in the checklist and act accordingly

Case No. 1:
You are the responsible physician for a 39-year-old female patient who underwent biopsy from breast imaging reporting and data system (BIRADs-IV) breast lesion. The result is invasive ductal carcinoma, grade III, and triple negative receptors.

Instruction:
Break the bad news to the patient.

Case No. 2:
You are asked to obtain an informed consent from a 44-year-old male patient who has low rectal cancer and finished his last session of neoadjuvant treatment 4 weeks ago.

Instruction:
Obtain informed consent.

Case No. 3:
You performed emergency right hemicolectomy to a 56-year-old male patient due to obstructing lesion (most likely colon cancer) at the ascending colon. Intra-operative the right ureter was difficult to identify and then you realized that it had been cut. The urology team joined the operation and repaired the injury.

Instruction:
Discuss what happened with the patient.

Case No. 4:
You are seeing a 43-year-old female patient whose thyroid fine needle aspiration (FNA) and lateral cervical lymph node FNA results just came as papillary thyroid cancer.

Instruction:
Break the bad news to the patient.

Case No. 5:
You are the surgeon on call who is seeing a 45-year-old male patient with strangulated right inguinal hernia.

Instruction:
Obtain informed consent.

Case No. 6:
You are asked to consult the vascular surgery team to join a laparotomy exploration for acute embolic mesenteric ischemia in a 66-year-old male patient.
Instruction:
Consult the vascular surgeon.

Case No.7:
You are called by the nurse to talk to the son of a 72-year-old male patient who is angry because his father was informed by the surgeon that he has colon cancer and he does not agree with telling the diagnosis to his father as this may make him depressed.
Instruction:
Talk to the patient's son.

Case No. 8:
You are asked by a 44-year-old female patient who had laparoscopic cholecystectomy 4 days ago about the reason she has bile fluid from the drain.
Instruction:
Explain to the patient what is going on.

Case No. 9:
You are the responsible surgeon for a 48-year-old female patient who underwent laparotomy exploration and emergency splenectomy following blunt abdominal trauma 1 week ago. She has persistent abdominal pain and the computed tomography (CT) scan showed retained gauze at the left upper quadrant.
Instruction:
Discuss what happened with the patient.

Case No. 10:
You are asked to obtain informed consent for total gastrectomy and D2 lymphadenectomy from a 41-year-old female patient who has gastric cancer.
Instruction:
Obtain informed consent.

Checklist

Section	Items	Done	Not done	Not applicable
Breaking bad news	Check all available information			
	Arrange some privacy			
	Ask the patient if he/she wants someone to be present			
	Find out how much the patient knows			
	Find out how much the patient wants to know			
	Reinforce the correct information the patient already knows			
	Give a warming shot			
	Give information in small parts			
	Use non-medical term			
	Check the reception and clarify			
	Repeat the important points			
	Listen to the patient's concerns			
	Observe the patient and give him/her time			
	Allow the patient to express his/her feeling			
	Discuss the plan			
	Invite questions			
	Mention what will come next			
	Thank the patient and close the session			

(continued)

Section	Items	Done	Not done	Not applicable
Informed consent	Greeting			
	Introduce him/herself to the patient			
	Establish the patient's knowledge about the procedure			
	Know how much the patient wants to know about the procedure			
	Clarify the name of the procedure			
	Explain the details of the procedure			
	Explain the risk of the procedure			
	Explain the benefit of the procedure			
	Discuss the consequences of not having the procedure			
	Mention the recovery timeline			
	Mention if there is any alternative			
	Check the patient understanding			
	Invite further question			
	Thank the patient			
Consultation	Introduce self, role, and the team			
	Confirmed that he/she is talking to the correct person			
	State the patient name, hospital ID, and location			
	State the reason for the call			
	Mention why the patient is admitted and since when			
	Describe the hospital course if necessary			
	Give details of the current event			
	Describe the examination finding			
	State what investigation and interventions have been done			
	Clarify what would like to be done			
	Ask if any further investigation or management is needed			
	Thank the receipt			
Dealing with angry patient/ relative	Recognizing that the patient/relative is angry			
	Understanding why the patient/ the relative become angry			
	Keeping calm tone			
	Speaking slowly and clearly			
	Maintaining professional, relaxed posture			
	Ask open question to understand the focus of patient/ relative anger			
	Demonstrating active listening			
	Eye contact, verbal response			
	Avoiding interrupting the patient/relative			
	Empathizing with the patient/relative			
	Apologizing when error has happened			
	Thanking the patient for sharing their feeling			
	Encouraging questions and solutions			
	Closing the interview			

References

1. Mabrouk R. Breaking bad knews. CETL, Feedback opportunities, a training resource for healthcare professionals. 2010.
2. Rachel Wamboldt NL. Communication skills for OSCES. Banbury: Scion Publishing; 2017.
3. Shahid S, Thomas S. Situation, background, assessment, recommendation (SBAR) communication tool for handoff in health care – a narrative review. Safety in Health. 2018;4(1):7.
4. 2021. Available from https://geekymedics.com/dealing-angry-patients-relatives/

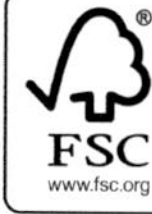

MIX
Papier aus verantwortungsvollen Quellen
Paper from responsible sources
FSC® C105338

If you have any concerns about our products,
you can contact us on
ProductSafety@springernature.com

In case Publisher is established outside the EU,
the EU authorized representative is:
Springer Nature Customer Service Center GmbH
Europaplatz 3, 69115 Heidelberg, Germany

Printed by Libri Plureos GmbH
in Hamburg, Germany